Hematology—refer

Measurement	:al
White cell count (WCC)	[illegible]
Red cell count	Males: 4.6–6 × 10^6/mm^3 Females: 3.9–5.6 × 10^6/mm^3
Hemoglobin (Hb)	Males: 13.5–18 g/dL Females: 11.5–16 g/dL
Hematocrit	Males: 40%–52% Females: 34%–46%
Mean cell volume (MCV)	Males: 80–100 pg Females: 79–98 pg
Mean cell hemoglobin (MCH)	25.4–34.6 fL
Mean cell hemoglobin concentration (MCHC)	Males: 31%–37% Females: 30%–36%
Neutrophils	1.8–8 k/μL 40%–75% WBC
Lymphocytes	1–5 k/μL 20%–45% WBC
Eosinophils	0.0–0.6 k/μL 1%–6% WBC
Basophils	0.0–0.2 k/μL 0–1% WBC
Monocytes	0–0.1 k/μL 2%–10% WBC
Platelet count	150–450 × 10^3/mm^3
Reticulocyte count	0.5%–1.5%
Erythrocyte sedimentation rate (ESR)	Depends on age
Prothrombin time (PT) (factors I, II, VII, X)	11–15 seconds
Activated partial thromboplastin time (aPTT) (VIII, IX, XI, XII)	25–39 seconds
D-dimers1	<0.5 mg/L

1 D-dimer assay may be useful as a screening test for thromboembolic disease; see Perrier A, et al. (1999). Non-invasive diagnosis of venous thromboembolism in outpatients. *Lancet* **353** 190. However, the reference range does depend on the assay—check with your hematology lab.

Reproduced with permission from Longmore ML, Wilkinson IB, Rajagopalan S (2004). *Oxford Handbook of Clinical Medicine*, 6th ed Oxford: Oxford University Press.

Useful Web sites

Description	Web address (URL)
Centers for Disease Control and Prevention	www.cdc.gov
Centers for Medicare and Medicaid Services	www.cms.hhs.gov
ClinicalTrials.gov	www.clinicaltrials.gov
Electronic Orange Book	www.fda.gov/cder/ob
Food and Drug Administration	www.fda.gov
FDA Postmarket Drug Safety Information for Patients and Providers	www.fda.gov/cder/drugSafety.htm
Institute for Safe Medication Practices	www.ismp.org
The Joint Commission	www.jointcommission.org
MedWatch	www.fda.gov/medwatch
Merck Manual	www.merck.com/pubs/
National Association of Boards of Pharmacy (NABP)	www.nabp.net
National Comprehensive Cancer Network	www.nccn.org
National Institutes of Health	www.nih.gov

American Association of Poison Control Centers

Poison control centers are open 24 hours, 7 days a week. Poison centers are staffed by pharmacists, physicians, nurses, and toxicology specialists. The Poison Help hotline is 1-800-222-1222.

Oxford American Handbook of
Clinical Pharmacy

Published and forthcoming Oxford American Handbooks

Oxford American Handbook of Clinical Medicine
Oxford American Handbook of Anesthesiology
Oxford American Handbook of Clinical Dentistry
Oxford American Handbook of Clinical Diagnosis
Oxford American Handbook of Critical Care
Oxford American Handbook of Emergency Medicine
Oxford American Handbook of Nephrology and Hypertension
Oxford American Handbook of Obstetrics and Gynecology
Oxford American Handbook of Oncology
Oxford American Handbook of Otolaryngology
Oxford American Handbook of Pediatrics
Oxford American Handbook of Psychiatry
Oxford American Handbook of Pulmonary Medicine
Oxford American Handbook of Rheumatology
Oxford American Handbook of Surgery

Oxford American Handbook of Clinical Pharmacy

Edited by

Michelle W. McCarthy, Pharm.D.

Director, Drug Information Services
Department of Pharmacy Services
University of Virginia Health System
Charlottesville, Virginia

Denise R. Kockler, Pharm.D., BCPS

Director, Drug Information Services
Department of Pharmacy Services
Virginia Commonwealth University Health System
Richmond, Virginia

with

Philip Wiffen
Marc Mitchell
Melanie Snelling
Nicola Stoner

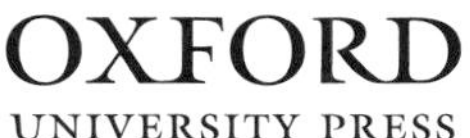
OXFORD
UNIVERSITY PRESS

OXFORD
UNIVERSITY PRESS

Oxford University Press, Inc. publishes works that further
Oxford University's objective of excellence
in research, scholarship and education.

Oxford New York

Auckland Cape Town Dar es Salaam Hong Kong Karachi
Kuala Lumpur Madrid Melbourne Mexico City Nairobi
New Delhi Shanghai Taipei Toronto

With offices in

Argentina Austria Brazil Chile Czech Republic France Greece
Guatemala Hungary Italy Japan Poland Portugal
Singapore South Korea Switzerland Thailand Turkey Ukraine Vietnam

Published by Oxford University Press Inc.
198 Madison Avenue, New York, New York 10016

www.oup.com

Oxford is a registered trade mark of Oxford University Press

Library of Congress Cataloging-in-Publication Data

Oxford American handbook of clinical pharmacy/edited by Michelle W. McCarthy,
Denise R. Kockler ; with Philip Wiffen ... [et al.].
p. ; cm. —(Oxford American handbooks)
Adapted from: Oxford handbook of clinical pharmacy/Philip Wiffen ... [et al.]. 2007
Includes bibliographical references and index.

ISBN 978–0–19–537510–7 (flexicover : alk. paper)

1. Hospital pharmacies—Handbooks, manuals, etc. 2. Pharmacy—Handbooks,
manuals, etc. 3. Clinical pharmacology—Handbooks, manuals, etc. I. McCarthy,
Michelle W., 1970- II. Kockler, Denise R., 1968- III. Wiffen, Phil. IV. Oxford
handbook of clinical pharmacy. V. Title: Handbook of clinical pharmacy. VI. Series:
Oxford American handbooks.

[DNLM: 1. Pharmaceutical Services—Handbooks. 2. Pharmacology,
Clinical—methods—Handbooks. QV 735 O975 2009]
RS152.O94 2009
615'.1—dc22 2009002713

9 8 7 6 5 4 3 2 1

Printed in China
on acid-free paper

Preface

Clinical pharmacy practice involves optimization of medication therapy and promotion of health, wellness, and disease prevention. Clinical pharmacists practice in many different settings and numerous specialty areas and are essential members of the healthcare team.

This book was developed to share essential knowledge relating to clinical pharmacy practice in a pocket-sized reference. The topics covered are those in which pharmacists have an impact on patient outcomes and decision making. The information within the chapters is provided in manageable amounts and includes recommended further readings if more detailed information is needed.

The contributors are many of our colleagues and peers who have established themselves as experts in their practice area and make positive contributions to the practice of pharmacy and patient care on a daily basis. We thank each of them for their dedication to the completion of this project.

We hope that the first Oxford American Handbook of Clinical Pharmacy will be a useful resource for practicing pharmacists, pharmacy students, and pharmacy residents.

Acknowledgments

We are extremely grateful to our families and friends who provided unending encouragement, support, and understanding:

Sean, Liam, and Ryan McCarthy,
Eddie Wilson,
Melanie Mayberry
Janet, Kim, and Steven Kozella,
Patricia Fulco

Contents

Detailed contents

Contributors

Brian Baird, PharmD, BCPS
Clinical Pharmacy Specialist
Drug Information
Virginia Commonwealth University
Health System
Richmond, Virginia

Kathleen A. Bledsoe, PharmD, BCPS
Clinical Pharmacy Specialist
Neurosciences
University of Virginia
Health System
Charlottesville, Virginia

Trisha N. Branan, PharmD
Critical Care Clinical Pharmacist
Medical College of Georgia
Health System
Augusta, Georgia

Kelly L. Branham, PharmD, MBA
Critical Care Pharmacy Resident
Virginia Commonwealth
University Health System
Richmond, Virginia

Stacey Baker Pattie, PharmD, BCPS
Clinical Pharmacy Specialist
Internal Medicine
University of Virginia
Health System
Charlottesville, Virginia

Ericka L. Breden, PharmD, BCPP, CGP
Clinical Pharmacy Specialist
Psychiatry
Clinical Assistant Professor
Pharmacy and Psychiatry
Virginia Commonwealth
University Health System
Richmond, Virginia

William D. Cahoon, Jr., PharmD, BCPS
Clinical Pharmacy Specialist
Acute Care Cardiology
Virginia Commonwealth
University Health System
Richmond, Virginia

Susan B. Cogut, PharmD
PGY2-Drug Information Resident
University of Virginia Health
System
Charlottesville, Virginia

Kristin W. Cox, PharmD
Clinical Pharmacy Specialist
Pediatrics
Virginia Commonwealth
University Health System
Richmond, Virginia

Kathlene DeGregory, PharmD, BCOP
Clinical Pharmacy Specialist
Hematology/Oncology
University of Virginia Health
System
Charlottesville, Virginia

Zachariah Deyo, PharmD
PGY1-Pharmacy Resident
Virginia Commonwealth
University Health System
Richmond, Virginia

Karen Eckmann, PharmD
PGY1-Pharmacy Resident
Virginia Commonwealth
University Health System
Richmond, Virginia

Frank A. Fulco, MD, RPh
Hospitalist and Assistant Professor
Associate Program Director
Virginia Commonwealth University Internal Medicine Residency
McGuire Veterans Affairs Medical Center
Richmond, Virginia

Jason C. Gallagher, PharmD, BCPS
Clinical Assistant Professor
Clinical Specialist
Infectious Diseases
Temple University
Philadelphia, Pennsylvania

Jorie A. Glick, PharmD
PGY1-Pharmacy Resident
Virginia Commonwealth University Health System
Richmond, Virginia

Tina M. Grof, PharmD
Clinical Pharmacy Specialist
Emergency Medicine
Charleston Area Medical Center
Charleston, West Virginia

Michelle Hobbs, PharmD
Coordinator
Investigational Drug Services
University of Virginia Health System
Charlottesville, Virginia

Jessica L. Johnson, PharmD
PGY1-Pharmacy Resident
University of Virginia Health System
Charlottesville, Virginia

Julie J. Kelsey, PharmD
Clinical Pharmacy Specialist
Women's Health
University of Virginia Health System
Charlottesville, Virginia

Mika Raye Kessans, PharmD
PGY2-Hematology/Oncology Pharmacy Resident
Virginia Commonwealth University Health System
Richmond, Virginia

Denise R. Kockler, PharmD, BCPS
Director, Drug Information Services
Department of Pharmacy Services
Virginia Commonwealth University Medical Center
Richmond, Virginia

Lynn Limon, PharmD
Staff Pharmacist
Virginia Commonwealth University Health System
Richmond, Virginia

Lena M. Maynor, PharmD, BCPS
Clinical Assistant Professor
West Virginia University School of Pharmacy
Morgantown, West Virginia

Michelle W. McCarthy, PharmD
Director, Drug Information Services
Department of Pharmacy Services
University of Virginia Health System
Charlottesville, Virginia

Lauren K. McCluggage, PharmD, BCPS
Assistant Professor of Clinical Pharmacy
University of the Sciences in Philadelphia
Philadelphia College of Pharmacy
Philadelphia, Pennsylvania

Nicole L. Metzger, PharmD, BCPS
Clinical Assistant Professor of Pharmacy Practice
Mercer University College of Pharmacy and Health Sciences
Atlanta, Georgia

Laura Morgan, PharmD, BCPS
Assistant Professor
Virginia Commonwealth University School of Pharmacy
Richmond, Virginia

Katie Muzevich, PharmD, BCPS
Critical Care Pharmacy Resident
Virginia Commonwealth University Health System
Richmond, Virginia

Ian Orensky, PharmD,MS
Supervisor, Pharmacy Services
Virginia Commonwealth University Health System
Richmond, Virginia

Amber G. Ormsby, PharmD
Critical Care Pharmacy Resident
University of Virginia Health System
Charlottesville, Virginia

Leah W. Paige, PharmD
Clinical Pharmacist
University of Virginia Health System
Charlottesville, Virginia

Shaila Patel, PharmD
PGY1-Pharmacy Resident
University of Virginia Health System
Charlottesville, Virginia

Patricia Pecora Fulco, PharmD, BCPS, FASHP
Clinical Pharmacy Specialist
Internal Medicine/HIV
Clinical Assistant Professor of Pharmacy, Assistant Professor of Internal Medicine
Division of Infectious Diseases
Virginia Commonwealth University
Virginia Commonwealth University Health System
Richmond, Virginia

Nathan Powell, PharmD
PGY1-Pharmacy Resident
University of Virginia Health System
Charlottesville, Virginia

Whitney D. Raper, PharmD
PGY1-Pharmacy Resident
University of Virginia Health System
Charlottesville, Virginia

Shelby Raynor, PharmD Candidate
Shenandoah University
Bernard J. Dunn School of Pharmacy
Winchester, Virginia

S. Rutherfoord Rose, PharmD, FAACT, DABAT
Professor of Emergency Medicine
Director, Virginia Poison Center
Virginia Commonwealth University Health System
Richmond, Virginia

Katharine A. Sheldon, PharmD, MS
Supervisor
Inpatient Pharmacy Services
Virginia Commonwealth University Health System
Richmond, Virginia

Chrissie V. Shirley, PharmD
Critical Care Pharmacy Resident
University of Virginia Health System
Charlottesville, Virginia

David Volles, PharmD, BCPS
Clinical Pharmacy Specialist Surgery
University of Virginia Health System
Charlottesville, Virginia

Donna M. White, RPh, CDE
Clinical Pharmacy Specialist Ambulatory Care
University of Virginia Health System
Charlottesville, Virginia

Nikki M. Yost, PharmD, BCOP
Clinical Pharmacist Hematology/Oncology
The Nebraska Medical Center
Omaha, Nebraska

Nancy S. Yunker, PharmD, BCPS
Assistant Professor of Pharmacy
Virginia Commonwealth University School of Pharmacy
Richmond, Virginia

Symbols and abbreviations

↑	increased
↓	decreased
>	greater than
<	less than
≥	greater than or equal to
≤	less than or equal to
°	degrees
5-HT	serotonin
AACE	American Academy of Clinical Endocrinologists
ABC	airway, breathing, and circulation
ABW	actual body weight
ACC	American College of Cardiologists
ACCP	American College of Chest Physicians; American College of Clinical Pharmacy
ACE	angiotensin-converting enzyme
AChR	acetylcholine receptor
ACIP	Advisory Committee on Immunization
ACLS	advanced cardiovascular life support
ACS	acute coronary syndrome
ACV	assist controlled ventilation
AD	Alzheimer's disease
ADA	American Diabetes Association
ADC	automated distribution cabinet
ADE	adverse drug event
ADHF	acute decompensated heart failure
ADLs	activities of daily living
ADM	automated dispensing machine
ADP	adenosine diphosphate
ADR	adverse drug reaction
AED	automated external defibrillator
AF	atrial fibrillation
AFB	acid-fast bacilli
AG	anion gap
AHA	American Heart Association
ALI	acute lung injury
ALT	alanine aminotransferase
AMA	American Medical Association

ANA	antinuclear antibody
APAP	acetaminophen
APhA	American Pharmacists Association
aPPT	activated partial thrombin time
AR	allergic rhinitis
ARB	angiotensin receptor blocker
ARDS	acute respiratory distress syndrome
ASHP	American Society of Health-System Pharmacists
AST	aspartate aminotransferase
AUC	area under the plasma concentration curve
AV	arteriovenous; atrioventricular
BB	beta-blocker
BCAA	branched-chain amino acid
bid	twice daily
BiPAP	bilevel positive airway pressure
BLS	basic life support
BMD	bone mineral density
BMI	body mass index
BMP	basic metabolic profile
BMR	basal metabolic rate
BMS	bare metal stent
BNP	B-type natriuretic protein
BP	blood pressure
BPH	benign prostatic hyperplasia
BUN	blood urea nitrogen
CABG	coronary artery bypass grafting
CAM	complementary and alternative medicine
CA-MRSA	community-acquired methicillin-resistant Staphylococcus aureus
CAP	community-acquired pneumonia
CAPD	continuous ambulatory peritoneal dialysis
CAVD	continuous arteriovenous hemodialysis
CAVH	continuous arteriovenous hemofiltration
CBC	complete blood count
CBER	Center for Biologics Evaluation and Research
CBT	cognitive-behavioral therapy
CBZ	carbamazepine
CC	chief complaint
CCB	calcium channel blocker
CD	controlled drug; Crohn's disease
CDC	Centers for Disease Control and Prevention
CDER	Center for Drug Evaluation and Research

CDS	clinical decision support
CF	cystic fibrosis
CFTR	cystic fibrosis transmembrane conductance regulator
CGMP	current good manufacturing practices
CI	confidence interval
CIN	contrast-induced nephropathy
CMV	controlled mechanical ventilation
CNS	central nervous system
CO	cardiac output
CO2	carbon dioxide
COC	combined oral contraception
COMT	catechol-O-methyltransferase
COPD	chronic obstructive pulmonary disease
COW	computer on wheels
CPAP	continuous positive airway pressure
CPOE	computerized prescriber/physician order entry
CPR	cardiopulmonary resuscitation
CR	controlled release
CrCl	creatinine clearance
CRP	C-reactive protein
CSF	cerebrospinal fluid
CTC	common toxicity criteria
CVC	central venous catheter
CVD	cardiovascular disease
CVP	continuous venous pressure
CVS	cardiovascular system
CVVHDF	continuous venovenous hemodiafiltration
CYP450	cytochrome P450
DA	dopamine
DBP	diastolic blood pressure
DES	drug-eluting stent
DH	drug history
DHA	docosahexaenoic acid
DI	drug information
DIC	disseminated intravascular coagulation
DIPS	drug interaction probability score
DM	diabetes mellitus; dermatomyositis
DMARD	disease-modifying antirheumatic drug
DMD	disease-modifying drug
DMSO	dimethylsulfoxide
DNR	do not resuscitate
DRI	Dietary Reference Index

DSHEA	Dietary Supplement Health and Education Act
DTI	direct thrombin inhibitor
DTR	deep tendon reflex
DUE	drug-use evaluation
DVT	deep vein thrombosis
DXA	dual X-ray absorptiometry
EBM	evidence-based medicine
EC	enteric-coated
ECF	extracellular fluid
ECG	electrocardiogram
ED	emergency department
EEG	electroencephalogram
EF	ejection fraction
ELBW	extremely low birth weight
eMAR	electronic medication administration record
EMG	electromyography
ESA	erythropoiesis stimulating agent
ESBL	extended-spectrum beta-lactamases
ESR	erythrocyte sedimentation rate
FDA	Food and Drug Administration
FD&C	Food, Drug and Cosmetic Act
FFP	fresh frozen plasma
FGA	first-generation antipsychotic
FH	family history
G6PD	glucose 6-phosphate dehydrogenase
GABA	G-aminobutyric acid
GAD	generalized anxiety disorder
GCA	giant cell arteritis
GCP	good clinical practice
GCS	Glascow Coma Score
GERD	gastroesophageal reflux disease
GFR	glomerular filtration rate
GGT	G-glutamyl transferase
GI	gastrointestinal
GMP	good manufacturing practice
GNR	gram-negative rod
GOR	glucose oxidation rate
GTN	glyceryl trinitrate
H2RA	histamine-2 receptor antagonist
HAART	highly active antiretroviral therapy
HAP	hospital-acquired pneumonia
HAV	hepatitis A virus

Hb	hemoglobin
HbA1C	glycosylated hemoglobin
HBIG	hepatitis B immunoglobulin
HBV	hepatitis B virus
HCP	health-care personnel
HCV	hepatitis C virus
HD	hemodialysis
HDF	hemodiafiltration
HDL	high-density lipoprotein
HE	hepatic encephalopathy
HEENT	head, eyes, ears, nose, throat
HF	hemofiltration
HFOV	high-frequency oscillation ventilation
HHS	Health and Human Services
Hib	Haemophilus influenza type B
HIPAA	Health Information Portability and Protection Act
HIV	human immunodeficiency virus
HPA	hypothalamic–pituitary–adrenal (axis)
HPV	human papillomavirus
HRS	hepatorenal syndrome
HSCT	hematopoietic stem cell transplant
HSV	herpes simplex virus
HTN	hypertension
IABP	intra-aortic balloon pump
IBD	inflammatory bowel disease
IBW	ideal body weight
ICF	intracellular fluid
ICS	inhaled glucocorticosteroids
ICU	intensive care unit
IFN	interferon
Ig	immunoglobulin
IM	intramuscular
IMV	intermittent mandatory ventilation
IND	Investigational New Drug
INR	international normalized ratio
IO	intraosseous
IOM	Institute of Medicine
IP	investigational product
IPA	International Pharmaceutical Abstracts
IR	immediate release
IRB	institutional review board
ISMP	Institute of Safe Medication Practice

ISS	injury severity score
IV	intravenous
J	Joule
JCAHO	Joint Commission of Accreditation of Healthcare Organizations
K+	potassium
kcal	kilocalorie
LBW	lean body weight
LDH	lactate dehydrogenase
LDL	low-density lipoprotein
LES	lower esophageal sphincter
LFT	liver function test
Li	lithium
LMT	lamotrigine
LMWH	low-molecular-weight heparin
LV	left ventricular
LVEF	left ventricular ejection fraction
MALT	mucosa-associated lymphoid tissue
MAOI	monoamine oxidase inhibitor
MAP	mean arterial pressure
MARS	molecular absorbent recirculating system
MDI	metered-dose inhaler
MDS	monitored dose system
mEq	milliequivalent
MG	myasthenia gravis
MHV	mechanical prosthetic heart valve
MI	myocardial infarction
MIC	minimum inhibitory concentration
MMF	mycophenolate mofetil
MMR	measles, mumps, rubella (vaccine)
MMSE	Mini Mental Status Exam
mOsm	milliosmole
MRI	magnetic resonance imaging
MRSA	methicillin-resistant Staphylococcus aureus
MS	multiple sclerosis
MSD	material safety data
MSE	Mental Status Exam
MSL	medical science liaison
MSSA	methicillin-susceptible Staphylococcus aureus
MTM	medication therapy management
mTOR	mammalian target of rapamycin
MW	molecular weight

NAC	N-acetylcysteine
NCCN	National Comprehensive Cancer Network
NCEP	National Cholesterol Education Program
NCI	National Cancer Institute
NDA	New Drug Application
NDC	National Drug Code
NE	norepinephrine
NG	nasogastric
NIH	National Institutes of Health
NMDA	N-methyl-D-aspartate
NNH	number needed to harm
NNT	number needed to treat
NOS	not otherwise specified
nPEP	nonoccupational post-exposure prophylaxis
NPSG	National Patient Safety Goals
NSAID	nonsteroidal anti-inflammatory drug
NSTEMI	non-ST-segment elevation myocardial infarction
NTG	nitroglycerin
O2	oxygen
OCD	obsessive-compulsive disorder
OG	orogastric
OHRP	Office of Human Rights Protection
OI	opportunistic infection
OTC	over the counter
PABA	para-amino benzoic acid
PaCO2	partial pressure of carbon dioxide in arterial blood
PaO2	partial pressure of oxygen in arterial blood
PAP	patient assistance program
PAR	perennial allergic rhinitis
PB	phenobarbitol
PC	percutaneously; presenting complaint
PCI	percutaneous coronary intervention
PCP	primary care physician; pneumocystis pneumonia
PCR	polymerase chain reaction
PCWP	pulmonary capillary wedge pressure
PD	Parkinson's disease
PE	pulmonary embolism
PEA	pulseless electrical activity
PEEP	positive end-expiratory pressure
PEG	percutaneous endoscopic gastroscopy
PEP	post-exposure prophylaxis
PhRMA	Pharmaceutical Research and Manufacturers of America

PHT	phenytoin
PICC	peripherally inserted central catheter
PM	polymyositis
PMH	past medical history
PML	progressive multifocal leukoencephalopathy
PMN	polymorphonuclear leukocyte (count)
PMR	patient medical records
PMS	premenstrual syndrome
PN	parenteral nutrition
PNS	peripheral nervous system
PO	per os (by mouth)
PONV	postoperative nausea and vomiting
PPI	proton pump inhibitor
ppm	parts per million
PR	per rectum (by the rectum)
PRM	primidone
PRN	pro re nata (as required)
PSV	pressure support ventilation
PT	prothrombin time
P&T	pharmacy and therapeutics
PTH	parathyroid hormone
PTSD	post-traumatic stress disorder
PTT	partial thromboplastin time
PUD	peptic ulcer disease
qid	four times daily
RA	rheumatoid arthritis
RAAS	renin–angiotensin aldosterone system
RASS	Richmond Agitation and Sedation Scale
RBC	red blood cells
RCRA	Resource Conservation and Recovery Act
RCT	randomized control trial
RF	rheumatoid factor
RSV	respiratory syncytial virus
SABA	short-acting beta-agonist
SAD	social anxiety disorder
SAR	seasonal allergic rhinitis
SBP	systolic blood pressure
SC	subcutaneously
SCA	sudden cardiac arrest
SCCM	Society of Critical Care Medicine
SGA	subjective global assessment; second-generation antipsychotic

SH	social history
SIADH	syndrome of inappropriate antidiuretic hormone
SIMV	synchronous intermittent mandatory ventilation
SJS	Stevens–Johnson syndrome
SL	sublingual
SLE	systemic lupus erythematosus
SNRI	serotonin–norepinephrine reuptake inhibitor
SOAP	subjective, objective, assessment, and plan
SOB	shortness of breath
SP	specific phobia
SR	sinus rhythm; sustained release
SRI	serotonin reuptake inhibitor
SSRI	selective serotonin reuptake inhibitor
STD	sexually transmitted disease
STEMI	ST-segment elevation myocardial infarction
T3	triiodothyronine
T4	thyroxine
TB	tuberculosis
TBW	total body weight
TCA	tricyclic antidepressant
TDM	therapeutic dose/drug monitoring
TEN	toxic epidermal necrolysis
TENS	transcutaneous electronic nerve stimulation
TFT	thyroid function test
TG	triglycerides
THR	total hip replacement
TIA	transient ischemic attack
tid	three times daily
TIPS	transjugular intrahepatic portosystemic shunt
TITRS	title, introduction, text, recommendation, & signature
TKR	total knee replacement
TLS	tumor lysis syndrome
TM	traditional medicine
Tmax	time to maximum drug concentration
TMP-SMX	trimethoprim-sulfamethoxazole
TNF	tumor necrosis factor
tPA	tissue plasminogen activator
TPN	total parenteral nutrition
TSH	thyroid-stimulating hormone
UA	unstable angina
UC	ulcerative colitis
U&E	urea and electrolytes

UFH	unfractionated heparin
ULN	upper limits of normal
USP	U.S. Pharmacopeia
VAC	vacuum-assisted closure
VAERS	Vaccine Adverse Event Reporting System
VAS	visual analogue scale
VF	ventricular fibrillation
VLCD	very-low-calorie diet
VPA	valproic acid
VRE	vancomycin-resistant enterococci
VRSA	vancomycin-resistant staphylococcus aureus
VT	ventricular tachycardia
VTBI	volume to be infused
VTE	venous thromboembolism
VV	venovenous
v/v	volume in volume
v/w	volume in weight
XR	extended release
WBC	white blood cells
WHO	World Health Organization
w/v	weight in volume
w/w	weight in weight

Chapter 1

Adherence

Denise R. Kockler

Introduction

Adherence (or compliance) to a medication regimen is defined as the extent to which patients take their medications as prescribed.

Compliance implies a paternalistic relationship between the doctor (or other health-care professional) and the patient, with little, if any, discussion or negotiation.

Adherence recognizes a shared role between provider and patient in decision making and has become the preferred term by health-care providers.

Importance of adherence

Globally, the World Health Organization (WHO) estimates that approximately 50% of patients taking medications for chronic conditions are nonadherent, which often results in worsened disease, decreased functionality, reduced quality of life, and early mortality. In the United States, nonadherence affects all age groups, both genders, and all socioeconomic levels. Additionally, it has been estimated that medication nonadherence results in approximately $177 billion annually in direct and indirect health-care costs.[1]

Because of the significance of medication nonadherence, the WHO has published an evidence-based guideline for health-care providers, managers, and policy makers to improve strategies for medication adherence: *Adherence to Long-Term Therapies: Evidence for Action.*

Adherence rates

Individual rates of medication adherence are often reported as the percentage of the prescribed doses of the medication actually taken by the patient over a specified period.

- Adherence rates are reported as being higher for acute conditions than for chronic conditions.
- Adherence rates are generally higher in clinical trials than in the general population.
- A standard rate for what is considered "adequate adherence" has not been established.

Reasons for nonadherence

Numerous studies have attempted to identify the causes of non-adherence and many factors have been identified (see Table 1.1). Different factors are relevant to different diseases or settings. The reasons for nonadherence generally fall into two categories:

- Unintentional: simply forgetting
- Intentional: influenced by patients' beliefs regarding medications or disease state

Differences between unintentional and intentional adherence have been reported in the elderly population, with more than 66% of nonadherence being considered intentional.[2]

Table 1.1 Factors reported to affect adherence

- Ability to attend appointments
- Age
- Beliefs about medicines
- Complexity of regimen
- Concerns about confidentiality
- Cost, payment, insurance
- Cultural practices or beliefs
- Depression
- Drug-level monitoring
- Educational status
- Frequency of doses
- Gender
- Health beliefs and attitudes (toward self and others)
- Impact on daily life
- Language barriers (if the patient's first language is different from that of health-care professional)
- Lifestyle (chaotic)
- Literacy
- Manual dexterity
- Race, ethnicity
- Side effects (past or current experience)
- Satisfaction with health care
- Self-esteem
- Socioeconomic status

1 Sabate E, ed. (2003). *Adherence to Long-Term Therapies: Evidence for Action*. Geneva: World Health Organization. Available at: http://www.who.int/chp/knowledge/publications/adherence_report/en/index.html

2 Cooper JK, Love DW, Raffoul PR (1982). Intentional prescription nonadherence (noncompliance) by the elderly. *J Am Geriatr Soc* **30**:329–333.

Adherence measures

Methods of measuring adherence can be divided into direct or indirect (see Table 1.2). Unfortunately, none of these methods are absolute, but each has advantages and disadvantages.

Table 1.2 Methods of measuring adherence

Test	Advantages	Disadvantages
Direct methods		
Directly observed therapy	Most accurate	Patients can hide pills in the mouth and then discard them; impractical for routine use
Measurement of the level of medicine or metabolite in blood	Objective	Variations in metabolism and "white-coat adherence" can give a false impression of adherence; expensive
Measurement of the biologic marker in blood	Objective; in clinical trials, can also be used to measure placebo	Requires expensive assays and collection of bodily fluids
Indirect methods		
Patient questionnaires, patient self-reports	Simple; inexpensive; the most useful method in the clinical setting	Susceptible to error with increases in time between visits; results are easily distorted by the patient
Pill counts	Objective, quantifiable, and easy to perform	A prescription refill is not equivalent to ingestion of medication; requires a closed pharmacy system
Rates of prescription refills	Objective; easy to obtain data	A prescription refill is not equivalent to ingestion of medication; requires a closed pharmacy system
Assessment of the patient's clinical response	Simple; generally easy to perform	Factors other than medication adherence can affect clinical response
Electronic medication monitors	Precise; results are easily quantified; tracks patterns of taking medication	Expensive; requires return visits and downloading data from medication vials
Measurement of physiologic markets (e.g., heart rate in patients taking beta-blockers)	Often easy to perform	Marker may be absent for other reasons (e.g., increased metabolism, poor absorption, lack of response)

Table 1.2 (*Contd.*)

Test	Advantages	Disadvantages
Patient diaries	Help to correct for poor recall	Easily altered by patient
When the patient is a child, questionnaire for caregiver or teacher	Simple; objective	Susceptible to distortion

Osterberg L, Blaschke T (2005). Adherence to medication. *N Engl J Med* **353**:487–497.

Strategies to improve adherence

The National Council on Patient Information and Education (NCPIE) has developed a U.S. consensus on 10 national priorities that may have the greatest impact on improving the state of patient adherence.[1] These priorities include the following:

- Elevate patient adherence as a critical health-care issue.
- Agree on common adherence terminology that will unite all stakeholders.
- Create a public–private partnership to mount a unified national education campaign to make patient adherence a national health priority.
- Establish a multidisciplinary approach to adherence education and management.
- Immediately implement professional training and increase the funding for professional education on patient medication adherence.
- Address the barriers to patient adherence for patients with low health literacy.
- Create the means to share information about best practices in adherence education and management.
- Develop a curriculum on medication adherence for use in medical schools and allied health-care institutions.
- Seek regulatory changes to remove roadblocks in adherence assistance programs.
- Increase the federal budget and stimulate rigorous research on medication adherence.

Numerous strategies (see Table 1.3) have been used to attempt to improve medication adherence, but there is little evidence that any of these strategies are effective long term.

1 National Council on Patient Information and Education (2007). *Enhancing Prescription Medicine Adherence: A National Action Plan.* Available at: http://www.talkaboutrx.org/enhancing prescription medicine adherence.pdf

Table 1.3 Medication adherence strategies

- Recognize poor adherence
  - Identify nonadherence markers (missed appointments and refills)
  - Unresponsive to medication
  - Inquire about adherence barriers (non-confrontational)
- Stress the significance of the regimen and the effect of adherence
- Discuss patient's feelings about their ability to adhere to the regimen, design supports to promote adherence (if necessary)
- Provide easy, clear instructions and simplify the regimen (if feasible)
- Promote utilization of a medication-taking system (i.e., pillboxes, electronic compliance devices, refill reminders)
- Listen to the patient, and modify the regimen in accordance with the patient's needs
- Obtain help from support personnel/systems (family members, friends, and community services)
- Emphasize desirable behavior and results
- Consider longer-acting medication formulations when adherence is uncertain
  - Susustained-release medications
  - Depot injections
  - Transdermal medications

Osterberg L, Blaschke T (2005). Adherence to medication. *N Engl J Med* **353**:487–497.

Adherence counseling

Pharmacists involved in adherence counseling should ideally employ the communication skills discussed in Chapter 5 (p. 68).

The American Society of Health System Pharmacists (ASHP) has established guidelines for educating and counseling patients about medications.[1] These guidelines include four core process steps that should be considered when patients are receiving new medications or returning for refills:

1. Develop appropriate relationships with the patients with regard to practice setting and stage in the patient's health-care management.
   - Introduce yourself as the pharmacist.
   - Determine the patient's primary spoken language.
   - Explain the purpose and expected length of the sessions.
   - Obtain the patient's agreement to participate.
2. Evaluate the patient's knowledge base for his or her health problems and medications, physical and mental capability to use the medications appropriately, and attitude toward the health problems and medications.
   - Ask open-ended questions about the purpose of each medication.
   - Determine what the patient expects from taking the medication.
   - Ask the patient to describe or show how he or she will use (or has been using) the medication.
   - Ask the patient to describe problems with and concerns or uncertainties about their medications.
3. Use oral and visual information (aids or demonstrations) to fill deficits in patient knowledge and understanding of the medication.
   - Open medication containers to show color, size, shape, and markings on oral solids.
   - Show dosage marks on measuring devices for oral liquids and injectables.
   - Demonstrate assembly and use of administration devices (e.g., inhalers).
   - Provide written documentation as supplemental communication to help with patient recall.
4. Verify patients' knowledge and understanding of medication use.
   - Ask patients to describe or show how they will use their medications and identify their effects.
   - Observe patients' medication-use capability and accuracy, and note their attitudes toward following their medication regimens and monitoring plans.

When counseling patients, specific content for an educating and counseling session have been developed (see Table 1.4) and should be considered. Not all of the content parameters will be used for each counseling session; rather, the decision to discuss specific information should be based on the pharmacist's professional judgment.

Table 1.4 Education and counseling content

Basic information

- Drug name (generic and trade name), strength, and formulation
- How it works—nontechnical explanation
- Why it is important to keep taking the treatment correctly

Using the treatment

- How much to use—e.g., number of tablets
- How often to use—e.g., twice daily, about 12 hours apart
- Special information—e.g., with food or drink plenty of water
- Storage—e.g., in the original container, in the refrigerator, or expiration date

Side effects

- Common side effects—e.g., when they might occur and what to do about them
- Managing side effects—e.g., taking drugs with food might reduce nausea or over-the-counter drug treatments
- Serious side effects—e.g., what to do and whether to contact the clinic (provide a phone number, if appropriate), local doctor, or hospital

Drug interactions

- Any drugs that the patient should avoid or be cautious with—in particular, mention over-the-counter medicines, herbal and traditional medicines, and recreational drugs

Other

- Availability
- Cost (per month or per year)
- Monitoring—e.g., frequency of tests and costs of tests

1 American Society of Health-System Pharmacists (1997). ASHP guidelines on pharmacist-conducted patient education and counseling. *Am J Health Syst Pharm* **54:**431–434.

Chapter 2

Adverse drug reactions and drug interactions

Michelle W. McCarthy

Introduction

Medication misadventure refers to any iatrogenic hazard or incident associated with medications; adverse drug events (ADEs), adverse drug reactions (ADRs), and medication errors are classified under this term. ADEs refer to any injury caused by medication and includes all ADRs and medication errors that result in harm to a patient. Medication errors will be discussed in Chapter 4.

ADRs are a frequent cause of morbidity and mortality in institutionalized patients as well those residing in the community. ADRs have a significant cost both financially and in terms of quality of life. Because many ADRs are undetected, unreported, and untreated, the exact frequencies are unknown. Studies of ADRs have identified the following:

- ADRs may occur in up to 28% of hospitalized patients.
- ADRs are responsible for 8%–15% of hospital admissions.
- ADRs occur in up to 20% of the ambulatory population receiving medication.
- ADRs result in annual costs of $5–7 billion for the health-care system.

Definitions of ADRs

A number of definitions for ADRs exist and are provided below.

World Health Organization (WHO): "A drug-related event that is noxious and unintended and occurs at doses used in humans for prophylaxis, diagnosis or therapy of disease or for the modification of physiological function."

Food and Drug Administration (FDA): A serious adverse event (relating to drugs or devices) in which "the patient outcome is death, life-threatening (real risk of dying), hospitalization (initial or prolonged), disability (significant, persistent or permanent), congenital anomaly, or required intervention to prevent permanent impairment or damage."

American Society of Health-System Pharmacists (ASHP): A significant ADR is any unexpected, undesired, or excessive response to a drug that

- Requires discontinuation of the drug
- Requires changing drug therapy
- Requires modifying the dose (except for minor dosage adjustments)
- Necessitates hospital admission
- Prolongs stay in a health-care facility
- Necessitates supportive treatment
- Significantly complicates diagnosis
- Negatively affects prognosis, or
- Results in temporary or permanent harm, disability or death.

Side effects are defined by ASHP as an "expected, well-known reaction resulting in little or no change in patient management; an effect with predictable frequency," and an effect with which intensity and occurrence are related to the dose.

Drug withdrawal, drug-abuse syndromes, accidental poisonings, and drug-overdose complications should not be classified as ADRs. Most ADR definitions also exclude therapeutic failure.

Pharmacists have an important role in monitoring, detecting, evaluating, documenting, and reporting ADRs and in intervening and providing educational feedback to prescribers, other health-care providers, and patients. Pharmacists in organized health-care settings should develop comprehensive, ongoing programs for monitoring and reporting ADRs.[1]

1 ASHP provided guidelines on ADR monitoring and reporting. American Society of Hospital Pharmacy. *Am J Health Syst Pharm* 1995;**52**:417–419.

Classification of ADRs

ADRs may be classified according to mechanism, severity, and probability.

Mechanism of ADRs

Various mechanisms for ADRs have been described. These are related to the pharmacologic or pharmacodynamic effects of drugs and can be a way to classify the type of reaction.

- *Idiosyncrasy:* an uncharacteristic response of a patient to a drug, usually not occurring on administration
- *Hypersensitivity:* a reaction, not explained by the pharmacologic effects of the drug, caused by altered reactivity of the patient and generally considered to be an allergic manifestation
- *Intolerance:* a characteristic pharmacologic effect of a drug produced by an unusually small dose, so that the usual dose tends to induce a massive overreaction
- *Drug interaction:* an unusual pharmacologic response that could not be explained by the action of a single drug, but was caused by two or more drugs
- *Pharmacologic:* a known, inherent pharmacologic effect of a drug, directly related to dose

Severity of ADRs

One ADR classification system from Karch and Lasagna,[1] two prominent ADR researchers, classifies severity as follows:

- *Minor:* no antidote, therapy or prolongation of hospitalization required
- *Moderate:* requires a change in drug therapy, specific treatment, or an increase in hospitalization by at least 1 day
- *Severe:* potentially life threatening, causing permanent damage or requiring intensive medical care
- *Lethal:* directly or indirectly contributes to the death of the patient

The FDA classifies an ADR as serious if it results in death, is life threatening (real risk of dying), requires initial or prolonged hospitalization, causes significant, persistent or permanent disability or congenital anomaly, or requires intervention to prevent permanent impairment or damage.

Probability of ADRs

It is difficult to prove cause and effect with ADRs. However, a number of tools have been developed to determine the probability that a particular drug caused an adverse event. The Naranjo algorithm (see Table 2.1) is widely accepted and incorporates the following definitions.

- *Definite* = score ≥9; 1) follows a reasonable temporal sequence from administration of the drug or in which the drug level has been established in body fluids or tissues; 2) follows a known response pattern to the suspected drug; and 3) is confirmed by improvement with drug withdrawal and reappearance upon rechallenge.

- *Probable* = score of 5–8; 1) follows a reasonable temporal sequence from administration of the drug; 2) follows a known response pattern to the suspected drug; 3) is confirmed by withdrawal but not by exposure to the drug; and 4) could not be reasonably explained by the known characteristics of the patient's clinical state.
- *Possible* = score of 1–4; 1) followed a temporal sequence after the drug's administration; 2) possibly followed a recognized pattern of the suspected drug; and 3) could be explained by characteristics of the patient's disease.
- *Doubtful* ≤0 and is likely related to factors other than the drug.

Table 2.1 Naranjo ADR Causality Scale

	Yes	No	Do not know
1. Are there previous conclusive reports of this reaction?	+1	0	0
2. Did the adverse event appear after the suspected drug was administered?	+2	–1	0
3. Did the adverse reaction improve when the drug was discontinued or a specific antagonist administered?	+1	0	0
4. Did the adverse reaction reappear when the drug was readministered?	+2	–1	0
5. Are there alternative causes (other than the drug) that could on their own have caused the reaction?	–1	+2	0
6. Did the reaction reappear when a placebo was given?	–1	+1	0
7. Was the drug detected in the blood (or other fluids) in concentrations known to be toxic?	+1	0	0
8. Was the reaction more severe when the dose was increased or less severe when the dose was decreased?	+1	0	0
9. Did the patient have a similar reaction to the same or similar drugs in any previous exposure?	+1	0	0
10. Was the adverse event confirmed by any objective evidence?	+1	0	0
Total score			

Reprinted by permission from Macmillan Publishers Limited: *Clinical Pharmacology & Therapeutics*. Naranjo CA, et al. (1981). A method for estimating the probability of adverse drug reactions. *Clin Pharmacol Ther* **30**:239–245, Copyright 1981.

1 Karch FE, Lasagna L (1977). Toward the operational identification of adverse drug reactions. *Clin Pharmacol Ther* **21**:247–254.

Adverse reactions: drug or disease?

Determining whether or not a symptom is an ADR can be difficult, especially if the patient has multiple comorbidities. Questions to ask are as follows:

- Is there another explanation for the symptom (e.g., is it disease related)?
- Is this a previously reported adverse effect of this drug? How common is it? This is harder to assess for new drugs because there is less information available.
- Does the time frame for ADR development make sense? If there is published literature on the ADR, does it describe a temporal relationship between the drug and the event?
- Is the dose excessive? Check serum levels if available. Check renal function—was the dose too high if renal function is impaired?
- Does the symptom resolve on stopping the drug or reducing the dose (dechallenge)?
- Does the symptom recur on restarting the drug (rechallenge)? Rechallenge may not be practical especially for idiosyncratic and serious reactions.

Factors predisposing to ADRs

Factors that predispose to ADRs are many and varied. Some are related only to specific disease–drug interactions. However, the following factors are generally considered to increase patient risk:

- Advanced (geriatric) or young age (pediatric)
- Organ impairment (hepatic, renal)
- Polypharmacy
- Previous history of ADRs

Helping patients understand the risk of ADRs

Terms such as *common* and *uncommon* are used to describe levels of risk of ADRs in patient information leaflets and summaries of product characteristics. The terms are standardized by the WHO according to the reported frequency found in clinical trials, for example (see Table 2.2), but patients routinely overestimate the level of risk that these terms are intended to imply.

The following strategies should help in communicating risk to patients:

- Avoid using verbal descriptors such as "common."
- Use frequencies rather than percentages—e.g., 1 person in every 1000 rather than 0.1%.
- Use the same denominator throughout—i.e., 1 in 1000 and 10 in 1000 rather than 1 in 1000 and 1 in 100.
- Give both positive and negative information—e.g., 95 out of 100 patients did not get the side effect and 5 patients did.
- Give information about baseline risk, e.g.:
  - The risk of deep vein thrombosis (DVT) in nonpregnant women who are not taking the combined oral contraceptive (COC) is 5 cases per 100,000 women per year.
  - The risk of DVT in pregnancy is 60 cases per 100,000 pregnancies.
  - The risk of DVT in women taking the COC is 15–25 cases per 100,000 per year.

Table 2.2 Terminology as standardized by the World Health Organization (WHO)

WHO terminology	Level of risk
Very common	>10%
Common (frequent)	>1 to <10%
Uncommon (infrequent)	>0.1 to <1%
Rare	>0.01 to <0.15
Very rare	<0.01%

Source: http://www.who-umc.org/DynPage.aspx?id=22684

Reporting ADRs

Significant underreporting of ADRs exists and as a result can lead to delays in identifying important reactions. The FDA MedWatch program is a voluntary reporting system by health-care providers; however, pharmaceutical manufacturers are required to report all adverse events to the FDA. Possible reasons for not reporting ADRs are listed in Table 2.3. Pharmacists should attempt to address these and encourage medical, nursing, and pharmacy colleagues to report ADRs.

The FDA accepts reports of ADRs associated with medical devices, prescription and over-the-counter (OTC) drugs, and dietary supplements from consumers and any type of health-care professional. The FDA's MedWatch program accepts reports by phone, FAX, mail, and online submission.[1] Adverse reactions and other problems associated with vaccines should be reported to the Vaccine Adverse Event Reporting System (VAERS), which is maintained by the FDA and the Centers for Disease Control and Prevention (CDC).[2]

Institution-specific ADR programs may be developed to monitor, report, and prevent ADRs. Pharmacists are in an excellent position to oversee such programs. ASHP and Joint Commission for Accreditation of Healthcare Organizations (JCAHO) standards are useful references for program development. Additionally, the pharmacy literature contains many articles regarding successful ADR programs.

1 http://www.fda.gov/medwatch/index.html
2 http://www.fda.gov/cber/vaers/vaers.htm

Table 2.3 Reasons for failure to report ADRs

1. Failure to detect the reaction because of a low level of suspicion
2. Fear of potential legal implications
3. Lack of training on drug therapy
4. Uncertainty about whether the drug caused the reaction
5. Lack of clear responsibility for reporting
6. Time and paperwork required to find and complete reports
7. Lack of financial incentive to report
8. Unfamiliar with reporting procedure
9. Desire to publish the report
10. Fear that a useful drug will be removed from the market
11. Complacency and lethargy
12. Guilty feelings because of patient harm
13. Reaction not considered serious enough to warrant reporting

Drug interactions

Drug interactions occur when the effect of a drug is altered by the co-administration of any of the following:

- Another drug
- Food
- Drink

The outcome of this is as follows:

- Frequently clinically insignificant
- Sometimes beneficial
- Occasionally potentially harmful

Mechanisms of drug interactions

Interactions can be caused by pharmacokinetic (i.e., handling of the drug in the body is affected) or pharmacodynamic (i.e., related to the pharmacology of the drug) mechanisms. Sometimes the interaction can be caused by more than one mechanism, although usually one mechanism is more significant. Most interactions are caused by the mechanisms listed below.

Pharmacokinetic mechanisms

Absorption

One drug will increase or decrease the absorption of another. This occurs most often when one drug or compound interacts with another—by adsorption, chelation, or complexing—to form a product that is poorly absorbed. This effect can be beneficial (e.g., activated charcoal adsorbs certain poisons) or problematic (e.g., antacids and tetracyclines).

Changes in gastric pH affect absorption of certain drugs—e.g., ketoconazole and itraconazole require an acidic environment to be absorbed, thus proton-pump inhibitors can reduce absorption and an acidic drink such as fruit juice or soft drinks (especially cola) will increase absorption.

Most drugs are absorbed from the upper part of the small intestine. Thus, changes in gut motility potentially affect absorption. Usually the total amount absorbed is unaffected, but the rate of absorption might be altered. This is seen with metoclopramide, which can speed up the rate of absorption of analgesics.

Distribution

Many drugs are bound to proteins in the serum. Only free (unbound) drug is active. Protein binding is a competitive effect, so one drug can displace the other from protein-binding sites. This interaction is only an issue with highly protein-bound drugs and is only significant if most of the drug remains in the plasma rather than being distributed into tissues (i.e., a low volume of distribution).

Displacement of drug from protein-binding sites often causes only a small "blip" in drug levels before equilibrium is restored (because the free drug is also now available for metabolism and excretion), but it could be significant for drugs with a narrow therapeutic index (e.g., warfarin).

Metabolism

Most clinically significant pharmacokinetic interactions are the result of metabolism. Induction or inhibition of the cytochrome P450 (CYP450) system leads to changes in drug levels. CYP450 represents a large group of isoenzymes; drugs are rarely metabolized by a single enzyme, although one usually predominates.

Equally, drugs can induce or inhibit several enzymes and some drugs can induce some enzymes and inhibit others (e.g., efavirenz). In addition, some (but not all) enzyme inhibitors or inducers can induce or inhibit their own metabolism.

When only two drugs are involved, the effect is fairly easy to predict, even if each drug is likely to affect the metabolism of the other. However, if three or more drugs, all of which are inducers or inhibitors, are involved, the effect is almost impossible to predict, and this type of combination should be avoided if possible.

The full effects of enzyme induction and inhibition do not occur immediately.

- Enzyme induction takes about 2–3 weeks to develop and wear off.
- Enzyme inhibition takes only a few days.

Thus, it might be necessary to delay dose adjustment or perform therapeutic drug monitoring (TDM) until a few days (inhibition) or at least a week (induction) after starting or stopping the offending drug(s).

An emerging area of study is drug interactions involving induction or inhibition of p-glycoprotein. This probably includes interactions involving an increase in bioavailability because it affects drug metabolism in the gut wall—e.g., grapefruit juice increases levels of cyclosporine by inhibiting gut-wall metabolism.

Excretion

Some drugs interfere with excretion (usually renal) of other drugs. If both drugs are excreted by the same active transport system in the kidney tubule, the excretion of each drug is decreased by the other. This might be used as a beneficial effect—e.g., probenecid has been used to prolong the half-life of penicillin—or problematic—e.g., methotrexate and nonsteroidal anti-inflammatory drugs (NSAIDs).

Pharmacodynamic interactions

These interactions occur if the pharmacological effects of two drugs are additive or opposing:

- *Additive*—the desired or adverse effects of the two drugs are the same. This can be beneficial or potentially harmful (e.g., ↑ sedation with alcohol plus hypnotics).
- Synergism—a form of additive effect. In this instance, the combination of the two drugs has a greater effect than just an additive effect (e.g., ethambutol ↑ the effectiveness of other drugs for tuberculosis).
- Antagonism—at the receptor level (e.g., a beta-blocker should be prescribed with caution to an asthmatic patient who uses a beta-agonist inhaler) or because of opposing effects (e.g., the desired effects of diuretics could be partly opposed by fluid retention caused by NSAIDs).

Predicting drug interactions

- Are the desired or adverse effects of the two drugs similar or opposing?
- If there is no information available for the drugs in question, are there reports of drug interactions for other drugs in the same class?
- Are both drugs metabolized by the liver? If so, by which enzymes? Information on which drugs are metabolized by which CYP450 enzymes might be listed in the summary of product characteristics and can also be found at: http://medicine.iupui.edu/flockhart/table.htm
- Drugs that are predominantly renally cleared are unlikely to interact with enzyme inducers and inhibitors.

Managing drug interactions

- Check whether or not the drug combination is new.
- If the patient has already been taking the drug combination, has he or she tolerated it? If yes, there is probably no need to change therapy, although monitoring might be required.
- Is the interaction potentially serious (e.g., significant risk of toxicity or ↓ drug effect)? If so, seek alternatives.
- Is the interaction potentially of low-to-moderate significance? If so, it might only be necessary to monitor for side effects and therapeutic effect, or arrange for TDM.
- Remember that some drugs in the same class can have different potentials to cause interactions (e.g., ranitidine vs. cimetidine).
- Remember that interactions occur when a drug is started, and unwanted effects can occur when a drug is discontinued.
- The elderly are at greater risk of drug interactions because of polypharmacy and impaired metabolism and excretion. Additive effects can be a particular problem in this population.
- Be aware of high-risk drugs and always check for potential interactions with these drugs.
    - Enzyme inhibitors and inducers (e.g., erythromycin, rifampin, phenytoin, and protease inhibitors)
    - Drugs with a narrow therapeutic index (e.g., warfarin, digoxin, lithium, phenytoin, and theophylline)
- Remember that interactions can occur with nonprescription drugs, which the patient might not tell you about.
    - Complementary and alternative medicines (dietary supplements, herbal, or homeopathic medicines)
    - Over-the-counter medicines
    - Recreational drugs, including alcohol, tobacco, and drugs obtained by other means, such as over the Internet.

Recently, the Drug Interaction Probability Scale (DIPS) was developed to guide evaluation of drug interaction causation in a specific patient. This tool was modeled after the Naranjo causality scale for ADRs (see Table 2.1) but modified to reflect the difference between a single drug event and a drug–drug interaction. The DIPS is provided in Table 2.4.

The *object drug* refers to the drug affected by the interaction. The *precipitant drug* is the drug that causes the interaction.

The following scores correlate with the probability of an interaction:

- Highly probable >8
- Probable: 5–8
- Possible: 2–4
- Doubtful: <2

Table 2.4 Drug interaction probability scale

	Yes	No	Do not know
1. Are there previous credible reports of this interaction in humans?	+1	–1	0
2. Is the observed interaction consistent with the known interactive properties of the precipitant drug?	+1	–1	0
3. Is the observed interaction consistent with the known interactive properties of the object drug?	+1	–1	0
4. Is the event consistent with the known or reasonable time course of the interaction (onset and/or offset)?	+1	–1	0
5. Did the interaction remit upon dechallenge of the precipitant drug with no change in the object drug? (If no dechallenge, use Unknown or NA and skip Question 6)	+1	–2	0
6. Did the reaction reappear when the precipitant drug was readministered in the presence of continued use of the object drug?	+2	–1	0
7. Are there reasonable alternative causes for the event?	–1	+1	0
8. Was the object drug detected in the blood or other fluids in concentrations consistent with the proposed interaction?	+1	0	0
9. Was the drug interaction confirmed by any objective evidence consistent with the effects on the object drug (other than drug concentrations from Question 8)?	+1	0	0
10. Was the interaction greater when the precipitant drug dose was increased or less severe when the precipitant drug dose was decreased?	+1	–1	0
Total score			

Consider clinical conditions, other interacting drugs, lack of adherence, and risk factors (e.g., age, inappropriate doses of object drug). NO presumes that enough information was presented such that one would expect any alternative causes to be mentioned. When in doubt, use Unknown or N/A.

Horn JR, Hansten PD, Chan LN (2007). Proposal for a new tool to evaluate drug interaction cases. *Ann Pharmacother* **41**:674–680. Reprinted with permission from *The Annals of Pharmacotherapy*, Copyright 2007, Harvey Whitney Books Co.

Chapter 3

Anaphylaxis

Denise R. Kockler

Symptoms and signs of anaphylaxis

Anaphylaxis is defined as a severe, acute systems hypersensitivity event produced by IgE-mediated release of chemicals from mast cells and basophils. Theoretically, prior exposure to the agent is required. The reaction is not dose or route related; however, anaphylaxis to an injected antigen is more frequent, severe, and rapid in onset.

Agents commonly causing anaphylaxis include the following:

- Drugs, e.g., penicillins, aspirin
- Insect stings, e.g., wasp and bee venoms
- Food, e.g., nuts

Urticaria and angioedema are the most common symptoms and signs of anaphylaxis. The absence of these symptoms suggests the reaction may not be anaphylaxis (see Table 3.1).

Airway edema, bronchospasm, and shock are life threatening and immediate emergency treatment is usually required.

The onset of symptoms following parenteral antigen (including stings) is usually within 5–30 minutes. With oral antigen, there is often a delay. Symptoms usually occur within 2 hours but may be immediate and life threatening. A late-phase reaction may also occur with recurrence of symptoms after apparent resolution. Recurrence is a fairly frequent phenomenon and health-care workers should be aware of this. Patients should not be discharged too quickly as they may require further treatment.

Table 3.1 Signs and symptoms of anaphylaxis

Frequent	Rare
Urticaria	Headache
Angioedema	Rhinitis
Dyspnea, wheeze	Substernal pain
Nausea, vomiting, diarrhea, abdominal cramping	Itching without rash Seizure
Flushing	
Upper airway edema	

Treatment of anaphylaxis

Anaphylaxis is a life-threatening condition; therefore, rapid recognition and treatment is essential. The first response is to secure the airway and lay the patient flat to reduce hypotension. If the patient cannot tolerate a supine position (because this can worsen breathing difficulties), a semi-recumbent position is preferable.

In hospital and some community settings (e.g., home intravenous [IV] antibiotic therapy), it might be appropriate to keep an "anaphylaxis kit" for emergency use, which contains the following essential drugs:

- Adrenaline (epinephrine)
- Antihistamines (usually diphenhydramine injection and ranitidine injection)
- Steroids (usually hydrocortisone injection)

Acute-phase reaction

Epinephrine

In adults, a dose of 0.01 mg/kg epinephrine (1:1000 solution, up to 0.5 mg per single dose; may repeat dose at 5-minute intervals) should be immediately administered subcutaneously (SC) or intramuscularly (IM) if the patient is showing clinical signs of shock, airway swelling, or breathing difficulty (stridor, wheezing, and cyanosis).

IV epinephrine is hazardous and should only be administered in the hospital setting. The IV route is preferred if there are concerns about IM absorption; however, time should not be wasted looking for IV access in the event of vascular compromise.

For IV epinephrine administration, use a dilution of at least 1:10 000 and administer the injection over several minutes. The 1:1000 solution is never used intravenously. In the community, patients and caregivers can be taught to administer epinephrine using an auto-injector device, such as an EpiPen® (see Table 3.2). Note that this device contains a residual volume after use and patients should be informed about this. Trainer pens are available from the manufacturers.

Last-phase reaction

Diphenhydramine

In adults, a dose of 1–2 mg/kg (up to 50 mg) diphenhydramine is administered IM or slow IV push after severe attacks to block histamine-1 receptors and help prevent relapse. It should be administered IM or by slow IV push to ↓ the risk of exacerbating hypotension.

Table 3.2 Epinephrine for self-administration (IM only)

EpiPen® auto-injector: adults and children (>30 kg body weight), dose is 0.3 mg of epinephrine
EpiPen® Junior: children (15–30 kg body weight), dose is 0.15 mg of epinephrine

H2-blockers
In adults, a dose of 50 mg ranitidine or 20 mg famotidine is administered by slow IV push after severe attacks to block histamine-2 (H2) receptors and help prevent relapse.

Hydrocortisone sodium succinate
In adults, a dose of 100 mg hydrocortisone is administered by IM or slow IV push after severe attacks and repeated every 2–4 hours to block the late-phase reaction and help prevent relapse.

Additional treatment

Provide symptomatic and supportive care as needed: inhaled albuterol or terbutaline or IV aminophylline can be used to treat bronchospasm, with oxygen (O_2) or other respiratory support given as needed. Crystalloid infusion (e.g., 0.9% sodium chloride) and vasoactive agents or inotropes (e.g., norepinephrine or dopamine) might be needed to treat severe hypotension.

All patients treated initially in the community should be transferred to the hospital for further treatment and observation.

Late sequelae

Patients should be warned of the possibility of symptom recurrence and, if necessary, kept under observation for up to 24 hours. This is especially applicable in the following circumstances:

- Past history of a recurrence (biphasic reaction)
- Severe reaction, with slow onset
- Possibility that the allergen could still be absorbed (e.g., oral administration)
- Past history of asthma or a severe asthmatic component to the reaction

Further reading

Guidelines for the diagnosis and management of anaphylaxis: an updated practice parameter is available from the National Guideline Clearinghouse at: http://www.guidelines.gov/summary/summary.aspx?ss=15&doc_id=6887&nbr=004211&string=anaphylaxis

Prevention of anaphylaxis

The risk of an anaphylactic reaction can be reduced by good drug history-taking and antigen avoidance.

- Check the patient's drug history for reports of allergy. If necessary, clarify the details of the reaction with the patient or a relative. A previous history of a mild penicillin-associated rash in infancy might not be a contraindication to future use, but bronchospasm would be.
- Instruct patients who have had anaphylactic reactions to food to read food ingredient labels to identify foods that should be avoided.
- Counsel patients with anaphylaxis to medications about all cross-reacting medications that should be avoided.
- Guide patients to specialists to obtain information about allergen immunotherapy.
- Advise patients with severe allergies to carry some form of warning information (e.g., medical alert bracelet).
- Advise patients with severe allergies to carry the self-injectable epinephrine with them at all times.
- Some drugs (e.g., NSAIDs and angiotensin-converting enzyme [ACE] inhibitors) can exacerbate or increase the risk of a reaction. Avoid concomitant use of these drugs in situations where the patient could be exposed to the allergen (e.g., desensitization).
- Remember that patients with peanut allergies should avoid medications containing arachis oil (e.g., ipratropium bromide metered dose inhaler, micronized progesterone in oil). Additional drug–food allergies are discussed in Chapter 10.

Chapter 4

Clinical pharmacy skills

Michelle W. McCarthy

Clinical pharmacy definition

Clinical pharmacy is defined by the American College of Clinical Pharmacy as "a health science discipline in which pharmacists provide patient care that optimizes medication therapy and promotes health, wellness, and disease prevention. The practice of clinical pharmacy embraces the philosophy of pharmaceutical care [see Chapter 12]; it blends a caring orientation with specialized therapeutic knowledge, experience, and judgment for the purpose of ensuring optimal patient outcomes. As a discipline, clinical pharmacy also has an obligation to contribute to the generation of new knowledge that advances health and quality of life."

Clinical pharmacists

"Clinical pharmacists care for patients in all health care settings. Clinical pharmacists

- Are experts in the therapeutic use of medications.
- Are a primary source of scientifically valid information and information on the safe, appropriate, and cost-effective use of medications.
- Routinely provide medication therapy evaluations and recommendations to patients and health-care professionals.
- Have in-depth knowledge of medications that is integrated with foundational understanding of biomedical, pharmaceutical, sociobehavioral, and clinical sciences.
- Apply evidence-based therapeutic guidelines as well as evolving sciences, emerging technologies and relevant legal, ethical, social, cultural, economic, and professional principles to achieve desired therapeutic goals.
- Assume responsibility and accountability for managing medication therapy in direct patient care settings, whether practicing independently or in collaboration or consultation with other health-care professionals."[1]

The American College of Clinical Pharmacy has developed a very complete list of competencies necessary for clinical pharmacists. These are clinical problem solving, judgment, and decision making; communication and education; medication information evaluation and management; management of patient populations; and therapeutic knowledge.

Further reading

Clinical pharmacist competencies. American College of Clinical Pharmacy. Available at: http://www.accp.com/docs/positions/whitePapers/CliniPharmCompTFfinalDraft.pdf

1 The definition of clinical pharmacy. *Pharmacotherapy* 2008; **28**:816–817.

Prescription screening and monitoring

Pharmacists collaborate with other health-care providers to ensure safe and effective drug therapy selection. This is accomplished by careful review of every drug order and prescription and evaluation of patient-specific information. In some settings, a heavy workload or lack of complete patient data may be barriers to the provision of comprehensive pharmaceutical care (see Chapter 12). The following discussion assumes all information is available, although it can be adapted to situations in which there are more limited data.

First impressions

Review the drug order or prescription and patient (if present). What does the prescription or record tell you about the patient?

- *Age*—think about special considerations in children (p. 202) and the elderly (p. 212)
- *Weight*—is the patient significantly overweight or underweight? Will you need to check doses according to weight?

Other charts can also provide important information—e.g., diet sheets, blood glucose monitoring, blood pressure (BP), and temperature.

What does observation of the patient tell you?

- Old, frail patients probably need dose adjustments because of low weight or poor renal function.
- Carefully evaluate medication doses for children and evaluate appropriateness of the formulation prescribed (p. 208).
- Unconscious patients cannot take drugs by mouth. Will you need to provide formulations that can be administered through a nasogastric or gastrostomy tube?
- Are IV fluids running? Consider fluid balance if other IV fluids will be used to administer drugs.
- If the patient's weight is not recorded, does the patient appear significantly overweight or underweight? If you have concerns, ask the patient if they know their weight, or weigh them.
- Is the patient pregnant or breastfeeding (pp. 194–201)?
- Could the patient's racial origin affect drug handling—e.g., there is a higher incidence of glucose 6-phosphate dehydrogenase (G6PD) deficiency in people of African origin (p. 220).

Review prescribed drugs

Check each drug prescribed. Newly prescribed drugs are the highest priority, but it is important to periodically review previously prescribed drugs.

- Are the dose, frequency, and route appropriate for the patient, their weight, and their renal function?
- What is the indication for the drug?
  - Is it appropriate for this patient?
  - Does it comply with local or national guidelines or formularies?
  - Could the drug be treating a side effect of another drug—if so, could the first drug be stopped or changed?

- Are there any potential drug interactions (p. 20)?
  - Are they clinically significant?
  - Do you need to get the interacting drug stopped or changed or just monitor for side effects?
- Is therapeutic drug monitoring (TDM) required?
  - Do you need to check levels or advise on dose adjustment?
  - Are levels being taken at the right time?
- Is the drug working?
  - Think about the signs and symptoms (including laboratory data and nursing observations) that should be monitored to check that the drug is producing the desired effect. Talk to the patient!
- Are any signs and symptoms due to side effects?
  - Do you need to advise a dose adjustment, a change in therapy, or symptomatic treatment of side effects? Remember that it is sometimes appropriate to prescribe symptomatic therapy in anticipation of side effects (e.g., antiemetics and laxatives for patients on opioids).
- Check that the patient is not allergic to or intolerant of any of the prescribed drugs. If allergies are indicated, it is important to determine what type of reaction occurred. Patients may state an allergy to a medication that was truly an adverse effect or intolerance (e.g., nausea from opioids).
- Ensure that you have looked at all prescribed drugs. Hospital records may have different sections for "as needed" and "once only" ("stat") drugs and IV infusions. Patients might have more than one record and some might have different charts for certain types of drugs (e.g., chemotherapy).

Review the patient's drug history

When patients are admitted to hospital, it is important that the drugs they normally take at home are continued, unless there is a good reason to omit them (see Medication Reconciliation section, p. 50).

- Check that the drugs that the patient usually takes are prescribed in the right dose, frequency, and form.
- Ideally, use a source of information that is different from the admission history:
  - Prior medical records or discharge summaries
  - Community pharmacy record
  - Primary care provider (PCP) records
  - Talk to the patient, relative, and/or caregiver.
  - Patient's medication history list
  - Talking to the patient often reveals drugs that might otherwise be overlooked (e.g., oral contraceptives, regular over-the-counter medicines, or herbal medicines).
- If there are any discrepancies between what has been prescribed and what the patient normally takes that you cannot account for, ensure that the doctors are aware of this. Depending on your local practice, it might be appropriate to record discrepancies on the patient's chart or in the medical notes.

Talk to the patient

Patients are an important source of information about their drugs, disease, and symptoms. Talk to them! You might find out important information that is not recorded in the medical notes or prescription chart. If you are reviewing charts at the bedside, always introduce yourself and explain your role and what you are doing.

It is a good idea to ask the patient if they have any problems with or questions about their medicines. If the patient is on many drugs or complex therapy, check their adherence by asking how they are managing their medicines at home.

Care plan

By completing the above steps, individualized monitoring and care plans can be developed. Prioritize high-risk patients and high-risk drugs (chemotherapy). An elderly patient with renal impairment who is taking multiple drugs is at higher risk of drug-related problems than a young, fit patient who is only taking one or two drugs. In some hospitals, a formal pharmaceutical care plan is written for each patient.

Screening discharge prescriptions

- Are all regular drugs from all prescription charts prescribed? If not, can you account for any omitted?
- Are timings correct and complete (e.g., diuretics to be taken in the morning)?
- Are any "as needed" drugs used frequently, and are they to be continued upon discharge?
- Are all the prescribed drugs actually needed on discharge (e.g., hypnotics)?
- Does the patient actually need a supply? They might have enough of their own supply on the ward or at home.
- Will the PCP need to adjust any doses or drugs after discharge? If so, is this clear on the prescription or discharge instructions?
- Is there any information that you need to pass on to the patient, caregiver, or PCP (e.g., changes to therapy or monitoring requirements)?
- Does the patient understand how to take the drugs, especially any new ones or those with special instructions (e.g., warfarin, p. 386)?
- Are adherence aids needed (Chapter 2)?

Pharmacist documentation in patient medical records (PMR)

Pharmacists should document in the PMR their professional actions that are intended to ensure safe and effective use of drugs that may affect patient outcomes. Information provided in the PMR will vary according to local practice but should include the following:

- Summary of patient's medication history on admission that includes medication allergies
- Oral and written consultations provided to other health-care providers regarding drug therapy selection and management
- Prescribers' oral orders received directly by the pharmacist
- Clarification of drug orders
- Adjustments made to drug dosage, dosage frequency, dosage form, or route of administration
- All drugs, including investigational drugs, administered
- Actual and potential drug-related problems that warrant surveillance
- Drug therapy monitoring findings, including the following:
  - Therapeutic appropriateness of the drug regimen, including route and method of administration
  - Therapeutic duplication in the drug regimen
  - Patient compliance with the prescribed regimen
  - Actual and potential drug–drug, drug–food, drug–laboratory test, and drug–disease interactions
  - Clinical and pharmacokinetic laboratory data pertinent to drug regimen
  - Actual and potential drug toxicity and adverse effects
  - Physical signs and clinical symptoms relevant to drug therapy
  - Drug-related patient education and counseling provided

All documentation should meet established criteria for legibility, clarity, lack of judgmental language, completeness, need for inclusion in the PMR, appropriate use of a standard format (e.g., SOAP [**S**ubjective, **O**bjective, **A**ssessment, and **P**lan] or TITRS [**T**itle, **I**ntroduction, **T**ext, **R**ecommendation, and **S**ignature]), and contact information (e.g., telephone or pager number).

Documentation of formal consultation solicited by other health-care providers may include direct suggestions or recommendations, as appropriate. Unsolicited informal consultations, clinical impressions, findings, suggestions, and indirect recommendations should be documented more subtly (e.g., "may want to consider").

Further reading

ASHP Guidelines on Documenting Pharmaceutical Care in Patient Medical Records. ASHP Best Practices. Available at: http://www.ashp.org

Understanding medical records

Each time a patient has a health-care encounter, a fairly standard assessment related to their physical examination is performed. The documentation of the encounter is recorded in the medical record.

Medical record documentation

Documentation in the medical record usually has the following format, although not every history includes every step:

- *General information* about the patient—name, age, gender, marital status, and occupation
- *Chief complaint (CC) or presenting complaint (PC)*—a statement of what symptoms or problems have led to the patient's admission or appointment, ideally using the patient's own words
- *History of present illness*—more detail about the symptoms (e.g., timing, whether they have occurred previously, whether anything improves or worsens them, severity and character)
- *Past medical history (PMH)*—does the patient have a past history of any medical complaint, including the following:
  - Previous hospital admission
  - Surgery
  - Chronic disease (e.g., diabetes mellitus or asthma)
- *Medication history*—the patient's current drugs and any drugs stopped recently are listed. Ideally, this should include any frequently used over-the-counter and herbal medicines. ADRs and allergies are also recorded here.
- *Social history (SH) and family history (FH)*—relevant details of the patient's occupation, home circumstances and alcohol and tobacco consumption are recorded. Significant information about the medical history of close family members is noted:
  - Whether parents and siblings are alive and well
  - Does anyone in the family have a medical problem related to the present illness?
  - If close family members have died, at what age and what was the cause of death?

All of the above information is found by asking the patient questions before the doctor examines the patient. This is known as "review of systems." Negative findings are recorded, in addition to positive findings.

- *Physical examination*—includes a general comment about what the patient looks like (e.g., pale, sweaty, or short of breath [SOB]).
- The doctor examines each *body system* in turn, recording what is found by looking, listening, and feeling. The clinician concentrates on any systems most relevant to the symptoms described by the patient. The following body systems are covered:
  - Head, ears, eyes, nose, and throat (HEENT)
  - Cardiovascular
  - Respiratory
  - Gastrointestinal (GI) system
  - Extremities
  - Skin

Laboratory values outside of normal values are also provided.

Much of the information is recorded using abbreviations and medical shorthand (see Table 4.1).

- *Assessment and plan*—based on the findings of the physical examination and history, the clinician draws a conclusion about the current diagnosis (Dx). If the diagnosis is not conclusive, several possibilities will be recorded (differential diagnoses). The plan for treatment, care, and further evaluations is recorded. The entry is signed and dated by the clinician who completes it. Contact information is also provided.

Other clinical information

The complete clinical record contains much more information than the medical notes. To get a complete picture of the patient's history and progress, you might need to use other information:

- Admission form (includes the patient's address, next of kin, and PCP details)
- Nursing notes
- Observation charts—e.g., temperature, BP, blood glucose levels, and fluid balance
- Laboratory data—might be paper copies in notes or on computer
- Notes from previous admissions or outpatient visits (including discharge summaries and clinic letters)

Problem-oriented medical record

In many instances, medical problems are presented in the medical charts or records in a standardized format such as the SOAP format. Under each problem, the following are included: subjective and objective data related to each problem, assessment, and plan. The SOAP format is summarized as follows:

- *Subjective*: the explanation or reason for the encounter, including patient-reported symptoms, previous treatments, medications, and adverse effects. This information is nonreproducilble because it is based on the patient's interpretation and recall of past events.
- *Objective*: summary of the physical examination, laboratory and diagnostic tests, pill counts, and pharmacy patient profile information. These data are measurable and reproducible.
- *Assessment*: description of problem, including conclusion or diagnosis that is supported by the subjective and objective data
- *Plan*: description of recommended or further workup, treatment, patient education, monitoring, and follow-up as it relates to the assessment

Table 4.1 Abbreviations commonly found in medical notes

ABG	arterial blood gases
ACTH	adrenocorticotrophic hormone
ADH	antidiuretic hormone
AF	atrial fibrillation
AFB	acid-fast bacilli
Ag	antigen
AIDS	acquired immune deficiency syndrome
ALL	acute lymphoblastic leukemia
AML	acute myeloid leukemia
ANF	antinuclear factor
APTT	activated partial thromboplastin time
ARDS	acute respiratory distress syndrome
ASD	atrial septal defect
AST	aspartate transaminase
A&W	alive and well
AXR	abdominal X-ray
Ba	barium
BBB	bundle branch block
bid	twice daily
BMT	bone marrow transplant
BP	blood pressure
BS	breath sounds, bowel sounds
BUN	blood urea nitrogen
Ca	carcinoma, cancer
CABG	coronary artery bypass graft
CAPD	continuous ambulatory peritoneal dialysis
CC	chief complaint
CF	cystic fibrosis
CHD	congestive heart disease
CHF	chronic heart failure; congestive heart failure
CLL	chronic lymphoblastic leukemia
CML	chronic myeloid leukemia
CMV	cytomegalovirus
CNS	central nervous system
C/O	complaining of
COPD	chronic obstructive pulmonary disease

Table 4.1 *(Contd.)*

CPAP	continuous positive airways pressure
CSF	cerebrospinal fluid
CSU	catheter specimen of urine
CT	computerized tomography
CVA	cerebrovascular accident
CVP	central venous pressure
CVS	cardiovascular system
CVVH	continuous venovenous hemofiltration
CXR	chest X-ray
D&C	dilatation and curettage
DDx	differential diagnoses (used if there is more than one possible diagnosis)
DH	drug history
DIC	disseminated intravascular coagulation
DM	diabetes mellitus
DNA	did not attend, or deoxyribose nucleic acid
D&V	diarrhea and vomiting
DVT	deep vein thrombosis
D/W	discussed or discussion with
Dx	diagnosis
EBV	Epstein–Barr virus
ECF	extracellular fluid
ECG	electrocardiogram
EEG	electroencephalogram
ELISA	enzyme-linked immunosorbent assay
EMU	early-morning urine
ENT	ear, nose, and throat
ESR	erythrocyte sedimentation rate
ERCP	endoscopic retrograde cholangiopancreatography
EUA	examination under anesthesia
FBC	full blood count
FEV1	forced expiratory volume in 1 second
FFP	fresh frozen plasma
FH	family history
FSH	follicle-stimulating hormone
FSH	family and social history
FVC	forced vital capacity

Table 4.1 (*Contd.*)

G6PD	glucose 6-phosphate dehydrogenase
GABA	G-aminobutyric acid
GFR	glomerular filtration rate
GGT	G-glutamyl transpeptidase
GH	growth hormone
GI	gastrointestinal
GTT	glucose tolerance test
GU	gastric ulcer, or genitourinary
GVHD	graft-versus-host disease
Hb	hemoglobin
HBV	hepatitis B virus
HCT	hematocrit
HCV	hepatitis C virus
HIV	human immunodeficiency virus
HLA	human leukocyte antigen
HPC	history of present condition (complaint)
HRT	hormone replacement therapy
HSV	herpes simplex virus
IBD	inflammatory bowel disease
IBS	irritable bowel syndrome
ICP	intracranial pressure
Ig	immunoglobulin
IHD	ischemic heart disease
IM	intramuscular
INR	international normalized ratio
IT	intrathecal
IV	intravenous
IVC	inferior vena cava
JVP	jugular venous pressure
LBBB	left bundle branch block
LFT	liver function tests
LH	luteinizing hormone
LP	lumbar puncture
LVF	left ventricular failure
MCHC	mean corpuscular hemoglobin concentration
MC&S	microscopy, culture, and sensitivities

Table 4.1 (*Contd.*)

MCV	mean corpuscular volume
MI	myocardial infarction
MVA	motor vehicle accident
NG	nasogastric
NKDA	no known drug allergies
N&V	nausea and vomiting
OA	osteoarthritis, or on admission
OCP	ova, cysts, parasites
O/E	on examination
OGTT	oral glucose tolerance test
PC	present complaint
PCP	Pneumocystis jirovecii pneumonia, or primary care provider
PCV	packed cell volume
PDA	patent ductus arteriosus
PE	pulmonary embolism
PEARL	pupils equal and reactive to light
PEEP	positive end-expiratory pressure
PEFR	peak expiratory flow rate
PID	pelvic inflammatory disease
PM	postmortem
PMH	past medical history
PR	per rectum, or pulse rate
PT	prothrombin time
PTH	parathyroid hormone
PTT	partial thromboplastin time
PUO	pyrexia of unknown origin
PV	per vagina, plasma volume, or papillomavirus
qid	four times a day
RA	rheumatoid arthritis
RBBB	right bundle branch block
RBC	red blood cell
RF	renal function
Rh	Rhesus
RS, RES	respiratory system
RTI	respiratory tract infection
RVF	right ventricular failure
S1 S2	heart sounds (first and second)

Table 4.1 (*Contd.*)

SIADH	syndrome of inappropriate diuretic hormone
SLE	systemic lupus erythematosus
SOB	shortness of breath
SOBOE	short of breath on exertion
ST	sinus tachycardia
SVC	superior vena cava
SVT	supraventricular tachycardia
TB	tuberculosis
TBG	thyroid binding globulin
TEE	transesophageal echocardiography
TFT	thyroid function tests
THR	total hip replacement
TIA	transient ischemic attack
TIBC	total iron binding capacity
tid	three times daily
TLC	tender loving care
TOP	termination of pregnancy
TPN	total parenteral nutrition
TRH	thyrotropin-releasing hormone
TSH	thyroid-stimulating hormone
TURP	transurethral resection of the prostate
UC	ulcerative colitis
URTI	upper respiratory tract infection
UTI	urinary tract infection
VF	ventricular fibrillation
VSD	ventricular septal defect
VT	ventricular tachycardia
WBC	white blood cell count

Further reading

Davis NM (2006). *Medical Abbreviations: 28,000 Conveniences at the Expense of Communications and Safety*. 13th ed. Huntingdon Valley, PA: Neil M. Davis Associates.

Medication review

Medication review is defined as a structured, critical examination of a patient's medicines by a health-care professional, reaching an agreement with the patient about treatment, optimizing the use of medicines, minimizing the number of medication-related problems, and avoiding wastage.

Regular medication review maximizes the therapeutic benefit and minimizes the potential harm of drugs. It ensures the safe and effective use of medicines by patients. Medication review provides an opportunity for patients to discuss their medicines with a health-care professional (see medication problem checklist, p. 263).

What does medication review involve?

- A structured, critical examination of a patient's medicines (prescription and other medicines, including alternatives) by a health-care professional
- Identification, management, and prevention of ADRs or drug interactions
- Minimizing the number of medication-related problems
- Optimizing the use of medicines
- Simplification of regimen
- Assurance that all drugs are appropriate and needed
- Avoidance of wastage
- Medication counseling
- Adherence counseling—to ensure that patients adhere to their drug regimens
- Assessment of ability to self-medicate
- Education of patient or caregiver—to help them understand their drugs better
- Education of the patient on safe and effective medication use
- Forum for suggesting effective treatment alternatives
- Recommendation of compliance aids

Principles of medication review

- Patients should have the opportunity to ask questions and highlight any problems with their medicines.
- Medication review should improve the impact of treatment for an individual patient.
- Any changes resulting from the review are agreed on by the patient.
- The review is documented in the patient's notes.
- The impact of any change is monitored.

Who to target

- Patients on multiple medications or complicated drug regimens
- Patients experiencing ADRs
- Patients with chronic conditions
- Elderly patients
- Nonadherent patients

Benefits of medication review

- Identification, management, and prevention of ADRs
- Ensures that patients have maximum benefit from their medicines
  - ↓ risk of drug-related problems
  - ↑ the appropriate use of medicines
- Improved clinical outcomes
- Cost-effectiveness
- Improved quality of life
- Optimizing therapy
  - Reduces waste of medicines
- Enables patients to maintain their independence
  - ↓ admissions to hospital
  - ↓ in drug-related deaths

Problems identified during a medication review

- Potential ADRs
- Potential interactions (drug–drug or drug–food)
- Suboptimal monitoring
- Adherence or lack of concordance issues
- Impractical directions
- Incorrect or inappropriate dosages
- Drugs no longer needed (e.g., one medication used to treat the side effects of another)
- Difficulties with using certain dose forms (e.g., inhaler or eye drops)

Recording medication reviews

- There is no universally agreed-upon way of documenting medication reviews.
- Local guidance for recording medication reviews needs to be followed.
- The minimum information that should be recorded is the following:
  - Current medication history
  - Problems identified
  - Advice given
  - Suggested time frame for the next medication review
  - Date, signature, name, and position

Medication reconciliation

Medication reconciliation is a process of comparing a patient's medication orders to all of the medications they have been taking. Reconciliation is performed to avoid medication errors such as dosing errors, drug interactions, omissions, and duplications.

Poor communication of medication information upon care transfer is associated with 50% of all medication errors and 20% of all ADRs. Medication reconciliation should be performed at every transfer of care in which new medications are ordered and existing orders are continued.

Medication reconciliation steps

1. *Obtain medication history.* The complete medication history obtained upon admission should include the name, indication, dose, route, frequency, and time of last dose of all prescription and over-the-counter medications and dietary supplements. Sources of information in addition to the patient may include visual inspection (if medications are brought with patient), family member or caregiver, previous medical history, and records from the PCP office and/or community pharmacy.
2. *Develop a list of medications to prescribe.* Once the list is complete, the prescriber should review and act upon each medication listed while determining the patient's admission medication orders.
3. *Compare the medications on the two lists.* Compare the prescribed admission medications to the medication history list and resolve any discrepancies.
4. *Make clinical decisions based on the comparison.* Each time a patient moves from one setting to another, the previous medication orders should be compared to new orders and plans for care, and any discrepancies should be resolved. Upon discharge, the reconciled admission list must be compared to the discharge orders and the most recent medication administration record. All differences must be reconciled before discharge.
5. *Share the list.* Communicate the complete list to the next provider of service when patients are transferred to other services, practitioners, or level of care within or outside the institution. The discharge medication list should be shared with the patient's PCP, and the patient should communicate the information to their community pharmacy.

Many types of practitioners, including pharmacists, nurses, and pharmacy technicians, may be involved in the medication reconciliation process.

Further reading

ASHP medication reconciliation toolkit. Available at: http://www.ashp.org/Import/PRACTICEANDPOLICY/PracticeResourceCenters/PatientSafety/ASHPMedicationReconciliationToolkit_1.aspx

My Medicine List™. Available at: http://www.ashpfoundation.org/MainMenuCategories/PracticeTools/MyMedicineList.aspx

Intervention monitoring

Clinical pharmacists can assess their impact on patient care by intervention monitoring. Some hospitals evaluate these data at regular intervals and present results internally or to the multidisciplinary team.

Data collection forms or electronic systems are used to collect the relevant data on a pharmacist's interventions to improve patient care. Examples of data collected for this purpose include the following:

- Patient details and demographics
- Area of work or specialization
- Written details of the intervention
- Date of intervention
- Other health-care professionals contacted
- Evidence used to support the intervention
- Who initiated the intervention—e.g., pharmacist, doctor, nurse, or patient
- Possible effect the intervention would have on patient care
- Outcome of the intervention
- Actual outcome on patient care that the intervention had
- Significance of intervention
- Category of intervention (see below for examples)

Examples of categories of pharmacist interventions in drug therapy include the following:

- Adverse drug event/ADR (potential or actual)
- Allergy
- Additional drug therapy required
- Medication error
- Therapeutic monitoring for toxicity or effectiveness
- Medication without indication
- Untreated condition or undertreated condition
- Minimal or no therapeutic effectiveness
- Compliance or drug administration issue
- Patient education
- Inappropriate or suboptimal dose, schedule, or route
- Therapeutic duplication
- Formulary adherence
- Drug–drug or drug–disease interaction
- Formulation
- Compatibility

Further reading

Hoth AB, Carter BL, Ness J, et al. (2007). Development and reliability testing of clinical pharmacist recommendation taxonomy. *Pharmacotherapy* **27**(5):639–646.

McDonough RP, Doucette WR (2003). Drug therapy management: an empirical report of drug therapy problems, pharmacists' interventions, and results of pharmacists' actions. *J Am Pharm Assoc* **43**(4):511–518.

Obtaining patient medication histories

Before taking a medication history from a patient, ensure that relevant information is obtained from the medical and nursing notes that might aid the process. Consider whether it is beneficial to have the patient's caregiver present, particularly for very young or old patients, for those who have difficulty communicating, or if the caregiver administers the medication. It is preferable that the medication history be conducted in an area where interruptions from visitors or other health-care professionals are minimized.

When taking the medication history, obtain details of the following:

- Drug name
- Dose
- Frequency
- Formulation
- Duration of treatment
- Indication
- Any problems with medication, such as with administration (e.g., inhaler), ADRs, or allergies
- Adherence to medications

It is essential that details of all types of medication be obtained for a medication history:

- Medicines prescribed by the PCP
- Medicines prescribed while hospitalized
- Over-the-counter medicines
- Alternative (e.g., herbal or homeopathic) medicines
- All forms of medicines (e.g., tablets, liquids, suppositories, injections, eye drops or ointments, ear drops, inhalers, nasal sprays, creams, and ointments)
- If a compliance aid (e.g., pill box) is used, who fills it?

Information obtained during medication histories may require verification if patients cannot remember the details of their medication or have not brought their medication with them. Medications can be verified by the following means:

- Checking against the personal supply
- Checking against PCP records
- Checking records of prescriptions used in the community
- Telephoning the PCP

During the medication history process, it is also useful to establish whether the patient has any drug allergies, including symptoms.

The following information from the medication history should be entered in the medical notes or other record according to local procedure:

- Date and time
- Medication list, including the above details
- Allergies
- Pharmacist recommendations
- Information provided to the patient as a result of this process
- Signature
- Name, profession, and contact information

Medication-use evaluation (MUE)

MUE is a performance-improvement method focused on evaluating and improving medication use processes to optimize patient outcomes. The goal of MUE is to improve patient quality of life through achievement of predefined, medication-related, therapeutic outcomes.

MUE may be performed on a medication or therapeutic class, disease state or condition, a medication-use process (prescribing, preparing and dispensing, administering, and monitoring) or specific outcomes. The MUE process can be carried out retrospectively, prospectively, or concurrently. MUE is used as a tool in areas where prescribing practice does not appear to be consistent with standards.

To ensure an effective MUE program, a multidisciplinary approach should be taken. Doctors and pharmacists should agree on the criteria, and accurate prescribing data should be collected. There should be critical evaluation of the data and an acceptable means of correcting any deficiencies in prescribing.

Medications or medication-use processes that meet one or more of the following criteria may be selected for evaluation:

- High potential for toxicity or ADRs or interaction with other medication, food, or diagnostic procedures that would result in a potential significant health risk
- Used in patient population at high risk for ADRs
- Affect a large number of patients or frequently prescribed
- Critical component of care for a specific disease, condition, or procedure (i.e., beta-blockers and aspirin following myocardial infarction)
- Potentially toxic or cause discomfort at normal doses
- Effective when used in a specific way
- Under consideration for formulary addition, retention, or deletion
- Suboptimal use has a negative effect on patient outcomes or system costs.
- High-cost medications

Steps to take in the MUE process include the following:

- Select a drug or therapeutic area for MUE.
- Determine objective, measurable criteria and standards of use for the target area if these are not set already.
- Design a sample data-collection sheet and pilot.
- Collect the prescribing data to evaluate current practice against the standards.
- Analyze the data.
- Evaluate the practice against the standards.
- Decide what intervention needs to be introduced to improve compliance with the agreed-upon criteria and action plan.
- Educate staff and introduce practice to correct any inappropriate prescribing.
- Evaluate the impact of the MUE.
- Communicate the results.

Benefits of MUE

- Confirms appropriate quality of prescribing, with respect to safety, efficacy, and cost to an organization
- Financial benefits with the ↓ of inappropriate drug use
- Improved quality of clinical pharmacy service, with respect to targeting clinical pharmacy activity and educational benefits
- Improves credibility of reports on drug expenditure
- Supports development, implementation, and monitoring of formularies

Pharmacist's role in MUE

- Develop a plan for MUE programs and processes consistent with the organization's overall goals and resource capabilities.
- Work collaboratively with prescribers and others to develop criteria for specific medications and to design effective medication-use processes.
- Review individual medication orders compared to MUE criteria.
- Manage MUE programs and processes.
- Collect, analyze, and evaluate patient-specific data to identify, resolve, and prevent medication-related problems.
- Interpret and report MUE finding and recommend changes in medication-use processes.
- Provide information and education based on MUE findings.

Further reading

ASHP Guidelines on Medication-Use Evaluation. ASHP Best Practices. Available at: http://www.ashp.org

Medication errors

Medication errors are defined as "any preventable event that may cause or lead to inappropriate medication use or patient harm while the medication is in the control of the health-care professional, patient, or consumer."[1] Medication errors are associated with significant unexpected drug-related morbidity and mortality. Errors in the medication-use process such as prescribing, dispensing, administering, and monitoring are responsible for 14% of drug-related deaths.

Medication management policies and procedures should be in place to minimize the risk of medication errors in the medication-use process. Pharmacists can play a prominent role in optimizing safe medication use and preventing medication errors.

Common causes of medication errors are the following:

- Ambiguous strength designation on labels or packaging
- Drug product nomenclature (look-alike or sound-alike names, use of lettered or numbered prefixes and suffixes in drug names)
- Equipment failure or malfunction
- Illegible handwriting
- Improper transcription
- Inaccurate dosage calculation
- Inadequately trained personnel
- Inappropriate use of abbreviations
- Labeling errors
- Excessive workload

The types and definitions of medication errors are provided in Table 4.2.

Pharmacists play a critical role in preventing medication errors. Pharmacists may prevent medication errors through the following activities:

- Participate in drug therapy monitoring and MUE activities to achieve safe, effective, and rational drug use.
- Recommend and recognize appropriate drug therapy by staying current with literature, consulting with other health-care professionals, and participating in continuing education programs
- Be available to prescribers and other health-care professionals to provide information about therapeutic drug regimens and correct medication use.
- Be familiar with the medication ordering system and drug distribution policies and procedures to provide for the safe distribution of all medications and supplies.
- Clarify confusing medication orders.
- Maintain an orderly work area and limit interruptions.
- Ensure accuracy of drug, labeling, packaging, quantity, dose, and instructions. This may involve checking of technical staff and automated devices, self-checking, and double-checking others.
- Dispense medications in ready-to-administer forms whenever possible.

1 National Coordinating Council for Medication Error Reporting and Prevention. Available at: http://www.nccmerp.org/aboutMedErrors.html

Table 4.2 Types and definitions of medication errors

Prescribing error	Incorrect drug selection (based on indications, contraindications, known allergies, existing drug therapy), dose dosage form, quantity, route, concentration, rate of administration, or instructions for use of a drug product ordered or authorized by prescriber; illegible prescription or medication order that led to errors that reach the patient
Omission error	Failure to administer an ordered dose to a patient before the next scheduled dose
Wrong-time error	Administration of the medication outside of a predefined time interval from scheduled administration time (each facility must establish the interval)
Unauthorized-drug error	Administration of a medication not authorized by a legitimate prescriber for the patient
Improper-dose error	Administration of a dose that is greater than or less than the amount ordered by the prescriber, or administration of duplicate doses to the patient (i.e., one or more dosage units from those that were ordered)
Wrong-dose form error	Administration of a drug product in a different form than that ordered by the prescriber
Wrong drug-preparation error	Drug product incorrectly formulated or manipulated before administration
Wrong administration-technique error	Inappropriate procedure or improper technique in administration of drug
Deteriorated-drug error	Administration of a drug that has expired or for which the chemical or physical dosage-form integrity has been compromised
Monitoring error	Failure to review a prescribed regimen for appropriateness and detection of problems, or failure to use appropriate clinical or laboratory data for adequate assessment of patient response to prescribed therapy
Compliance error	Inappropriate patient behavior regarding adherence to a prescribed medication error
Other medication error	Any medication error that does not fall into one of the above predefined categories

Originally published in *Am J Hosp Pharm* 1993; **50**:305–314.

- Use auxiliary labels that help in prevention of errors (e.g., shake well, not for injection).
- Ensure delivery of medications to the patient-care area in a timely fashion.
- Observe medication use in patient-care areas to ensure that dispensing and storage procedures are followed to optimize patient safety.
- Counsel patients or caregivers on appropriate medication use.
- Review preprinted medication order forms and computerized medication ordering screens.

Each institution must have a system for reporting errors. The system should be nonpunitive and focus on developing systems that minimize recurrence. Institutional reporting techniques may include the following:

- Anonymous self-reports
- Incident reports—errors are written up as legal reports and satisfy JCAHO requirements.
- Critical incident technique—observations and interviews of those involved in the error are used to analyze and identify weaknesses in the system.
- Disguised observation—observers are placed among health-care professionals to watch for errors.

Institutions should also involve numerous types of health-care providers in assessing and monitoring medication errors and in developing educational and interventional programs.

Medication errors should also be reported to national monitoring programs so that information shared can increase patient safety. National programs include the following:

- United States Pharmacopeia–Institute for Safe Medication Practice (USP-ISMP) accepts anonymous reports 24 hours/day. Call 1–800-23-ERROR or report the incident online, at: https://www.ismp.org/orderforms/reporterrortoISMP.asp
- MedMARx is subscription program for reporting errors and benchmarking errors between institutions. Go to: http://www.usp.org/hqi/patientSafety/medmarx/

Further reading

ASHP Guidelines on Preventing Medication Errors in Hospitals. ASHP Best Practices. Available at: http://www.ashp.org

Financial reports and budget statements

Pharmacists may be actively involved in analyzing and summarizing financial data provided within their institution. Reports are generally monthly or quarterly. At the end of the financial year, an annual finance report is usually produced. Reports are usually sent to the finance manager, clinical director, and manager of a clinical area.

The objectives of a financial report are as follows:

- Relevant and timely information
- Easy-to-understand and concise information
- Verifiable and complete numbers
- Format enables comparison.
- Reporting is consistent in form and content.
- Reports are adequate for the audience.
- Reports are periodic.
- Data are inclusive, analytical, and comparative.
- Assumptions are attached.

Financial reports should include the following elements:

- Statistical data
- Financial data
- Current period of assessment
- Actual vs. budgeted

The type of financial information that a pharmacist supplies is as follows:

- Overall drug expenditure for a financial year by month or quarter
- Actual drug expenditure to date
- Projected expenditure for that financial year and next financial year
- Comparison of expenditure with that of the previous financial year (e.g., by month, quarter or year)
- Analysis of expenditure by clinical areas, and inpatient, outpatient, and take-home medication.
- The top 20–50 high-expenditure drugs by month, quarter, or year
- High-expenditure therapeutic areas for a specified period of time (e.g., month, quarter, or year)
- Explanation of any areas of unexpected high expenditure
- Interpretation of financial information, detailing areas where cost-savings can be made
- Detail where cost-savings have already been achieved
- Interpretation of changes in expenditure or drug use
- Exceptions to previous trends

This information can be portrayed in a tabular or graphic form but should be presented in ways that are easy to interpret and should include a commentary.

It is helpful to determine what the recipient actually wants in the report before providing financial reports.

Additional resources

Tools for evaluating high-impact drugs: American Society of Health-System Pharmacists, at: http://www.ashp.org/Import/PRACTICEANDPOLICY/PracticeResourceCenters/Pharmaceutical-Reimbursement/StrategiesforSuccess/ToolsforEvaluatingHighImpactDrugs.aspx

Hospital budget statements

- The finance department often produces budget statements, which are useful for pharmacists to understand.
- Financial years vary from organization to organization; many are July 1 to June 30.
- The budget statement reflects the budget that is available and the financial position at a given point in a financial year.
- These budget statements include salary (pay), nonsalary (nonpay), and income budgets for a department or group of departments.
- Drug budgets make up the majority of the nonsalary budget.
- The drug-budget expenditure is based on the cost of the pharmacy drugs issued.
- Budget statements usually include the following information for each of the budgets:
- Total annual budget
- Budget available for the year to date
- Actual budget spent for the year to date
- Difference between the available budget and the actual budget spent (variance)
- Percentage of budget spent to date
- Forecast expenditure for the financial year
- Total financial position
- If a budget is overspent, it is usually represented as a positive number.
- If a budget is underspent, it is usually represented as a negative number.
- Finance department budget statements should be linked to financial reports prepared by pharmacy staff (see p. 60).
- Pharmacists might be asked for a breakdown of drug-expenditure information.

Patient assistance programs

Pharmacists and pharmacy technical staff may be involved in identifying lower-cost alternatives, reimbursement, or patient assistance programs (PAPs) for patients with difficulty affording drug therapy. PAPs provide prescription medications to patients who are either uninsured or under-insured. PAPs typically cover patients without prescription drug coverage who do not qualify for government assistance programs (e.g., Medicaid) and who are unable to pay for their prescription medications.

Each pharmaceutical manufacturer determines the criteria for eligibility based on annual income, family size, and insurance status. Many brand-name drugs are available at no cost through PAPs; another program exists offering generic drugs at a reduced cost if no brand-name program is available.

Patients may contact manufacturers to obtain application requirements. Additionally, pharmacists or pharmacy technicians may assist patients in applying for PAPs. A number of useful resources can be found:

- Partnership for Prescription Assistance (https://www.pparx.org/Intro.php)
- Needy Meds, Inc. (http://www.needymeds.org)
- ASHP and the Health Resources and Services Administration Pharmacy Services Support Center (PSSC) at the American Pharmacists Association (http://www.ashp.org/pap)

Drug and medication information services

The first U.S. drug information (DI) center was established in 1962 at the University of Kentucky Medical Center with the goals of serving as the source of selected, comprehensive DI for health-care professionals, educating health-care students, and influencing pharmacy students on their role as drug consultants. Between the 1960s and the 1990s there was a significant expansion in the number of U.S. DI centers.

DI centers were established in a number of locations including hospitals and health systems, chain drug stores, pharmaceutical-industry managed care organizations, and schools of pharmacy. Because of differences in definitions used by different authors, the exact current number of U.S. DI centers is unknown; various articles report from 81 to over 200.

Activities provided by DI specialists vary greatly and include responding to specific queries, managing formulary and nonformulary drug use, managing adverse drug reaction, medication error, and medication use evaluation programs, developing medication policies and drug use or therapeutic guidelines, managing drug shortages, and educating students and residents. Select U.S. centers provide medication information to patients and health-care professionals. Additionally, some U.S. DI centers have merged with poison control centers.

The provision of medication information is one of the fundamental professional responsibilities of pharmacists. Effective providers of medication information

- Perceive and evaluate medication information needs of patients and families, health-care professionals, and other personnel, and
- Use a systematic approach for medication information needs by effectively searching, retrieving, and evaluating the literature and communicating and applying the information to patient-care situations.

All pharmacists are capable of providing medication information. In using a systematic method, the individual is required to do the following:

- Identify the appropriate perspective (consider the educational level and professional training of the requester).
- Determine the need and urgency.
- Classify requests as patient-specific or not, in order to select the most appropriate resources.
- Obtain complete background information relating to the patient (age, organ function).
- Perform a systematic literature search that may include primary, secondary, and tertiary literature sources.
- Evaluate, interpret, and combine information from several sources.
- Anticipate the need for additional information (alternative treatments).
- Provide a response in the manner requested and most appropriate for the situation.
- Follow up to determine the impact of the response on patient outcomes or medication use practices and behaviors.
- Document the request, resources used, and response.

When responding to patient-specific requests, it is helpful to obtain the following background, based on the type of request:

- Drug details, including dose, route, formulation, brand and indication
- Patient details, including underlying condition, relevant laboratory results, age, weight, and past medical history
- ADRs—nature of reaction, timing of the event, other drugs, any dechallenge or rechallenge, and the outcome
- Pregnancy—number of weeks' gestation, whether or not the drug has already been taken by the mother, and indication
- Breastfeeding—age, weight, medical status of infant, indication for and anticipated duration treatment
- Drug interactions—which drugs or drug classes are involved, nature of the event, timing of drugs if a suspected interaction has already occurred

Responders should also determine the identity of the requester as well as contact information, urgency of the request, and type of response requested (written or verbal).

Further reading

ASHP Guidelines on Provision of Medication Information by Pharmacists. ASHP Best Practices. Available at: http://www.ashp.org

Chapter 5

Tips for professional conduct

Michelle W. McCarthy

Communication skills

Communication is a key skill for pharmacists. Every day pharmacists communicate with a variety of different groups:

- Patients and customers
- Other health-care professionals
- Drug company representatives
- Managerial staff

Depending on the audience and circumstances a different approach might be required, but the core skills are the same (see Tables 5.1 and 5.2).

Planning and preparation

Before any encounter, a certain amount of planning and preparation is required to establish a customer's requirements.

- Establish the most appropriate means of communication—this might be written, in the form of a letter, memo, or leaflet, or verbal, such as a conversation, seminar or oral presentation, or both.
- Know the subject—if necessary, do some background reading or research. Even if it means keeping a customer waiting, a quick reference search could mean that ultimately your message is accepted more readily because it is well informed.
- Know the audience—understanding their background, knowledge base, and requirements aids effective communication. Communicating with one person requires different strategies from those needed for communicating with a small or large group.
- Prepare the message—a simple, straightforward piece of information, such as dosage instructions, requires little, if any, preparation. However, a more complex message, such as the answer to a drug information inquiry, might require some preparation:
    - Be clear in your own mind about what message or messages you want to get across.
    - Break the message down into a series of points.
    - Structure message so ideas are presented in order of importance.
    - Provide a one- or two-sentence summary or conclusion at the end.
- Think ahead—try to anticipate any questions that might arise and be prepared with the information needed to answer them.

Delivering the message

Whether communicating in writing or verbally, the same rules apply:

- Use language appropriate to the audience—avoid jargon and complex terms; use simple, direct words.
- Avoid vague terms, e.g., "occasionally" or "frequently," because these may mean different things to different people.
- Check understanding by asking for feedback or questions.

Remember that verbal communication is made up of three aspects:

- 55% body language
- 38% tone of voice
- 7% words that make up the communication

Table 5.1 Barriers to good communication

Physical barriers

- Speech problems
- Hearing impairment
- Communicating in a language that is not the audience's first language or through a translator
- Visual impairment
- Learning difficulties
- Noisy or distracting environment

Emotional barriers

- Preconceptions and prejudice
- Fear
- Aggression

Table 5.2 Checklist of essential interpersonal skills to improve communication

- Body language
  - Be aware of body language when interacting with people.
  - Mirror body language.
  - Ensure that body language, tone, and words are sending out the same messages.
- Rapport with people
- Social poise, self-assurance, and confidence
- Tact and diplomacy
- Consideration of others
- Assertiveness and self-control
- High standards
- Ability to analyze facts and solve problems
- Tolerance and patience
- Ability to make good decisions
- Honesty and objectivity
- Organizational skills
- Good listening habits
- Enthusiasm
- Persuasiveness
- Ability to communicate with different types of people

Listening skills

An essential part of communication is listening (see Table 5.3). Not only does this ensure your own understanding, it shows interest and concern and empowers the respondent by enabling them to fully participate in the communication process.

The traditional active–passive roles of health-care professional talking and patient listening respectively are not conducive to good communication. Good listening (by both parties) ensures that the encounter has the mutual participation of health-care professional and patient. This should lead to the information elicited being more valuable; any message is more likely to be remembered and acted upon.

- Reflecting back—clarify your understanding by repeating back ("mirroring") information, but in paraphrase.
- Summarizing—"What I think I hear you saying is…."
- Body language
    - Use facial expressions and postures to show empathy.
    - Mirror facial expression.
    - Nod encouragingly.
    - Adopt a listening posture—as appropriate, lean toward the speaker while being careful to avoid invading their personal space.
    - Maintain eye contact.
    - Avoid signs of impatience or being in a hurry.
- Ask open-ended questions—e.g., how and why.
- Use closed questions, as appropriate–i.e., those with a "yes" or "no" response.
- Use silences appropriately.
    - Allow the speaker to finish what they want to say and avoid the temptation to jump in.
    - Do not interrupt or finish the speakers' sentences.
    - If necessary, allow a short period of silence to elapse, especially if the speaker is slow or hesitant in their speech.
    - Silences can be helpful in giving thinking time.
- Use verbal or nonverbal signals to show you are listening, and encourage the speaker—e.g., nodding and saying "yes" or "mm."
- If necessary, note key points while the other person is speaking but avoid scribbling throughout. Warn the speaker that you will be doing this so that they are prepared.
- In responding, avoid the following:
    - Exclamations of surprise, intolerance, or disgust
    - Expression of over-concern
    - Moralistic judgments, criticism, or impatience
    - Being defensive and getting caught up in arguments
    - Making false promises, flattery, or undue praise
    - Personal references to your own difficulties
    - Changing the subject or interrupting unnecessarily
    - Speaking too soon, too often, or for too long

Table 5.3 10 ways to become a better listener

- Schedule a time and place to listen
- Create comfort
- Avoid distractions
- State the reasons for the conversation
- Use nonverbal signals
- Use reflection, paraphrasing, and summarizing
- Listen for the message behind the emotions
- Be patient
- Write down any commitments
- Follow up

Questioning

Questioning is also an important skill for communicating effectively. As pharmacists, this often involves direct questioning of a colleague about a course of action or prescribing decision. However, when communicating with patients, a broader approach might be required to get all the information required.

- Use open questions to enable the respondent to elaborate and give new information, e.g., "how are you managing with your medications?"
- Phrasing questions in different ways often elicits different information—e.g., asking "do you have any problems with your medicines?" can elicit more information than asking "do you have any side effects?".
- Avoid leading questions, e.g., "you're not having any side effects, are you?", because usually the respondent will give the answer they think the questioner wants (in this case, "no").
- Closed questions can be used to establish specific information, e.g., "are you taking this medicine with food?"
- Be specific because the respondent might interpret certain terms differently than you—e.g., "are you taking these medicines regularly?" could mean to the respondent taking them once daily, once weekly, or once monthly.
- Avoid questions that the respondent might interpret as being judgmental or critical.
- As appropriate, ensure you understand the answer by paraphrasing it back to the respondent, e.g., "just to be clear, I think you are saying…"

Oral presentation skills

Pharmacists often make presentations to a variety of audiences. These can be both formal and informal. Below are some suggestions on how to prepare and effectively deliver an oral presentation.

- Know the expected duration of the presentation.
- Know the composition of the audience.
- Know the format—e.g., workshop or formal presentation.
- Know the facilities—e.g., availability of audiovisual aids.
- Prepare approximately one slide per 1–2 minutes of presentation.
- Are you expected to supply handouts to the audience? How many and what format is expected, e.g., a copy of slides or outline?
- Check whether you are expected to send the presentation slides in advance and, if so, the timelines for this.
- Plan and prepare your presentation.
- A presentation usually consists of three parts:
    - Tell the audience what you are going to talk about.
    - Talk about it.
    - Tell the audience what you told them.
- Always take a back-up option for the presentation—have the presentation saved on more than one USB port.
- Arrive at the presentation in plenty of time to ensure that the equipment can be tested or your presentation can be downloaded.
- Familiarize yourself with the venue and the equipment available—e.g., pointer or computer equipment.
- Ensure that you are not blocking the audience's view of your slides from where you are standing.
- Check that your slides are in focus.
- Look at the audience and NOT the screen!
- Make sure you look at ALL of the audience, so that they all feel included.
- Minimize how much you move around.
- Ensure that the audience can hear you.
- Introduce yourself, why you are presenting, and your background experience to the subject.
- Use a pointer to highlight important points of data; avoid overuse and excessive circling.
- Involve the audience by asking questions or for input, as appropriate.
- Ask the audience if they have any questions. Depending on the time and format, invite questions during the presentation and/or at the end.
- When responding to questions, consider repeating the question asked so that all audience members can hear the question and response and to ensure the question was understood.

Written communication skills

Pharmacists may be required to use written communication skills for many job functions. Examples may include the following:

- Drug expenditure analysis
- Evaluation of a new drug for formulary
- Proposal for a new project
- Article submitted for publication

A well-written and well-presented paper is more likely to be read and acted on than something that is messy and incoherent. Much of the guidance below also applies to writing business letters, e-mails, and memos (see Table 5.4).

Define the purpose

- What is the purpose and what are you trying to achieve? Is it simply to inform the reader or is some course of action expected?
- Use a title that describes the purpose or the content. As appropriate, write the purpose and objectives:
  - Purpose describes what you intend to do.
  - Objectives describe how you intend to achieve the purpose.

Content

The content should all be relevant to the title and purpose. Look through your notes and delete any unnecessary material.

- Ensure that the content is appropriate for the readership:
  - Who are the readers?
  - What do they already know about the subject?
  - How much time will they have to read the report?
  - Do they have certain expectations of the report or preconceptions about the subject?
  - Why are you submitting this report to them?
- What type of information will you be including and how is this best presented?
  - Drug expenditure report requires graphs and tables.
  - Review of papers is predominantly text.
- Review the information and classify it under headings or sections, following the suggested structure and the rules below:
  - Headings should follow a logical sequence:
    - — Problem, cause, solution
    - — Chronological order
    - — Priority, by urgency or need
    - — Drug review—follow standard headings, i.e., pharmacology, pharmacokinetics, indication, summary of clinical trials, safety including precautions, contraindications, warnings, and adverse effects, dosing and administration, potential for medication error, and recommended monitoring.
  - Headings should clearly tell the reader what that section is about.
  - Ensure content of each section is relevant to the heading.
  - Avoid repeating the same information in different sections.

Table 5.4 Report structure

The following is a suggested structure. Depending on the type of report, the structure can vary.

Title

Identification

Your name, department and contact details and the date

Distribution

It might be helpful to list the following:

- Those who need to take action
- Those for whom the report is for information only

Contents

Purpose and objectives

Summary or abstract

Introduction

- Provides the background and context of the report
- Explains why the report was written
- Gives terms of reference

Method or procedure

There should be sufficient information for the reader to understand what you did, without giving every detail.

Results or findings

Discussion

This is the main body of the report; use section headings here.

Conclusions

- A re-statement of the main findings
- Includes recommendations or proposals for future work

References

Use a standard system, such as the *American Medical Association Manual of Style*.

Appendices

These should include information that is useful to the reader but not essential on the first reading.

Glossary

Explain any unusual or scientific terms or unavoidable jargon.

Author name, date of preparation, review date. and page numbers.

Layout

A well-written document with informative content may be overlooked if it is difficult to read. A large amount of type crowded onto a page is difficult to read.

- Margins should be at least 1 inch all around. This gives the reader space to write notes and ensures that print on the left-hand side doesn't disappear into the binding.
- Avoid left and right justification. Left justification only creates spaces in the text, which is easier on the eye.
- Double or 1.5 spacing provides more white space but will increase the length of the document. Follow the spacing practice that is customary at your institution.
- Use subheadings as necessary to organize the paper. Review the Instructions for Authors from the journal to which you intend to submit the paper to determine subheadings.

Bullet points and numbering

Putting information into lists using bullet points or numbering has the following benefits:

- Makes it easier to read
- Has more impact
- Reduces the number of words

Most word-processing programs offer a selection of bullet points. Keep things simple and use one or two different types of bullet in your report.

Use a straightforward numbering system, e.g., 1, 1.1, 1.2, 1.2.1, and avoid over-numbering, e.g., 1.2.1.1.1.

Font

Use a font that is clear and easy to read. Avoid using capitals or underlining to highlight text; **boldface** type is easier to read than CAPITALS or underlining.

Paragraphs

A paragraph should cover only one point or argument. As a rule, it should be about seven or eight lines long and certainly no longer than 10 lines. The most important information should be in the first or last sentence of the paragraph.

Charts and tables

These should be used to convey information that might be too complex to describe in words. However, overuse or inappropriate use can divert the reader from the main message, making the paper confusing. When deciding whether to use a chart or table, consider the following points:

- Will it save words?
- Will it clarify things for the reader?
- Is the information to be presented quantifiable in some way?
- Will it help the reader to make comparisons?
- Will it help to illustrate a specific point?

In general, bar charts are the simplest charts to produce and suit most data. They are easier to interpret and less prone to be misleading than pie charts, graphs, or pictograms.

When using charts, consider, the following points:

- Give the chart a title.
- Make sure bars or axes start at zero.
- If comparing two charts, the axes should have the same scale.
- Label axes and bars.
- Show actual amounts on bars and pie chart slices.
- Use only two-dimensional versions—three-dimensional bars and slices can distort the relative proportions.
- Avoid overuse of color or shadowing, which might not reproduce clearly.
- Keep it simple!

Language

- Keep language simple and to the point.
- Use proper grammar and spelling.
- Avoid long sentences.
- Use active rather than passive sentences."Use acetaminophen regularly for pain" is preferable to "'Acetaminophen is to be used regularly for pain."
- Avoid double negatives as these can cause confusion. "Acetaminophen is not incompatible with breastfeeding" could easily be misinterpreted as "Acetaminophen is not compatible with breastfeeding."
- Only use common abbreviations without explanation, such as "e.g.". Where you wish to use an abbreviation, write the term in full the first time it is used, followed by the abbreviation—e.g., American Society of Health-System Pharmacists (ASHP). Thereafter, the abbreviation can be used.
- Avoid jargon and clichés.
- Avoid the first person (e.g., I, we, us).
- Avoid contractions.

Revision and editing

As much as 50% of the time spent writing a report should be devoted to revision and editing (see Table 5.5).

- Print the report and check for spelling mistakes and other obvious errors (do not just rely on computer spelling and grammar checks).
- Read the report out loud.
- Check punctuation.
- Work through the report using the editing checklist and revise, as necessary.
- Ask a colleague to read the report and make comments. Check that they interpret the information as you intended.

Table 5.5 Editing checklist

Purpose
Is the purpose clear?
Is the content at the right level for the reader?
If action is required as a result of the report, is this clear?
Content
Is the structure logical?
Do the conclusions follow the argument?
Are numerical data accurate and clearly presented?
Do graphs and tables achieve their purpose?
Have you quoted references and sources appropriately?
Language
Are paragraphs the right length?
Have unnecessary words, double negatives, contractions, first person, clichés and jargon been avoided?
Is spelling and punctuation correct?
Presentation
Are abbreviations and symbols explained and used consistently throughout?
Do page breaks fall at natural breaks in the text?
Are page numbers and footers included, as needed?
Does any of the text get lost on printing?
Does the report look professional?

Further reading

Cohen H (2006). How to write a patient case report. *Am J Health Syst Pharm* **63**:1888–1892.

Hamilton CW (2008). A stepwise approach to successful poster presentations. *Chest* **134**:457–459.

International Committee of Medical Journal Editors. Uniform Requirements for Manuscripts Submitted to Biomedical Journals: Writing and Editing for Biomedical Publication. Available at: http://www.icmje.org/

Assertiveness

Assertiveness is an essential skill that can be learned, developed, and practiced. Applying assertive strategies enables you to stand up for yourself and express yourself appropriately and constructively.

Definition of assertiveness

- Expressing thoughts, feelings, and beliefs in a direct, honest, and appropriate way
- Having respect for yourself and others
- Relating well to people
- Expressing your needs freely
- Taking responsibility for your feelings
- Standing up for yourself, if necessary
- Working toward a "win–win" solution to problems
- Ensuring that both parties have their needs met as much as possible

Assertive people effectively influence, listen, and negotiate so that others choose to cooperate willingly. Assertiveness promotes self-confidence, self-control, and feelings of positive self-worth, and it is the most effective means for solving interpersonal problems.

Assertive behavior

- When you differ in opinion with someone you respect, you can speak up and share your own viewpoint.
- You stand up for your rights or those of others no matter what the circumstances.
- You have the ability to correct the situation when your rights or those of others are violated.
- You can refuse unreasonable requests made by friends or co-workers.
- You can accept positive criticism and suggestions.
- You ask for assistance when you need it.
- You have confidence in your own judgment.
- If someone else has a better solution, you accept it easily.
- You express your thoughts, feelings, and beliefs in a direct and honest way.
- You try to work for a solution that, as much as possible, benefits all parties.
- You interact in a mature manner with those who are offensive, defensive, aggressive, hostile, blaming, attacking, or otherwise unreceptive.

Nonassertive behavior

- *Aggressive behavior* involves a person trying to impose their views inappropriately on others. It can be accompanied by threatening language and an angry, glaring expression, and communicates an impression of disrespect.
- *Submissive behavior* is the opposite of aggressive behavior. The person plays down their own needs and is willing to fit in with the wishes of others to keep the peace. It shows a lack of respect for the person's own needs and communicates a message of inferiority. It can be accompanied by passivity, nervousness, and lack of eye contact.

- *Manipulative behavior* occurs when a person seeks to ingratiate themselves with another through flattery and other forms of deceit. It can be accompanied by overattention.

Strategies for behaving more assertively

- Identify your personal rights, wants, and needs.
- Use "I" messages to give people complete information to address a problem. This should include three parts:
  - Behavior—what is it that the other person has done or is doing?
  - Effect—what is happening because of their behavior?
  - Feelings—what effect does their behavior have on your feelings?
- Be direct and express your request succinctly.
- Choose assertive words.
- Use factual descriptions.
- Avoid exaggerations.
- Express thoughts, feelings, and opinions reflecting ownership.
- Convey a positive, assertive attitude using the following communication techniques:
  - Maintain good eye contact.
  - Maintain a firm, factual, but pleasant, voice.
  - Pay attention to your posture and gestures.
    - Stand or sit erect, possibly leaning forward slightly, as a normal conversational distance.
    - Use relaxed, conversational gestures.
  - Listen, to let people know you have heard what they said.
  - Ask questions for clarification.
  - Look for a win–win approach to problem solving.
  - Ask for feedback.
- Evaluate your expectations and be willing to compromise.

Examples of assertive language

- I am….
- I think we should….
- I feel bad when….
- That seems unfair to me.
- Can you help me with this?
- I appreciate your help.

Leading meetings

To efficiently lead meetings, get the best results, and use time effectively, follow the tips below.

- Ensure that the agenda is understood in advance. Circulate a written agenda before the meeting, including the following points for each item to be discussed:
  - Topic
  - Duration
  - Responsibility
- Circulate any necessary or pertinent materials to be read before the meeting.
- The meeting should have a chairperson who ensures that the meeting runs smoothly and on time, allowing all participants to be involved.
- Be clear with the participants why the meeting is being held and what it will achieve.
- Ensure that at least two-thirds of the participants have a role in every topic on the agenda. Consider rearranging the agenda so that people do not waste time listening to a topic in which they have no active interest.
- Be clear what preparation is required in advance of the meeting.
- Always start and finish on time.
- Discourage deviations from the agenda and tangential topic discussions.
- Consider using a flip chart and record actions on it for all to see.
- Try to ensure that individuals record their actions before leaving, and do not wait for the arrival of the minutes.
- Minute taking depends on the culture of the organization. The material to be recorded, how it is recorded, and by whom may vary between meetings and institution.
- Minutes should be circulated as soon as possible after the meeting, ideally no longer than 2 weeks after the meeting.
- Do not hold meetings that are only informational. Minimize the use of meetings just to distribute information that could be circulated electronically.

Prioritizing

Pharmacists can be called upon to undertake a variety of tasks. Work often has to be prioritized to use time effectively and complete tasks in a timely manner. The ability to understand the priorities of others and to prioritize your own work is a very important skill to learn. Below are some tips on prioritizing.

- When deciding the priority of a particular task, consider both its importance (is it worth doing?) and its urgency (does it need to be done right now?).
  - If a task is both urgent and important, drop everything else and do it. It is preferable to take care of important tasks before they become urgent.
  - If a task is important but not urgent, get it done before time becomes short to avoid unnecessary stress.
  - If a task is urgent but unimportant, get it done as quickly as possible and without elaboration.
  - If a task is neither important nor urgent, don't waste time on it.
- When deciding whether to do a particular task, consider the number of people it affects and the cost of undertaking the task.
- Numbered daily checklists are often helpful.
- To understand the priorities of others you need excellent communication skills, especially the ability to ask good-quality questions. Listen to the answers and notice body language.
- Knowing where your plan fits into the plans of others is useful in predicting problems, solving problems, and influencing solutions.
- Knowing where your plan fits in your own organization's priorities ensures access to and release of resources.
- Figure 5.1 shows a useful tool for prioritizing your work—write tasks in the boxes according to whether they fit the labels.
  - Urgent and important tasks take first priority.
  - Important tasks that are not urgent take second priority.
  - Unimportant tasks that are also not urgent take lowest priority.

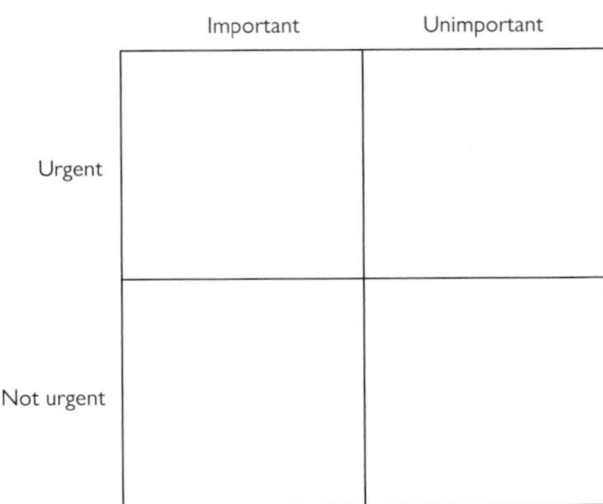

Figure 5.1 Tool for prioritizing work—write tasks in the boxes according to where they fit the labels.

Project planning

The purpose of a project plan is to determine and facilitate the achievement of a set of objectives, i.e., achievement of milestone objectives en route to achievement of goal objectives. Planning is done in the context of the stated mission of the organization and the vision of the organization.

Planning is about the following:
- Ensuring that every individual involved knows what to do, when, how, where, and why.
- Communicating the plans to those who need to be confident that the ambitions will be delivered to the specification required, on time, and within budget.
- Forecasting what might occur so that action can be taken to achieve the desired goal and avoid undesirable outcomes.
- Making decisions about actions that will be taken prior to and during anticipated situations.

A project plan needs to be broken down into tasks that need to be done, and then sequencing the tasks in a logical order. Tasks are actions. Accurate identification of the tasks is essential, as they are the basis of
- Developing schedules
- Identifying milestone.
- Implementing change plans
- Planning communication.
- Resource planning: human resources, materials, and machinery
- Monitoring
- Maintaining records
- Managing risk
- Measuring progress
- Forecasting remaining work

It can be useful to complete a one-page summary of each task, containing all the information needed to delegate the responsibility for completion of the task to one person, as each task is effectively a mini-project.

The quickest and most effective way to produce outline plans is to do it in five phases:
1. Describe the scope of the project.
2. Identify the tasks.
3. Schedule the tasks into a sensible order that will achieve the outcome of the plan.
4. Identify milestones. Milestones are the significant objectives to be achieved on the way to completing the project and serve as visible indications of progress. They enable people to know that the plan is being implemented without having to know the details.
5. Implement the plan.

When scoping the project, questions to be considered are as follows:
- Obtain a simple description.
- Why it is being considered?
- Where does it fit with other projects?
- What are the benefits to the organization?

- What are the downsides or penalties of not doing it?
- What are the major issues?
- What are the risks?
- What are the measures of success?
- What is the return on the investment? Obtain a summary for this.
- What are the names of key stakeholders and stakeholder groups?
- Get an indication of whether to invest resources in a project plan.

Software is available to help with project planning and the production of time flow charts.

Time management

Quick techniques for managing time include the following:

- The four R's of paperwork:
  - **R**ecycle (bin)
  - **R**efer (out-tray and delegation)
  - **R**espond
  - **R**ecord (file)
- Invest time, don't spend it.
- De-clutter
- Use a system for time management.
  - Use a list system to write down ideas, thoughts, and tasks as you think of them.
  - Touch each paper, e-mail, report only once.
  - Use a diary system.
  - Use a name-and-address system.
  - Bracket tasks, appointments, and travel time.
  - Set time limits, with interruptions.
  - Use "scrap time" wisely.
  - Take frequent, quick breaks to increase productivity.
  - Do the most important tasks first.
  - Or, do the fastest and easiest tasks first.
  - Demand completed work from your staff.
  - Communicate upward when you have problems:
    - — Description of problem
    - — List of possible solutions
    - — Recommended solution
    - — List of necessary resources
    - — Implementation of the solution

Ethical dilemmas

Medical ethics involves situations in which there are no clear courses of action. In some cases there may be a lack of scientific evidence, but more frequently moral, religious, or other values have a significant influence on decision making. Thus medical ethics differs from research ethics in that the latter is concerned with evaluating whether clinical trials are appropriate, safe, and in the best interests of the participants and/or the wider population. Many hospitals have medical ethics, in addition to research ethics committees.

The issues debated by medical ethics committees are many and varied. They might produce guidelines to cover certain issues, but frequently a committee does not give a definite answer and simply provides a forum for debate. Issues debated by medical ethics committees include the following:

- Consent to or refusal of treatment, especially for those unable to make decisions themselves—i.e., children or incapacitated adults
- End-of-life issues, such as do not resuscitate (DNR) orders, living wills, and withdrawal of treatment
- Organ donation and transplantation
- Contraception and abortion

Like most other health-care professionals, pharmacists are expected to conduct their professional (and to a certain extent their personal) lives according to ethical principles. The Code of Ethics for Pharmacists from the American Pharmacists Association and ASHP has eight core principles. These principles are based on moral obligations and virtues and are established to guide pharmacists in their duties to patients, health professionals, and society. The principles indicate that pharmacists are to

- Respect the covenantal relationship between the patient and pharmacist.
- Promote the good of every patient in a caring, compassionate, and confidential manner.
- Respect the autonomy and dignity of each patient.
- Act with honesty and integrity in professional relationships.
- Maintain professional competence.
- Respect the values and abilities of colleagues and other health professionals.
- Serve individual, community, and societal needs.
- Seek justice in distribution of health resources.

There are occasions when pharmacists are faced with dilemmas for which there is no clear course of action:

- The pharmacist's religious beliefs or moral values are in conflict with what is expected of them, e.g., over-the-counter sale of emergency hormonal contraception.
- There is no clear scientific or evidence-based treatment available, e.g., use of unlicensed or experimental treatments.
- Business or economic issues clash with patient or public interests.

In attempting to deal with these dilemmas, ethical decision making involves the following considerations:

- The values or beliefs that lie behind the dilemmas
- The reasons people give for making a moral choice
- Duty of care—to the patient, their family, and to other health-care professionals or yourself
- Medical law

In many instances there is not a right or wrong answer, and different people might make different—but equally justifiable—decisions based on the same set of circumstances.

Try not to deal with ethical dilemmas alone. Depending on the situation, it is advisable to discuss the situation with the following people:

- A colleague
- The multidisciplinary team
- Other interested parties, such as management, patient advocates, clergy, or legal advisers

Consider the following points:

- What are the patient's wishes? Ask yourself, "Do I know what the patient really wants?".
- What do the patient's relatives or representatives think? Are they adequately informed to make a decision? Do they have the patient's best interests at heart? (Remember that you need to have the patient's permission to discuss the situation with their family.)
- Would you be willing for a member of your own family to be subjected to the same decision-making process?
- Could the decision made in this situation adversely affect the treatment of other patients?
- Do issues of public health or interest outweigh the patient's rights?
- Is the decision or course of action legally defensible?
- Is the decision just and fair—e.g., are limited resources being used appropriately?

It is also important to remember the following points:

- "Do no harm" is a good basic principle, but sometimes some "harm" must be done to achieve a greater individual or public good.
- Ensuring patient health should include mental and spiritual health, in addition to physical health.
- Acting with compassion is not necessarily the same as acting ethically.

Working with medical staff

Medical hierarchy

In the United States, medical education is a lengthy process that involves undergraduate education, medical education and graduate medical education. Undergraduate education is the completion of a Bachelor's degree usually in an area of basic sciences such as biology or chemistry. Medical education or undergraduate medical education requires the completion of 4 years at an accredited school of medicine. The 4 years is a combination of preclinical and clinical activities. Graduates are awarded doctor of medicine (M.D.) degrees or doctor of osteopathic medicine (D.O.) degrees upon completion.

Before practicing independently as a physician, graduates must complete residency training or graduate medical education (GME). Medical residency programs are 3 to 7 years in duration, depending on the specialty. Family medicine, internal medicine, and pediatrics require 3 years of training, whereas general surgery requires 5 years.

Physicians who chose a highly specialized practice area such as gastroenterology, cardiology, and child and adolescent psychiatry complete 1 to 3 years of fellowship training. After completion of undergraduate, medical education, and graduate medical education, physicians must obtain a license to practice medicine.

The majority of U.S. physicians become board certified in their specialty area; however, this is a voluntary, optional process. Board certification ensures that the physician has been tested to assess his or her knowledge, skills, and experience in a specialty and is deemed qualified to provide quality patient care in that specialty. There two levels of certification through general medical specialties and subspecialties.

In academic medical centers, medical staff members work in teams that include individuals at various levels of training. The teams are led by attending or hospital physicians. Hierarchy for graduate medical education is based on the trainees' postgraduate training year (PGY).

Working with medical staff

- Communicate with the correct team of doctors—ideally, directly with the prescriber if a change in the prescription or medication order is required.
- Be aware of the medical hierarchy, and work with the appropriate physician.
- Be assertive.
- Be confident with your knowledge of the subject. If necessary, do some background reading.
- Try to anticipate questions and have answers ready.
- Explain succinctly.
- Repeat, if necessary.
- Understand and explore others' viewpoints.
- Be prepared with alternative suggestions.
- Come to a mutual agreement.
- Do not let yourself be bullied.

- Be honest.
- Acknowledge if you don't know, and be prepared to follow up.
- If necessary, walk away from a difficult situation and seek the support of a more experienced colleague.
- Occasionally, you might need a discussion with a more senior medical team member if you are unhappy with the response from the junior team member. This situation should be approached with tact and diplomacy.

Patient etiquette

When directly interacting with patients it is essential that pharmacists follow an appropriate code of conduct, as described below.

- Introduce yourself to the patient, stating your name and job title or role.
- Ask if it is convenient for you to speak to the patient about their medication.
- Check the patient's identity against the drug chart and notes:
  - Ask them their name.
  - If necessary, check their date of birth.
- Ask the patient how they would like to be addressed, e.g., by first name or Mrs. or Ms., or Mr.
- Explain what you will be doing—e.g., checking the medicine chart, taking a medication history, counseling patients on their new medicine. Use the term *medicine* rather than *drug* when talking to patients.
- Check whether the patient has any questions at the end of the consultation.
- If you are sorting out any problems with the medication, ensure that the patient is kept fully informed.
- Avoid consultations while patients are having their meals. If it is essential to speak to the patient at that time, check that it is acceptable with the patient to interrupt their meal.
- If patients have visitors present, check with the patient if it is all right to interrupt. If so, determine if it is acceptable with the patient for the visitor to be present during the consultation. If the patient does not want the visitors present, ask the visitors to return after a set period of time.
- If the curtains are around the patient's bed, check with the staff on the reason. If necessary, speak to the patient from outside the curtain to check whether it is all right for them to see you or whether you should return later.
- If the patient becomes distressed or is too ill, try to sort out the task with the help of the notes, staff, and/or relative or return later when the patient can be involved with the consultation.
- Be polite at all times.
- Respect the patient's privacy.

Working with distressed patients

Occasionally pharmacists might have interactions with patients who are distressed or agitated, for the one of the following reasons:

- Their diagnosis
- Difficulty in tolerating side effects
- Witnessing an upsetting event with another patient
- The behavior of visitors, other staff, or other patients

If faced with this situation, even the busiest pharmacist should try to spend some time comforting or supporting the patient as best they can. Spending even a little time with a distressed patient may bring them considerable relief from their distress.

- Do not ignore the patient, even if you are busy or unsure of how to deal with the situation. If you feel you cannot address the situation yourself, acknowledge the patient's distress and ask if they would like you to call another staff member.
- Ask the patient if they would like to talk to you about what is upsetting them.
- Listen to the patient and don't interrupt.
- Never say, "I know how you feel." Even if you have had to deal with the same situation yourself, it is presumptuous to state that you know how another person feels.
- If any misunderstandings or misconceptions are contributing to the patient's distress, try to correct these. If necessary, ask the medical team to talk to the patient.
- Answer any questions the patient has as honestly and openly as you can.
- Provide reassurance about symptoms that might be causing anxiety—e.g., pain can be controlled, narcotic treatment will not make them an addict, and side effects can be managed.
- If the patient's distress is caused by another colleague's behavior, do not offer any comment or judgment. Listen and make a noncommittal comment, such as "I'm sorry that's how you feel." As appropriate, suggest that they speak to a senior staff member.
- Remember that silence is often as helpful as conversation. Just sitting with a patient for a few minutes while they get their emotions under control can be very helpful.
- As appropriate, physical contact, such as holding the patient's hand or touching their arm, can be a source of comfort.
- Offer practical comfort, e.g., tissues, glass of water, a chair, or privacy.
- Don't avoid the patient or the incident next time you see them, but be careful not to get too emotionally involved. A simple question like "How are you today?" acknowledges the patient's previous distress and allows them to talk further if they wish.

Working with dying patients

Death is an almost daily occurrence in hospitals. Although in general, patients spend most of the final year of life at home, 90% of patients spend some time in the hospital and 55% die there.

As a pharmacist, you might not be as closely involved in the care of a dying patient as the nursing or medical staff, but it is still a situation that affects most pharmacists at some stage. Some pharmacists, such as those working in palliative care, oncology, or intensive care units, might frequently be involved in the care of both the dying patient and their family. Learning how to deal with your own feelings, in addition to those of the patient and their family, is important.

The patient

On being told that he or she is dying, a patient (or their relatives) usually goes through the following stages (although not all people go through every stage):

- Shock and numbness
- Denial
- Anger
- Grief
- Acceptance

It is important to let these processes happen while supporting the patient and family sensitively.

Providing information about the illness enables the patient and family to make informed decisions about medical care and personal and social issues; this is where you can help. Patients and relatives might perceive doctors as being too busy to answer their questions or be embarrassed to ask. A pharmacist might be perceived as having more medical knowledge (and being less busy!) than the nursing staff but being more approachable than the medical staff.

When talking to dying patients and answering their questions, bear the following points in mind:

- Be honest—don't give the patient false hope. Answer questions as honestly and openly as possible. If the patient asks you directly whether they are dying, it may not be appropriate to confirm this. An appropriate response might be to ask why they are asking you this or to inquire what they have been already told and then formulate an appropriate response.
- Be sensitive—some patients might want lots of information about their diagnosis and care, but others might not be interested. Respect the patient's need for privacy at a difficult time but do not be afraid of talking to a dying patient—sometimes patients can feel lonely and isolated, and a discussion lasting even a few minutes can be of real benefit. Remember that different cultures have different responses to death. Whatever your own views, respect patients' religious or secular beliefs.
- Be careful—patients might not wish family or friends to know the diagnosis or that they are dying, so be especially careful what you say if other people are present.

Patients often have questions about treatment:

- Will current treatment be continued or stopped?
- Can pain or other symptoms be controlled?
- Will they get addicted to narcotics?
- What happens if they can no longer take medication orally?

Answer these questions as fully as you can, without overloading the patient with information. Be practical with your information and remember that some cautions become irrelevant at this stage—e.g., do not insist on NSAIDs being taken with food if the patient is not eating. If you don't feel it is appropriate for you to answer a question, tactfully tell the patient that it would be better to ask someone more appropriate, e.g., the doctors. However, you could help the patient to formulate the question so that they feel better able to ask the doctors.

The information you provide will depend on the situation and your level of expertise. If you feel out of your depth, ask a senior colleague for advice.

Caregivers and relatives

Caregivers' and relatives' needs and questions will often be the same as the patient's and you might need to go over some issues more than once. If the patient is going to be cared for at home, there can be many practical questions and information needs that you can answer.

- A simpler (layman's) explanation of the diagnosis and symptom management (Often caregivers, relatives, and patients find it difficult to ask doctors for a simplified explanation.)
- Coping with (potentially complex) medication regimens
- Side effects and what to do about them
- What to do if the patient vomits soon after taking a dose
- Medicine storage
- Obtaining further supplies
- What to with unused medicines when the patient dies
- What to do if symptoms are not controlled
- What to do if the patient becomes too ill to take oral medicines

Yourself

It is important to recognize your own emotional needs, especially if your job means you are frequently involved in the care of dying patients or if a death is especially close to home. The patient or the circumstances of their illness or death might remind you of the death of a close relative or friend.

When a patient dies, you might experience various emotions:

- Sadness—a natural response to any death, but accept that it is a hazard of working in health care.
- Relief—a prolonged or distressing illness is over.
- Grief or loss—you might have become quite attached to the patient and/or their family.
- Guilt or inadequacy—if symptoms weren't controlled or the patient's death was unexpected.

It is important to find ways to cope with this. Talking to a colleague, hospital chaplain, or close friend might help, but patient confidentiality must be maintained.

If the patient is well known to the institutional or community pharmacy staff, the family might invite them to the funeral or memorial service. Attending the funeral can benefit health-care workers, in addition to giving the family support. Consider whether your attendance could breach confidentiality. Avoid wearing a uniform, remove identification badges and pagers, and consider whether wearing a symbol, such as a red or pink ribbon, would be inappropriate. If you are unsure whether it would be appropriate to attend, discuss this with a senior member of the staff or your manager.

Euthanasia

It is extremely unlikely that a patient would directly ask a pharmacist to assist them to die. However, you might be aware that a patient has expressed this desire to other staff. Whatever your personal view on the morality of euthanasia, you should treat the patient the same as any other patient.

Euthanasia is illegal in most countries. However, it is generally considered acceptable to give treatment that is adequate to control symptoms, even if this could shorten the duration of life, provided the primary intent is symptom control. If you have any concerns about the appropriateness of therapy or doses in this situation, you should discuss this with the prescriber and/or a senior colleague.

Chapter 6

Pharmacy automation

Ian Orensky

Pharmacy automation and technology

The 1999 Institute of Medicine (IOM) report *To Err Is Human* dramatically increased public awareness of the frequency and cost associated with adverse events in medicine. The IOM's shocking estimate that 98,000 persons die annually from medical errors served as a wake-up call for the U.S. health-care system to take steps toward reducing medical errors. This study concluded that in its current state, the provision of health care in the United States is a dangerous business where human error can and frequently does lead to harm.

Over the last decade, in response to public and regulatory pressure, health systems have refocused their efforts on patient safety initiatives, especially those that pertain to the medication management process. Several automated systems have been introduced that help health-care practitioners reduce human error during the prescribing, transcription, dispensing, and administration phases of the medication use process. These technologies are the following:

- Computerized physician order entry (CPOE) with clinical decision support (CDS)
- Automated storage and distribution systems
- Bar-coded medication administration systems (BCMA)
- "Smart" infusion pumps

The purpose of this chapter is to briefly describe the function of these four technologies and to provide an overview of how each automated system can improve one facet of the medication-use process.

Further reading

Kilbridge PM, Welebob EM, Classen DC (2006). Development of the leapfrog methodology for evaluating hospital implemented inpatient computerized physician order entry systems. *Qual Saf Health Care* **15**:81–84.

Kohn KT, Corrigan JM, Donaldson MS (1999). *To Err Is Human: Building a Safer Health System*. Washington, DC: National Academy Press.

Leape LL, Berwick DM (2005). Five years after *To Err Is Human*: What have we learned? *JAMA* **293**(19):2384–2390.

Schneider PJ (2007). Opportunities for pharmacy. *Am J Health Syst Pharm* **64**(9):S10–S16.

Computerized prescriber order entry (CPOE) and clinical decision support (CDS)

According to one estimate, approximately 39% of medication errors occur during the prescribing process, while another 12% of medication errors occur during the pharmacy order transcription and verification processes. Computerized prescriber order entry (CPOE) is one automated system used to help reduce errors during the prescribing and order transcription processes.

CPOE has been defined as an electronic application or suite of applications used by prescribers to order medications, laboratory tests, nursing orders, and consultation requests.

CPOE systems allow prescribers to accurately prescribe medications, labs and other tasks with little risk of transcription error due to illegibility or lack of completeness. With a CPOE system, a health-care facility can create customized, pre-composed order sentences that direct a prescriber toward the most common dose, route, frequency, or rate for a medication. Orders are typically organized alphabetically or by diagnosis.

Order sets help prescribers adhere to both formulary guidelines and evidence-based practices. Pre-composed order comments may also provide additional instructions to nursing or ancillary personnel during the administration phase. CPOE systems typically include real-time access to a patient's electronic health record (EHR) so that valuable laboratory values, vital signs, and active medication orders may be reviewed.

Clinical decision support (CDS) is a powerful set of tools that are incorporated into the CPOE system. CDS includes a number of functions directed at assisting physicians in making the best possible decisions regarding a patient's care. CDS includes automated pop-up warnings or timely information linked to drug selection, dosage, drug–drug and drug–food interactions, allergies, therapeutic alternatives and substitutions, existing duplicate orders, or the need for additional orders. Some CDS systems allow for dose-range checking and will alert the user if a dose is prescribed that is outside of preset dosing parameters.

CPOE systems often include or are interfaced with an electronic medication administration record (eMAR). The eMAR allows documentation of medication administration and may also include documentation of completed tasks by ancillary services. By implementing an electronic MAR, all disciplines have real-time access to all administration activities that have occurred for a given patient. In some facilities patient charging is linked to charting of various activities on the eMAR.

In many institutions, pharmacists are responsible for building medication products and order sentences that correspond to each formulary item. Pharmacists may also be tasked with building the warnings and alerts that are so vital to any CDS system. It is critical that pharmacists collaborate with their physician and nursing colleagues to develop disease-specific or service-specific order sets that are most appropriate for a given institution.

Pharmacy informaticists are a specialized group of pharmacy personnel that combine years of pharmacy experience with specialized information systems training. Pharmacy informatacists play a huge role in the implementation and maintenance of a CPOE system.

Mature CPOE systems should be able to alert the end users to the following problems:

- Therapeutic duplications
- Single and cumulative dosing limits
- True allergies and cross-sensitivities
- Contraindicated routes
- Drug–drug and drug–food interactions
- Contraindications and dose limit based on diagnosis, weight, age, or lab value
- Corollaries that prompt a user to perform another task

Benefits of CPOE include the following:

- Improved legibility of medication orders
- Less pharmacy follow-up to clarify medication orders
- Prescribing guidance (i.e., order sentences are available for most medications)
- Warnings that prospectively prevent medication errors or adverse drug reactions
- Integration of order entry, pharmacy verification, eMAR and billing components so information can be transferred quickly and accurately

Challenges with CPOE include the following:

- Excessive warnings cause alert fatigue, which makes prescribers less likely to respond appropriately to legitimate warnings.
- CPOE is very expensive to implement and upgrade.
- CPOE requires a great deal of resources from many disciplines to implement.
- Training can be difficult.
- CPOE requires continued resources from pharmacy to build products and order sets and to arrange them in a user-friendly format.
- Upgrades are required frequently.
- Downtime procedures must be established so medication orders can be placed and filled when the system is nonfunctional.
- The published literature is mixed on whether CPOE results in less medication errors.

Additional research on the effectiveness of CPOE is warranted. A large body of evidence shows statistically significant reductions in medication errors of all types after implementation of a CPOE system. However, most experts would agree that the research is less than ideal due to flaws in study design and design differences among CPOE systems. There is also evidence that CPOE may not be as effective at catching errors in some sensitive populations, such as pediatrics, because of design flaws and suboptimal human interface.

Further reading

Bates DW, Cullen DJ, Laird N (1995). Incidence of adverse drug events and potential adverse drug events—implications for prevention. *JAMA* **274**:29–34

Kilbridge PM, Welebob EM, Classen DC (2006). Development of the Leapfrog methodology for evaluating hospital implemented inpatient computerized physician order entry systems. *Qual Saf Health Care* **15**:81–84.

Sittig DF, Wright A, Osheroff JA, et. al. (2008). Grand challenges in clinical decision support. *J Biomed Inform* **41**:387–392.

Walsh KE, Landrigan CP, Adams WG, et al. (2008). Effect of computer order entry on prevention of serious medication errors in hospitalized children. *Pediatrics* **121**:421–427.

Wolfstadt JI, Gurwitz JH, Field TS, et al. (2008). The effect of computerized physician order entry with clinical decision support on the rates of adverse events: a systematic review. *J Gen Intern Med* **23**(4):451–458.

Automated storage and distribution systems

The term *automated distribution system* can be used to describe any of a number of mechanical medication distribution systems. The majority of automated distribution systems can be segregated into two categories: automated distribution cabinets (ADCs) or robotic pharmacy systems. Automated distribution systems have been increasingly adopted into institutional pharmacy practice. By 2005, 72% of American hospitals reported using ADCs, while 15% reported using robots.

Automated distribution cabinets

An *ADC* can be defined as a mechanical device intended for secure storage and distribution of medications and supplies, which collects, controls and maintains transactional information. ADCs allow pharmacy departments to further secure inventory in patient-care areas. Decentralizing the distribution system through the use of ADCs speeds up the medication distribution system and allows for quicker administration to the patient. ADCs are designed to help reduce errors at the distribution and administration phases of the medication administration process.

ADCs have also been called automated dispensing machines (ADMs). For the purposes of this section, the term *ADC* will be used preferentially because *dispensing* implies that a device is performing a function that only a pharmacist is legally and professionally qualified to do.

The benefits of ADCs include the following:

- ADCs reduce distributional responsibilities of the pharmacist so they can participate in a more clinical role.
- They increase distributional efficiency, which yields faster turnaround times for medication administration.
- They interface with a pharmacy computer system and/or CPOE system so that a medication profile is established.
- They prevent the removal of medications for a patient until an order has been verified by pharmacy (or is overridden).
- They control all aspects of the medication vending process including dosage form, dose, route and time(s) of administration.
- ADCs capture all transactions that occur at the cabinet and archives them for further review.
- They record all controlled-substance transactions including witnessing of waste and discrepancy resolution reasons.
- They allow the pharmacist to conduct proactive detection of controlled-substance diversion.
- User access to medications is limited by user type, location, and drug class.
- ADCs enable expiration-date checking for all medications stocked in the cabinets.
- Use of unit-dosed medications is encouraged, in accordance with The Joint Commission (TJC) regulations and the Institute of Safe Medication Practice (ISMP) recommendations.
- ADCs can be configured to support bar code–assisted refill.

- Pop-up warnings can alert the user to take precautions during the administration of potentially hazardous medications.
- Access to drug-information databases is provided at each ADC.

Some challenges of ADCs include the following:
- ADCs are expensive.
- Some drawer types do not prevent nurses from removing the wrong medication for a patient.
- Workarounds can nullify built-in safety functions.
- Training is intensive for pharmacy and nursing staff.
- Implementation requires significant personnel resource allocation.
- Overrides and discrepancies must be monitored by pharmacy.
- Mechanical failures do occur.
- Downtime procedures must be developed.

Robotic pharmacy systems

A robotic pharmacy system is a mechanical device that stores large quantities of bar code–repackaged medications, interfaces with a pharmacy computer system, and quickly and accurately picks only those medications that have been verified by the pharmacist. Most robotic pharmacy systems rely on a daily manual cart exchange system. Robots can be configured to fill first doses as well. Robots can integrate with ADCs to help reduce overall manual order filling and secure controlled substances that are not typically dispensed through a manual cart fill process.

Use of a robot can be very effective for reducing the overall pharmacy workload and can reduce picking errors significantly compared with the amount made in a manual picking system. Pharmacy robots are generally used by larger single and multisite pharmacy systems. Pharmacy robots specifically help reduce pharmacy dispensing and nurse administration errors when used in conjunction with bar code medication administration systems (BCMA).

Benefits of robotic pharmacy systems include the following:
- Distributional functions by the pharmacist are reduced.
- There is an extremely low picking error with bar code–labeled medications; in some states pharmacists are not required to check robot picks.
- They help with BCMA initiatives.
- Robots can be used to service multiple local facilities at one time if a transportation system is devised.

Challenges of robotic pharmacy systems include the following:
- An increased packaging burden does exist in comparison to that with ADCs or a manual picking system.
- Technicians must package and enter all medications into the robot prior to picks occurring.
- A robot is often run on midnight shift, requiring in some cases multiple persons to operate it during this undesirable time period.
- Mechanical failures do occur, so downtime procedures must be developed.

- There can be a significant gap between the time that the order entry or verification occurs and when a dose is ultimately sent out of the pharmacy.
- Robots are very expensive.
- Not all medications can be placed in a robot, so manual picks must still occur.
- A separate storage and accountability system must be developed for controlled substances.
- A pharmacist must check all bar code–packaged items prior to entering them into the robot, taking care to associate the correct product ID with a medication's NDC number.

Automated distribution systems and a culture of safety

One of the Institute of Medicine's primary recommendations in their follow-up report to the original 1999 IOM *To Err Is Human* was to increase technology in an effort to increase patient safety. However, regardless of the type of distribution system implemented by a hospital or health system, any benefits in safety can be completely mitigated if the end users do not use the machines properly and with patient safety in mind.

For example, even though an ADC may have profile functionality implemented, a nurse can still pull the wrong medication for a patient and administer it. If a pharmacy technician running a robot takes shortcuts to decrease workload, the wrong medication may end up in a patient's medication bin. A pharmacist can become distracted and check something incorrectly that is destined for an ADC.

In all three of these examples, a culture of safety, of not taking shortcuts, and of taking time to perform activities correctly can reduce errors when using this equipment. A culture of patient safety has to be at the basis of all of these technologies for them to work as intended.

Further reading

ASHP guidelines on the safe use of automated medication storage and distribution devices (1998). *Am J Health Syst Pharm* **55**:1403–1407.

Leape LL, Berwick DM (2005). Five years after *To Err Is Human*: what have we learned? *JAMA* **293**(19):2384–2390.

Pederson CA, Schneider PJ, Scheckelhoff DJ (2006). ASHP national survey of pharmacy practice in hospital settings: Dispensing and administration 2005. *Am J Health Syst Pharm* **63**:327–345.

Schneider PJ (2007). Opportunities for pharmacy. *Am J Health Syst Pharm* **64**(9):S10–S16.

Wikowski P (2007). Case study: novel ways automation enhances medication safety. *Am J Health Syst Pharm* **64**(Suppl 9):S21–S23.

Bar-coded medication administration

A *bar-coded medication administration (BCMA)* system is defined as a medication administration system that uses medication-specific bar codes and hand-held bar code scanners at the point of care to ensure the correct identity of the drug, dose, time of administration, route, and patient. The BCMA system is integrated with the pharmacy's stand-alone computer system or CPOE system. When a user scans their ID badge (or other identifier), the drug, and the patient's wristband, the user receives immediate feedback on whether the drug and dose are correct for administration or if there is an error.

A bar code is a visual representation of a unique series of characters that corresponds with only one specific drug entity. The bar code usually contains a medication's National Drug Code (NDC) number or other unique identifier (e.g., the medication order ID). Bar code errors occur far less frequently than manually typed errors (1:10,000,000 vs. 1:100, respectively). While most product bar codes are linear, two-dimensional (2-D) bar code types are becoming commonplace. Two-dimensional bar codes allow manufacturers to provide much more information than can be captured by a linear bar code using less space (e.g., lot number and expiration date).

BCMA systems are specifically meant to address medication errors during the administration process. When used correctly, BCMA systems have been shown to significantly reduce medication errors by 65%–86%. This is not surprising, considering that 38% of medication errors occur in the administration process, while only 2% of errors are detected at this stage using traditional means of administration.

According to a 2005 ASHP survey of pharmacy directors from across the United States, only 9.4% of hospitals had implemented a BCMA system. This may be in part due to the significant obstacles that health systems must overcome to successfully implement these programs.

Currently the FDA mandates that all medications in unit-dosed packages be labeled with a medication-specific bar code. In response to this regulation, drug manufacturers have complied, but the number of unit-dosed medications available has been reduced.

The increased cost and operational complexity of packaging and repackaging all medications dispensed from the pharmacy are significant barriers to successful implementation. Significant capital outlay must be in place to purchase adequate quantities of scanners and wireless laptops or computers on wheels (COWs). Successful implementation of a BCMA system also hinges on the availability of wireless infrastructure, which can often be costly.

Furthermore, workarounds to BCMA programs, such as photocopying patient wristbands or medication packaging and then scanning the bar code, circumvent the safety procedures inherent in the BCMA program. Nurses can also override the administration warnings, thus rendering the system ineffective. For these reasons, it is imperative that nursing staff be included in the initial design and implementation process so that workarounds can be dealt with proactively.

Benefits of BCMA include the following:

- There is a significant reduction in administration errors assuming proper use of the system.
- Staff training is relatively simple.
- Less employee resources are required to start up BCMA in comparison to those needed for CPOE or ADCs.

Challenges of BCMA include the following:

- BCMA has a high start-up cost, including equipment procurement and service contracts
- BCMA must be interfaced with the current CPOE or pharmacy computer system
- False alarms breed ambivalence to warnings.
- Scanning problems (packager or bar code on packaging) prevent scanning.
- Pharmacy employees must be designated to assist with increased packaging needs if the pharmacy is not currently using packaging with a bar code
- Additional bar code–capable packaging equipment may need to be purchased or outsourcing companies may be used.
- Wireless infrastructure may need to be installed.
- Continual maintenance of the bar code medication library is necessary.
- The health system must have a downtime procedure.
- Data collection and review should be conducted to help identify system errors.

Further reading

ASHP Foundation (2004). Implementing a Bar Coded Medication Safety Program: Pharmacists Tool Kit.

Cochran GL, Jones KJ, Brockman J, et al. (2007). Errors prevented by and associated with bar-code medication administration systems. *Jt Comm J Qual Patient Saf* **33**(5):293–301.

Koppel R, Wetterneck T, Telles JL, Karsh BT (2008). Workarounds to barcode medication administration systems: their occurrences, causes, and threats to patient safety. *J Am Med Inform Assoc* **15**:461–465

Neuenschwander M, Cohen MR, Valda AJ, et .al. (2003). Practical guide to bar coding for patient medication safety. *Am J Health Syst Pharm* **60**:768–779.

Computerized infusion pumps ("smart pumps")

It is widely known that administration errors are common in hospitals and are most difficult to intercept. The aim of smart pumps is to prevent administration errors that occur due to misprogramming of infusion pumps. This technology is incredibly important, considering that an estimated 90% of hospitalized patients receive at least one IV medication or fluid during their stay. By 2005, an estimated 32.2% of U.S. hospitals had implemented smart pumps and almost all had implemented them throughout their facilities.

Smart pumps are defined as IV infusion pumps with software that check programmed doses against preset limits specific to a drug or clinical location. These preset limits are often referred to as *guardrails.*

The user is first prompted to enter the patient's location or service that corresponds with the correct guardrail library. The user is then prompted to select the correct drug name, dose to be administered, volume to be infused (VTBI), patient weight (if applicable), and rate of infusion. If a user programs the pump with a dose or rate outside the preset parameters, the system will produce an alarm and prompt the user to correct the mistake.

The pump's user may either override an alert (soft limit) or not be allowed to continue (hard limit), depending on the preset limits. Most smart pumps may detect errors in programming such as dosing in the wrong units (e.g., mg/kg/min vs. mg/min), delivery of the entire VTBI over too short a period, or decimal place errors (e.g., 50mL/hr vs. 5mL/hr).

Multiple patient safety features are incorporated into the smart pumps. Drug libraries may use tall man lettering to help reduce the risk of users selecting the wrong drug from the database (e.g., DOPamine vs. doBUTamine). Some smart pump systems use bar code scanners to help reduce medication selection errors. On some pumps, labels scroll to show the current drug and infusion rates on the pump. Various lights show the user which modules are active or when pump rates have been overridden.

A least one brand of smart pumps can also be equipped with a nasal cannula that measures partial pressure of carbon dioxide (pCO_2). This can alert the nursing staff and stop the pump if a patient's pCO_2 is elevated due to reduced respiratory rate. This may be a very useful tool for reducing opiate infusion–related overdose.

Pharmacists may play a large role in the implementation and updating of pump drug libraries. Pharmacists are often tasked with developing each hospital's unique drug guardrails. Pharmacists can also help collect and analyze quality assurance data for purposes of refining the drug library (e.g., number and type of false alarms).

Data collected by the pumps include time, date, drug, concentration, rate programmed by the user, volume infused, limit exceeded (upper or lower), and the user's response to any warning. Data can be collected from the pumps and downloaded for further review. Some smart pumps can be outfitted with wireless capabilities such that real-time updates and data downloads can be executed without connecting the pump directly to a PC.

The literature on smart pump efficacy is not as encouraging as expected. One study suggested that only 4% of IV administration errors were caught by smart pump technology. Specific errors not caught by smart pumps included medications being administered to the wrong patient or a dose administered at the wrong rate, but within accepted parameters.

Further reading

Husch M, Sullivan C, Rooney D, et al. (2005). Insights from the sharp end of intravenous medication errors: implications for infusion pump technology. *Qual Saf Health Care* **14**:80–86.

Nuckols TK, Bower AG, Paddock SM, et. al. (2007). Programmable infusion pumps in ICUs: an analysis of corresponding adverse drug events. *J Gen Intern Med* **23** (Suppl 1):41–45.

Wilson K, Sullivan M (2004). Preventing medication errors with smart infusion technology. *Am J Health Syst Pharm* **61**:177–183.

Chapter 7

Clinical trials

Michelle Hobbs
Michelle W. McCarthy

Phases of clinical trials

New drug development occurs with four phases of clinical trials.

Phase I trials

Phase I trials assess the maximum tolerated dose and toxicity of a drug used for the first time in humans. They are primarily concerned with the safety, pharmacokinetics, and pharmacodynamics of the drug. The drug is usually administered as a single, low dose, and then the dose and duration are gradually increased depending on the side effects experienced by the volunteers.

Phase I trials usually only involve small numbers of participants and are usually undertaken in healthy volunteers, unless it is unethical (e.g., cytotoxic drugs must be tested in cancer patients). Phase I studies provide information on the tolerability o f a range of doses of the drug, early dose–response relationships, and pharmacokinetics.

Phase II trials

Phase II trials are usually the first time that patients are exposed to the drug (with the exception of anti-cancer drugs). These trials assess the efficacy of a treatment and define the therapeutic dose range and dosing regimen for a specific indication, with minimum side effects. They also produce additional information on safety, pharmacokinetics, and pharmacodynamics in the presence of the disease process.

Relatively small numbers of patients are studied under close supervision, usually by specialized investigators. Phase II studies are usually just a trial of the drug and provide information on the small range of doses that should be used in phase III studies. Phase II studies do not assess the drug's efficacy versus that of another agent.

Phase III trials

Phase III studies assess real outcomes in a variety of patients approximating the population of patients who will receive the drug once it is marketed. Phase III trials are undertaken in large numbers of patients, often in multiple centers. Their aim is to compare new treatments with existing treatments and to demonstrate long-term safety and tolerance.

Phase IV trials

These studies are performed after a product license is obtained. Their main aim is to either investigate the incidence of relatively rare ADRs or compare drugs with standard treatments, often to extend the range of approved indications.

Trial design, randomization, and blinding (phase III and IV studies)

The most robust trials include blinding and randomization.

- Randomized controlled trials form the cornerstone of phase III testing.

- *Controlled clinical trials* compare a test treatment with another treatment. Comparisons in controlled trials can be with either retrospective patients who have the same disease (historical controls) or a prospective control group.
- *Prospective clinical trials* can be designed as parallel or crossover studies.
  - *Parallel studies* assign patients to receive one of the study treatments and two or more groups of patients continue in the study in parallel.
  - *Crossover studies* assign both of the treatments to one group of patients. They receive one treatment for a period of time and, following a wash-out period, the same patients receive the second treatment.
- *Randomized trials* assign treatments to successive patients in a predetermined manner that results in patients having an equal chance of receiving any of the study options. Randomized trials aim to show that one treatment is superior to another, and they avoid investigator bias. There are several practices of randomization:
  - *Simple randomization* assigns equal numbers of patients to each group.
  - *Unequal randomization* can be used—e.g., if experience is required in a larger number of patients receiving a new treatment.
  - *Stratification* is used to avoid bias if a large difference in responses between groups is expected; separate randomization lists, containing different disease categories, are used. That is, if a patient factor could affect the patient response, stratification ensures equal allocation of patients with this factor to both treatment groups. Stratification occurs before randomization.
- In *randomized controlled trials*, patients are randomly allocated to either the new drug or an existing recognized treatment with which it is being compared. These trials are often blinded and there are two levels of blinding:
  - *Single-blind study*—the subject or investigator does not know which treatment has been administered.
  - *Double-blind study*—neither the subject nor the investigator knows which treatment has been given. This is the preferred type of study. Controlled, randomized, double-blind, parallel-group studies are the reference standard for comparing treatments.

There can be problems with blinding in a clinical trial.

- If the drugs have obvious differences, e.g., IV vs. oral forms
- When ADRs are associated with one arm of the trial
- Ethical issues of withholding information from patients on the exact treatment they are receiving

When trials are blinded, mechanisms are in place to ensure individuals can be unblinded in the case of emergencies.

Further reading

Di Giovanna I, Hayes G (eds) (2001). *Principles of Clinical Research*. Guildford, CT: Wrightson Biomedical Publishing.

Licensing

Before a clinical trial that uses a new drug or hopes to add an indication for an existing drug starts, the following authorizations and approvals must be obtained:

- Clinical trial authorization in the form an IND number (Investigational New Drug) from a competent authority. In the United States this is the Food and Drug Administration (FDA).
  - The competent authority must consider the application within 30 days (maximum).
  - The competent authority must notify the sponsor within 30 days if there are grounds for refusal.
- Approval from the investigator's local institutional review board (IRB). This board may be local to the investigator's institution, or for those sites without a local IRB there are regional and professional IRBs that may be used.
- Trials using already marketed or approved drugs that will not seek an additional indication for that drug need only obtain IRB approval; an IND is not needed.

U.S. Food and Drug Administration

- Clinical trials are guided by the Food, Drug and Cosmetic Act of 1938 and the Food and Drug Modernization Act of 2007.
- These acts enforce controls on the preparation and testing of clinical trial materials (investigational products [IPs]) on humans.
- The FDA directive on good clinical practice (GCP) in clinical trials provides a legal framework and regulates standards for clinical trials.
- The FDA enforces these standards in the United States and worldwide for those facilities importing drugs into the United States by performing inspections of GCP and good manufacturing practice (GMP).
- The following requirements must be met before commencement of a clinical trial:
  - Justification for human use
  - A detailed protocol that clearly defines procedures necessary to carry out the trial
  - Approval of the local IRB
- Failure to comply with the FDA clinical trials directive is a criminal offense.
- The conduct of clinical trials must follow these requirements:
  - The sponsor must notify the FDA and their IRB of the conclusion of the trial.
  - If the trial terminates early, the sponsor must notify the FDA and the investigator, who must then notify the IRB in a timely manner.
  - The FDA can suspend or terminate any trial if there are doubts about the safety or scientific validity.
- In summary, the regulations set standards for the following reasons:
  - To protect clinical trial participants
  - To establish IRBs
  - The manufacture, import, and labeling of IPs
  - Manufacture and labeling of drugs compliant with GMP
  - Provision for quality assurance of clinical trials and IPs
  - Safety monitoring of patients participating in trials
  - Procedures for reporting and recording ADRs and events through the U.S. FDA Medwatch Program
- GCP documents for undertaking clinical trials include the following:
  - CDER (Center for Drug Evaluation and Research) guidance documents, located at: www.FDA.gov/CDER/

Further reading

American Society of Health-System Pharmacists (1998). ASHP guidelines on clinical drug research. *Am J Health Sys Pharm* **55**:369–376.

ASHP Guidelines on Clinical Drug Research

Receipt of supplies

- Ensure that all clinical trial supplies are received from an approved supplier.
- Clinical trial supplies must be prepared in a FDA-approved facility using GMP.
- Clinical trial supplies manufactured outside the United States must be imported into the United States with FDA approval usually through the IND application.

Storage and handling

- The pharmacy department should manage all clinical trial medication.
- Clinical trial materials must be kept in a separate and secure storage area, with sufficient room to ensure that there is no confusion between trial materials.
- The designated pharmacist should ensure that the formulation, presentation, and storage of clinical trial medications are appropriate.
- Clinical trial medication must be dispensed against appropriate prescription forms, which have been agreed on by the trial investigators and pharmacy department. Each clinical trial drug prescription must contain enough information to identify the correct trial to ensure the dispensation of the correct clinical trial medication.
- The pharmacy department should be involved in the reconciliation and disposal of unused medication. Guidance is available from the institutional quality-assurance document on waste disposal.

Labeling, packaging, and stability issues

- All medication must be suitably labeled to comply with current labeling requirements for IPs, as outlined in Code of Federal Regulations (CFR) Title 21 Section I Part 312 (21 CFR 312).
- Pharmacists, and those working under their supervision, do not need to hold a manufacturing license to repackage or change the packaging of clinical trial materials, if this is done in a hospital or health center for patients of that establishment.

Documentation and records

- The pharmacy department must keep appropriate records of the dispensing of clinical trial drugs and detailed drug accountability. Clinical trial documentation should be retained in the pharmacy for the life of the trial, and may be destroyed 2 years after approval or withdrawal of the IND or longer per sponsor request.
- All training, if required by the sponsor, must be documented and available for inspection.
- Records of storage conditions must be kept.
- Clinical trial randomization codes should be held in the pharmacy department. Arrangements for the codes to be broken outside of normal pharmacy working hours must be made. Criteria for code breaking should be available and records made in the relevant trial documentation.
- Departmental standard operating procedures must be in place, which are suitably version-controlled and reviewed at regular intervals.

Charging for clinical trials

- The pharmacy department should have a standard method of charging for clinical trials. These charges are typically the responsibility of the investigator, but each institution should follow their standard procedures.
- Arrangements should be made for the levy of prescription charges in accordance with current guidance.
    - Prescription charges may not be passed on to the patient for IND products without prior approval of the FDA.

Further reading

American Society of Health-System Pharmacists (1998). ASHP guidelines on clinical drug research. *Am J Health Syst Pharm* **55**:369–376.

Institutional review boards (IRBs)

The FDA ensures that there are local ethics committees, institutional review boards (IRBs), for human subject protection, that must approve all clinical trials at their affiliated site. For those sites too small for their own IRB there are regional and professional IRBs that can provide the required oversight usually for a fee.

OHRP

The Office of Human Rights Protections (OHRP) is the entity empowered by the Department of Health and Human Services (HHS) to

- Protect the rights, health, and safety of subjects involved in research conducted or supported by HHS.
- Help to ensure that such research is carried out in accordance with the regulations outlined in 45 CFR 46.
- Provide clarification and guidance.
- Develop educational programs and materials.
- Maintain regulatory oversight.

Composition of IRB

- 12–18 members (lay and medical)
- Balanced age and gender distribution
- Subcommittees encouraged
- Lead reviewers suggested
- Quorum of seven members stipulated and defined
- Co-opted members allowed, as defined, to ensure that the balance of the committee is maintained

Rule of IRBs

Ethics committees consider the following:

- The relevance of the clinical trial and trial design
- Whether the evaluation of the anticipated benefits and risks is satisfactory and conclusions are justified
- The protocol
- The suitability of the investigator and supporting staff
- The investigators brochure
- The quality of the facilities
- The consent form and patient information sheet
- The procedure to be followed for obtaining informed consent
- Justification for research on persons incapable of giving informed consent
- The arrangements for the recruitment of subjects
- Provision for indemnity or compensation in the event of injury or death
- Insurance or indemnity to cover the liability of the investigator and sponsor
- The arrangements for rewarding or compensating investigators and trial subjects, including the amount, and the relevant aspects of any agreement between the sponsor and the site

Further reading

American Society of Health-System Pharmacists (1998). ASHP guidelines on clinical drug research. *Am J Health Syst Pharm* **55**:369–376.

Pharmacists advising IRBs

Pharmacists advising ethics committees should be able to use their pharmaceutical expertise to advise on the following issues:

- Quality assurance
- GCP issues
- GMP issues
- Storage
- Issues surrounding drug administration, e.g., blinding
- Monitoring ADRs
- Clinical trial design and randomization
- IND arrangements for the trial
- Safety and efficacy of any drugs involved
- Appropriateness of the proposed dosage regimens
- Appropriateness of the formulation
- The method of monitoring compliance with drug regimens
- Patient education
- Probability of a continuing supply of medications for 2 years following the trial

Gene therapy

The development of genetically modified viruses and advances in cloning and sequencing the human genome have offered the opportunity to treat a wide variety of diseases using gene therapy. The term *gene therapy* applies to any clinical therapeutic procedure in which genes are intentionally introduced into human cells.

Gene therapy clinical trials have been undertaken in cystic fibrosis, cancer, cardiac disease, HIV, and inherited genetic disorders. Preparation of gene therapy products is a pharmaceutical preparation process that should be carried out under the control of a pharmacist in suitable facilities to minimize the risk of microbiological contamination and medication errors.

Gene therapy can be divided into two main categories: gene replacement or addition. *Gene replacement* tends to be used for monogenic diseases, in which a single "faulty" gene can be replaced with a normal gene.

For example, an abnormal cystic fibrosis transmembrane conductance regulator (CFTR) gene can be replaced in cystic fibrosis. Currently, the majority of gene-therapy clinical trials use a *gene-addition* strategy for cancer, whereby a gene or genes can be added to a cell to provide a new function, e.g., tumor-suppresser genes to cancer cells.

For gene therapy to be successful, a therapeutic gene must be delivered to the nucleus of a target cell, where it can be expressed as a therapeutic protein. Genes are delivered to target cells by vectors, in a process called *gene transfer*. The greatest challenge to gene therapy is finding a vector that can transfer therapeutic genes to target cells specifically and efficiently. Gene transfer vectors can be broadly divided into nonviral and viral systems. Nonviral vectors, such as liposomes, have limited efficiency.

Genetically modified viruses have proved to be the most efficient way of delivering DNA. Viruses are merely genetic information protected by a protein coat. They have a unique ability to enter (infect) a cell delivering viral genes to the nucleus using the host-cell machinery to express those viral genes. A variety of viruses have been used as vectors, including retroviruses, herpes viruses, and adenoviruses.

Many viral vectors have been genetically modified so that they cannot form new viral particles and so are termed *replication-deficient* or *replication-defective*. Replication-deficient viruses have had the viral genes required for replication and the pathogenic host response removed. This prevents the virus from replicating and thus the potential for the therapeutic virus to reverse back to a pathogenic virus. The deleted genes are replaced by a therapeutic gene, thus allowing the delivery and expression of the therapeutic gene without subsequent spread of the virus to surrounding cells.

Future gene-therapy vectors will be able to replicate under genetically specified conditions.

There are potential infectious hazards with gene therapy, which include possible transmission of the vector to hospital personnel. Gene therapy products should be manipulated in pharmacy aseptic areas, because of the uncertain effects of specific genes on normal human cells, potential for operator sensitization on repeated exposure, and potentially infective nature of some products.

Consideration must be given to protect both the product and the staff handling these agents. Some gene-therapy agents might require handling in negative-pressure isolators in separate, specific aseptic facilities.

A risk assessment should be made for each product, with input from the lead investigator or biological safety officer, because they should have a good understanding of molecular biology and virology.

Further reading

Gene Therapy Fact Sheet. U.S. Department of Energy Office of Science. Available at: http://www.ornl.gov/sci/techresources/Human_Genome/medicine/genetherapy.shtml

Genetics Science Learning Center. University of Utah. Available at: http://learn.genetics.utah.edu/content/tech/genetherapy/

Chapter 8

Evidence-based medicine

Michelle W. McCarthy
Zachariah Deyo
Karen Eckmann

Evidence-based medicine (EBM) and clinical pharmacy

Evidence-based medicine (EBM) is increasingly becoming the standard practice. Although it is probably more widely practiced in primary care, the following definitions of EBM can be adapted for clinical pharmacy.

Definition of EBM

Sackett et al. define EBM as the conscientious, explicit, and judicious use of current best evidence in making decisions about the care of individual patients.[1] The authors go on to state that the practice of EBM requires the integration of individual clinical expertise with the best available external clinical evidence from systematic research.

A second definition comes from the McMaster University Web site:

> EBM is an approach to health care that promotes the collection, interpretation, and integration of valid, important, and applicable patient-reported, clinician-observed, and research-derived evidence. The best available evidence, moderated by patient circumstances and preferences, is applied to improve the quality of clinical judgements.[2]

Evidence-based clinical pharmacy

Borrowing the Sackett definition above, a definition for clinical pharmacy might be as follows: evidence-based clinical pharmacy is the conscientious, explicit, and judicious use of current best evidence in making decisions about the care of individual patients.

Evidence-based clinical pharmacy fits well with the concept of pharmaceutical care (see Chapter 12). Clinical pharmacists must keep abreast of developments in their chosen specialty, but also apply clinical developments to patient circumstances and preferences.

Strengths of evidence

A hierarchy of evidence (see Table 8.1) is helpful in assessing the strength of evidence of a particular study. Currently, there are a number of grading systems that are useful for identifying the level of evidence available and as a tool for categorizing recommendations made in clinical guidelines. Examples of grading systems from the American College of Chest Physicians and American College of Cardiology/American Heart Association may be found in the Appendix (p. 770).

Some evidence tables regard large randomized trials as level I evidence. Evidence from levels IV and V should not be discounted if that is the only information available. Conversely, recommendations should not be made on level V evidence if level I or II evidence is available.

1 Sackett DL, Rosenberg WM, Gray JA, Haynes RB, Richardson WS (1996). Evidence-based medicine: what it is and what it isn't. *BMJ* **312**:71–72.

2 McMaster University. http://hiru.mcmaster.ca

Table 8.1 Type and strength of efficacy evidence

I.	Strong evidence from at least one systematic review of multiple well-designed randomized controlled trials
II.	Strong evidence from at least one properly designed randomized controlled trial of appropriate size
III.	Evidence from well-designed trials without randomization, single-group, cohort, time series, or matched case-controlled studies
IV.	Evidence from well-designed nonexperimental studies from more than one center or research group
V.	Opinions of respected authorities, based on clinical evidence, descriptive studies, or reports of expert committees

Statistical vs. clinical significance

Statistical significance is typically identified when the *p* value is <0.05. *P* values <0.05 do not indicate a greater degree of statistical significance. Statistical significance does not guarantee that that the finding is important or meaningful when applied to clinical practice. Large trials or large meta-analyses have the potential to find very small statistically significant differences between groups. An important consideration when interpreting significant findings is assessment of how clinically significant the finding is.

Clinical significance refers to a value judgment people make when determining the meaningfulness of the magnitude of an intervention effect.

For example, if an expensive medication was found to significantly decrease systolic blood pressure (SBP) by an average of 2 mmHg, it is important to consider the clinical merit of the intervention. Are there any important health benefits to a patient of a decrease in SBP of 2 mmHg? Would it be worth investing in an expensive intervention if it delivered such a minimal decrease in SBP? Are there any less expensive medications available that produce greater decrease in BP?

Well-conducted, rigorous, randomized controlled trials should identify the number of participants necessary to detect a difference between groups that is determined to be clinically significant (sample size calculations). Sample size calculations should be performed prior to study initiation and reflect the number of subjects completing the study. Authors should enroll more patients than necessary to account for dropouts.

Sample size calculations should take the following factors into consideration:

- Alpha: the probability of having a type I error; maximum acceptable value = 0.05
- Beta: the probability of having a type II error; maximum accepted value = 0.02
- Delta: the expected difference between the study groups

The value chosen for delta should be supported by prior clinical trial results. For example, when comparing a new antihypertensive to a well-established drug, researchers may be looking for a difference in BP of 10 mmHg between the two agents. The smaller the difference (delta) the investigators hope to find, the larger the study sample size will need to be.

Odds ratios and relative risk

What is an odds ratio?

The number needed to treat (NNT) is a very useful way of describing the benefits (or harms) of treatments, both in individual trials and in systematic reviews. Few studies report results using this easily interpretable measure. NNT calculations, however, come second to working out whether an effect of treatment in one group of patients is different from that found in the control groups.

Many studies, particularly systematic reviews, report their results as odds ratios or as a decrease in odds ratios. Odds ratios are also commonly used in epidemiological studies to describe the probable harm an exposure might cause.

Calculating the odds

The odds of an event occurring are calculated as the number of events divided by the number of nonevents. For example, 24 pharmacists are on call in a major city. Six pharmacists are called. The odds of being called are 6 divided by 18 (the number who were not called), or 0.33. An odds ratio is calculated by dividing the odds in the treated or exposed group by the odds in the control group.

In general, epidemiological studies try to identify factors that cause harm—those with odds ratios >1. For example, case–control studies investigating the potential harm of giving high doses of calcium-channel blockers to treat hypertension might use odds ratios.

Clinical trials typically look for treatments that decrease event rate, and that have odds ratios of <1. In these cases, a percentage decrease in the odds ratio is often quoted instead of the odds ratio itself. For example, the Fourth International Study of Infarct Survival (ISIS-4) reported a 7% decrease in the odds of mortality with captopril treatment, rather than reporting an odds ratio of 0.93.

Relative risks

The risk (or probability) of being called in the example above is 6 divided by 24 (the total number on call), or 0.25 (25%). The relative risk is also known as the "risk ratio," and if reporting positive outcomes, such as improvement, it can be called "relative benefit."

Risks and odds

In many situations in medicine, we can get a long way in interpreting odds ratios by pretending that they are relative risks. When events are rare, risks and odds are very similar.

For example, in the ISIS-4 study, 2231 out of 29,022 patients in the control group died within 35days: a risk of 0.077 [2231/29,022] or an odds of 0.083 [2231/(29,022 – 2231)]. This is an absolute difference of 6 in 1000, or a relative error of approximately 7%. This close approximation holds true when we talk about odds ratios and relative risks, providing the events are rare.

Why use an odds ratio rather than relative risk?

If odds ratios are difficult to interpret, why don't we always use relative risks instead? There are several reasons for continuing with odds ratios, most of which relate to the superior mathematical properties of odds ratios. Odds ratios can always take values between zero and infinity, which is not the case for relative risks.

The range that relative risk can take, therefore, depends on the baseline event rate. This could obviously cause problems if we were performing a meta-analysis of relative risks in trials with greatly different event rates. Odds ratios also possess a symmetrical property: if you reverse the outcomes in the analysis and look at good outcomes rather than bad outcomes, the relationships have reciprocal odds ratios. This, again, is not true for relative risks.

Odds ratios are always used in case–control studies, where disease prevalence is not known: the apparent prevalence depends solely on the ratio of sampling cases to controls, which is totally artificial. To use an effect measure that is altered by prevalence in these circumstances would obviously be wrong, so odds ratios are the ideal choice. This, in fact, provides the historical link with their use in meta-analyses: the statistical methods routinely used are based on methods first published in the 1950s for the analysis of stratified case–control studies. Meta-analytical methods are now available that combine relative risks and absolute risk reductions, but more caution is required in their application, especially when there are large variations in baseline event rates.

A fourth point of convenience occurs if it is necessary to make adjustments for confounding factors using multiple regression. When measuring event rates, the correct approach is to use logistic regression models that work in terms of odds and report effects as odds ratios. Thus odds ratios are likely to be in use for some time, so it is important to understand how to use them.

Of course, it is also important to consider the statistical significance of an effect, in addition to its size: as with relative risks, it is easy to spot statistically significant odds ratios by noting whether their 95% confidence intervals do not include 1, which is analogous to a <1 in 20 chance (or a probability of <0.05 or gambling odds of better than 19:1) that the reported effect is solely owing to chance.

Formula to calculate an odds ratio

$$\text{Odds ratio} = \frac{\text{exposure odds in cases}}{\text{exposure odds in control}}$$

Where odds ratio = 1, this implies no difference in effect.

Formula to calculate a relative risk

$$\text{Odds ratio} = \frac{\text{risk on treatment}}{\text{risk on control}}$$

Where risk ratio = 1, this implies no difference in effect.

Types of data

Statistical tests are selected on the basis of type of data being presented. Clinical data can be grouped into three or four categories: nominal, ordinal, interval, and ratio. However, interval and ratio data can be combined and classified and continuous data.

Nominal data

Nominal data are those that fall into one of several groups: male or female, dead or alive, complete response, partial response, no response, or disease progression.

Ordinal data

Ordinal data are those that are ranked. These may have a numeric value associated with them: 5 = strongly agree, 4 = agree, 3 = neutral, 2 = disagree, and 1 = strongly disagree. However, the numeric value has no clinical meaning and should not be averaged.

Interval and ratio or continuous data

These data are those that fall along a continuum: BP in mmHg, age in years, weight in kg, serum levels (mg/dL).

A discussion of statistical analysis and the assumptions made when certain statistical tests are used is beyond the scope of this handbook. However, a few of the most common statistical tests used, according to the type of data, are listed below.

- Nominal data: chi-squared test, Fisher's exact test
- Ordinal data: Mann–Whitney U test, Wilcoxon rank sum test
- Continuous data: Student *t*-test, analysis of variance, Mann–Whitney U test (for nonparametric)

Descriptive statistics

A number of terms are commonly used to describe data from an experimental study. *Mean, median,* and *mode* refer to the center of distribution of the data, whereas *variance* and *standard deviation* illustrate the spread of data from the center of distribution.

The mean of a sample, represented by the symbol $\overline{X}$, is the average of all data points. The mean can only be calculated with continuous data (p. 134). The equation to calculate the mean is:

$$\overline{X} = \frac{x_1 + x_2 + \ldots + x_n}{n}$$

The median of a sample is the center point in a set of data when the data is arranged in numerical order. In a sample with an even number of observations, the central two observations can be summed and divided in half to calculate the median. The median can be determined from all numerical data, including ordinal and continuous (p. 134).

The mode of a sample is the value that occurs with greatest frequency. This measure can be used with all types of data and is most useful in nominal data (p. 134) when the value is categorical (e.g., male or female).

E.g., Sample data in a study on weight gain (lbs): {8, 3, 9, 1, 7, 5, 2, 5, 4, 5, 100, 1}

The first step is to rearrange the data in ascending order: {1, 1, 2, 3, 4, 5, 5, 5, 7, 8, 9, 100}.

$$\text{Mean: } \overline{X} = \frac{1+1+2+3+4+5+5+5+7+8+9+100}{12} = \frac{150}{12} = 12.5 \text{ lbs}$$

$$\text{Median: } \frac{5+5}{2} = 5 \text{ lbs}$$

Mode: 5 lbs

As illustrated by this example, the mean can be affected by extreme values in the data, called *outliers*, and is therefore often a less accurate representation of the center of distribution than the median.

The **variance** of a sample, represented by the symbol $\mathbf{S^2}$, is a measure of how much each observation varies from the center of the distribution.

The equation to calculate variance is:

$$S^2 = \frac{(x_1-\overline{X})^2 + (x_2-\overline{X})^2 + \ldots (x_n-\overline{X})^2}{n-1}$$

The **standard deviation**, represented by *S*, is calculated by taking the square root of the variance.

$$S = \sqrt{S^2}$$

The variance has no unit of measurement and the standard deviation is expressed in the same units as the mean.

Whereas the standard deviation is used to describe the variation within a sample, the **standard error of the mean** can be used to describe the potential variation of the mean itself. If multiple random samples of observations are drawn from a population, the population mean can be estimated by averaging the means of each sample. The standard error of the mean, represented by SEM, can be calculated as shown:

$$\text{SEM} = \frac{S}{\sqrt{n}}$$

Using the above data set as an example, the variance, standard deviation, and standard error of the mean are calculated as follows:

$$S^2 = (1 - 12.5)^2 + (1 + 12.5)^2 + \ldots (100 - 12.5)^2/12 - 1 = 8425/11 = 765.9$$

$$S = \sqrt{765.9} = 27.7 \text{ lbs}$$

$$\text{SEM} = \frac{27.7}{\sqrt{12}} = 8.0$$

Mean difference and the standardized mean difference

Analyses of continuous data often show the difference between the means of the groups being compared. In a meta-analysis, this can involve either comparing the mean difference of trials in two groups directly if the unit of measurement of the outcome is the same (e.g., if height is the outcome of interest and all trials measure height in centimeters), or standardizing the outcome measure and comparing the difference between the standardized means if different assessment scales are used to measure subjective conditions, such as mood, depression, or pain.

In a meta-analysis of continuous data, if an experimental intervention has an identical effect as a control (or comparison), the mean difference or standardized mean difference is = 0.6. If the lower limit of a confidence interval around a mean difference or standardized mean difference is >0, the mean of the experimental intervention group is significantly greater than that of the control group. Similarly, if the upper limit of the confidence interval is <0, the mean of the experimental intervention is significantly lower than the control. In confidence intervals that cross 0, there is no significant difference between the means of the groups being compared.

Consider the output from a Cochrane review that compared the effect of very low–calorie diets (VLCDs) with other interventions for weight loss in patients with type 2 diabetes mellitus (see Fig. 8.1). In this case, weight loss is measured in kilograms, so there is no need for standardization. As can be seen in Figure 8.1, the meta-analysis of the two trials[1,2] indicated that the mean difference in weight between the management with a VLCD and other interventions is –2.95 kg. This suggests that patients with type 2 diabetes mellitus on a VLCD are, on average, 2.95 kg lighter than patients with type 2 diabetes mellitus on the comparison interventions. However, the range of the 95% confidence intervals (CI) includes 0, which indicates that the difference in weight loss between the two groups is not statistically significant.

1 Wing RR, Marcus MD, Salata R, Epstein LH, Miaskiewicz S, Blair EH (1991). Effects of a very-low-calorie diet on long-term glycemic control in obese type 2 diabetic subjects. *Arch Intern Med* **151**: 1334–1340.

2 Wing RR, Blair E, Marcus M, Epstein LH, Harvey J (1994). Year-long weight loss treatment for obese patients with type II diabetes: does including an intermittent very-low-calorie diet improve outcome? *Am J Med* **97**: 354–362.

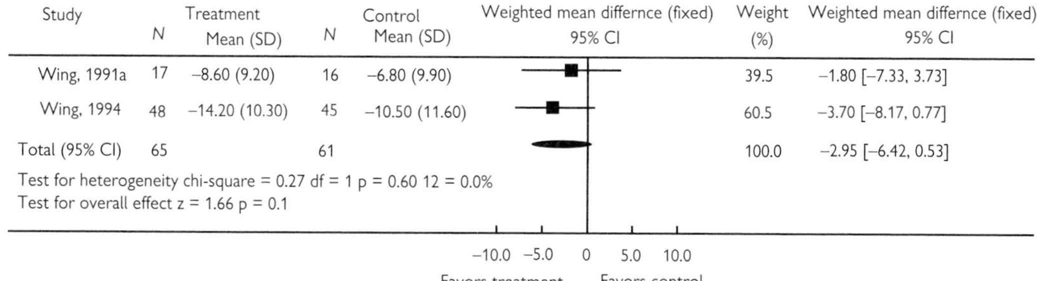

Review: Long-term non-pharmacological weight loss interventions for adults with type 2 diabetes mellitus
Comparison: 01 VLCD vs different intervention (1–10: fixed models. 11–20: random models. rho = 0.75)
Outcome: 01 weight loss (kg)
Study
Treatment N Mean (SD)
Control N Mean (SD)
Weighted mean differnce (fixed) 95% CI
Weight (%)
Weighted mean differnce (fixed) 95% CI
Wing, 1991a 17 −8.60 (9.20) 16 −6.80 (9.90) 39.5 −1.80 [−7.33, 3.73]
Wing, 1994 48 −14.20 (10.30) 45 −10.50 (11.60) 60.5 −3.70 [−8.17, 0.77]
Total (95% CI) 65 61 100.0 −2.95 [−6.42, 0.53]
Test for heterogeneity chi-square = 0.27 df = 1 p = 0.60 12 = 0.0%
Test for overall effect z = 1.66 p = 0.1
−10.0 −5.0 0 5.0 10.0
Favors treatment
Favors control

Figure 8.1 Meta-analysis of a very-low-calorie diet (VLCD) vs. other interventions for weight loss in patients with type 2 diabetes mellitus.

L'Abbé plots

L'Abbé plots are named after a paper by Kristen L'Abbé and colleagues and are an extremely valuable contribution to understanding systematic reviews. The authors suggest a simple graphical representation of the information from trials. Each point on a L'Abbé scatter plot represents one trial in the review.

L'Abbé plots are a simple and effective way to present a series of results, without complex statistics. The proportion of patients achieving the outcome with the experimental intervention is plotted against the event rate in the control group. Even if a review does not show the data in this way, it is relatively simple to determine this, if the information is available.

For treatment, trials in which the experimental intervention was better than the control are in the upper-left section of the plot, between the *y*-axis and the line of equality. If the experimental intervention was no better than the control, the point falls on the line of equality, and if the control was better than the experimental intervention, the point is in the lower-right section of the plot, between the *x*-axis and the line of equality (Fig. 8.2).

For prophylaxis, this pattern is reversed. Because prophylaxis decreases the number of bad events, e.g., death after myocardial infarction following the use of aspirin, we expect a smaller proportion of patients harmed by treatment than in the control group. So if the experimental intervention is better than the control, the trial results should be between the *x*-axis and the line of equality.

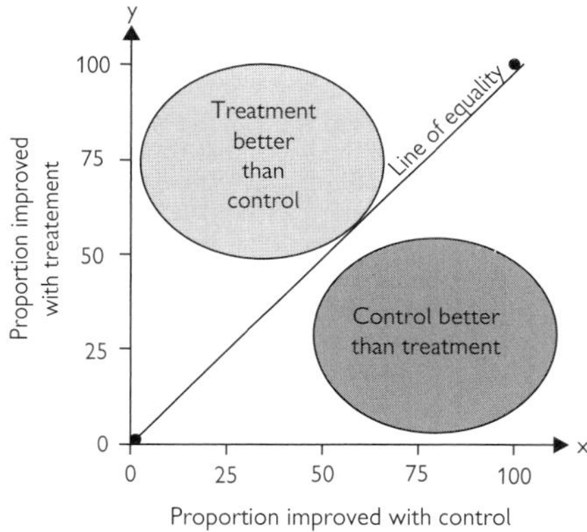

Figure 8.2 L'Abbé plot for treatment.

Assessing the quality of randomized studies

Assessment tools for randomized studies are widely available and all have problems, because they do not cover all the issues that could be considered to be important. This simple method picks up on the main issues of randomization, blinding, and patient withdrawal from studies (see Table 8.2). The maximum quality score is 5 if all the criteria are fulfilled.

In addition, a more general appraisal tool is presented in Table 8.3. It picks up details from the scoring system described in Table 8.2.

Table 8.2

Is the study randomized?	**Score**
Yes	1
Is the randomization appropriate?	
Yes—e.g., random number tables	1
No—e.g., alternate patients, date of birth, or hospital number	–1
Was the study double blind?	
Yes	1
Was blinding correctly carried out?	
Yes—e.g., double dummy	1
No—e.g., treatments did not look identical	–1
Were withdrawals and dropouts described?	
Yes	1

Jadad A, Moore RA, Carroll D, et al. (1996). Assessing the quality of reports of randomized clinical trials: is blinding necessary? *Control Clin Trials* **17**:1–12.

Table 8.3 Assessment tool for a randomized trial

Was the method of randomization appropriate (e.g., computer generated)?			
Was the study described as "double blind"? And was the method of blinding adequate (e.g., double dummy, or identical tablets)?			
Was the trial sensitive, i.e., able to detect a difference between treatment groups, e.g., use of a placebo, or additional active groups?			
Were baseline values for each treatment group adequate for trialists to measure a change following treatment?			
Were the groups similar at the start of the trial?			
Similar patients?			
Diagnostic criteria clearly stated?			
Similar baseline measures?			
Was the size of the trial adequate?			
How many patients were there in each group?			
Were outcomes clearly defined and measured appropriately?			
Were they clinically meaningful?			
Were they primary/surrogate outcomes?			
Were the outcome data presented clearly?			
If multiple tests were conducted, were single positive results inappropriately presented?			
Quality score			
Randomization	**Double-blinding**	**Withdrawals/drop outs**	**Total score**

Jadad A, Moore RA, Carroll D, et al. (1996). Assessing the quality of reports of randomized clinical trials: is blinding necessary? *Control Clin Trials* **17**:1–12.

Critical appraisal of systematic reviews

Systematic reviews are considered to be the best level of evidence if they are well conducted and evaluate a number of randomized trials. They can be particularly useful when seeking to answer clinical questions. However, they are only reliable if the process of the review has followed rigorous scientific principles.

Authors should explicitly state the topic being reviewed and have made a reasonable attempt to identify all the relevant studies. The following 10 questions help in that assessment (see Table 8.4). If the study fails either of the first two questions, it is not worth proceeding further.

Table 8.4 10 questions to make sense of a review

For each question, answer: Yes, No, or Don't Know

A. Are the results of the review valid?

1. Did the review address a clearly focused issue (e.g., the population, intervention, and/or outcomes)?
2. Did the authors look for the appropriate sort of papers?

- Check that the authors looked for randomized controlled trials or had clear reasons for including other types of studies.

Is it worth continuing?

3. Do you think the relevant important studies were included?

- Look for search methods, use reference list, unpublished studies, and non-English language articles.

4. Did the authors do enough to assess the quality of the studies included?

- This would routinely be in the form of an assessment tool for randomized controlled trials.

5. If the results of studies were combined, was it reasonable to do so?

B. What are the results?

6. What is the overall result of the review?

   Is there a clear numerical expression?

7. How precise are the results?

   What were the confidence intervals?

C. Will the results help my local situation?

8. Can the results be applied locally?
9. Were all important outcomes considered?
10. Are the benefits worth the harms and costs?

Oxman AD, Cook DJ, Guyatt GH (1994). Users' guide to the medical literature. VI. How to use an overview. *JAMA* **272**(17): 1367–1371.

Critical assessment of papers

A vast amount of biomedical literature is published each year. However, increasing quantity does not always correlate with increasing quality. As drug therapy experts, pharmacists are highly trained in the evaluation of biomedical literature. In many situations a quick read-through is all that is needed. However, if the information gleaned from the paper is going to be used to decide on treatment options or might be used to support a formulary application, a more thoughtful approach is required.

Although the information provided here specifically relates to critically evaluating a clinical trial, the same process, adapted to the content, can be used for other types of clinical studies.

It is not necessary to be a statistician or an expert in trial design to critically evaluate a paper. A full critical evaluation should take all the following points into account.

Title

Does this accurately reflect the content of the paper? Ideally, the title should state the question under investigation, rather than potentially biasing readers by declaring the results. Cryptic titles are a popular way of attracting readers' attention. Titles that are too obscure may reflect that the authors are not experts in this topic area. Before progressing, consider how useful this trial is in the clinical setting. If it is too esoteric, it might not be worth reading any further!

Authors

Authors should be from professions and institutions appropriate to the subject studied. Be cautious with paper solely authored by pharmaceutical-industry employees who have a vested interest in a positive finding. Multicenter studies should list key authors and acknowledge other participants at the end. Is a statistician listed as an author or acknowledged? This should provide reassurance that the statistics are correct.

Journal

Never assume that because a paper is published in a reputable journal that it describes a well-designed and valid trial. However, be more cautious of papers from obscure journals or supplements.

The introduction

This should give relevant, appropriately referenced background information, building logically to the study topic. If the introduction is waffley or irrelevant, ask yourself if the authors really know what they are writing about.

Method

A well-written method should give sufficient information for another person to reproduce the study. The information given should include the following:

- Type of study (e.g., randomized controlled trial, cohort, or case study)
- Numbers involved, ideally including details of powering

- Patient selection and randomization—details of patient demographics should be given and the baseline characteristics of each group should be roughly the same (and should be acknowledged if not).
- Inclusion and exclusion criteria—consider whether these are appropriate. It is important to validate exclusion criteria to determine applicability in the clinical setting. A study of a new antihypertensive that excludes patients with diabetes may have limited value in clinical practice.
- Outcome measurements—by now, the question the authors are trying to answer should be clear. The factors used to measure the outcome should be appropriate and, if possible, directly related to the question. Be cautious of surrogate markers. In many clinical settings, it might be unethical or too invasive or take too long to use the target outcome. However, check that the surrogate marker closely reflects the target outcome as a whole and not just one aspect of it.
- An appropriate comparator drug should be used at its standard dose. Any new drug should be tested against standard therapy. If a drug is compared with placebo or an outdated or rarely used drug, ask yourself why. With the exception of the study treatment, all other interventions should be the same. For example, if two smoking-cessation therapies are being compared, lifestyle interventions (counseling) should be offered to all participants in each group.
- Randomization ensures that each patient has an equal and independent chance of receiving the treatments being studied. Proper randomization techniques include computer-generated numbers, lottery systems, etc. Determining treatment on the basis of medical record numbers, phone numbers, etc. does not ensure proper randomization.
- Blinding in clinical trials prevents bias by limiting those aware of the interventions to which subjects are receiving. Open-label studies are not blinded; both subjects and investigators are aware of the treatments. This may be acceptable when the outcome measure is objective. In single-blind studies, one group (either the subjects or investigators) is unaware of the treatment being received. This method may be used when the treatments being compared are offered in two different settings (inpatient vs. outpatient). Double-blinding, the standard, is when both investigators and subjects are unaware of treatment assignment. To ensure that blinding remains intact, all therapies received should be identical in frequency, appearance, etc. The double-dummy method is used to maintain blinding. For example, if an IV therapy is being compared to a subcutaneous therapy, both patients will receive therapy intravenously (either control or intervention) and subcutaneously (either control or intervention).
- Crossover trials may be used to limit the number of patients needed as each patient receives all interventions being studied, thereby serving as their own control. If the diseases being studied could improve with time without treatment (especially if self-limiting or seasonal), a crossover trial is inappropriate. An adequate washout period between treatments is essential.

- Washout periods are also needed when patients with chronic diseases who were previously maintained on other therapies are included in the trial. These are often classified as "single-blind, placebo run-in" periods. It is important to ensure that the period is of an adequate duration for any maintenance therapy to be eliminated from the patient's system.
- The details of statistical tests should be given—the tests should be appropriate to the type of data presented (see types of data, p. 134). Beware of trials that use numerous statistical tests. Why are so many tests needed? Is it that there is nothing to prove?

Results

Results should answer the question originally asked and be easy to comprehend.

- Graphs and tables should be relevant and clear. If there are too many graphs and tables the authors may be having difficulty proving their point! Watch for labeling of axes on graphs. Sometimes labeling is skewed (e.g., not starting at zero) to give more impressive results.
- If means are quoted, the variance and/or median should also be quoted. This helps determine whether the mean is a true "average" or whether extreme values have skewed the results.
- The results might be statistically significant, but are they clinically significant? Results presented as odds ratios, relative risks, or NNT are generally easier to apply in a clinical setting.

Discussion

This should logically build from the results to answer the original question, one way or another. If the authors make statements such as "further study is required" ask yourself why. Is this because the original study design was unsuitable?

- The authors should compare their study findings to those of other studies performed on the same topic. Differences in findings should be explained satisfactorily.
- Be cautious of overly bold words such as "superior," "profound," "remarkable," etc. Such language is not appropriate for biomedical literature.

Conclusion

This should correlate with the study objective and be supported by the data presented to give a definite final answer. If the conclusion is indecisive, was there any point to the study in the first place or were the authors just "paper chasing"?

Bibliography

This should be up to date and relevant. Beware of too many references from obscure journals or excessive self-citation. You should be able to satisfactorily follow up statements made in the rest of the paper by reference to the original papers quoted.

Acknowledgments

Look for any specialists not in the author list, which might provide reassurance if you had any doubts about the authors' expertise in any angle of the study. Watch out for funding or sponsorship from parties with a vested interest in the outcome of the study (notably the pharmaceutical industry); however, many investigations are supported by the pharmaceutical industry.

Further reading

Glasser SP, Howard G (2006). Clinical trial design issues: at least 10 things you should look for in clinical trials. *J Clin Pharmacol* **46**:1106–115.

Useful references for pharmacists

The following Web sites are useful evidence-based references that may be of assistance to clinical pharmacists:

- Bandolier's library of knowledge Web site: http://www.medicine.ox.ac.uk/bandolier/booth/booths/pharmacy.html
- InfoPOEMS: www.essentialevidenceplus.com
- National Guidelines Clearinghouse: http://www.guidelines.gov/
- Evidenced-based medicine tutorial: http://www.hsl.unc.edu/Services/Tutorials/EBM/welcome.htm
- Links to EBM resources: http://library.ncahec.net/ebm/pages/resources.htm

The number needed to treat (NNT) and number needed to harm (NNH)

The *number needed to treat (NNT)* is a measure of clinical significance and changes the viewpoint from "does a treatment work?" to "how well does a treatment work?". This concept is widely used and instrumental not only in its own right but also in enabling direct comparisons of treatments. The league table of treatments from the Oxford Pain Research Unit illustrates the value of such an approach (see Fig. 8.3). Ideally, we would want an NNT of 1. Although there are treatments that meet this criteria—e.g., anesthetic agents—in practice NNT are >1 for the reasons explained below.

The *NNT* is defined as follows: the number of people who must be treated for one patient to benefit. The NNT is expressed in terms of a specific clinical outcome and should be shown with confidence intervals.

Calculating the NNT for active treatments

The NNT calculation is received from the understanding of risk ratios (see Fig. 8.4). Although the NNT is the reciprocal of the absolute risk reduction, it is not necessary to understand this concept to calculate the NNT; a worked example is included so that the process is transparent. The equation is quite simple and it is easy to calculate the NNT in published trials using a pocket calculator.

The NNT was initially used to describe prophylactic interventions. The *NNT for prophylaxis* is given by the following equation:

> 1/(proportion of patients benefiting from the control intervention minus the proportion of patients benefiting from the experimental intervention),

and the *NNT for active treatment* is given by the following equation:

> 1/(proportion by patients benefiting from the experimental intervention minus the proportion of patients benefiting from the control intervention)

From the equation in Figure 8.4 it should be apparent that any response in the control arm leads to an NNT that is >1. People often ask what a good NNT is; it depends on whether the NNT is for treatment—ideally in the range 2–4—or prophylaxis—the NNT is generally larger. Issues such as toxicity have an influence, including cost. For example, an inexpensive and safe intervention that prevents a serious disease but has an NNT of 100 might well be acceptable.

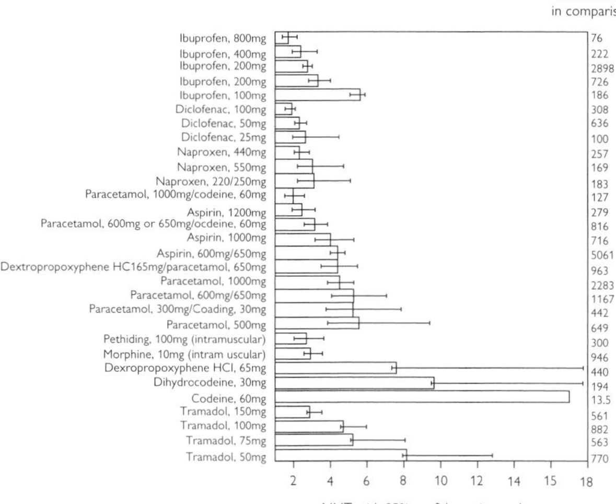

Figure 8.3 League table of NNT to produce ≥50% pain relief for 4–6 hours compared with placebo in patients with pain of moderate or severe intensity.

	Controls	Active treatment
Number of patients improved = clinical end point	N_{con} Imp_{con}	N_{act} Imp_{act}

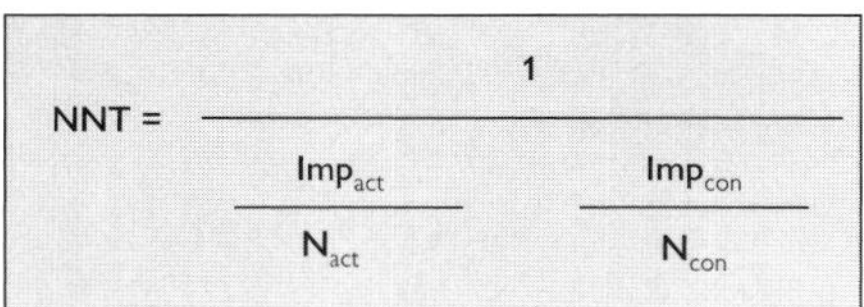

$$\text{NNT} = \frac{1}{\dfrac{Imp_{act}}{N_{act}} \quad \dfrac{Imp_{con}}{N_{con}}}$$

Figure 8.4 Number needed treat (NNT).

Using the NNT to express harm

The number needed to harm (NNH) can also be helpful, in addition to the NNT. The NNH is calculated using a similar formula derived from data for adverse events rather than those for desired effect (see Fig. 8.5).

	Controls	Active treatment
Number of patients	N_{con}	N_{act}
AE-number with the adverse	AE_{con}	AE_{act}

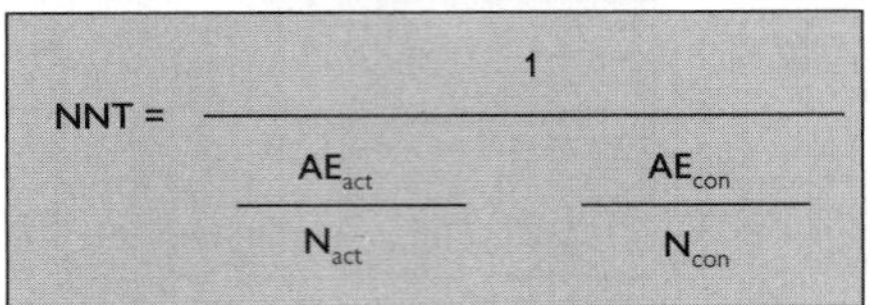

$$NNT = \frac{1}{\dfrac{AE_{act}}{N_{act}} \qquad \dfrac{AE_{con}}{N_{con}}}$$

Figure 8.5 Number needed to harm (NNH).

Confidence intervals

Most pharmacists are aware of *p* values in terms of an answer being significant (in a statistical sense) or not. However, the use of *p* is increasingly redundant and new methods of reporting significance have emerged The most common method is the confidence interval (CI), which enables us to estimate the margin of error.

If, for example, we measured BP in 100 adults, we could derive a mean result. If we then took a further 100 adults and repeated the experiment, we would arrive at a similar but not equal, figure. The confidence interval, expressed as a percentage, enables calculation of the margin of error and tells us how good our mean is. Generally, the figure is set at 95% so we can be confident that the true mean lies somewhere between the upper and lower estimates (see Fig. 8.6). Expressed a different way, there is only a 5% chance of the result being outside the calculated limits.

The statistics involved are derived from a range of 1.96 standard deviations above and below the point estimated. For a 99% confidence interval, the figure of 2.58 standard deviations is used.

Calculating confidence intervals

Although the CI formulas are available in standard statistics works, there are a number of confidence interval calculators on the Internet. These require the calculated point estimate and the number of samples to derive the confidence interval at a given percentage.

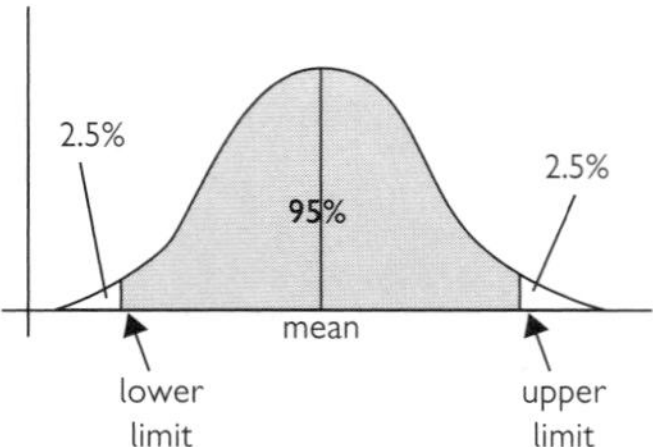

Figure 8.6 Illustration of data incorporated within a 95% confidence interval.

Validity

Validity is the extent to which a study measured what it intended to measure. Validity can be classified as internal and external.

Internal validity

Internal validity correlates to the quality of the study design and can only be applied to the specific study in question. The key question in internal validity is whether observed changes can be attributed to the intervention (i.e., the cause) and not to other possible causes.

External validity

External validity is the ability to apply clinical trial results in practice. Studies that possess external validity have results that can be applied directly to patient care.

Chapter 9

Herbal medications

Lauren K. McCluggage

Overview of herbal medications

Herbal medications are part of a broader category of complementary and alternative medicine (CAM) or traditional medicine (TM). The World Health Organization (WHO) published a report defining these terms as well as conventional medicine.[1]

- *Herbal medications* are preparations (extractions, powders, oils, resins, etc.) that include one or more herbal materials processed from crude plant material such as leaves, fruit, bark, stems, roots, etc.
- *CAM* is a compilation of medical practices that are not considered part of the country's dominant medical system and include herbal medications, acupuncture, chiropractic care, folk medicine, etc.
- *Traditional medicine* is practice that includes the use of herbal, animal, and mineral products and spiritual techniques for the treatment, diagnosis, and prevention of diseases.
- *Conventional medicine* is medical practice using biomedical and scientifically proven treatments.

The use of CAM and herbal medications is large. In 1997, $30 billion (CAM) and $5 billion (herbal medicines) were spent by the U.S. population on these treatments.[2] Common reasons for increases in use of herbal medication include use in patients with chronic, noncurable diseases, use in diseases associated with pain and discomfort, and the expense and availability of conventional medicine compared to that of herbal medications.[3]

In 2002, approximately 19% of U.S. adults reported using herbal medications in the previous 12 months.[3] These adult users were characterized as being women and patients with higher education levels, regardless of race or ethnicity. Of the patients using herbal medicines in combination with conventional medicines, most were not informing their physicians of herbal product use.

Pharmacists must balance the risk vs. benefit when evaluating herbal products. Because of the lack of clinical studies supporting herbal-medication claims, true efficacy is often not known. However, risks have been reported with herbal product use and include adverse effects, drug interactions, product contamination or adulteration, and incorrect plant specimen use.

1 World Health Organization (2000). General guidelines for methodologies on research and evaluation of traditional medicine. Accessed August 12, 2008, from: http://whqlibdoc.who.int/hq/2000/WHP_EDM_TRM_2000.1.pdf

2 Center for Food Safety and Applied Nutrition. Food and Drug Administration (2007). The use of CAM in the United States. College Park, MD. Accessed August 12, 2008, from: www.cfsan.fda.gov/~dms/supplement.html

3 Banres PM, Powell-Griner E, McFann K, Nahin Rl (2004). Complimentary and alternative medicine use among adults: United States 2002. *Adv Data* **343**:1–19.

Legislation of herbal medications

Dietary Supplement Health and Education Act

In 1994, the U.S. Congress passed the Dietary Supplement Health and Education Act (DSHEA) to ensure that safe dietary supplements would remain available to consumers.[1] The DSHEA amended the federal Food, Drug and Cosmetic Act (FD&C), which had required all new ingredients including dietary supplements to be approved by the FDA prior to marketing. Key elements of the DSHEA include the following:

- Reclassification of dietary supplements so that pre-marketing evaluation is not needed.
- The manufacturer is responsible for determining safety of products and ensuring that there is not a greater than reasonable harm if the product is taken as directed.
- Safety information does not need to be presented to the FDA.
- The label of dietary products can state the effect on body structure, function, or overall effect, but cannot claim to prevent, cure, treat, or diagnose a disease.
- The label must state that the claim is not endorsed by the FDA.
- All ingredients of the product must be listed on the label.
- The FDA can remove harmful or adulterated products from the market after it is proven to be such, at the cost and time of FDA.

Dietary Supplement and Nonprescription Drug Consumer Protection Act

In 2006, the Dietary Supplement and Nonprescription Drug Consumer Protection Act was passed by Congress to ensure reporting of serious adverse events caused by nonprescription drugs or dietary supplements.[2] Under this act, the manufacturer is responsible for reporting to the FDA any serious adverse event. All of the adverse events are to be reported through MedWatch, and the FDA is responsible for reviewing reports.

Dietary Supplement Current Good Manufacturing Practices

In June 2007, the FDA established current good manufacturing practices (CGMP) for dietary supplements including herbal medicines.[3] Under this rule, manufacturers are responsible for the following:

- Maintaining a safe and effective physical plant
- Using equipment appropriate for the task
- Instituting quality-control measures
- Maintaining batch production records
- Ensuring appropriate temperature, humidity, light, and sanitation to maintain quality of the product
- Keeping a record of any complaint related to CGMP

All manufacturers of herbal medicines must meet these standards by June 2010. Manufacturers may get an exemption for components of the product that do not affect the end product. Therefore, it is possible that not all of the ingredients in a given product will meet the CGMP.

1 Center for Good Safety and Applied Nutrition. Food and Drug Administration. Dietary Supplement Health and Education Act of 1994. December 1995. College Park, MD. Accessed May 23, 2008, from: http://www.cfsan.fda.gov/~dms/dietsuppl.html

2 Food and Drug Administration. Dietary Supplement and Nonprescription Drug Consumer Protection Act. December 2006. Accessed August 12, 2008, from: http://www.fda.gov/opacom/laws/p1109462.html

3 Center for Food Safety and Applied Nutrition. Food and Drug Administration. Dietary supplement current good manufacturing practices (CGMPs) and interim final rule (IFR) facts. June 25, 2007. Accessed August 12, 2008, from: http://cfsan.fda.gov/~dms/dscgmps6.html

Herbal medications of current interest

Top herbal medications

Over 20,000 herbal medications and natural products are available in the United States and have been used to treat various organ systems (see Table 9.1). Data from the 2002 National Health Interview Survey showed that echinacea, Asian ginseng, ginkgo biloba, garlic, St. John's wort, peppermint, ginger, and soy were the most commonly used herbal medications in the United States.[1]

Information regarding the evidence for these herbal medicines' effectiveness is presented below,[2] and general information for these products and others is presented in Table 9.2.

Echinacea

The data supporting the use of echinacea for treating the common cold are diverse and not standardized. Trials used different species and

Table 9.1 Herbal medication uses by organ system

Organ system	Herbal medicine
Cardiovascular	Garlic, ginkgo, grape seed/pine bark, hawthorn, horse chestnut seed extract
Digestive	Chamomile, ginger, licorice, milk thistle, peppermint, plantago, senna
Immune stimulant	Andrographis, echinacea, eleuthero, ginseng, green tea
Genitourinary	African plum, saw palmetto, uva-ursi
Nervous	Butterbur, feverfew, huperzine, St. John's wort, valerian
Respiratory tract	Bitter orange, slippery elm
Skin and mucous membranes	Aloe vera gel, goldenseal, Melissa (lemon balm), tea tree oil, witch hazel
Women's health	Black cohosh, black currant oil, borage seed oil, chastetree berry, evening primose oil, soy

Data from: Hume AL, Strong KM (2006). Botanical medicines. In: Berardi RR, Kroon LA, McDermott JH, Newton GD, Oszko MA, et al. (eds). *Handbook of Nonprescription Drugs*. 15th ed. Washington DC: American Pharmacists Association, pp. 1103–1136.

1 National Center for Health Statistics. National Health Interview Survey (NHIS). Accessed August 12, 2008, from: www.cdc.gov/nchs/about/major/nhis/hisdesc.htm

2 Natural medicines comprehensive database [Internet]. Stockton, California: Therapeutic Research Faculty. August 2008. Available at: http://www.naturaldatabase.com

Table 9.2 General information about commonly used herbal medications

Herbal drug	Use(s)	Proposed mechanism of action	Dose	Other considerations
Black cohosh	• Treat PMS and dysmenorrhea • Reduce menopausal symptoms such as hot flashes	• May have estrogen-like activity • Suppresses leutenizing hormone secretion	40 mg bid	• Not recommended longer than 6 months • May relieve vasomotor symptoms • Effect on breast cancer, osteoporosis and cardiovascular risk is not known
Chamomile	• Reduce anxiety and insomnia • Relieve GI spasms	• Contains flavonoids, which are active component • Benzodiazepine receptor binding ligand	1:1 liquid extract in 45% alcohol: 1–4 mL tid	• Allergic reactions reported esp. if patient has ragweed allergy • Sedation is additive with other therapies
Echinacea	• Treat and prevent colds • Stimulate immune system	• Increases phagocytosis and lymphocyte activity • Anti-inflammatory	Product specific	• Not recommended for longer than 8 weeks • Can worsen asthma
Evening primrose oil	• Treat symptoms of PMS and menopause	• Active component likely linoleic acid	2–4 g daily	• Evidence is controversial • Side effects include headache, nausea and diarrhea
Feverfew	• Prevent migraines • Relieve dysmenorrhea • Improve inflammatory processes	• Inhibits prostaglandin synthesis • Analgesic properties	50–100 mg daily	• Rapid withdrawal may cause "post-feverfew syndrome"— anxiety, headaches, and insomnia • Must be taken daily for migraine prevention • Not used for migraine treatment

Table 9.2 (Continued)

Herbal drug	Use(s)	Proposed mechanism of action	Dose	Other considerations
Garlic	• Lower cholesterol • Treat hypertension • Prevent stomach and colon cancer	• Antioxidant and antiplatelet activity • Smooth muscle relaxant and vasodilator • HMG-CoA reductase inhibitor	600–1200 mg daily for hypertension and hyperlipidemia	• Odorless preparations have less of the active component • Enteric coating ensures proper absorption
Ginger	• Decrease GI upset and nausea • Reduce postsurgical nausea	• Serotonin antagonist at 5-HT3 receptor in ileum • Anti-inflammatory	1–2 g 1 hour prior to surgery 250 mg tid for nausea	• Toxicity include sedation and arrhythmias • Adverse effects include gas, heartburn, and bloating
Ginkgo biloba	• Enhance memory • Treat or prevent dementia	• Antioxidant • Increases blood circulation by decreasing viscosity • Regulates vascular smooth muscle	120–240 mg daily in 2–3 divided doses	• Uncooked seeds contain ginkgotoxin, which can cause seizures
Ginseng	• Stimulate immune system • Improve blood glucose and blood pressure control	• Increases cortisol concentrations • Stimulates natural killer cells	200–600 mg/day	• Limit use to 3 months • May cause sleep disturbances • Avoid large amounts of caffeine

Hawthorn	• Treat heart failure • Improve hypertension • Treat coronary heart disease	• Anti-inflammatory properties • Lipid-lowering properties	160–1800 mg/day in divided doses	• May decrease dyspnea and fatigue • No mortality or morbidity data
Horse chestnut	• Improve symptoms of chronic venous insufficiency • Decrease leg edema	• Seeds contain aescin, which reduces venous capillary permeability • Anti-inflammatory • Weak diuretic activity	300 mg bid	• May increase bleeding when in combination with warfarin • Can turn urine red • Can cause kidney or liver damage
Licorice	• Treat stomach ulcers • Relieve constipation	• Glycyrrhizin and glycyrrhetinic acid prevent degradation of prostaglandins in the gastric mucosa • Antioxidant activity	200–600 mg of glycyrrhizin daily Maximum duration is 4–6 weeks	• Can cause sodium and water retention and hypokalemia • Avoid in patients with cardiovascular or renal disorders
Milk thistle	• Protect the liver	• Seeds contain silymarin • Antioxidant, anti-inflammatory activity • Inhibits mitochondrial damage	12–15 g	• GI side effects are common, including nausea, diarrhea, and fullness • Cross-sensitivity to ragweed allergy
Peppermint	• Reduce nausea and indigestion • Treat headaches • Improve irritable bowel syndrome	• Direct relaxing on GI smooth muscle • Inhibits potassium depolarization in intestine	0.2–0.4 mg tid on an empty stomach	• Avoid in patients with preexisting GI disorders • May decrease absorption of iron

Table 9.2 *(Contd.)*

Herbal drug	Use(s)	Proposed mechanism of action	Dose	Other considerations
Saw palmetto	• Treat benign prostatic hyperplasia	• May inhibit 5α reductase • Local antiandrogenic and anti-inflammatory effects on prostate	320 mg daily either once or twice a day	• Symptom improvement was similar to that seen with finasteride • No long term data
Soy	• Decrease cholesterol • Relieve menopausal symptoms • Improve bone marrow density	• Isoflavones bind α and β estrogen receptors	Menopausal symptoms: 34–120 mg/day of isoflavones	• Causes nausea, bloating, and constipation
St. John's wort	• Treat depression and anxiety	• Active components, hypericin and hyperforin, inhibit serotonin, dopamine, and norepinephrine reuptake	500–1050 mg daily of hypericum in three divided doses with meals	• May cause photosensitivity • Avoid in patients with psychiatric illness—bipolar and schizophrenia • May have withdrawal effect after chronic use
Valerian	• Treat anxiety and insomnia	• Binds with GABA receptor in CNS	400–900 mg 0.5 to 1 hr before bedtime	• Can cause excitability with high doses • Takes weeks for effect • Hepatotoxic

Hume AL, Strong KM (2006). Botanical medicines. In: Berardi RR, Kroon LA, McDermott JH, Newton GD, Oszko MA, Popovich NG, et al. (eds). *Handbook of Nonprescription Drugs*. 15th ed. Washington, DC: American Pharmacists Association, pp. 1103–1136.

Natural medicines comprehensive database [Internet]. Stockton, California: Therapeutic Research Faculty. August 2008. Available at: http://www.naturaldatabase.com

preparations as well as differing patient populations. Due to these limitations, evaluating the literature regarding echinacea's effectiveness for treating the common cold is contradictory.

The greatest benefit was seen if patients started therapy when symptoms first appeared and continued it for 7–10 days; this led to a decrease in severity and duration by 10%–30%. Concerning prevention, data currently do not support echinacea use.

Echinacea has not shown efficacy for the treatment or prevention of herpes simplex virus (HSV) or influenza.

Asian ginseng

In otherwise healthy middle-aged adults, ginseng has been reported to increase mental capabilities in abstract thinking, arithmetic, and reaction time; however, it does not enhance patients' memories.

Few data support the use of ginseng for decreasing blood glucose, although one trial found that 200 mg of ginseng daily decreased fasting blood glucose and hemoglobin A1C in type 2 diabetics.

Ginseng is ineffective in improving athletic performance, decreasing menopausal symptoms, or improving general sense of well-being.

Currently there is no sufficient-quality data to assess ginseng's effect on cancer, bronchitis, influenza, common cold, or congestive heart failure.

Ginkgo biloba

Lower doses of ginkgo (120–240 mg/day) appear to improve memory and cognitive speed in healthy young to middle-aged adults. For elderly adults, the benefit of ginkgo has only been shown in patients with mild to moderate memory impairment.

Evidence does support the benefit of ginkgo for improving symptoms of Alzheimer's disease, vascular dementia, and mixed dementia. Gingko stabilizes or improves social functioning and cognitive function moderately. It has been suggested that the effect of ginkgo is equivalent to 5 mg of donepezil for mild to moderate Alzheimer's disease. Evidence does not support the use of ginkgo for prevention of dementia.

Garlic

At doses of 300–900 mg/day, garlic has been shown to slow the decrease in aortic elasticity and slow development of atherosclerosis. Also, garlic supplementation can decrease blood pressure by 2%–7% if taken for 4 weeks.

While dietary garlic intake may decrease one's risk of colorectal and gastric cancer, supplementation does not seem to confer the same benefit.

Previous literature did show a benefit of garlic on lowering total cholesterol, LDL, and triglycerides, but these studies were flawed and not reproducible. An analysis of high-quality studies evaluating garlic's effect on cholesterol found there was no significant benefit to garlic therapy.

St. John's wort

Multiple studies have examined the effect of St. John's wort on depression. Overall, St. John's wort is better than placebo and as effective as tricyclic antidepressants and selective serotonin reuptake inhibitors (SSRIs). Specific symptoms that were improved include mood, anxiety, somatic symptoms, and insomnia. Although the studies show that St. John's wort may be as effective as traditional therapies, it is associated with many drug interactions and the long-term effect is not known.

Peppermint

When peppermint oil was added to barium enemas, colonic spasms decreased without an effect on the diagnostic test. Peppermint oil taken orally before the barium enema was also effective.

In dyspepsia, peppermint oil in combination with caraway oil appeared to decrease feelings of fullness and gastrointestinal spasms. Other combinations that include peppermint oil are effective for reducing acid reflux, nausea, emesis, and epigastric pain.

When applied topically to the head, peppermint oil has been shown to relieve tension headaches.

One study of the use of peppermint oil capsules for irritable bowel syndrome found benefit in reducing symptoms; another trial did not.

Ginger

For pregnant women experiencing morning sickness, ginger supplementation reduced the severity of nausea and vomiting more than placebo and comparably to vitamin B_6.

One gram of ginger taken 1 hour prior to surgery was shown to decrease the incidence of 24-hour postoperative nausea and vomiting, but not 3-hour postoperative nausea and vomiting.

Ginger does not appear to be effective for treatment of motion sickness. The data regarding the use of ginger for chemotherapy-induced nausea and vomiting are conflicting, and currently ginger is not recommended for this.

Soy

When soy protein is used as a substitute for dietary protein, it decreases total cholesterol and LDL. More specifically, soy appears to decrease total cholesterol by up to 7% and LDL cholesterol, up to 10%. The products evaluated contained 15–135 g/day of soy protein and 40–318 mg/day of isoflavones, and a dose–response effect was not seen.

Most studies that have examined soy's effect on menopausal symptoms, specifically hot flashes, have used supplements that contain 34–120 mg of isoflavones. At this dose, evidence showed a decrease in frequency and severity of hot flashes. When compared with estrogens, one study found soy to be less effective while another showed it to be similar in effect. Of note, it took up to 2 months for the full effect of soy supplementation to be seen.

For soy to have an effect on bone mineral density (BMD), doses of 80–90 mg of isoflavones must be taken daily. The data show an increase in BMD and decrease in bone turnover in perimenopausal and postmenopausal females. The benefit was not seen in adolescent or premenopausal females. There are some conflicting data that do not support the use of soy for BMD. Some of the variance in evidence may be due to only about 50% of females being "equol producers," which means they can convert isoflavone to the estrogenic component, equol.

Soy's preventative effect on endometrial cancer, lung cancer, prostate cancer, breast cancer, and thyroid cancer is based on epidemiological evidence that compares Asians with the Westerners. More controlled studies are needed before a benefit can be determined.

Safety and adverse effects

It has been reported that the incidence of adverse effects with herbal medications has increased. Reasons for this increase include the rise in herbal medication consumption and lack of product standardization. An abbreviated list of adverse reactions is shown in Table 9.3.

Although an herbal medicine by one manufacturer may be deemed safe, that does not imply that all products with that component are safe. Herbal medicines can differ in quality for a number of reasons[1]:

- Variation of species of herb
- Environmental factors
- Timing of harvest
- Plant part used
- Storage conditions and processing techniques
- Adulteration with other herbal products or conventional medicine
- Quantity of active ingredient

United States Pharmacopeia (USP)

Herbal medications can have two different USP-verified marks if submitted and shown to meet criteria.[2]

USP-verified dietary supplements

A manufacturer of herbal medications can voluntarily submit their finished product to the USP for inspection. If the product passes USP testing, it is given the verified mark. In order to pass the tests, the product must show the following:

- The final product contains the specified dose.
- All the ingredients listed are contained.
- It does not contain harmful contaminants.
- It undergoes proper degradation and absorption in humans.
- Good manufacturing practices were followed.

USP-verified dietary supplement ingredient

Active and inactive ingredients used to manufacture herbal medications can be verified similarly to the final product. This verification is helpful for manufacturers of final herbal products when determining the quality of ingredients to purchase. In order for ingredients to receive this verification, they must show the following:

- Consistency between batches
- Contain the stated strength, quality, purity, and identity of product
- Good manufacturing practices were followed.
- Contamination does not exceed the acceptable amount.

Table 9.3 Adverse reactions associated with herbal medications

Adverse reaction	Herbal medication
Cardiotoxicity	Aconite root tuber, ginger, licorice root, ma huang
Cross-sensitivity with ragweed	Arnica, calendula, dandelion, echinacea, feverfew, German chamomile, goldenrod, March blazing star, milk thistle, mugwort, pyrethrum, stevia, tansy, wormwood oil, yarrow
Gastrointestinal (nausea, emesis, dyspepsia, etc.)	Echinacea, ephedra, evening primrose oil, garlic, ginger, milk thistle, soy
Hepatotoxicity	Borage, calamus, chaparral, Chinese herbs, coltsfoot, echinacea, germander, kava rhizome, kombucha, life root, mahuang, pennyroyal, sassafras, skullcap, soy, valerian
Neurotoxicity	Aconite root tuber, ginkgo seed or leaf, kava rhizome, mahuang, pennyroyal
Renal toxicity	Chinese yew, hawthorn, impila root, pennyroyal, star fruit
Sedation	Chamomile, ginger, St. John's wort, valerian

Data from:

Boullata JI, Nace AM (2000). Safety issues with herbal medicine. *Pharmacotherapy* **20**(3):257–269.

De Smet PA (2002). Herbal remedies. *N Engl J Med* **347**(25):2046–2056.

Hume AL, Strong KM (2006). Botanical medicines. In: Berardi RR, Kroon LA, McDermott JH, Newton GD, Oszko MA, Popovich NG, et al. (eds). *Handbook of Nonprescription Drugs*. 15th ed. Washington DC: American Pharmacists Association, pp. 1103–1136.

Natural medicines comprehensive database [Internet]. Stockton, CA: Therapeutic Research Faculty. Accessed August 20, 2008, from: http://www.naturaldatabase.com

1 Boullata JI, Nace AM (2000). Safety issues with herbal medicine. *Pharmacotherapy* 20(3):257–269.

2 U.S. Pharmacopeia. USP Verified 2008. Rockville, MD. Accessed August 26, 2008, from: http://www.usp.org/USPVerified/

Drug interactions

Information regarding herbal–drug interactions is limited. Most data are from case reports, case series, pharmacologic information, animal studies, and, seldom, randomized trials. Although the information is not of the highest quality, it is improving and growing in quantity, since patients continue to combine herbal medications with conventional therapy.

Another cause of the lack of interaction information or the variation in the current information is the lack of product standardization.[1] It is possible for two tablets from the same bottle to contain differing herbal components and doses.

Table 9.4 contains information regarding common drug and herbal interactions. Note that this list is not all-inclusive, and care needs to be taken to check for interactions for any patient taking any herbal therapy.

Table 9.4 Conventional and herbal medication interactions

Conventional medicine	Herbal medicine	Interaction effect on conventional medicine
Antidepressants	St. John's wort	Increased risk of serotonin syndrome
Anticoagulants and antiplatelet agents (warfarin, aspirin, clopidogrel, etc.)	Chamomile, evening primrose oil, fenugreek, feverfew, garlic, ginseng, ginkgo, horse chestnut	Enhanced effect and higher risk for bleeding
	Ginseng (American), St. John's wort	Decreased effect
Anticonvulsant therapy	Borage, evening primrose oil, wormwood	Decreased effect
Antihypertensives	Black cohosh, garlic	Enhanced effect
CNS depressants	Chamomile, hops, passion flower, valerian	Increased effect
Digoxin	Hawthorn, licorice, uzara root	Increased effect and toxicity
Hypoglycemic agents	Chromium, garlic, ginseng, fenugreek	Enhanced effect
Immunosuppressants	Echinacea, licorice	Decreased effect
Iron	Chamomile, feverfew, peppermint, St. John's wort	Decreased absorption

1. Boullata JI, Nace AM (2000). Safety issues with herbal medicine. *Pharmacotherapy* **20**(3):257–269.

Table 9.4 (*Contd.*)

Conventional medicine	Herbal medicine	Interaction effect on conventional medicine
Levothyroxine	Horseradish, kelp	Decreased effect due to thyroid suppression
MAO-I	Ginseng, licorice, passion flower, St. John's wort, yohimbine	Increased effect and risk of serotonin syndrome
NNRTI and Protease inhibitors	Milk thistle	Decreased effect
Oral contraceptive agents	St. John's wort	Decreased effect
Saquinivir	Garlic	Decreased AUC
Substrates of 2C19	Ginkgo	Increased concentration
Subtrates of 2C9 and 1A2	St. John's wort	Decreased concentration
	Ginkgo	Increased concentration
Substrates of 2D6	Ginkgo, ginseng	Increased concentration
Substrates of 3A4	Garlic, St. John's wort	Decreased concentration

Data from:

Boullata JI, Nace AM (2000). Safety issues with herbal medicine. *Pharmacotherapy* **20**(3):257–269.

De Smet PA (2002). Herbal remedies. *N Engl J Med* 347(25):2046–2056.

Gardiner P, Phillips R, Shaughnessy AF (2008). Herbal and dietary supplement–drug interactions in patients with chronic illnesses. *Am Fam Physician* **77**(1):73–78.

Miller LG (1998). Herbal medicinals: selected clinical considerations focusing on known or potential drug–herb interactions. *Arch Intern Med* **158**(20):2200–2211.

Skalli S, Zaid A, Soulaymani R (2007). Drug interactions with herbal medicines. *Ther Drug Monit.* **29**(6):679–686.

Special considerations

- Patients often do not tell health-care professionals about their herbal-medication use. Ask patients specifically about use of herbal medications or CAM.
- Information regarding the efficacy of herbal medications is currently limited and care needs to be taken to check for safety, efficacy, and interactions.
- Currently, standards for the manufacturing of herbal medications are lacking; therefore, actual product contents are unknown.
- Recommend using USP-certified herbal medications since these have undergone a standardization and certification process.
- Many herbal therapies interfere with surgical medications and procedures. Advise patients to stop herbal-medication therapy approximately 2 weeks prior to surgery.

Further references

- Natural Standard: Herb and Supplement Reference
- National Center for Complementary and Alternative Medicine
- Office of Dietary Supplements

Chapter 10

Patient management issues

Denise R. Kockler
Katie Muzevich
Jorie A. Glick
Julie J. Kelsey
Kristin W. Cox
Nicole L. Metzger
Susan B. Cogut

Introduction to liver disease

Liver dysfunction is a general term that encompasses a number of hepatic disorders (see Table 10.1). Approximately 2.5 million people in the United States are affected by liver disease. In 2004, the Center for Disease Control and Prevention (CDC) reported that chronic liver disease and cirrhosis were the 12th leading cause of mortality.

Biochemical markers, collectively referred to as *liver function tests* (LFTs), are used to characterize the origin and extent of liver dysfunction (see Table 10.2).

Table 10.1 Hepatic disorders

Hepatocellular injury	Damage to the main cells of the liver (hepatocytes)
Hepatitis	Inflammation of the liver, a type of hepatocellular injury. Could be caused by viruses, drugs, or other agents, or could be idiosyncratic
Cirrhosis	Chronic, irreversible damage to liver cells, usually caused by alcohol or hepatitis C. If the remaining cells cannot maintain normal liver function (compensated disease), ascites, jaundice, and encephalopathy can develop (decompensated disease).
Cholestasis	Reduction in bile production or bile flow through the bile ducts
Liver failure	Severe hepatic dysfunction in which compensatory mechanisms are no longer sufficient to maintain homeostasis. Could be acute and reversible or irreversible, e.g., end-stage cirrhosis

Table 10.2 Common liver function tests

	Normal values	Type of injury if value is increased
Alanine aminotransferase (ALT)	<40 units/L	Hepatocellular injury
Aspartate aminotransferase (AST)	<40 units/L	Hepatocellular injury
Alkaline phosphatase	50–120 units/L	Cholestasis
γ-glutamyl transferase (GGT)	<30 units/L	Cholestasis
Lactate dehydrogenase (LDH)	<200 units/L	Variable
Bilirubin, total	0.3–1 mg/dL	Variable
Bilirubin, direct (conjugated)	≤0.4	Hepatobiliary disease

Drug use in liver disease

Liver disease may alter the pharmacokinetic and pharmacodynamic properties of drugs, since the liver is the primary site of drug metabolism. In most cases, metabolism leads to inactivation of a drug, although some drugs have active metabolites (e.g., morphine) or require metabolism to be activated (e.g., cyclophosphamide).

Because the liver has large functional reserve, dose modification or drug selection is not usually necessary. However, special consideration of dose modifications and drug selections are required in the following situations:

- **Hepatotoxic drugs**—regardless of whether hepatotoxicity is dose related (e.g., methotrexate) or idiosyncratic (e.g., indomethacin, phenytoin), these drugs are more likely to cause toxicity in patients with liver disease. Therefore, these drugs should be avoided if possible.
- **Protein binding**—the liver is the main source of synthesis of plasma proteins (e.g., albumin). As liver disease progresses, plasma protein levels fall. With less protein available for binding, more free drug is available, which can lead to increased effects and toxicity, especially if the therapeutic index is narrow or the drug is normally highly protein-bound (e.g., phenytoin). If albumin levels are decreased, therapeutic drug monitoring may be used to assess serum drug concentration.
- **Anticoagulants or drugs that cause bleeding**—the liver is the main source of synthesis of clotting factors, thus there is an increased risk of bleeding as liver function worsens. Anticoagulants (e.g., warfarin) should be avoided and drugs that increase bleeding risks (e.g., NSAIDs) should be used with caution in patients with liver disease. Additionally, intramuscular (IM) injections should be avoided in these patients because of possible hematoma risk.
- **Liver failure**—patients with clinical signs of liver failure (e.g., significantly deranged liver enzymes, ascites, or profound jaundice) usually have altered drug handling. In addition, drugs that may worsen the condition should be avoided.
  - Hepatic encephalopathy could be precipitated by certain drugs. Avoid all sedative drugs (including opioid analgesics), drugs causing hypokalemia (including loop and thiazide diuretics), and drugs causing constipation.
  - Edema and ascites could be exacerbated by drugs that cause fluid retention (e.g., NSAIDs and corticosteroids). Drugs with high sodium content (e.g., soluble or effervescent formulations, some antacids) should also be avoided.

Further reading

Ozer J, Ratner M, Shaw M, Bailey W, et al. (2008). The current state of serum biomarkers of hepatotoxicity. *Toxicology* **245**:194–205.

Drug dosing in liver disease

The effects of liver disease and its impact on the various aspects of drug disposition are diverse and often unpredictable. Drug clearance does not increase in a linear fashion as liver function worsens. Some quantitative metabolic markers (e.g., antipyrine, galactose, monoethylglycine-xylide) can be used to assess liver damage; however, the Child–Pugh score classification is often used clinically to assess the severity of liver disease and to adjust drug dosing (see Table 10.3).

Some drugs that should be avoided with Child–Pugh class C (severe liver disease) include the following:[1]

- Abacavir
- Atazanavir
- Caspofungin
- Darifenacin
- Fosamprenavir
- Galantamine
- Pilocarpine tablets
- Sildenafil
- Solifenacin
- Vardenafil
- Voriconazole

Primary factors affecting drug clearance

Hepatic blood flow

Hepatic blood flow may be altered in liver disease because of cirrhosis (fibrosis inhibits blood flow), hepatic venous outflow obstruction (Budd–Chiari syndrome), or portal vein thrombosis. Even in the absence of liver disease, hepatic blood flow may be decreased in cardiac failure or if BP is significantly decreased (e.g., in shock).

Table 10.3 Child–Pugh classification

	1 point	2 points	3 points
Bilirubin (mg/dL)	<2	2–3	>3
Albumin (g/dL)	>3.5	2.8–3.5	<2.8
Prothrombin time proglongation (seconds)	1–3	4–6	>6
Ascites	None	Mild	Refractory
Encephalopathy	None	Mild (grades 1–2)	Severe (grades 3–4)

Child classes: A (mild), 5–6 points; B (moderate), 7–9 points; C (severe), 10–15 points

Pugh RN, Murray-Lyon IM, Dawson JL, Pietroni MC, et al. (1973). Transection of the oesophagus for bleeding oesophageal varices. *Br J Surg* **60** :646–649. Reprinted with permission of Blackwell Publishing.

1 Spray JW, Willett K, Chase D, et al. (2007). Dosage adjustment for hepatic dysfunction based on Child-Pugh scores. *Am J Health Syst Pharm* **64**, 690–693.

Clearance (see Table 10.4)

The clearance of drugs highly metabolized by the liver (high extraction/high clearance drugs) is directly related to blood flow. When these drugs are administered orally, their first-pass metabolism is significantly decreased (if hepatic blood flow is decreased) and so bioavailability is increased.

Administration by nonenteral routes, especially IV administration, avoids the effect of first-pass metabolism and allows for bioavailability to be unaffected. The effect of liver impairment on the clearance of these drugs is thus fairly predictable, being directly related to hepatic blood flow. Drug doses should be titrated according to clinical response and side effects.

Table 10.4 High-, intermediate-, and low-extraction drugs

High-extraction drugs		
Dose at 10%–50% normal for oral administration		
Dose at 50% normal for IV administration		
Increased dose interval in portal systemic shunting		
• Bromocriptine • Buspirone • Chlorpromazine • Cyclosporine • Doxepin • Fluorouracil • Fluvastatin • Idarubicin • Imipramine • Isosorbide dinitrate • Labetalol	• Levodopa • Lovastatin • Mercaptopurine • Metoprolol • Midazolam • Morphine • Nicardipine • Nitroglycerin • Promethazine • Propoxyphene	• Propranolol • Quetiapine • Selegiline • Sertraline • Sildenafil • Sirolimus • Sumatriptan • Tacrolimus • Venlafaxine • Verapamil
Intermediate-extraction drugs		
• Amiodarone • Atorvastatin • Azathioprine • Carvedilol • Ciprofloxacin • Clozapine • Codeine • Diltiazem • Erythromycin	• Etoposide • Felodipine • Fluphenazine • Haloperidol • Itraconazole • Lidocaine • Medroxyprogesterone • Meperidine	• Methylphenidate • Mirtazapine • Nifedipine • Nortriptyline • Olanzapine • Omeprazole • Paroxetine • Pravastatin • Simvastatin
Low-extraction drugs with high protein-binding		
Dose at 50% normal (all routes)		
Increased dose interval		
• Ceftriaxone • Chlordiazepoxide • Clarithromycin • Clindamycin • Diazepam • Gemfibrozil • Glipizide	• Lansoprazole • Lorazepam • Methadone • Mycophenolate mofetil • Oxazepam • Phenytoin	• Prednisolone • Rifampin • Tamoxifen • Temazepam • Trazodone • Valproic acid • Zolpidem

Metabolism (see Table 10.4)
Drugs that are poorly metabolized (low extraction/low clearance drugs) are unaffected by changes in hepatic blood flow. Clearance of these drugs is affected by a variety of other factors. Drug doses should be titrated according to clinical response and side effects.

Decreased hepatocellular surface area (see Table 10.4)
Extensive liver cell damage can occur in both acute and chronic liver disease. High-extraction drugs are metabolized less efficiently; therefore doses should be decreased because peak plasma levels are increased. Low-extraction drugs will have decreased systemic clearance, leading to delayed elimination. Thus the dose should remain the same but the dosing interval should be increased.

When liver disease is present, many factors must be considered when dosing medications. General guidelines for prescribing in liver disease are listed in Table 10.5.

Other considerations in liver disease

Portal systemic shunting
If cirrhosis or portal hypertension is present, collateral venous circulation may develop, which bypasses the liver. This means that drugs absorbed by the gastrointestinal (GI) tract may directly enter the systemic circulation. Thus, there is minimal first-pass metabolism of high-extraction drugs and peak concentrations are increased. For both high-extraction and low-extraction drugs, the half-life is prolonged; therefore, the dosing interval should be increased (see Table 10.4).

Cholestasis
In cholestasis, substances normally eliminated by the biliary system accumulate, including some drugs eliminated by bile salts (e.g., rifampin). Because lipid absorption is dependent on bile salt production, it is possible that a decrease in absorption of lipid-soluble drugs may occur.

In cholestasis, bile salts accumulate in the blood. This could increase bioavailability of protein-bound drugs because of competition for binding sites.

Table 10.5 General guidelines for prescribing in liver disease

- Avoid hepatotoxic drugs (note that many herbal medicines are potentially hepatotoxic).
- If possible, use renally cleared drugs.
- Monitor closely for side effects of hepatically cleared drugs.
- Avoid drugs that increase the risk of bleeding.
- Avoid sedating drugs if there is a risk of encephalopathy.
- Avoid constipating drugs if there is a risk of encephalopathy.
- In moderate or severe liver impairment, consider the following options:
    - Decrease the dose of highly metabolized drugs.
    - Increase the dose interval for all hepatically cleared drugs.
- If albumin levels are low, consider decreasing the dose of highly protein-bound drugs.
- Drugs that affect electrolyte balance should be used cautiously and monitored carefully.
- Consider using older, well-established drugs if there are data for use in liver impairment.
- Start with the lowest possible dose and increase cautiously, according to response or side effects.

Further reading

Delcò F, Tchambaz L, Schlienger R, Drewe J, et al. (2005). Dose adjustment in patients with liver disease. *Drug Saf* **28**,529–545.

Pugh RN, Murray-Lyon IM, Dawson JL, Pietroni MC, et al. (1973). Transection of the oesophagus for bleeding oesophageal varices. *Br J Surg* **60**,646–649.

Hepatorenal syndrome

Hepatorenal syndrome (HRS) is defined as a reversible "functional" renal impairment that occurs in those with advanced liver disease and is associated with significant morbidity and mortality. It is characterized by an intense renal vasoconstriction that results in reduced renal perfusion and a very low glomerular filtration rate (GFR). HRS can be divided into two clinical types (see Table 10.6).

Factors associated with HRS

- Spontaneous bacterial peritonitis (SBP); ascites fluid with polymorphonuclear leukocyte (PMN) count of 250 or greater (regardless of positive or negative culture results)
- GI bleeding with hypovolemic shock
- Severe urinary sodium retention
- Spontaneous dilutional hyponatremia
- Mean arterial blood pressure <80 mmHg

Diagnosis

The diagnosis of HRS is one of exclusion and based on predefined criteria established by the International Ascities Club (IAC) (see Box 10.1).

Management of HRS

General measures

- Maintain renal perfusion.
    - Correct hypovolemia—human albumin is the preferred agent (avoid 5% dextrose in water because it may exacerbate hyponatremia).
    - Maintain blood pressure—if necessary, using vasopressors.
- Consider and correct other causes of renal failure.
    - Stop diuretics and all potentially nephrotoxic drugs.
    - Start empiric broad-spectrum antimicrobials, consider possible septic source and perform blood cultures.
    - Avoid paracentesis without colloid administration.

Table 10.6 Clinical HRS types

Type I	• Rapid progression
	• Median survival less than 14 days
	• 100% increase of initial serum creatinine to a level >2.5 mg/dL OR 50% reduction of the initial 24-hour creatinine clearance to a level <20 mL/min in less than 14 days
Type II	• Slower progression
	• Median survival approximately 6 months
	• Refractory ascities often present
	• Moderate, steady renal failure with serum creatinine >1.5 mg/dL

Box 10.1 Diagnostic criteria of HRS

*Major criteria**
- Chronic or acute liver disease with advanced hepatic failure and portal hypertension
- Low glomerular filtration rate, as indicated by serum creatinine of >1.5 mg/dL or 24-hour creatinine clearance <40 mL/min
- Absence of shock, ongoing bacterial infection, and current or recent treatment with nephrotoxic drugs. Absence of GI fluid losses (repeat vomiting or intense diarrhea) or renal fluid losses (weight loss >500 g/day for several days in patients with ascites without peripheral edema or 1000 g/day in patients with peripheral edema)
- No sustained improvement in renal function (decrease in serum creatinine to 1.5 mg/dL or less or increase in creatinine clearance to 40 mL/min or more) following diuretic withdrawal and expansion of plasma volume with 1.5 L isotonic saline
- Proteinuria <500 mg/dL and no ultrasonographic evidence of obstructive uropathy or parenchymal renal disease

Additional criteria
- Urine volume <500 mL/day
- Urine sodium <10 mEq/L
- Urine osmolality greater than plasma osmolality
- Urine red blood cells <50 per high power field
- Serum sodium concentration <130 mEq/L

***All** major criteria are necessary for diagnosis of HRS.

Arroyo V, Gines P, Gerbes AL, et al. (1996). Definition and diagnostic criteria of refractory ascites and hepatorenal syndrome in cirrhosis. Hepatology 23(1):164–176. Reprinted with permission of John Wiley & Sons, Inc.

Pharmacological therapy

Prevention

Limited data have been reported for patients with SBP. Administration of albumin 1.5 g/kg upon diagnosis, and then 1 g/kg after 48 hours, in addition to antibiotics has decreased HRS incidence and hospital mortality.

Management
- Systemic vasoconstrictors
- Vasopressin analogues (Ornipressin and Terlipressin; not approved in the United States)
- Somatostatin analogue (Octreotide)
  - Usual dose: 100 mcg subcutaneously (SC) three times daily
  - Adverse effects: hyper/hypoglycemia, cholelithiasis, cardiovascular
- α-adrenergic analogue (Midodrine)
  - Usual dose: 2.5 to 10 mg PO three times daily (dose reduce in renal insufficiency, start with 2.5 mg)
  - Adverse effects: hypertension
- Albumin

Nonpharmacological therapy

- Transjugular intrahepatic portosystemic shunts (TIPS)—clinical trials have not shown a survival advantage.
- Institute renal-replacement therapy.
    - Because of the poor prognosis, the decision to start dialysis should not be taken lightly and only instituted if other organs are functioning well.
    - Continuous hemodialysis is required because intermittent therapy can lead to significant disturbance of hemodynamics and intracranial pressure.
    - Renal-replacement therapy is usually necessary until liver function improves.
    - Molecular adsorbent recirculating system (MARS) is a form of dialysis that removes albumin-bound toxins. Early studies have shown improved survival over that for hemofiltration.
- Expedited liver transplantation is the only proven treatment option for HRS.

Further reading

Arroyo V, Gines P, Gerbes AL, et al. (1996). Definition and diagnostic criteria of refractory ascites and hepatorenal syndrome in cirrhosis. *Hepatology* **23**:164–176.

Turban S, Thuluvath PJ, Atta MG (2007). Hepatorenal syndrome. *World J Gastroenterol* **13**,4046–4055.

Wadei HM, Mai ML, Ahsan N, et al. (2006). Hepatorenal syndrome: pathophysiology and management. *Clin J Am Soc Nephrol* **1**:1066–1079.

Drugs in renal impairment

Renal impairment can affect all aspects of drug disposition, including absorption, distribution, metabolism, and elimination. The pharmacokinetic alterations associated with renal impairment must be considered when individualizing drug therapy.

Absorption

Drug absorption from the GI tract may be impaired by multiple factors in patients with renal impairment. These factors include edema of the GI tract, slowed gastric transit, vomiting, and diarrhea. Administration of phosphate-binding antacids can also decrease the absorption of certain drugs by forming insoluble complexes that cannot be absorbed through the GI tract. While drug absorption is generally decreased in renal impairment, several drugs have been shown to have increased bioavailability secondary to reduced first-pass hepatic metabolism.

Distribution

The volume of distribution may be significantly increased or decreased in patients with renal impairment because of changes in extracellular fluid status and protein binding. Edema and ascites can increase the volume of distribution of highly water-soluble and protein-bound drugs and decrease the volume of distribution of lipid-soluble and low protein-bound drugs. The opposite effect is seen in patients with dehydration or muscle wasting.

Plasma protein binding is altered in uremic patients because of a decrease in serum albumin concentration, structural alterations in albumin, and displacement of drugs by organic acids. The binding of acidic drugs is significantly reduced, resulting in increased active drug, whereas the binding of basic drugs usually remains normal, but may be slightly decreased or increased. This alteration in binding can be especially significant for drugs with a narrow therapeutic index.

Metabolism

Renal impairment may have substantial effects on nonrenal metabolism, depending on the metabolic pathway involved. Hydrolysis, reduction, and acetylation are generally slowed, whereas glucuronidation, sulfation, and oxidation occur at normal rates in renal impairment. The reduction in nonrenal clearance is proportional to the reduction in glomerular filtration rate (GFR).

Patients on chronic therapy may experience accumulation of metabolites and/or parent compounds. Some common drugs with active metabolites that may accumulate in renal failure include acetaminophen, allopurinol, azathioprine, codeine, meperidine, morphine, sulfonamides, procainamide, and theophylline.

Excretion

The net renal clearance (CL) of a drug depends on the GFR, tubular secretion, and reabsorption:

$$CL_{renal} = (GFR \times f_u) + CL_{secretion} - CL_{reabsorption}$$

As glomerular filtration decreases with increased nephron destruction, the renal clearance of drugs is decreased substantially. Drugs that depend on renal tubular secretion via active transport systems will be excreted more slowly in patients with renal impairment.

Assessing renal function

Renal function is assessed by measuring the GFR. The normal range of GFR values in adults is 100–140 mL/min. An estimate of the GFR can be made by measuring or calculating the creatinine clearance (CrCl) rate. Creatinine is a by-product of muscle metabolism that is excreted primarily by glomerular filtration. Thus, measuring the rate of creatinine clearance provides an estimate of GFR; however, it requires a 24-hour urine collection. The Cockroft and Gault equation estimates the rate of creatinine clearance without a 24-hour urine collection:

$$\text{CrCl} = \frac{(140 - \text{age}) \times \text{weight (kg)} \times 0.85 \text{ (if female)}}{72 \times \text{SCr (mg/dL)}}$$

This equation may over- or underestimate creatinine clearance by up to 20%.

For patients who weigh more than 30% above their ideal body weight (IBW), the IBW should be used rather than actual body weight (ABW).

For men, IBW = 50.0 kg + 2.3 kg x (the # of inches over 5 feet tall).

For women, IBW = 45.5 kg + 2.3 kg × (the # of inches over 5 feet tall).

Remember that serum creatinine is a function of muscle mass, which may be decreased in elderly, emaciated, or debilitated patients or may be increased in athletes.

Estimating the GFR assumes stable renal function with a constant serum creatinine. For adult patients with unstable renal function or acute renal failure, the GFR can be estimated using the Modification of Diet in Renal Disease (MDRD) equation:

$$\text{GFR} = 186.3 \times (\text{SCr})^{-1.154} \times (\text{age})^{-0.203} \times 1.212 \text{ (if African American)} \times 0.742 \text{ (if female)}$$

This equation takes into account the patient's serum creatinine, age, race, and gender.

For children with stable renal function, CrCl can be estimated using the Schwartz equation:

$$\text{CrCl} = \text{K} \times \frac{\text{Length in (cm)}}{\text{SCr (mg/dL)}}$$

Where the K = constant of proportionality that is age specific (see Table 10.7).

This equation may not provide an accurate estimate of GFR for infants less than 6 months of age, or for those with severe starvation or muscle wasting. The normal range of CrCl standardized to body surface area increases with age and stabilizes at one year (see Table 10.8).

Table 10.7 Age-specific constant of proportionality

Age	K
Low birth weight ≤1 year	0.33
Full-term ≤1 year	0.45
2–12 years	0.55
Female 13–21 years	0.55
Male 13–21 years	0.70

Originally published in Schwartz GJ, Brion LP, Spitzer A (1987). The use of plasma creatinine concentration for estimating glomerular filtration rate in infants, children and adolescents. *Pediatrics Clinics of North America* **34**(3):571–590. Copyright Elsevier 1987.

Table 10.8 Normal CrCl for those 12 months of age and younger

Age	Normal range of CrCl (mL/min/1.73m2)
5–7 days	45– 55
1–2 months	60–70
5–8 months	75–100
9–12 months	75–95

Taketomo CK, Hodding JH, Kraus DM (2008). *Pediatric Dosage Handbook*, 15th ed. Hudson: Lexi-Comp, p. 2075. Reprinted with permission of Lexi-Comp, Inc.

Dosage adjustment in renal failure

The kidney is involved in the metabolism and excretion of many drugs and their active metabolites. If drug therapy is not individualized for patients with renal impairment, accumulation and toxicity may occur. Drugs for which the kidney is the major site of elimination pose the greatest problem in clinical practice. The ideal drug for use in patients with renal impairment has the following characteristics:

- <25% excreted unchanged in the urine
- No active or toxic metabolites
- Not highly protein bound
- Minimally affected by fluid balance
- Not nephrotoxic

For drugs that do not meet these criteria, dose adjustment is usually necessary. The initial or loading dose for patients with normal extracellular fluid volume does not need to be adjusted. For patients with excess extracellular fluid, such as those with edema or ascites, a larger initial dose may be required. Similarly, a smaller initial dose may be needed in patients who are severely debilitated or dehydrated.

When subsequent doses are required, the maintenance dose should also be adjusted on the basis of renal function. There are two methods of dose reduction that can be used alone or in combination for adjusting the maintenance dose:

- Interval extension—the same dose is given at a longer dosing interval
- Dosage reduction—a smaller dose is given at the same dosing interval

Recommendations for maintenance dosing are published in many reference sources (see Further reading, p. 193). Additional dosage adjustments may be required in patients who are receiving concomitant therapy that interacts with or inhibits drug metabolism.

Whenever possible, nephrotoxic drugs should be avoided in patients with renal impairment. Adjusting the dose of medications in renal impairment cannot guarantee therapeutic efficacy and lack of toxicity. Patients should be monitored carefully for efficacy and adverse effects. When possible, serum drug concentrations should be evaluated. Remember that renal function may improve or deteriorate over time, and doses should be adjusted accordingly.

Drug dosing in dialysis

Patients undergoing dialysis require further consideration for dose adjustment. There are four types of renal replacement therapy commonly used (see Chapter 15, Renal Replacement Therapy, p. 408):

- Intermittent hemodialysis (HD)
- Continuous ambulatory peritoneal dialysis (CAPD)
- Continuous arteriovenous hemodialysis (CAVD)
- Continuous arteriovenous hemofiltration (CAVH)

Each method removes toxins from the blood by diffusion or osmosis across a semipermeable membrane into a dialysis solution. Depending on the type of dialysis, certain drugs may be substantially removed. In patients on HD, supplemental doses after the dialysis session may be required; however, scheduling doses after HD can prevent the need for supplemental doses.

CAVH and CAVD are continuous processes; therefore, doses do not need to be scheduled around dialysis sessions. In general, HD is more effective than PD at removing drugs; however, there are many dialysis-related and drug-related factors that affect dialysis drug clearance.

Dialysis-related factors affecting drug clearance

- Duration of dialysis
- Blood flow rate in dialyzer
- Type of dialyzer membrane
- Pore size
- Flow rate of dialysate
- Solute composition of dialysate
- Temperature of dialysate
- pH of dialysate

Drugs that have a low molecular weight, volume of distribution, and protein binding and a high degree of water solubility are most likely to be removed by dialysis.

Drug-related factors affecting drug clearance

- Molecular weight
- Protein binding
- Volume of distribution
- Water solubility
- Degree of ionization

Recommendations for dosage adjustments based on the type of dialysis are published in many references (see Further reading, p. 193). Dose adjustment can also be made on the basis of the theoretical GFR of the dialysis technique (see Table 10.9). Adjusting the dose of medications based on the theoretical GFR or published recommendations cannot guarantee therapeutic efficacy and lack of toxicity. Patients should be monitored closely for drug response and toxicity.

Table 10.9 Theoretical GFR in renal replacement therapy

Renal replacement therapy	Typical theoretical GFR achieved (mL/min)
HD during dialysis	150–160
HD between dialysis periods	0–10
CAVD	15–20
CAVH	10
CAPD (4 exchanges daily)	5–10

Further reading

Aronoff GR, Bennett WM, Berns JS, et al. (eds) (2007). *Drug Prescribing in Renal Failure: Dosing Guidelines for Adults and Children, American College of Physicians*, 5th ed.

Ashley C, Currie A (eds) (2004). *The Renal Drug Handbook*, 2nd ed. Radcliffe Medical Press.

Cockroft DW, Gault MH (1976). The estimation of creatinine clearance from serum creatinine concentration. *Nephron* **16**:31–38.

Munar MY, Singh H (2007). Drug dosing adjustments in patients with chronic kidney disease. *Am Fam Physician* **10**:1487–1496.

Swan SK, Bennett WM (1992). Drug dosing guidelines in patients with renal failure. *West J Med* **156**:633–638.

Drugs in pregnancy

A *teratogen* is a substance, organism, physical agent, or deficiency state capable of inducing abnormal structure or function, such as gross structural abnormalities, functional deficiencies, intrauterine growth restriction, behavioral aberrations, or fetal demise.

Teratogenic effects usually only occur when the fetus is exposed during a critical period of development. Even then, not all fetuses exposed will be affected—e.g., only 20% of fetuses exposed to thalidomide developed congenital abnormalities. Later drug exposures may lead to functional deficiencies or growth restriction.

Other possible causes

- The congenital anomaly rate is approximately 3%–4% of live-born infants. Of these, about 10% are caused by environmental factors (drugs, diseases, infections, chemicals, etc.), ~20% are related to genetic factors, and the rest are unknown.
- Maternal morbidity or an acute exacerbation/relapse of a disease could present a higher risk to the fetus than the drug.
- Exposure to multiple agents or to environmental toxins may increase the rate of anomalies.
- Smoking and alcohol use during pregnancy can lead to congenital abnormalities, growth retardation, spontaneous abortion, and preterm delivery.

Drug characteristics

- Most drugs cross the placenta via passive diffusion, however, they can cross by facilitated diffusion or active transport.
- High-molecular-weight drugs do not cross the placenta—e.g., heparins and insulin.
- Nonionized, lipophilic drugs cross the placenta to a greater extent than ionized, hydrophilic drugs.
- Highly protein-bound drugs cross the placenta to a much less degree.
- The placenta contains CYP450 enzymes and can conjugate drugs, so little drug may enter the fetal circulation (e.g., prednisone).
- A drug can cause fetal toxicity without crossing the placenta—e.g., any drug that causes vasoconstriction of the placental vasculature.

Timing

- If the drug is taken during the first 12 days post-conception (pre-embryonic phase), there is an "all-or-nothing" effect—i.e., if most cells are affected this leads to spontaneous loss, and if a few cells are affected this leads to cell repair or replacement and a normal fetus.
- Exposure during the first trimester (especially weeks 3–11) carries the greatest risk of congenital abnormalities.
- The cerebral cortex and renal glomeruli continue to develop during the second and third trimester and are still susceptible to damage.
- Shortly before or during labor there is a risk of maternal complications (e.g., NSAIDs and maternal bleeding) or neonate complications (e.g., opioids and sedation).

The FDA has created five categories for all approved medications that indicate the risk associated with the induction of birth defects. Keep in mind that drug-risk ratings may be different, depending on the trimester.

Risk-factor ratings in pregnancy[1]

- **A.** Controlled trials in women showed no risk to the fetus in the first trimester (and no evidence of risk in second or third trimesters) or a remote possibility of fetal harm.
- **B.** Animal-reproduction trials did not report a fetal risk, but no controlled trials in pregnant women OR animal-reproduction trials reported an adverse effect (other than decrease in fertility), but these results were not confirmed in controlled trials in women in the first trimester (and no evidence of risk in second or third trimesters).
- **C.** Animal trials have revealed adverse effects to the fetus (teratogenic or embryocidal or other); however, there are no controlled trials in women, or trials in women and animals are not available. Drugs should only be given if potential benefit outweighs the potential risk to fetus.
- **D.** There is positive evidence of human fetal risk, but benefits of use in pregnant women may be acceptable despite the risk.
- **X.** Animal and human trials have shown fetal abnormalities or evidence of fetal risk based on human experience or both, and the risk of the drug in pregnant women clearly outweighs any possible benefit. The drug is contraindicated in women who are or may become pregnant.

The FDA has proposed major changes to prescription drug labeling for pregnancy. The changes would eliminate the current pregnancy risk categories (A, B, C, D, X). The labeling would include pregnancy subsections that would have three principle components:

- Fetal risk summary (characterizes the risk of four types of developmental abnormalities: structural anomalies, fetal and infant mortality, impaired physiological function, alterations to growth)
- Clinical considerations (inadvertent exposure, prescribing decisions for pregnant women, drug effects during labor or delivery)
- Data section (detailed human and animal data)

Other components of the product labeling include

- Pregnancy exposure registries
- General statement about background risk

Several agents are unsafe in pregnancy and should be avoided (see Table 10.10), whereas others have a good safety record (see Table 10.11). One should refer to the FDA product labeling and additional information about drug safety in pregnancy that is listed in the Further Reading of this section.

1 Center for Drug Evaluation and Research, FDA (2008). Summary of proposed rule on pregnancy and lactation labeling. www.fda.gov/CDER/regulatory/pregnancy_labeling/summary.htm

Table 10.10 Some drugs that should be avoided* in pregnancy

Drugs known to cause congenital malformations	
• Older anticonvulsants	• Lithium
• Cytotoxics	• Retinoids (systemic)
• Androgens	• Warfarin
Drugs that can affect fetal growth and development	
• ACE inhibitors (after 12 weeks)—fetal or neonatal renal failure	
• Barbiturates, benzodiazepines, and opioids (near term)—drug dependence in fetus	
• NSAIDs (third trimester)—premature closure of ductus arteriosus	
• Tetracyclines (after 12 weeks)—abnormalities of teeth and bone	
• Warfarin—fetal or neonatal hemorrhage	

* Note that if the benefit clearly outweighs the risk (e.g., life-threatening or pregnancy-threatening disease), these drugs can be used in pregnancy. However, if the drug holds a category X rating, it is contraindicated in women who are or may become pregnant.

Table 10.11 Some drugs that have a good safety record in pregnancy

- Analgesics: acetaminophen
- Antacids containing aluminum, calcium, or magnesium
- Antibacterials: penicillins, cephalosporins, erythromycin, clindamycin, and nitrofurantoin (avoid near term)
- Antiemetics: doxylamine, meclizine, and promethazine
- Antifungal agents (topical and vaginal): clotrimazole and nystatin
- Antihistamines: chlorpheniramine and loratadine
- Asthma: bronchodilator and steroid inhalers (avoid high doses in the long term), and short-course oral steroids
- Corticosteroids (topical, including nasal and eye drops)
- Insulin
- Laxatives: bulk forming, senna, and docusate
- Levothyroxine
- Methyldopa
- H2 blockers (ranitidine, famotidine)

Other considerations

- Presence or absence of teratogenic effects in animals does not necessarily translate to the same effects in humans. Most studies use higher doses in animals than would be used in humans.
- Drugs associated with abnormalities at high doses for long durations during the first trimester might be lower risk at lower doses during the second or third trimester (e.g., fluconazole).
- If treatment cannot be avoided during pregnancy, use established drugs that have good evidence of safety. Sometimes a lack of reports of teratogenicity for a well-established or frequently used drug can be taken as evidence of safety.
- Some teratogenic effects are dose related. Higher doses or combining more than one drug with the same effect may increase the risk.
- Consider non-drug treatments (e.g., acupressure wrist bands for morning sickness) or whether treatment can be delayed until after pregnancy.

Maternal considerations

- Maternal pharmacokinetics change during pregnancy; doses or frequency may need to be adjusted, or monitoring may need to be performed more often.
- Remind the mother that some over-the-counter, herbal, and vitamin products should be avoided in pregnancy.

Further reading

Briggs GG, Freeman RK, Yaffe SJ (eds) (2008). *Drugs in Pregnancy and Lactation*, 8th ed. Philadelphia: Lippincott Williams and Wilkins.

Shepard TH (ed.) (1995). *Catalog of Teratogenic Agents*, 7th ed. Baltimore: John Hopkins University Press.

Motherisk, www.motherisk.org

REPROTOX (subscription required, available through MicroMedex)

TERIS (subscription required, available through MicroMedex)

Drugs in breastfeeding

Breastfeeding has many advantages over bottle-feeding, including decreases in the risk or severity of diarrhea and in the occurrence of many infectious diseases (e.g., respiratory tract infections, otitis media, bacteremia, bacterial meningitis, botulism, urinary tract infections, necrotizing enterocolitis, and delayed sepsis) and other various diseases (diabetes, lymphoma, leukemia, obesity, asthma, and ulcerative colitis). Because of an increase in breastfeeding, a 21% reduction in postneonatal mortality (>28 days old) has been reported in the United States.

Even if the mother is taking a drug that is excreted in breast milk it may be better to continue breastfeeding. However, a couple main questions to consider include the following:

- Do the drugs affect milk production (negatively)?
- Is the drug excreted into breast milk in quantities that are clinically significant?
- Do these drug levels pose any threat to the infant's health?

To answer these questions, the following factors must be considered.

Drug effects on lactation

- Galactagogues increase milk supply.
  - Dopamine antagonists: metoclopramide
- Drugs that decrease milk supply
  - Dopaminergic agents: bromocriptine, amantadine
  - Estrogens
  - Diuretics

Factors that affect drug transfer into breast milk

Maternal drug plasma level

This is usually the most important determinant of breast milk drug levels. Drugs enter the breast milk primarily by diffusion. For most drugs, the higher the maternal dose, the higher the drug level in the breast milk. Diffusion of drug between plasma and milk is a two-way process and is concentration dependent.

At peak maternal plasma levels (T_{max}), drug levels in breast milk are also at their highest. As the level of the drug in the plasma falls, the level of the drug in breast milk also falls as drug diffuses from the milk back into the plasma. Drugs that only have a short half-life only appear in breast milk for a correspondingly short time.

- During the first 4 days after delivery, drugs diffuse more readily into the breast milk because there are gaps between the alveolar cell walls in mammary capillaries. These gaps permit enhanced access for most drugs, in addition to immunoglobulins (Ig) and maternal proteins. This results in increased drug levels in breast milk during the neonatal stage. After the first 4–7 days, these gaps close.
- Some drugs pass into breast milk by an active process, such that the drug is concentrated in the milk. This occurs with iodides, especially radioactive iodides, making it necessary to interrupt or stop breastfeeding.

Lipid solubility of the drug

Fat-soluble drugs (e.g., benzodiazepines, opioids, and many other CNS-active drugs) preferentially dissolve in the lipid globules of breast milk. As a general rule, increased lipid solubility leads to increased penetration into milk.

Milk pH levels

Breast milk has a lower pH than that of blood. Thus, drugs that are weak bases (e.g., propranolol), become ionized in milk and less likely to diffuse back into the plasma. This can lead to accumulation in the breast milk of these drugs. Conversely, weakly acidic drugs (e.g., penicillins) tend not to accumulate in breast milk.

Molecular size and molecular weight of the drug

As a general rule, "bulky" drugs do not diffuse across capillary walls because the molecules are simply too big to pass through the gaps.

Drug protein-binding

Highly protein-bound drugs (e.g., phenytoin and warfarin) do not normally pass into breast milk in significant quantities because only free, unbound drug diffuses across the capillary walls. If the drug is displaced by a second drug, this could (at least temporarily) increase milk levels of the first drug.

To help decrease the risk of drug exposure to breastfed infants, knowledge of lactation risk categories for drugs (see Box 10.2) and general principles should be considered (see Box 10.3).

The FDA has proposed including information about breastfeeding risk for prescription drug labeling. The labeling would include breastfeeding subsections that would have three principle components:

- Risk summary (if applicable, a breastfeeding compatibility statement; effect on milk production, if drug is present in human milk and how much, effect of drug on breastfed child)
- Clinical considerations (ways to minimize exposure, potential drug effects and monitoring of effects, dosing adjustments)
- Data (overview of clinical data on which risk summary and clinical considerations are based)

Infant factors

- Bioavailabilty—drugs that are destroyed in the gut or are not absorbed orally (e.g., insulin and aminoglycosides), should not cause any adverse effect because the infant's absorption of the drug is negligible, if any. However, these drugs can sometimes have a local effect on the infants gut causing GI symptoms, such as diarrhea.
- Infant status—must be taken into account. If the baby is premature or ill, they might be less able to tolerate even small quantities of a drug. Consider whether drug side effects could exacerbate the infant's underlying disease. For example, opioids in breast milk may be a higher risk for a baby with respiratory problems than a healthy baby.

Box 10.2 Dr. Hale's lactation risk categories*

- *L1 (safest)*: Drug taken by a large number of breastfeeding women without an observed increase in adverse effects to the infant. Controlled trials in breastfeeding women fail to demonstrate a risk to the infant and the possibility of harm to the breastfeeding infant is remote; or the product is not orally bioavailable in an infant.
- *L2 (safer)*: Drug evaluated in a limited number of breastfeeding women without an increase in adverse effects to the infant; and/or evidence of a demonstrated risk that is likely to follow use of this medication in a breastfeeding woman is remote.
- *L3 (moderately safe)*: No controlled trials in breastfeeding women; however, the risk of untoward effects to a breastfed infant is possible; or, controlled trials show only minimal non-threatening adverse effects. Drugs should only be given if the potential benefit justifies the potential risk to the infant. (Newly approved medications without published data for breastfeeding are automatically categorized as an L3, regardless of how safe they may be).
- *L4 (possibly hazardous)*: Positive evidence of risk to a breastfed infant or to breast milk production, but the benefits from use in breastfeeding mothers may be acceptable despite the risk to the infant (e.g., drug is needed in a life-threatening emergency or for a serious disease for which safer drugs cannot be used or are ineffective)
- *L5 (contraindicated)*: Trials in breastfeeding women have demonstrated a significant and documented risk to the infant based on human experience, or it is a medication that has a high risk of causing significant damage to an infant. The risk of using the drug in breastfeeding women clearly outweighs any possible benefit from breastfeeding. The drug is contraindicated in women who are breastfeeding an infant.

*Currently, the FDA does not have risk ratings for drug use in breastfeeding.
Reprinted with permission from: Hale TW (ed). (2008). *Medications and Mother's Milk*, 13th ed. Pharmasoft Publishing.

- **Metabolism and excretion** of some drugs is altered in infancy, especially in premature infants who have immature renal and hepatic function. Thus, the drug effects can be greater than expected because the clearance of the drug is decreased. This can be especially true for drugs with a long half-life.
- **Drugs often administered to infants**—e.g., acetaminophen, are generally safe if absorbed in breast milk. Better agents to use have a relative infant dose of <10% of the maternal dose on a mg/kg/day basis.

Other factors to consider

- Some mothers and healthcare workers assume that because the infant was exposed to the drug during pregnancy, it will be safe in breast feeding. However, in pregnancy it is the maternal organs that clear the drug from the infant's circulation, but during breastfeeding the infant is clearing the drug. In addition, some adverse effects, such as respiratory depression, are not important during pregnancy but become relevant after delivery.

Box 10.3 General principles to decrease risk to breastfed infants

- Consider whether non-drug therapy is possible.
- Can treatment be delayed until the mother is no longer breastfeeding?
- Use drugs where safety in breastfeeding has been established
- Keep the maternal dose as low as possible
- Use drugs with a local effect (e.g., inhalers, creams, or drugs not absorbed orally, such as nystatin).
- Use drugs with a short half-life.
- Avoid polypharmacy—additive side effects and drug interactions potentially increase the risk.
- Advise the mother to breastfeed when the level of the drug in breast milk will be lowest. This is usually just before the next dose is due.
- Administer the drug prior to the infant's longest sleep to have lower amounts in breast milk.
- Alternate feeding for a couple of feedings after the dose is taken may be needed.
- Withhold breastfeeding temporarily—advise mother to pump and save milk ahead of time so that it can be used while breastfeeding is temporarily being suspended.

- Some mothers are resistant to using conventional medicines during breastfeeding because of perceived risks and decide to use alternative therapies. Mothers should be reminded that herbal or homeopathic medicines might be excreted in breast milk and cause adverse effects on the infant.
- Some drugs can reduce milk supply, such as systemic sympathomimetics (pseudoephedrine or phenylephrine) or sedating antihistamines. These drugs taken on a frequent schedule will have a more pronounced effect.
- Sometimes breastfeeding might have to be interrupted or stopped completely if there is no alternative to administering a potentially risky drug. For short courses, it might be possible to stop breastfeeding temporarily. Using a breast pump and discarding the pumped milk until such time as it is safe to resume breastfeeding should encourage continued breast milk production.

Further reading

Briggs GG, Freeman RK, Yaffe SJ (eds.) (2008). *Drugs in Pregnancy and Lactation*, 8th ed. Philadelphia: Lippincott, Williams & Wilkins.

Center for Drug Evaluation and Research, FDA (2008). Summary of proposed rule on pregnancy and lactation labeling. www.fda.gov/CDER/regulatory/pregnancy_labeling/summary.htm

Hale TW (ed.) (2008). *Medications and Mother's Milk*, 13th ed. Pharmasoft Publishing.

U.S. National Library of Medicine. Drugs and Lactation Database (LactMed). Available at: http://toxnet.nlm.nih.gov/cgi-bin/sis/htmlgen?LACT

Medicines for children: introduction

Children represent a significant proportion of patients in both primary and secondary care. It is important to remember that children are not small adults, nor are they a homogenous group. Drug handling in children can be quite different from that in adults and can also be different at different ages.

For medical and pharmaceutical purposes, children are often grouped according to age (see Table 10.12). Not only do medication regimens vary depending on the child's age, certain medications have age contraindications (e.g., avoid tetracycline use in children ≤8 years).

Pediatric patients are at increased risk of medication errors secondary to variations in weight, body surface area, and organ maturation. These age-based differences impact pharmacokinetic and pharmacodynamic properties of the medication. Other reasons that children are at increased risk of medication errors or adverse drug reactions are as follows:

- The medication-use process in children is detailed and labor intensive. Children require individualized dose calculations that increase the risk of math, decimal, and fractional errors (mg vs. g). Preparing medications for children requires more medication handling and manipulation to provide precise doses.
- Many dosage forms and concentrations required for pediatric medication administration are not commercially available. Hence, children often require the use of compounded preparations and are more likely to have medications administered by alternate routes (e.g., IV form given orally).
- Most marketed medications are not FDA approved for use in children. Published information regarding dosing, pharmacokinetics, efficacy, safety, and clinical use of medications in children are lacking.
- Children have a limited ability to communicate medication efficacy or side effects with health-care providers. Dosage instructions given to caregivers are often misunderstood or ambiguous.

Several organizations, including the American Academy of Pediatrics and the Institute of Safe Medication Practices, have published guidelines to prevent medication errors in children.[1–3] The role of pharmacists in preventing these errors is included in their recommendations.

1 Levine SR, Cohen MR, Blanchard NR, et al. (2001). Guidelines for preventing medication errors in pediatrics. *J Pediatr Pharmacol Ther* **6**:426–442.

2 American Academy of Pediatrics (2003). Prevention of medication errors in the pediatric inpatient setting. *Pediatrics* **112**:431–436.

3 The Joint Commission (2008). Sentinal event alert: preventing pediatric medication errors. Issue 39, April 11, 2008. Available at: www.jointcommission.org

Table 10.12 Age classifications

Term	Definition
Gestational age	Time from conception to birth
Postnatal age	Time from birth to present
Postmenstrual age	Gestational age + Postnatal age
Premature	Born before 37 weeks gestation
Term	Born 37–42 weeks gestation
Neonate	≤4 weeks*
Infant	1 month–1 year
Child	1–12 years
Adolescent	12–18 years

* If premature, add the number of weeks premature, e.g., if born 2 weeks premature, the baby is considered a neonate until 6 weeks old.

Medicines for children: pharmacodynamics and pharmacokinetics

Virtually all pharmacokinetic parameters change with age. An understanding of how drug handling changes with age is essential to avoid toxicity or underdosing.

Absorption

Newborns have a prolonged gastric-emptying time. Because GI absorption is slower in newborns and infants than in adults, it may take longer for them to achieve maximum plasma levels. Lower levels of gastric acid in newborns might decrease absorption of weak acids (e.g., phenobarbital). Drugs that bind to calcium and magnesium should not be given at the same time as milk feeds. Drug absorption approaches adult values by 6–12 months.

Intramuscular absorption requires muscle movement to stimulate blood flow so absorption may be reduced or slower in newborns that have decreased muscle mass and are relatively immobile.

Topical absorption of agents is enhanced in neonates and infants because the skin is thinner and more hydrated. This age group also has a proportionally larger body surface area for weight than older children. Thus, topical agents applied over a large area can provide a significant systemic dose.

Distribution

Total body water decreases with age:

- Premature—80% of body weight
- Newborn and infants—70% of body weight
- Children—60%–65% of body weight
- Adults—60% of body weight

This affects the volume of distribution of water-soluble drugs, and higher doses per kilogram might be required for premature or newborn infants.

In neonates, the blood–brain barrier is more permeable than in older children. Hence, neonates are more susceptible to the central nervous system (CNS) effects of certain medications.

Protein binding

In young infants and neonates, protein binding of drugs is decreased. Less protein stores and decreased binding capacity result in an increase in unbound medication. This increase in free fraction of drug can result in toxicity even with normal or low plasma concentrations of total drug. Highly protein-bound drugs can also displace bilirubin from albumin in neonates, resulting in hyperbilirubinemia (e.g., ceftriaxone).

Metabolism

Premature and newborn infants metabolize drugs more slowly than adults, secondary to immature metabolic enzymes. Each of the phase I and phase II enzymes has a unique maturation profile. Most liver enzymes are mature by 1 year of age.

Young children actually have a faster rate of metabolism, which decreases to adult levels with increased age. An increase in liver mass as a percentage of body mass in young children may contribute to their increased metabolic capacity. Thus, doses of highly metabolized drugs are proportionally lower per kilogram for neonates and infants and higher for young children.

As the child grows, doses should be frequently recalculated not only to allow for differing rates of drug metabolism but also to allow for increases in height and weight.

Elimination

Nephrogenesis is complete by 36 weeks gestational age but is functionally immature in premature infants and neonates. Neonatal GFR is usually ~30% of the adult rate and reaches adult values by 1 year of life. Dosing intervals may need to be extended in neonates to prevent accumulation and toxicity.

Creatinine clearance in children can be estimated using the Schwartz equation (see Drugs in Renal Impairment, p. 188). After infancy, plasma clearance of some drugs is significantly increased because of both increased hepatic elimination (as above) and increased renal excretion.

Medicines for children: licensing

Up to 60% of prescribing for children is unlicensed or off-label—i.e., the drug is not licensed for that age range, route, dose, or indication. Research on prescribing for children is limited because of the complexity and expense of pediatric clinical trials and the lack of financial or legal incentives for manufacturers. Several voluntary initiatives have been introduced by the FDA to encourage the pharmaceutical industry to submit pediatric labeling information.

- In 1994, the FDA changed regulations to allow adult efficacy data to be extrapolated to children for certain medications when the indication for use is similar. Manufacturers only have to complete pharmacokinetic dosing studies in children to achieve pediatric labeling.
- The FDA Modernization Act (1997) provides a financial incentive to manufacturers who complete pediatric studies on medications that the FDA considers essential. The FDA grants a 6-month extension on existing patents once studies are submitted that lead to improved labeling for children.
- The Pediatric Final Rule (1998) was a mandatory regulation requiring pediatric studies for new medications in which significant use or benefit in children was expected. The U.S. Circuit Court of Appeals for the District of Columbia, however, struck down the Final Rule in 2002, contending that the FDA could not mandate pharmaceutical companies to conduct pediatric studies.
- The Best Pharmaceuticals for Children Act (2002) supports the continued use of the financial incentives to manufacturers that complete pediatric clinical trials.

The above initiatives have led to over 100 medications with new or revised pediatric labeling. Despite this improvement, the use of off-label medications in children continues to be widespread.

There are many concerns with using off-label medications in children; however, off-label use does not imply improper or illegal use. In most situations, off-label drug use is not considered research and does not require special consent. Decisions about whether institutional review or written consent is required depend on the degree of risk, deviation from standard practice, and/or if research is involved.

Prescribing FDA-approved medications for unapproved uses should be based on all available data. Practitioners that choose to prescribe off-label medications are encouraged to publish their observations and to report any adverse events to the drug manufacturer or directly to the FDA.

Off-label medication use in children may be beneficial, ineffective, or harmful. Clinical studies of new and existing medications are required to confirm efficacy and safety in medications in children and to minimize off-label use.

Medicines for children: calculating children's doses

A reputable reference source should be used for children's doses. Different sources quote doses in different ways, and it is important to be clear how the dose is calculated to avoid the risk of overdose. Doses are usually quoted as follows:

- The total dose in mg/kg body weight per day, and the number of doses it should be divided into
- The individual dose in mg/kg body weight per dose, and the number of doses that should be given each day

Most doses are based on weight, although doses based on body surface area (BSA) are more accurate because this takes into account the child's overall size (see Table 10.13). BSA dosing is more frequent for drugs if accurate dosing is critical (e.g., cytotoxic drugs). Nomograms for calculating BSA can be found in pediatric drug handbooks, or the following equation can be used:

$$\text{Body surface area } (\text{m})^2 = \sqrt{\frac{\text{body weight (kg)} \times \text{height (cm)}}{3600}}$$

When calculating pediatric doses, adult maximum doses should not be exceeded unless indicated by drug monitoring or the clinical situation is known to alter drug disposition. In premature infants and neonates, dosing regimens are often calculated using gestational, postnatal, and/or postmenstrual age as well as weight to account for changes in organ maturation and volume of distribution.

When there are no published doses in pediatric drug references, health-care providers need to refer to primary literature to determine whether the medication has ever been used in children, at what doses, and for what indications. When it is impossible to find a published pediatric dose for a drug, the initial dose can be estimated from the adult dose as a proportion of adjusted body weight or BSA (see Table 10.14). Whether to use BSA or body weight depends on the patient's age and the volume of distribution and/or metabolic pathway of the drug.[1] Doses should be titrated according to clinical response, as necessary.

1 Bartelink IH, Rademaker CMA, Schobben AF, et al. (2006) Guidelines on pediatric dosing on the basis of developmental physiology and pharmacokinetic considerations. *Clin Pharmacokinet* **45**:1077–1097.

Table 10.13 Approximate surface area and weight*

	Weight (kg)	Surface area (m^2)
Newborn	3	0.2
6 months	7	0.38
1 year	10	0.49
3 years	15	0.64
5 years	20	0.76
9 years	30	1.06
12 years	40	1.34
14 years	50	1.5
Adult	70	1.73

* Note: many children in developing countries might only weigh 60%–80% of the average weight

Table 10.14 Estimating children's doses as a proportion of adult doses

Child dose = Adult dose x (Body $weight_{child}$ / Body $weight_{adult}$)
Child dose = Adult dose x (BSA_{child} / BSA_{adult})

Data from Bartelink, IH, Rademaker CMA, Schobben AF, et al. (2006) Guidelines on pediatric dosing on the basis of developmental physiology and pharmacokinetic considerations. *Clin Pharmacokinet* **45**:1077–1097.

Further reading

Phelps SJ, Hak EB (eds.) (2007). *Pediatric Injectable Drugs*, 8th ed. American Society of Health-System Pharmacists, Inc.

Taketomo CK, Hodding JH, Kraus DM (eds.) (2007). *Pediatric Dosing Handbook*, 14th ed. Lexi-Comp, Inc.

Young TE, Mangum B (eds) (2008) *Neofax*, 13th ed. Thomson Healthcare.

Medicines for children: adherence

Counseling on medicine use and adherence issues is important for children. Parents might be familiar with taking medicines themselves, but this doesn't mean they will be able to cope with giving medicines to their child, especially if they are distressed by the child's diagnosis or the child is uncooperative. The toddler age group is often the most difficult because at this age children can be uncooperative but lack the language ability and insight needed for parents to reason with them.

- Wherever possible and within the child's level of understanding, pharmacists should aim to involve the child in discussions about their medicines.
- Explain to the child in simple terms why they need to take their medicine, allowing for any limitations on disclosure of the diagnosis—e.g., a child may not have been told they have HIV but might have been told that they need medicine to help them fight infection.
- Ideally, counseling about medicine use and adherence should involve both parents (or two caregivers), especially if the therapy is complex and/or long term. As appropriate, school nurses should be involved.
- Help parents to think ahead about how medicines will be administered during the school day or during a school or youth organization event. Tailoring the regimen to once-daily or twice-daily dosing helps avoid drug administration during school hours.
- The most appropriate delivery form should be selected. Most parents find an oral syringe easy to use but most children object to using them. Once measured, the medicine may be transferred to a spoon.
- Parents and caregivers might find it easier to give the medicine mixed with a small amount of food or drink. They should be taught how to do this correctly so that the child takes the full dose. Medicines should not be added to feeding bottles because the full quantity might not be taken.
- Provide parents with strategies on how to administer medications to children (see Box 10.4). Whenever possible, give children choices about the medication process (e.g., "What would you like to drink before or after taking your medicine?")
- Encourage parents to involve the child in the administration process. From quite a young age (and with appropriate supervision and support), children can be taught to measure doses of liquid medicines, make up a weekly medication box, or even self-administer insulin.
- Adolescents might wish to discuss their medicines without their parents present. Nonadherence among adolescents is a common way of expressing independence and requires sensitive handling.
- Be aware that some patient information leaflets might be for indications other than the one for which the medicine is being used.

Box 10.4 Tips on making medicines more palatable

- Chill the medicine (but do not freeze it).*
- Take the medicine through a straw.
- Use an oral syringe to direct the medicine toward the back of the mouth and away from the tongue (and, therefore, away from the highest concentration of taste buds).
- Chocolate disguises many flavors—try mixing the medicine with a small amount of chocolate milk, spread or syrup.*
- Coat the tongue and roof of the mouth with a spoonful of peanut butter or maple syrup before taking the medicine.
- Suck an ice cube or Popsicle® immediately before taking the medicine.
- Brush teeth after taking the dose.
- Consume strongly flavored food or drink after the dose, e.g. citrus fruit, Kool-Aid®, orange juice, grape juice, flavored crackers.*
- Crushed tablets may be mixed with soft foods that do not require chewing, e.g. applesauce, yogurt, ice cream, pudding. *
- Ask your doctor or pharmacist about using flavor additives such as FLAVORx®.

* Check drug compatibility and storage temperature requirements.

Further reading

Clinical Reference System: Helping Children Swallow Medicines (2008). Elsevier, Inc. Available from: www.mdconsult.com

Gardiner P, Dvorkin L (2006). Promoting medication adherence in children. *Am Fam Physician* **74**:793–798.

Web site of the Pediatric Pharmacy Advocacy Group: www.kidsmeds.info

Medicines for elderly people: introduction

Elderly people are high consumers of prescription and over-the-counter (OTC) medicines. Adverse drug reactions (ADRs) can have significant medical and safety consequences for older adults. In the United States, the number of persons ≥65 years of age is expected to double from the year 2000 (approximately 35 million) to 2030 (approximately 71 million persons).[1] Because of the potential ADRs and the growth in the elderly population, an increase in health-care costs is anticipated.

Much prescribing for elderly people is done as "repeats," and without regular review, this can frequently lead to inappropriate or unnecessary therapy, including prescribing for "diseases" that are actually ADRs.

Elderly people are at increased risk of medication-related problems:

- Increased risk of ADRs (many preventable) caused by polypharmacy, drug interactions, and changes in pharmacokinetics and pharmacodynamics
- Underprescribing of some medicines, e.g., thrombolysis in MI
- Nonadherence
- Repeat medicines not being reviewed, leading to unnecessary long-term therapy and stockpiling
- Difficulty accessing the pharmacy

In 1991, Beers et al. published the first set of explicit criteria for determining inappropriate medication use in nursing home residents. Since then these criteria have been revised and updated (2002). The criteria now include 48 individual drugs or drug classes (see Table 10.15) to be avoided in older persons. The potential related concerns, 20 diseases or conditions, and the drugs to avoid prescribing for older persons with these diseases or conditions are also included in the Beers criteria.[2]

Some controversy exists over these criteria since they address only the prescribing of inappropriate medications, not the underprescribing of clinically indicated drugs and other drug-management issues (e.g., drug–drug interactions). The latest update of the Beers criteria for potentially inappropriate drugs for elderly people is available at: www.archinte.ama-assn.org/cgi/content/full/163/22/2716

1 Centers for Disease Control and Prevention (2003). Public health and aging: trends in aging—United States and worldwide. *MMWR Weekly* **52**(06);101–106. Available at: http://www.cdc.gov/mmwr/preview/mmwrhtml/mm5206a2.htm

2 Fick DM, Cooper JW, Wade WE, et al. (2003). Updating the Beers criteria for potentially inappropriate medication use in older adults. *Arch Intern Med* **163**:2716–2724.

Table 10.15 Drugs to avoid in patients ≥65 years*

Analgesic/anti-inflammatory
- Indomethacin (including SR)
- Ketorolac
- Long-term use of full-dose, longer half-life, non–COX-selective NSAIDs: naproxen, oxaprozin, and piroxicam
- Meperidine
- Pentazocine
- Propoxyphene and propoxyphene combination products

Cardiovascular
- Amiodarone
- Clonidine
- Digoxin (should not exceed 0.125 mg/day, except when treating atrial arrhythmias)
- Disopyramide
- Doxazosin
- Ethacrynic acid
- Guanadrel
- Methyldopa and methyldopa-hydrochlorothiazide
- Reserpine
- Short-acting dipyridamole
- Short-acting nifedipine
- Ticlopidine

Diabetic agents
- Chlorpropamide

Gastrointestinal
- Cimetidine
- Gastrointestinal antispasmodic drugs: dicyclomine, hyoscyamine, propantheline, belladonna alkaloids, and clindinium-chlordiazepoxide
- Long–term use of stimulant laxatives: bisacodyl, cascara sagrada, Neoloid, except when used with opiate analgesic
- Mineral oil
- Trimethobenzamide

Muscle relaxants
- Muscle relaxants, antispasmodics: methocarbamol, carisoprodol, chlorzoxazone, metaxalone, cyclobenzaprine, oxybutynin (do not consider oxybutinin XL)
- Orphenadrine

Psychotropics
- Amitriptyline, chlordiazepoxide-amitriptyline, perphenazine-amitriptyline
- Amphetamines, anorexic agents
- Barbiturates (except phenobarbital), except when used for seizures control
- Benzodiazepines (short-acting): doses >3 mg lorazepam; >60 mg oxazepam; >2 mg alprazolam; >15 mg temazepam; >0.25 mg triazolam
- Benzodiazepines (long-acting): chlordiazepoxide, chlordiazepoxide-amitriptyline, clidinium-chlordiazepoxide, diazepam, quazepam, halazepam, chlorazepate
- Doxepin
- Ergot mesyloids, cyclandelate
- Fluoxetine, daily dose
- Flurazepam
- Guanethidine
- Meprobamate
- Mesoridazine
- Thioridazine

Respiratory/allergy
- Anticholinergics & antihistamines: chlorpheniramine, diphenhydramine, hydroxyzine, cyproheptadine, promethazine, tripelennamine, dexchlorpheniramine
- Diphenhydramine

*Includes drugs currently approved in the United States.

Drug–drug interactions may cause life-threatening consequences in elderly patients who often take several medications for multiple diseases. It has been reported that 91% of community-dwelling U.S. adults 65 years of age or older took at least 1 drug per week, with 51% taking 5 or more drugs per week and 12% taking 10 or more drugs per week.[3]

To decrease the chance of drug–drug interactions occurring in elderly patients, the following interventions should be considered:

- Simplify the drug regimen (i.e., number of drugs and dosing intervals).
- Initiate drugs at low doses and then titrate slowly.
- Ask about side effects and complaints.
- Remember that signs and symptoms of drug interactions in elderly patients may be different from those in younger patients. Such symptoms may be associated with aging (e.g., weakness, confusion, loss of appetite).
- Encourage patients to fill their prescriptions at a single pharmacy.
- Help patients keep an updated medication list, and have them carry it with them at all times.
- Conduct a regular medication profile review.

Further reading

Beers criteria are available at: http://archinte.ama-assn.org/cgi/content/full/163/22/2716

3 Kaufman DW, Kelly JP, Rosenberg L, et al. (2002). Recent patterns of medication use in the ambulatory adult population of the US: The Slone Survey. *JAMA* **287**:337–344.

Medicines for elderly people: pharmacokinetics and pharmacodynamics

Physiological changes that occur with age affect drug pharmacokinetics and pharmacodynamics. Predicting at what age these changes become significant is almost impossible because people age at different rates, depending on environmental, social, and other factors. However, the pharmacist should be aware of pharmacokinetic and pharmacodynamic differences that exist in elderly persons so that drug dosing can be monitored and adjusted appropriately.

Absorption

Aging rarely has a significant effect on absorption. Delayed gastric emptying increases time to peak concentrations (T_{max}) but is rarely clinically significant. Decreases in the production of gastric acid can lead to decreased absorption of drugs that require an acid environment for absorption (e.g., itraconazole), but can slightly increase the amount absorbed of drugs that are broken down by gastric acid (e.g., penicillins).

Increased regional blood flow might decrease the rate of absorption of drugs administered by the IM or SC route, but the total amount absorbed is the same.

Distribution

- Lean body mass decreases with age, leading to increased levels of drugs distributed in the muscle (e.g., digoxin).
- Adipose tissue increases up to age 85 years, leading to increased tissue levels and thus prolonged duration of the effect of lipid-soluble drugs (e.g., diazepam). Patients >85 years tend to lose adipose tissue.
- The decrease in total body water leads to an increase in the serum concentration of water-soluble drugs (e.g., gentamicin and digoxin).
- Decreased serum albumin leads to increased levels of free drug for highly protein-bound drugs (e.g., phenytoin). In the acute phase, homeostatic mechanisms usually counteract the increased drug effects. Increased level of free drug also means increased amounts for clearance, so the effect is rarely significant in the long term.

Metabolism

Elderly people can have up to a 40% decrease in hepatic blood flow. Drugs with high first-pass metabolism can be significantly affected (see Drug Use in Liver Disease, p. 181). There may be up to a 60% decrease in metabolism of some drugs, such as NSAIDs and anticonvulsants, leading to increased concentrations, duration of action, and possibly accumulation.

Excretion

The natural aging process between the ages of 20 and 80 years lead to a 30%–35% loss of functioning of glomeruli, with a consequent loss of normal renal function of up to 50%. Serum creatinine levels may be normal or near normal because of decreased muscle mass, but creatinine clearance will be decreased. Acute illness and dehydration can cause a rapid decline in renal function, which can be exacerbated by the use of potentially nephrotoxic drugs (e.g., aminoglycosides, NSAIDs, cyclosporine).

It is advisable to calculate the creatinine clearance (using the Cockroft and Gault equation; see p. 189) for any patient >65 years who is prescribed renally cleared or potentially nephrotoxic drugs.

Pharmacodynamic changes

As the body ages, there is a natural loss of function at a cellular level, leading to increased or decreased drug sensitivity. Changes in receptor–drug interactions can occur (e.g., there is a decreased response to both B-adrenoceptor agonists and B-adrenoceptor antagonists).

Homeostatic responses can be blunted in old age (e.g., postural hypotension is more likely to be caused by blunting of reflex tachycardia, and cardiac failure may result from fluid overload caused by overenthusiastic rehydration or NSAIDs combined with decreased cardiac output and renal function).

There is increased susceptibility to CNS effects of drugs. Even drugs not normally associated with CNS effects can cause such symptoms in elderly people (e.g., H2 antagonists and diuretics). These effects can occur without changes in kinetics, probably because of increased CNS penetration or altered drug response.

For example, confusion and disorientation are more common in elderly people receiving benzodiazepines, antidepressants, and NSAIDs, even at standard doses. In addition, changes in kinetics can lead to CNS effects not usually seen in younger people—e.g., decreased renal function can lead to confusion associated with increased levels of drugs, such as ciprofloxacin and acyclovir.

Medicines for elderly people: medication review

Regular medication review is an essential, but often overlooked, aspect of care of elderly patients. Prioritize those patients at highest risk of medication-related problems:

- Taking four or more drugs.
- Recently discharged from hospital
- Taking "high-risk" medicines: (see Beers criteria reference, p. 213).
  - Hypnotics—drowsiness and falls
  - Diuretics—dehydration, renal failure, and confusion caused by hypokalemia
  - NSAIDs—fluid retention and GI bleeds
  - Antihypertensives—falls resulting from postural hypotension
  - Digoxin—nausea and vomiting, confusion could be missed as signs of toxicity
  - Warfarin—bruising and bleeding

Other factors that can increase the risk of medication-related problems include the following:

- Social—lack of home support
- Physical—poor vision, hearing, and dexterity
- Mental—confusion, depression, and difficulty understanding instructions

Elderly patients are often high users of OTC medicines, thus the pharmacist should be aware of this. OTC drugs can:

- Be unnecessary
- Increase the risk of drug interactions
- Increase the risk of additive side effects
- Be an indicator for ADRs to other medicines (e.g., high antacid consumption could point to NSAID-induced gastric irritation)

Medication reviews should include partners and caregivers (formal and informal) if possible and the results should be fed back to the relevant health-care workers. If patients are attending the clinic for a review, they should be asked to bring all medications with them ("brown bag review"). This enables the pharmacist to check for the following:

- Stockpiling
- Out-of-date medicines
- Problems with reading or interpretation of medicine labels
- Strategies for self-administration (e.g., marking containers or transferring medicines to other containers)
- Problems with manipulation (e.g., opening bottle caps or using technologically difficult products, such as inhalers or eye drops)
- Use of OTC or herbal medicines

Glucose 6-phosphate dehydrogenase (G6PD) deficiency

G6PD is an enzyme that produces reduced glutathione, which protects red blood cells against oxidant stress. G6PD deficiency is an X-linked genetic disorder. Thus men are either normal or deficient, whereas women are normal, deficient, or intermediate.

G6PD deficiency is the most common human enzyme defect, affecting over 400 million persons worldwide. The highest prevalence is in Africa, Southern Europe, the Middle East, South East Asia, and Oceania. Because of migration, prevalence in North and South America as well as parts of Northern Europe has emerged. Areas where G6PD deficiency and *Plasmodium falciparum* malaria are endemic have parallel occurrence, which suggests that G6PD deficiency confers resistance against malaria.

Fortunately, most G6PD-deficient individuals remain clinically asymptomatic throughout their lives. The most common clinical manifestation is acute hemolytic anemia, often in response to one of the following trigger events:

- Infection
- Fava (broad) beans
- Oxidizing drugs

An acute hemolytic attack is generally characterized by fatigue, back pain, anemia, and jaundice. In most cases, the attack is self-limiting, although adults (but rarely children) can develop renal failure.

Considerations in G6PD deficiency

- Patients in at-risk groups should be tested for G6PD deficiency.
- Patients with severe deficiency should not be prescribed highly oxidizing drugs (see Table 10.16), and drugs with a lower risk should be prescribed with caution.
- The risk and severity of hemolytic anemia are almost always dose related. Thus, even severely deficient patients can tolerate low doses of these drugs, if there is no alternative.

Treatment of a hemolytic attack

- Withdraw drug.
- Maintain high urine output.
- Give red blood cell transfusion, if indicated.

Table 10.16 Drugs to be used with caution in G6PD deficiency

Drugs with definite risk of hemolytic anemia in most G6PD-deficient patients (avoid)

- Dapsone and other sulfones
- Methylthioninium chloride (methylene blue)
- Nalidixic acid
- Nitrofurantoin
- Primaquine
- Quinolones
- Rasburicase
- Sulfonamides

Drugs with possible risk of hemolytic anemia in some G6PD-deficient patients (caution)*

- Aminosalicylic acid
- Amodiaquine
- Ascorbic acid
- Aspirin (doses >1 g/day)
- Chloramphenicol
- Chloroquine**
- Dimercaprol
- Hydroxychloroquine
- Isoniazid
- Levodopa
- Menadione (water-soluble vitamin K derivatives)
- Penicillins
- Probenecid
- Pyrimethamine
- Quinidine
- Quinine**
- Streptomycin

* Use with caution; low doses are probably safe.

** Acceptable to treat acute malaria at usual doses.

Further reading

G6PD Deficiency Favism Association: http://www.g6pd.org/favism/english/index.mv?pgid=intro

Drug use in celiac disease

Celiac disease is a multisystem, autoimmune disorder that is attributable to permanent gluten intolerance in genetically predisposed individuals. It affects approximately 1% of the general population in the United States, and is three times more common in women than in men. Celiac disease is associated with maldigestion and malabsorption of nutrients, vitamins, and minerals within the gastrointestinal tract, specifically the proximal small intestine.

Risk factors

- First-degree relative of patients with celiac disease
- Down syndrome
- Autoimmune disease (e.g., type 1 diabetes, Hoshimoto's thyroiditis)

Signs and symptoms (classic)

Children

- Diarrhea
- Abdominal distension
- Failure to thrive

Adolescents and adults

- Diarrhea
- Constipation
- Weight loss
- Weakness
- Short stature
- Flatus
- Abdominal pain
- Vomiting

Signs and symptoms (atypical)

- Iron deficiency
- Anemia
- Osteoporosis

Treatment

- Adherence to a gluten-free diet (avoidance of wheat, rye, barley, and their derivatives)
- Supplements for nutritional deficiencies (e.g., multivitamin, iron, calcium and vitamin D)

Six core elements for managing individuals with celiac disease have been identified by the National Institutes of Health Consensus Development Panel and are listed in Table 10.17.

Table 10.17 Elements for managing celiac disease

C	Consultation with a skilled dietitian
E	Education about celiac disease
L	Lifelong adherence to a gluten-free diet
I	Identification and treatment of nutritional deficiencies
A	Access to an advocacy group
C	Continuous long-term follow up

* Use with caution; low doses are probably safe.

** Acceptable to treat acute malaria at usual doses.

Further reading

Celiac Disease Foundation: www.celicac.org/

Niewinski MM (2008). Advances in celiac disease and gluten-free diet. *J Am Diet Assoc* **108**:661–672.

Drug use in acute porphyria

Porphyrias are rare metabolic disorders that develop from inherited or acquired enzyme defects within the heme biosysnthesis pathway. Prophyrias are classified as hepatic (acute or chronic) or erythropoietic. Classification is dependent on the predominate site of porphyrin production (see Table 10.18).

Common symptoms and signs

- Gastrointestinal
  - Abdominal pain
  - Vomiting
  - Constipation
  - Diarrhea
- Neurological
  - Pain (extremities, back, chest, neck, head)
  - Paresis
  - Respiratory paralysis
  - Mental symptoms
  - Seizures
- Cardiovascular
  - Tachycardia
  - Systemic arterial hypertension

Common triggers

- Endogenous or exogenous steroid hormones
- Medications (barbiturates, sulfonamide antibiotics; see Table 10.19)
- Starvation (crash diets)
- Smoking
- Metabolic stress (surgery, infections)
- Pregnancy

Table 10.18 Classification of porphyrias

Hepatic	Erythropoietic
ALA-D-deficient porphyria*	Erythropoietic protoporphyria
Acute intermittent porphyria*	Congenital erythropoietic porphyria
Variegate porphyria*	
Hereditary coproporphyria*	
Porphyria cutanea tarda	

* Acute; the others are considered chronic.

Table 10.19 Major drugs considered unsafe and safe in acute porphyrias*

Unsafe	Safe
Alcohol	Acetaminophen
Barbiturates†	Aspirin
Carbamazepine†	Atropine
Carisoprodol†	Bromides
Clonazepam (high dose)	Cimetidine
Danazol†	Erythropoietins**
Diclofenac and possibly other NSAIDs†	Gabapentin
Ergots	Glucocorticoids
Estrogens†,‡	Insulin
Ethchlorvynol†	Narcotic analgesics
Glutethimide†	Penicillin and derivatives
Griseofulvin†	Phenothiazines
Mephenytoin	Ranitidine†,**
Meprobamate (also mebutamate and tybutamate)†	Streptomycin
Phenytoin†	
Primidone†	
Progesterone and synthetic progestins†	
Pyrazinamide†	
Pyrazolones (aminopyrine and antipyrine)	
Rifampin†	
Succinimides (ethosuximide and methsuximide)	
Sulfonamide antibiotics†	
Valproic acid	

* More extensive list of drugs and their status are available in texts and Web sites (such as www.porphyriafoundation.com and www.porphyria-europe.com).

† Porphyria is listed as a contraindication, warning, precaution, or adverse effect in U.S. labeling for these drugs. For drugs listed as unsafe, absence of such cautionary statements in U.S. labeling does not imply lower risk.

‡ Estrogens have been regarded as harmful, mostly from experience with estrogen–progestin combinations and because they can exacerbate porphyria cutanea tarda. Although evidence that they exacerbate acute porphyrias is weak, they should be used with caution. Low doses of estrogen (e.g., transdermal) have been used safely to prevent side effects of gonadotropin-releasing hormone analogue s in women with cyclic attacks.

** Although porphyria is listed as a precaution in U.S. labeling, these drugs are regarded as safe by other sources.

Anderson KE, et al. (2005). Recommendations for the diagnosis and treatment of the acute porphyrias. Ann Intern Med 142:439–450. Reproduced with permission of the American College of Physicians.

Treatment (Supportive and symptomatic)

- Symptom and complication treatment
- Carbohydrates (10% glucose infusion; at least 300 g daily)
- Hemin intravenous (Panhematin)
  - Dose: 1–4 mg/kg/day IV for 3–14 days; in severe cases may repeat dose no earlier than 12 hours; maximum of 6 mg/kg in 24 hours
  - Adverse effects: phlebitis, acute renal failure, increased prothrombin time (PT), thrombocytopenia

Prevention

- Education
- Identification of triggers
- Avoidance of alcohol, smoking and medications that may induce exacerbations (see Table 10.19).
- Adequate nutrition

Further reading

American Porphyria Foundation: http://www.porphyriafoundation.com/index.html

Drug and food allergies

Food allergy is defined as an abnormal IgE immune response, which is triggered by a food protein. These abnormal responses may lead to life-threatening reactions in patients. In the United States, approximately 6% to 8% of children less than 3 years of age and 4% of adults have food allergies. The most common types of food allergies in these two patient populations differ (see Table 10.20).[1]

A food component may be a part of various medications; thus, pharmacists must conduct a detailed history for food allergies to avoid administration of these agents to patients with an interacting food allergy. Select drugs with food components are listed below.[2]

Egg

- Clevidipine injection
- Fat emulsion
- Influenza vaccine
- Interferon alfa-n3
- Measles and mumps vaccines
- Measles-mumps-rubella (MMR) vaccine
- Propofol
- Verteporfin
- Yellow fever vaccine

Fish

- Protamine

Iodine

- Amiodarone (tablet/injection)
- Potassium iodide

Milk protein

- Cefditoren pivoxil

Papaya

- Crotalidae polyvalent immune Fab
- Digoxin immune Fab (ovine)

Peanut oil

- Dimercaprol
- Ipratropium/albuterol meter dose inhaler (MDI)
- Micronized progesterone in oil
- Soy isoflavones

Table 10.20 Common food allergies in adults and children

Adults	Children
• Shellfish (e.g., shrimp, crayfish)	• Eggs
• Peanuts	• Milk
• Tree nuts (e.g., walnuts)	• Peanuts
• Fish	• Tree nuts
• Eggs	

* Acute; the others are considered chronic.

Sesame oil

- Dronabinol
- Fluphenazine decanoate
- Haloperidol decanoate
- Nandrolone decanoate

Soy lecithin

- Clevidipine injection
- Fat emulsion
- Liposomal doxorubicin
- Propofol
- Soy isoflavones

1 U.S. Department of Health and Human Services, National Institute of Health, National Institute of Allergy and Infectious Diseases Food Allergy: An Overview. NIH Publication No. 07–5518. July 2007. Available at: www.niaid.nih.gov

2 Hofer KN, McCarthy MW, Buck ML (2003). Possible anaphylaxis after propofol in a child with food allergy. *Ann Pharmacother* **37**:398–401.

Drug therapy for enteral feeding tubes

The administration of medication to patients with enteral feeding tubes can be challenging. Prior to drug administration, certain considerations must occur: tube type (see Chapter 15, Enteral Feeding, p. 462) tube location in the GI tract, site of drug action and absorption, effects of food on drug, continued need for medication (availability of different formulations), and the consequences of withdrawal or administration delay. If an improper drug administration technique is used, complications such as tube obstruction, increased toxicity, or reduced efficacy may occur.

Several oral medications should not be crushed (sustained-release, enteric-coated, or microencapsulated products). Crushing destroys the sustained-released and microencapsulated properties, resulting in erratic blood levels. Additionally, enteric coatings do not crush well. Instead, they break apart into small pieces that that clump together when mixed with water and may clog the feeding tube. A detailed list of oral dosage forms that should not be crushed or chewed is available at: http://www.ismp.org/tools/DoNotCrush.pdf

Administering medications to patients with feeding tubes[1]

- Determine if each medication is currently necessary; discontinue or interrupt therapy if possible.
- Use alternate routes of administration, if appropriate (i.e., buccal, intramuscular, intravenous, intraosseous, transdermal, topical, nebulized, rectal, subcutaneous, sublingual, etc.).
- Consider where the drug is absorbed, its site of action, incompatibilities, and food effects on drug absorption.
- Determine medication dosage form (consider cost, ease of use, and risk of adverse events).
  - Oral liquid: dilute with 15–30 mL sterile water or enteral formula if hyperosmolar
  - Oral immediate-release tablet: crush to fine powder and mix with 15–30 mL of sterile water
  - Oral immediate-release capsule: open capsule and crush capsule contents to fine powder and mix with 15–30 mL of sterile water
  - Oral soft gelatin capsule: remove liquid contents with a needle and syringe, then mix with 15–30 mL of sterile water (e.g., acetazolamide, nifedipine)
  - IV liquid preparation: draw dose into an amber oral syringe prior to administration
- Hold enteral feeds 30 minutes before and after administration if the drugs are to be administered on an empty stomach (adjust enteral feeding rate to maintain daily nutrition goals).
- The feeding tube should be flushed with 30 mL of sterile water before and after drug administration.
- Administer each drug separately (do not mix drugs). Flush with 30 mL of sterile water between each drug administration.

Drug-specific issues

- *Phenytoin suspension:* 50%–75% reduction in serum levels when given with enteral nutrition. Hold tube feedings 2 hours before and after each dose and flush the tube before and after each phenytoin dose.
- *Fluoroquinolones* (ciprofloxacin, levofloxacin, moxifloxacin): give enterally via large-bore feeding tube, crush tablets, and mix with 20–30 mL of sterile water prior to administration. Hold tube feedings 2 hours before and 4 hours after administration. Ciprofloxacin suspension should not be administered via the feeding tube. It has a thick consistency that may clog the tube, and since it is an oil-based suspension it does not mix well with water.
- *Warfarin:* reductions in absorption may occur, because enteral feeding solutions may bind warfarin. Vitamin K is present in many of the enteral formulas; therefore, doses of warfarin might need to be adjusted (monitor INR).

Unclogging a feeding tube (medication-related)[1]

- Before starting the unclogging process, remove any remaining enteral feeding that is in the tube.
- Remove the obstruction as follows:
  - Warm water: slowly inject 5 mL of warm sterile water into tube and clamp for 5–10 minutes. Unclamp tube, apply gentle pressure, and attempt suctioning. If tube is unclogged, flush with water until clear, then resume enteral feeds.
  - Alkalinized enzyme solution: 1 crushed sodium bicarbonate 324 mg tablet and 1 crushed pancrealipase (Viokase) tablet (or 1 teaspoon of Viokase powder), add 5–15 mL of warm sterile water. Slowly inject mixture into tube and clamp for 5–10 minutes. If tube is unclogged, flush with sterile water until clear, then resume enteral feeds.

1 Beckwith MC, Feddema SS, Barton RG, et al. (2004). A guide to drug therapy in patients with enteral feeding tubes: dosage form selection and administration methods. *Hosp Pharm* **39**:225–237.

Patients with altered GI tracts and bariatric surgery

Pharmacists will encounter patients with altered gastrointestinal (GI) tracts in their clinical practice, most commonly as a result of bariatric surgery or short bowel syndrome (SBS). These patients require careful evaluation, medication selection and dosing, and monitoring.

There are several bariatric surgery procedures that produce weight loss. The Roux-en-Y gastric bypass and the biliopancreatic diversion are two surgical procedures that result in intestinal malabsorption, which may lead to nutritional deficiencies requiring supplementation and monitoring.

Small bowel resection may lead to SBS, which is characterized by the malabsorption of electrolytes, nutrients, and fluids. Major complications of SBS are dehydration and malnutrition, which may be managed via dietary interventions, supplementation, and pharmacologic agents.

Bariatric surgery

Background

Indications for bariatric surgery

- Body mass index (BMI) ≥40 kg/m^2 without comorbidities
- BMI ≥35 kg/m^2 without obesity-associated comorbidities

Bariatric surgical procedures

- Adjustable gastric banding
- Gastroplasty
- Vertical restrictive gastrectomy
- Roux-en-Y gastric bypass
- Biliopancreatic diversion with or without duodenal switch

Routine supplementation and screening post-surgery

- Multivitamin daily
- Calcium citrate with vitamin D
  - 1200–2000 mg/day + 400–800 units/day
- Folic acid
  - 0.4 mg/day
- Elemental iron for menstruating women
  - 40–65 mg/day
- Vitamin B_{12}
  - Oral: ≥350 mcg/day
  - Intramuscular: 1000 mcg/months or 3000 mcg/ every 6 months

Nutritional deficiencies by procedure

- The majority of nutritional deficiencies are seen with Roux-en-Y gastric bypass and biliopancreatic diversion procedures (see Table 10.21).

Table 10.21 Nutritional complications by procedure

Bariatric procedure	Nutritional complications	Treatment	Monitoring
Roux-en-Y gastric bypass	1. Iron deficiency 2. B_{12} deficiency 3. Protein deficiency 4. Calcium and vitamin D deficiency 5. Nephrolithiasis 6. Thiamine (B_1) deficiency	1. Iron supplementation: 150–300 mg of oral elemental iron daily with vitamin C 2. Oral vitamin B_{12} 350 mcg/day or parenteral B_{12} 1000 mcg/month 3. Protein supplementation (≥60 g/day) 4. Oral calcium: oral ergocalciferol or cholecalciferol 5. Hydration, probiotics, & low oxalate diet 6. Parenteral vitamin B_1 100mg/day for 7–14 days	1. CBC and iron studies 2. Annual vitamin B_{12} evaluation 3. Bone density 4. Signs and symptoms of nephrolithiasis 5. Neurological symptoms
Biliopancreatic diversion with duodenal switch	1. Iron deficiency 2. B_{12} deficiency 3. Protein deficiency 4. Calcium and Vitamin D deficiency 5. Nephrolithiasis 6. Vitamin A deficiency 7. Thiamine (B_1) deficiency	1. Iron supplementation: 150–300 mg of oral elemental iron daily with vitamin C 2. Oral vitamin B_{12} 350 mcg/day or parenteral B_{12} 1000 mcg/month 3. Protein supplementation (80–120 g/day) 4. Oral calcium: oral ergocalciferol or cholecalciferol 5. Hydration, probiotics, & low oxalate diet 6. Vitamin A 5,000–10,000 units/day or fat-soluble vitamin supplement 7. Parenteral vitamin B_1 100mg/day for 7–14 days	1. CBC and iron studies 2. Annual vitamin B_{12} evaluation 3. Bone density 4. Signs and symptoms of nephrolithiasis 5. Vision 6. Neurological symptoms

Data from: Mechanick JI, Kushner RF, Sugarman HJ, et al. (2008). Executive summary of the recommendations of the American Association of Clinical Endocrinologists, The Obesity Society, and American Society for Metabolic and Bariatric Surgery medical guidelines for clinical practice for the perioperative, nutritional, metabolic, and nonsurgical support of the bariatric surgery patient. *Endocr Pract* **14**, 318–36.

Monitoring

- Patients who undergo Roux-en-Y gastric bypass or biliopancreatic diversion require laboratory monitoring every 3–6 months of the first year and every 3–12 months thereafter, depending on complications.
- Laboratory monitoring may include the following:
    - Complete blood count (CBC), electrolytes, iron studies, vitamin measurements (B_{12}, 25-hydroxyvitamin D, fat-soluble vitamins), liver function tests, lipid profile, coagulation profile, intact parathyroid hormone, evaluation for nephrolithiasis and metabolic bone disease

Miscellaneous complications

- Diarrhea
    - Celiac sprue, bacterial overgrowth, *Clostridium difficile*, steatorrhea
- Ulceration
    - Avoid NSAIDs
    - *Helicobacter pylori* evaluation
- Gallbladder
    - Treatment: Ursodiol 300 mg twice daily for 6 months
    - Cholecystectomy for cholelithiasis
- Bacterial overgrowth
    - Treatment: Metronidazole or probiotic supplementation with *Lactobacillus*
- Incisional hernias
    - Asymptomatic hernias can be repaired 12–18 months post-procedure.
    - Incarcerated or umbilical hernias with abdominal pain require emergent intervention to prevent bowel ischemia.
- Bowel obstruction
    - Conduct emergent evaluation of cramping abdominal pain to avoid serious complications.
    - Exploratory laporatomy or laproscopy may be indicated.
- Malnutrition
    - Patient may require hospitalization for volume resuscitation and parenteral nutrition.

Short bowel syndrome

Background

- The small intestine absorbs protein, carbohydrates, fat-soluble vitamins, bile salts, vitamin B_{12}, fluids, and electrolytes.
- Significant small intestine resection (<200 cm of remaining bowel) reduces the absorptive surface area and impairs digestion, which results in short bowel syndrome.
- Disorders that cause severe malabsorption may also result in SBS.

Common etiologies

Adults

- Inflammatory bowel disease
- Superior mesenteric artery occlusion or thrombosis
- Volvulus
- Trauma
- Retroperitoneal tumor excision

Neonates and children
- Necrotizing enterocolitis
- Intestinal atresia

Complications
- Malnutrition
- Diarrhea
- Hypovolemia
- Electrolyte abnormalities (hypocalcemia, hypomagnesemia)
- Vitamin deficiencies (A, D, E, and B_{12})
- Hypergastrinemia
- Intestinal dysmotility
- Bacterial overgrowth
- Nephrolithiasis

Bowel adaptation
- Acute phase: 4 weeks post-surgery
- Adaptation phase: 1–2 years post-surgery
- Commonly requires nutritional supplementation with enteral and parenteral feeding
- Maintenance phase: following the adaptation phase
- Patient-specific nutritional supplementation required

Treatment (see Table 10.22)

Adverse effects of long-term parenteral nutrition
- Cholelithiasis secondary to biliary stasis
- Liver failure
- Catheter-related infections and sepsis
- Small bowel atrophy

Table 10.22 Complications, monitoring, and treatment of short bowel syndrome

Complications	Monitoring	Treatment
Bacterial overgrowth	LFTs	Broad-spectrum antimicrobials
Diarrhea	Electrolytes, volume status, frequency of bowel movements	NPO, IV fluid and electrolyte resuscitation. May start loperamide or diphenoxylate once patient is able to tolerate oral intake
High jejunostomy output	Electrolytes, volume status	IV fluid and electrolytes, restrict hypotonic fluids to <500 mL/day, increase sodium intake, ingest glucose-saline solution, octreotide*
Hypergastrinemia	Acid reflux	IV proton pump inhibitors or H2 antagonists. May transition to PO once able to tolerate
Hypocalcemia	Calcium concentrations, bone density	PO calcium 800–1200 mg/day
Malabsorption/ malnutrition	Electrolytes, volume status, weight	**Acute phase**: Initially, NPO and long-term CVC for TPN. Introduce enteral feeding once able to tolerate **Adaptation phase**: Transition to oral/enteral feeding and wean TPN, if possible. Consider recombinant growth hormone (r-hGH) **Maintenance phase**: Target 45–60 kcal/kg/day divided into small meals. Supplement electrolytes, vitamins, and trace elements
Nephrolithiasis	BUN, SCr, pain, hematuria	Restrict dietary oxelate. Administer PO calcium. Avoid vitamin C in TPN
Vitamin B_{12} deficiency	Vitamin B_{12} level	Intranasal or parenteral vitamin B_{12} supplementation

BUN, blood urea nitrogen; CVC, central venous catheter; LFTs, liver function tests; NPO, no food or drink; PO, by mouth; SCr, serum creatinine; TPN, total parenteral nutrition.

* Tachyphylaxis occurs with prolonged use.

Data from:

Misiakos EP, Macheras A, Kapetanakis T, et al. (2007). Short bowel syndrome: current medical and surgical trends. *J Clin Gastroenterol* **41**:5–18.

Steiger E (2006). Guidelines for pharmacotherapy, nutritional management, and weaning parenteral nutrition in adult patients with short bowel syndrome: introduction. *J Clin Gastroenterol* **40** (Suppl 2):S73–S74.

Pharmacogenomics

Medication responses can differ between patients. These response differences are often greater among populations than between patients. From 20% to 95% of patient variability may be due to genetic factors that are considered a lifetime constant.

In pharmacogenomics, the genome-wide approach is used to explain the inherited basis of differences between persons in medication effects. Genetic polymorphisms that influence drug disposition include the following:

- Drug transporters (e.g., P-glycoprotein)
- Drug-metabolizing enzymes (e.g., CYP3A enzymes)
- Drug targets/receptors (e.g., β_2 adrenoreceptor)

Additionally, there are polymorphisms in genes encoding proteins that are neither direct targets of medications nor involved in their disposition, but rather in disease or treatment modification (e.g., prothrombin and factor V: increased risk of deep-vein and cerebral-vein thrombosis with oral contraceptives).

Use of pharmacogenetic testing helps individualize medicine regimens. It enables practitioners to make better decisions about therapy to avoid, treatment failures, and medication adverse effects.

Further reading

Evans WE, McLeod HL (2003). Pharmacogenomics—drug disposition, drug targets, and side effects. *N Engl J Med* **348**(6):538–549.

Transdermal drug therapy

Transdermal drug delivery systems are pharmaceutical preparations that, when applied to intact skin, deliver the active ingredient(s) to the systemic circulation through passive diffusion. These preparations have some advantages over oral preparations (avoiding GI absorption and hepatic first-pass metabolism, obtaining a controllable and sustained plasma level, and improving patient compliance) and intravenous therapies (avoiding intravenous access and risk of infection).

Types of transdermal drug delivery systems[1]

Reservoir membrane-modulated

Drug is contained in a reservoir between an impermeable backing layer and a microporous rate-controlling membrane. The rate of drug release is determined by polymer, membrane layer thickness, and drug properties (molecular size, lipophilic or hydrophilic). Active drug cannot penetrate the backing layer, thus the rate-controlling membrane is the only mechanism for drug release. An example of this type of transdermal patch is fentanyl (Duragesic).

Microreservoir membrane-modulated

Drug is contained in several, smaller drug reservoirs. Its design is similar to the drug reservoir membrane-modulated system. An example of this type of transdermal patch is clonidine (Catapres-TTS).

Drug-in-adhesive layer design

Drug is homogeneously mixed into a polymer-based adhesive and is then applied to an impermeable backing. Sometimes an additional non-drug infused adhesive layer may be incorporated to improve skin contact or to serve as a rate-controlling layer. An example of this type of transdermal patch is lidocaine (Lidoderm).

Matrix patch

Drug is equally distributed into a layer of polymer matrix and then attached to an impermeable backing with a peripheral adhesive or adhesive layer completing the system (similar to a drug-in-adhesive layer system). An example of this type of transdermal patch is estradiol (Vivelle-Dot).

Cutting transdermal drug delivery systems

In general, most transdermal dug delivery systems should not be cut. Altering the system may cause unpredictable delivery rates and efficacy. However, since the drug-in-adhesive layer patch design uses a homogeneous mixture as well as diffusion control (directly proportional to the surface area of the patch in contact with the skin) for drug delivery, cutting or altering the patch size can be done safely (e.g., lidocaine patch).

1 Ball AM, Smith KM (2008). Optimizing transdermal drug therapy. *Am J Health Syst Pharm* **65**:1337–1346.

Contrast media

Contrast media are agents used to enhance the visibility of structures within the body, and can be categorized as iodinated or non-iodinated as well as being high osmolar, low osmolar or isomolar. Allergic reactions (mild to severe) and toxicities (e.g., contrast-induced nephropathy) may occur when these agents are administered.

Allergic reactions may range from mild (flushing) to severe (cardiac arrest) in nature. Therefore, before contrast media are administered, screening for allergies specifically (iodine, shellfish) is essential.

Contrast-induced nephropathy (CIN) is often defined as an increase in serum creatinine (0.5 mg/dL increase or a 25% increase from baseline) occurring within the first 24 hours after contrast exposure and peaking up to 5 days afterward.

Risk factors for developing CIN[1]

- Chronic kidney disease (particularly when diabetes is also present), GFR <60 mL/min/1.73 m^2
- Intra-arterial administration of contrast, ionic high-osmolality agents (compared to low-osmolality agents)
- Higher contrast volumes (>100 mL)
- Intra-arterial administration of iodinated contrast (compared to intravenous administration)
- Multiple administration (<2 weeks between administrations)

Management of patients receiving iodinated contrast media[1]

- GFR ≥60 mL/min
  - Discontinue metformin or any metformin-containing medication
  - Good clinical practice
- GFR 30–50 mL/min
  - Discontinue metformin or any metformin-containg medication, NSAIDs, other nephrotoxic drugs
  - Volume expansion (intravenous isotonic crystalloid 1–1.5 mL/kg/hr, 3–12 hours before and 6–24 hours after procedure)
  - Limit contrast volume to <100 mL
  - Consider pharmacological treatment (no adjunctive medical treatment has proven efficacious in reducing CIN; however, some agents that have been studied and deserve further evaluation include acetylcysteine, theophylline, statins, ascorbic acid, prostaglandin E1)
  - Obtain a serum creatinine before discharge or within 24–72 hours
- GFR <30 mL/min
  - Hospital admission
  - Nephrology consultation
  - Dialysis planning
  - Other strategies as for GFR 30–59 mL/min
  - Serial serum creatinine and electrolytes

1 Laskey W (ed.) (2006). Contrast-induced nephropathy: clinical insights and practical guidance—a report from the CIN Consensus Working Panel. *Am J Cardiol* 98 (6 Suppl 1):1–78.

Principles of extravasation

An *extravasation* is the inadvertent administration of intravenously administered vesicants into tissue, causing tissue damage. Extravasations are estimated to occur in 0.1%–6% of peripheral IV infusions and 0.3%–4.7% of implanted port infusions.

Signs and symptoms

- Pain, burning, swelling, erythema, loss of blood return, skin necrosis

Risk factors

- Age (young or elderly)
- Limited clinician experience in administering IVs
- Distractions during IV infusion
- Large-gauge catheters
- Unsecured IV devices
- High vesicant potential of medication infused

Medications at high risk for causing extravasations

- Chemotherapeutic agents
- Concentrated electrolyte solutions
- Vasoconstrictors
- Hyperosmotic solutions

If left undiagnosed or inappropriately treated, extravasation of chemotherapy can cause necrosis and functional loss of the tissue and limb.

Prevention of extravasations

- Avoid areas of joint flexion for IV sites.
- Use smallest-gauge catheter possible.
- Use central IV lines for infusing hyperosmolar medications.
- Confirm positive blood return through catheter.
- Anchor catheter to minimize movement.
- Counsel patient on signs and symptoms of extravasation.
- Monitor patient for pain during infusion.
- Assess infusion site for erythema or swelling for early signs of extravasation.
- Stop infusion with any suspicion for extravasation.

Vesicant potential of chemotherapeutic agents

Vesicants

- Cisplatin (>20 mL of 0.5 mg/mL)
- Dactinomycin
- Daunorubicin
- Doxorubicin
- Epirubicin
- Idarubicin
- Mechlorethamine
- Melphalan
- Mitomycin
- Paclitaxel
- Vinblastine
- Vincristine
- Vindesine
- Vinorelbine

Irritants

- Carmustine
- Cisplatin (>20 mL of 0.5 mg/mL)
- Dacarbazine
- Daunorubicin
- Daunorubicin liposomal
- Etoposide
- Floxuridine
- Irinotecan
- Mitoxantrone
- Oxaliplatin
- Topotecan

Non-vesicants

- Aldesleukin
- Asparaginase
- Bleomycin
- Cladribine
- Cyclophosphamide
- Cytarabine
- Fludarabine
- Gemcitabine
- Gemtuzumab
- Ifosfamide
- Methotrexate
- Pentostatin
- Rituximab
- Thiotepa
- Trastuzumab

Further reading

Hadaway L (2007). Infiltration and extravasation. *Am J Nurs* **107**:64–72.

Sauerland C, Engelking C, Wickham R, Corbi D (2006). Vesicant extravasation part I: mechanisms, pathogenesis, and nursing care to reduce risk. *Oncol Nurs Forum* **33**:1134–1141.

Schulmeister L (2007). Extravasation management. *Semin Oncol Nurs* **23**:184–190.

Wickham R, Engelking C, Sauerland C, Corbi D (2006). Vesicant extravasation part II: evidence-based management and continuing controversies. *Oncol Nurs Forum* **33**:1143–1150.

Management of extravasations in adult patients

The following are recommendations for management of extravasations. Institution-specific policies should be followed, if available.

- Stop infusion immediately.
- Remove peripheral catheter or flush central venous catheter affected.
- Apply warm or cold compresses for 15–30 minutes every 4–6 hours for 24–48 hours (see Table 10.23).
  - Heat increases drug distribution into tissue; this is useful for vinca alkaloids.
  - Cold causes vasoconstriction and localization of drug to a limited area, useful for hyperosmolar fluids.
- Elevate extravasated limb.
- Notify physician.
- Administer antidote if appropriate (see Use of Antidotes for Extravasations and Table 10.23).
- Document details of event (e.g., date and time of extravasation, estimated volume of extravasated medication, infusion settings, catheters involved, description of blood return prior to infusion, patient-reported symptoms, description of affected site, interventions, etc.).
- Document extravasation to risk management per institution policy.
- Consult surgery if necessary.

Antidotes for extravasations

Phentolamine

- Use: vasoconstrictor extravasations
- Mechanism of action: α_1-receptor antagonist
- Dose: 5–10 mg subcutaneously around affected area within 12 hours of extravasation

Hyaluronidase

- Use: extravasations of various agents
- Mechanism of action: hydrolyzes hyaluronic acid found in connective tissue, leading to diffusion and absorption of injected fluids
- Dose: 1–6 mL of 150 unit/mL solution through IV line or multiple subcutaneous injections totaling 150 units around extravasation site

Topical dimethylsulfoxide (DMSO)

- Use: extravasations of various agents
- Mechanism of action: increases skin permeability, promotes absorption of vesicants, scavenges free radicals
- Dose: apply 1–2 mL of 50%–100% DMSO to skin twice the size of extravasated area. Repeat every 4–8 hours for 7–14 days.

Sodium thiosulfate

- Use: mechlorethamine or concentrated cisplatin (>20 mL of 0.5 mg/mL) extravasations
- Mechanism of action: forms non-toxic thioesters excreted into urine

- Dose: inject 2 mL of 1/6 molar solution for each mg of mechlorethamine or 100 mg of concentrated cisplatin

Dexrazoxane

- Use: anthracycline extravasation
- Mechanism of action: decreases free radical formation
- Dose: administer IV in away from extravasated site (e.g., opposite arm). Infuse 1000 mg/m^2 day 1, 1000 mg/m^2 day 2, 500 mg/m^2 day 3 (max. 2000 mg/day). Reduce dose in impaired renal function. Do not use concurrently with DMSO.

Follow-up care

- If IV therapy is to be continued on the same day as an extravasation incident, avoid using the limb where the extravasation has occurred.
- Monitor extravasation site. If it is not ulcerated, it may continue to be used.
- Inform risk management of outcome per institution policy.

Further reading

Bertelli G, Gozza A, Forno GB, Vidili MG, Silvestro S, Venturini M, et al. (1995). Topical dimethylsulfoxide for the prevention of soft tissue injury after extravasation of vesicant cytotoxic drugs: a prospective clinical study. *J Clin Oncol* **13**:2851–2855.

Boyle DM, Engelking C (1995). Vesicant extravasation: myths and realities. *Oncol Nurs Forum* **22**:57–67.

Dorr RT (1990). Antidotes to vesicant chemotherapy extravasations. Blood Rev **4**:41–60.

Hadaway L (2007). Infiltration and extravasation. *Am J Nurs* **107**:64–72.

Rudolph R, Larson DL (1987). Etiology and treatment of chemotherapeutic agent extravasation injuries: a review. *J Clin Oncol* **5**:1116–1126.

Sauerland C, Engelking C, Wickham R, Corbi D (2006). Vesicant extravasation part I: mechanisms, pathogenesis, and nursing care to reduce risk. *Oncol Nurs Forum* **33**:1134–1141.

Schulmeister L (2007). Extravasation management. *Semin Oncol Nurs* **23**:184–190.

Wickham R, Engelking C, Sauerland C, Corbi D (2006). Vesicant extravasation part II: evidence-based management and continuing controversies. *Oncol Nurs Forum* **33**:1143–1150.

Treatment of extravasations in adult patients

Table 10.23 Antidote and compress temperature for extravasated agents

Drug	Antidote	Compress
Aminophylline	Hyaluronidase	Cold
Calcium	Hyaluronidase	Cold
Carboplatin	Sodium thiosulfate	Cold
Carmustine	Sodium bicarbonate	Cold
Cisplatin	Sodium thiosulfate	Cold
Cyclophosphamide	Sodium thiosulfate	Cold
Dacarbazine	Sodium thiosulfate	Cold
Dactinomycin	Topical DMSO	Cold
Daunorubicin	Dexrazoxane or topical DMSO	Cold
Dextrose	Hyaluronidase	Cold
Dobutamine	Phentolamine	Warm
Docetaxel	Hyaluronidase, topical DMSO	Warm or cold
Dopamine	Phentolamine	Warm
Doxorubicin	Dexrazoxane or topical DMSO	Cold
Doxycycline	N/A	Cold
Epinephrine	Phentolamine	Warm
Epirubicin	Dexrazoxane or topical DMSO	Cold
Erythromycin	N/A	Cold
Etoposide	Hyaluronidase	Warm
Fluorouracil	Topical DMSO	Cold
Idarubicin	Dexrazoxane or topical DMSO	Cold
Mechlorethamine	Sodium thiosulfate	Cold
Mitomycin C	Topical DMSO	Cold
Mitoxantrone	Topical DMSO	Cold

Table 10.23 (*Contd.*)

Drug	Antidote	Compress
Norepinephrine	Phentolamine	Warm
Oxaliplatin	Sodium thiosulfate	Warm
Paclitaxel	Hyaluronidase or normal saline	Warm or cold
Phenylephrine	Phentolamine	Warm
Penicillin	Hyaluronidase	Cold
Potassium	Hyaluronidase	Cold
Promethazine	N/A	Cold
Sodium bicarbonate	Hyaluronidase	Cold
Streptozocin	Topical DMSO	Cold
Vancomycin	Hyaluronidase	Cold
Vinblastine	Hyaluronidase	Warm
Vincristine	Hyaluronidase	Warm
Vinorelbine	Hyaluronidase	Warm

Further reading

Bertelli G, Gozza A, Forno GB, Vidili MG, Silvestro S, Venturini M, et al. (1995). Topical dimethylsulfoxide for the prevention of soft tissue injury after extravasation of vesicant cytotoxic drugs: a prospective clinical study. *J Clin Oncol* **13**:2851–2855.

Boyle DM, Engelking C (1995). Vesicant extravasation: myths and realities. *Oncol Nurs Forum* **22**:57–67.

Hurst S, McMillan M (2004). Innovative solutions in critical care units. *Dimens Crit Care Nurse* **23**:125–128.

Rudolph R, Larson DL (1987). Etiology and treatment of chemotherapeutic agent extravasation injuries: a review. *J Clin Oncol* **5**:1116–1126.

Wickham R, Engelking C, Sauerland C, Corbi D (2006). Vesicant extravasation part II: evidence-based management and continuing controversies. *Oncol Nurs Forum* **33**:1143–1150.

Chapter 11

Pharmaceutical calculations

Susan B. Cogut

Concentrations

Pharmaceutical preparations consist of a number of different ingredients in a vehicle; ingredients can be solid, liquid, or gas. *Concentration* is an expression of the ratio of the amount of an ingredient to the amount of product.

Concentrations are expressions of ratios that can represent

- Amount strength
- Percentage strength
- Ratio strength
- Parts per million

Amount strength

A preparation contains 900 mg of sodium chloride dissolved in water to make a final volume of 100 mL. The concentration of this solution can be written as an amount strength in units of 900 mg/100 mL, 9 mg/mL, 0.9 g/100 mL, or 9 g/L.

Percentage strength

Percentage in pharmaceutical calculations is quantified as the amount of ingredient in 100 parts of the product.

- % w/v expresses the number of grams of solid constituent in 100 mL of solution (e.g., 900 mg of sodium chloride in 100 mL of water = 0.9 g in 100 mL = 0.9% w/v sodium chloride).
- % v/v expresses the number of mL of a liquid constituent in 100 mL of solution (e.g., 25 mL sodium benzoate in 100 mL = 25% v/v sodium benzoate).
- % w/w expresses the number of grams of a solid constituent in 100 g of preparation (e.g., 0.5 g procaine in 100 g = 0.5% w/w procaine).

Ratio strength

Ratio strengths are the ratio of the quantity of the agent to the quantity of the total preparation. A ratio strength of 1:50 is read as follows:

- 1 part in 50 parts
- 1 in 50
- 1 g in 50 mL (if w/v)
- 1 mL in 50 mL (if v/v)
- 1 g in 50 g (if w/w)

If w/v, v/v, or w/w is not designated in the ratio strength, the type of preparation is assumed on the basis of its components.

Parts per million (ppm)

When the ratio of ingredient to product is very small, the concentration is expressed by ppm.

1 ppm weight in volume = 1 g in 1,000,000 mL
1 ppm weight in weight = 1 g per 1,000,000 g
1 ppm volume in volume = 1 mL in 1,000,000 mL

Example calculation

How many milliliters of a 1:50 w/v solution are required to make 500 mL of a 0.02% w/v solution?

$$500 \text{ mL} \times \frac{0.02 \text{ g}}{100 \text{ mL}} = 0.1 \text{ g}$$

$$0.1 \text{ g} \times \frac{50 \text{ mL}}{1 \text{ g}} = 5 \text{ mL}$$

Moles and millimoles

A *mole* (mol) is the molecular weight of a substance in grams. Molecular weight is expressed as grams per mole (g/mol).

Example. The molecular weight of sodium chloride is 58.5 g/mol and consists of one sodium ion and one chloride ion in a molecule of sodium chloride:

- 1 mol sodium ion weighs 23 g.
- 1 mol chloride ion weighs 35.5 g.

Moles can be expressed with SI prefixes:

- 1 mol contains 1000 millimoles (mmol).
- 1 mmol contains 1000 micromoles (μmol).
- 1 μmol contains 1000 nanomoles (nmol).
- 1 nmol contains 1000 picomoles (pmol).

Example. How many mmol of sodium chloride are contained in a liter of sodium chloride 0.9% w/v?

$$1\ \text{L} = 1000\ \text{mL}$$

$$1000\ \text{mL} \times \frac{0.9\ \text{g}}{100\ \text{mL}} = 9\ \text{g}$$

$$9\ \text{g} \times \frac{1\ \text{mol}}{58.5\ \text{g}} = 0.154\ \text{mol} = 154\ \text{mmol}$$

Milliequivalents and milliosmoles

Milliequivalents

A *milliequivalent* (mEq) is a unit that reflects chemical activity based on valence. *Valence* is equal to ion charge (e.g., Na = 1, phosphate = 1, Ca = 2, carbonate = 2).

$$\text{mEq} = \text{mg} \times \frac{\text{valence}}{\text{molecular weight}}$$

or,

$$\text{mg} = \text{mEq} \times \frac{\text{molecular weight}}{\text{valence}}$$

Example. How many grams of potassium citrate are needed to make 1.5 L of a 2 mEq potassium/mL solution? (molecular weight [MW] potassium citrate = 324; valence potassium = 3)

$$1.5 \text{ L} \times \frac{1000 \text{ mL}}{1 \text{ L}} \times \frac{2 \text{ mEq}}{1 \text{ mL}} = 3000 \text{ mEq}$$

$$3000 \text{ mEq} \times \frac{324}{3} = 324{,}000 \text{ mg}$$

$$324{,}000 \text{ mg} \times \frac{1 \text{ g}}{1000 \text{ mg}} = 324 \text{ mg}$$

Milliosmoles

A *milliosmole* (mOsm) is a unit that reflects osmotic activity of a substance.

$$\text{mOsm} = \text{mg} \times \frac{\text{number of species}}{\text{molecular weight}}$$

or,

$$\text{mg} = \text{mOsm} \times \frac{\text{molecular weight}}{\text{number of species}}$$

The number of species is equal to the number of ions produced when a compound completely dissociates (e.g., NaCl = 2, KPO4 = 2).
Osmolarity is an expression of concentration in mOsm/L.

Example. How many mOsm are in 500 mL of dextrose 5% in water and 0.9% sodium chloride (D5W/NS)? (MW dextrose = 180; MW NaCl = 58.5) What is its osmolarity?

$$500 \text{ mL} \times \frac{5 \text{ g}}{100 \text{ mL}} \times \frac{1000 \text{ mg}}{1 \text{ g}} = 25{,}000 \text{ mg}$$

$$25{,}000 \text{ mg} \times \frac{1}{180} = 139 \text{ mOsm (from D5W)}$$

$$500 \text{ mL} \times \frac{0.9 \text{ g}}{100 \text{ mL}} \times \frac{1000 \text{ mg}}{1 \text{ g}} = 4500 \text{ mg}$$

$$4500 \text{ mg} \times \frac{2}{58.5} = 154 \text{ mOsm (from NS)}$$

Total mOsm in 500 mL D5W/NS = 139 + 154 = 293 mOsm

$$1 \text{ L} \times \frac{1000 \text{ mL}}{1 \text{ L}} \times \frac{293 \text{ mOsm}}{500 \text{ mL}} = 586 \text{ mOsm/L}$$

Practical issues involving pharmaceutical calculations

- Pay attention to units.
- Double-check your work.
- Check if the answer is logical.

Preparing dilutions

- Ensure correct choice of diluent.
- Correctly express the concentration of the diluted product on the label.

Example 1. Calculate the amount of benzalkonium chloride 50% w/v solution needed to prepare a 150 mL of a solution of benzalkonium chloride 10% w/v.

$$150\text{ mL} \times \frac{10\text{ g}}{100\text{ mL}} = 15\text{ g}$$

$$15\text{ g} \times \frac{100\text{ mL}}{50\text{ g}} = 30\text{ mL}$$

30 mL of benzalkonium chloride solution 50% w/v must be diluted to 150 mL to produce a 10% w/v solution.

Example 2. Calculate the quantity of potassium permanganate 0.25% w/v solution that is required to produce 100 mL of a 0.0125% w/v solution of potassium permanganate.

$$100\text{ mL} \times \frac{0.0125\text{ g}}{100\text{ mL}} = 0.0125\text{ g}$$

$$0.0125\text{ g} \times \frac{100\text{ mL}}{0.25\text{ g}} = 5\text{ mL}$$

5 mL of potassium permanganate solution 0.25% w/v must be diluted to 100 mL with water to produce a 0.0125% w/v solution.

Pharmaceutical calculations involving infusion rates

Many infusion rate calculations involve converting units such as mcg/kg/min into mL/hr.

Example 1. A patient requires a parenteral loading dose of 0.5 mg of digoxin. Digoxin is available as an injection containing 250 mcg/mL. How many milliliters of injection are needed for the required dose?

$$0.5 \text{ mg} = 500 \text{ mcg}$$

$$500 \text{ mcg} \times \frac{1 \text{ mL}}{250 \text{ mcg}} = 2 \text{ mL}$$

Example 2. Dobutamine is available as a standard concentration of 250 mg in 50 mL 5% dextrose solution. What infusion rate (in mL/hr) is needed to deliver 5 mcg/kg/min for a 70 kg patient?

$$70 \text{ kg} \times \frac{5 \text{ mcg}}{\text{kg*min}} \times \frac{60 \text{ min}}{1 \text{ hr}} \times \frac{1 \text{ mg}}{1000 \text{ mcg}} \times \frac{50 \text{ mL}}{250 \text{ mg}} = 4.2 \text{ mL/hr}$$

Pharmaceutical calculations involving infusion rates

Chapter 12

Pharmaceutical and patient-centered care

Katharine A. Sheldon
Michelle W. McCarthy

The concepts of patient-centered and pharmaceutical care

Between 1860 and the 1960s the scope of pharmacy services in the United States was largely devoted to manufacturing, compounding, and dispensing medications. The earliest published reference to pharmaceutical care was by Donald Brodie, who stated that "the ultimate goal of the services of pharmacy must be the safe use of drugs by the public.... [T]he mainstream function of pharmacy is clinical in nature, one that may be identified accurately as drug-use control."[1]

The concept of clinical pharmacy and drug information services emerged in the mid- to late-1960s, which allowed pharmacists to focus on patient-centered care. In 1989, pharmacy leaders from all practice settings gathered at the second Pharmacy in the 21st Century Conference and proposed a new philosophy in pharmacy practice: pharmaceutical care.

Pharmaceutical care definition

In 1990, Hepler and Strand published the most frequently cited definition of pharmaceutical care, which has been endorsed by both the American Pharmacists Association (APhA) and the American Society of Health-System Pharmacists (ASHP). Hepler and Strand described pharmaceutical care as "the responsible provision of drug therapy for the purpose of achieving definite outcomes that improve a patient's quality of life."[2]

Pharmaceutical care is a philosophy of practice that promotes a systemic approach to optimize therapeutic outcomes and improve quality of life for the patient. A key belief in pharmaceutical care is the pharmacist accepts personal responsibility for the outcomes of the patient. As stated by Hepler and Strand, the most important component of pharmaceutical care is that "the fundamental goals, processes, and relationships ... exist regardless of the practice setting."[2]

Pharmaceutical care is an interdependent process through which a pharmacist collaborates with health professionals in designing, implementing, and maintaining a therapeutic plan that will produce specific outcomes for the patient. This process, with the patient's participation, involves three major functions:

- Identifying potential and actual drug-related problems
- Resolving actual drug-related problems
- Preventing drug-related problems.[2]

Patient-centered care

Patient-centered care, like pharmaceutical care, involves a greater emphasis on individual patients and less involvement in the distributive aspects of practice. Through patient-centered care the pharmacist has an

1 Brodie DC, Benson RA (1976). The evolution of the clinical pharmacy concept. *Drug Intell Clin Pharm* **10**:506–510.

2 Hepler CD, Strand LM (1990). Opportunities and responsibilities in pharmaceutical care. *Am J Health Syst Pharm* **47**:533–543.

opportunity to provide individualized care by supplementing basic pharmacotherapeutic knowledge with the patient's understandings of and beliefs, attitudes, and behaviors toward health, disease, and medications.

The patient-centered care approach requires pharmacists to understand medications as their patients experience them. Pharmaceutical care is applied to each patient in his or her social and educational contexts. This approach requires a considerable degree of openness between the pharmacist and patient. Six strategies to improve openness include listening, acknowledging, wondering, recognizing, questioning, and reflecting.

Further reading

Committee on Quality of Health Care in America, Institute of Medicine (2001). *Crossing the Quality Chasm: A New Health System for the 21st Century*. Washington, DC: National Academy Press.

De Oliveira DR, Shoemaker SJ (2006). Achieving patient centeredness in pharmacy practice. *J Am Pharm Assoc* **46**:56–66.

Hepler CD, Strand LM (1990). Opportunities and responsibilities in pharmaceutical care. *Am J Health Syst Pharm* **47**:533–543.

Higby GJ (1997). American pharmacy in the twentieth century. *Am J Health Syst Pharm* **54**:1805–1815.

Core elements of pharmaceutical care

Certain elements describe a standardized method that all pharmacists should perform when providing pharmaceutical care to individual patients. The following elements or guidelines have been developed to standardize pharmaceutical care in any practice setting:

- Collect and organize patient-specific information (e.g., demographic, medical, medication therapy, behavioral, social/economic, etc.).
- Determine the presence of medication-therapy problems.
- Summarize the patient's health-care needs.
- Design a pharmacotherapeutic regimen.
- Design a monitoring plan.
- Develop a pharmacotherapeutic regimen and corresponding monitoring plan in collaboration with the patient and other health professionals caring for the patient.
- Initiate the pharmacotherapeutic regimen.
- Monitor the effects of the pharmacotherapeutic regimen.
- Redesign the pharmacotherapeutic regimen and monitoring plan.

Provision of pharmaceutical care necessitates monitoring and revising the regimen as the patient's conditions and needs change, documenting the results, and assuming responsibility for the pharmacotherapeutic effects. The pharmacist is responsible for achieving outcomes that improve the patient's quality of life. The outcomes sought are as follows:

1. Cure of a patient's disease.
2. Elimination or reduction of a patient's symptomatology.
3. Arresting or slowing of a disease process.
4. Prevention of a disease or symptomatology.

Further reading

American Society of Health-System Pharmacists (1996). ASHP guidelines on a standardized method for pharmaceutical care. *Am J Health Syst Pharm* **53**:1713–1716.

American Society of Hospital Pharmacists (1993). ASHP statement on pharmaceutical care. *Am J Health Syst Pharm* **50**:1720–1723.

Medication problem checklist

After patient-specific information has been collected, the patient's information must be assessed to identify any medication therapy problems. The following list describes a range of potential medication problems that could be encountered:

- Medications without medical indications.
- Medical conditions for which there are no medications prescribed.
- Medications prescribed inappropriately for a particular medical condition.
- Inappropriate medication dose, dosage form, schedule, route of administration, or method of administration.
- Therapeutic duplication.
- Prescribing of medications to which the patient is allergic.
- Actual and potential adverse drug events.
- Actual and potential adverse clinically significant drug–drug, drug–disease, drug–nutrient, and drug–laboratory test interactions.
- Interference with medical therapy by social or recreational drug use.
- Failure to receive the full benefit of prescribed medication therapy.
- Problems arising from the financial impact of medication therapy on the patient.
- Lack of understanding of the medication therapy by the patient.
- Failure of the patient to adhere to the medication regimen.

Checklists and other methods can be used to identify and document medication therapy problems. The method selected should be used consistently among patients and be proactive in nature.

Further reading

American Society of Health-System Pharmacists (1996). ASHP guidelines on a standardized method for pharmaceutical care. *Am J Health Syst Pharm* **53**:1713–1716.

Pharmaceutical care economics

Health-care costs continue to rise, forcing health-care payers to become concerned and to scrutinize reimbursement to health systems and health-care providers. Health-system administrators continue to be faced with increasing costs, not only operational and supply costs, but also from regulatory mandates. Now more than ever, pharmacists can demonstrate their value to patient care. Over 300 studies have been published since 1996 evaluating the economic impact of clinical pharmacy and pharmaceutical care.

A number of benefits from clinical pharmacy services and interventions have been published in the literature. The clinical pharmacy services that have been associated with decreased cost include in-service education, drug information, drug protocol management, and admission drug histories. One study found that each full-time clinical pharmacist was associated with a decrease of approximately $22,000 in drug costs per hospital.

In addition to the above services, drug-use evaluation, adverse drug reaction management, pharmacist participation on cardiopulmonary resuscitation teams, and pharmacist participation on medical rounds has been shown to decrease patient mortality rates. More recent publications have found further support for the positive economic benefit of clinical pharmacy services: for every $1 invested in clinical pharmacy services, a $4.81 reduction in cost or other economic benefits is derived.

It is evident that clinical pharmacy services and pharmaceutical care provide added value, through either direct cost savings or cost avoidance. Pharmacists are encouraged to continue quantifying and publishing the economic and health-outcome benefits of their services and interventions.

Further reading

Bond CA, Raehl CL (2007). Clinical pharmacy services, pharmacy staffing and hospital mortality rates. *Pharmacotherapy* **27**(4):481–493.

Bond CA, Raehl CL, Franke T (1999). Clinical pharmacy services, pharmacist staffing, and drug costs in United States hospitals. *Pharmacotherapy* **19**(12):1354–1362.

Bond CA, Raehl CL, Pitterle ME, et al. (1999). Health care professional staffing, hospital characteristics, and hospital mortality rates. *Pharmacotherapy* **19**(2):130–138.

De Rijdt T, Willems L, Simoens S (2008). Economic effects of clinical pharmacy interventions: a literature review. *Am J Health Syst Pharm* **65**:1161–1172.

Perez A, Doloresco F, Hoffman JM, et al. (2009). Economic evaluations of clinical pharmacy services: 2001–2005. *Pharmacotherapy* **29**:128.

Standards for research

Pharmaceutical care is an obvious research area for pharmacists, but there has been a great deal of variability in design and conduct of research in this area. The recommendations below are provided as an aid to those who read pharmaceutical-care literature and to those who undertake research in pharmaceutical care.

A review of pharmaceutical care by Kennie et al.[1] led the authors to make recommendations aimed at improving the quality of further research:

- Pharmacists must exercise discipline when using the term *pharmaceutical care*.
- Database systems should take measures to ensure that pharmaceutical-care research literature can be correctly and easily extracted.
- A standard reporting method should be adopted that clearly describes the pharmaceutical-care process in the research methodology.
- Randomized controlled studies should be conducted to measure the effect of the provision of pharmaceutical care.
- Pharmaceutical-care research should contain a clear description of the pharmacy practice setting and patient demographics.
- Consistent methods for data collection for different practice sites should be created and validated.
- Informed consent should be obtained for all patients involved in pharmaceutical research, and the procedure should be stated.
- A pharmacist's qualifications and/or certification in providing pharmaceutical care should be addressed and described.
- Pharmaceutical-care research should not only emphasize the evaluation of patient outcomes, but must also first evaluate the structures that exist for the provision of pharmaceutical care.
- The three aspects of evaluation (i.e., structure, process, and outcome) should be linked when assessing the quality of pharmaceutical care.
- The economic impact of pharmaceutical care should be evaluated.
- Standards for pharmaceutical-care research should be developed and accepted by the profession.
- Further pharmaceutical-care research needs to be conducted, with an emphasis on community-based pharmacy.
- A pharmaceutical-care research network should be developed to coordinate efforts and identify areas where research is required.
- Research should be conducted to determine the feasibility and extent of implementing pharmaceutical care in various practice sites.

The authors concluded that few studies have evaluated the provision of pharmaceutical care in a defined population, and identified that there is a need for more research in this area.

Further reading

Plumridge RJ, Wojnar-Hortan RE (1998). A review of the pharmacoeconomics of pharmaceutical care. *Pharmacoeconomics* **14**(2):175–189.

1 Kennie NR, Schuster BG, Einarson TR (1998). Critical analysis of the pharmaceutical care research literature. *Ann Pharmacother* **32**:17–26.

Future practice goals

Leaders of both ASHP and the American College of Clinical Pharmacy (ACCP) have identified their vision for pharmacy practice in the future. ASHP developed the 2015 Health-System Pharmacy Initiative to improve the practice of health-system pharmacy practice by making health-system medication use more effective, scientific, and safe. The 2015 Initiative includes 6 goals and 31 objectives with thresholds for achievement.

The six goals are as follows:

- Increase the extent to which pharmacists help individual hospital inpatients achieve the best use of medications.
- Increase the extent to which health-system pharmacists help individual nonhospitalized patients achieve the best use of medications.
- Increase the extent to which health-system pharmacists actively apply evidence-based methods to the improvement of medication therapy.
- Increase the extent to which pharmacy departments in health systems have a significant role in improving the safety of medication use.
- Increase the extent to which health systems apply technology effectively to improve the safety of medication use.
- Increase the extent to which pharmacy departments in health systems engage in public health initiatives on behalf of their communities.

ASHP offers many resources to assist in achieving the goals and objectives of the 2015 Initiative, including a self-assessment tool and success stories (available at: www.ashp.org/2015.)

ACCP's recommendations regarding practice focus on the roles and training of those in direct patient care. All ACCP position papers can be found at: http://www.accp.com/govt/positionPapers.aspx.

Pharmacy workforce

Articles by Bond and Raehl[1–3] have suggested that increasing the number of clinical pharmacists is associated with a decrease in the total cost of care. The current demand for pharmacists in most institutions far outweighs the available supply.

A number of initiatives have been aimed at defining the long-term vision for the pharmacy workforce in institutions. As pharmacist shortages prevail and the complexity of drug therapy problems increase, institutions will need highly qualified pharmacy staff members (pharmacists and technicians). Both ASHP and ACCP have developed recommendations for the future pharmacy workforce.

- "ASHP Long Range Vision for Pharmacy Workforce in Hospitals and Health Systems" is one document that may be helpful as institutions plan their long-term staffing goals and requirements.
- The ACCP white paper "Vision for Pharmacy's Future Roles, Responsibilities, and Manpower Needs" also addresses the expected changes in practice as well as the evolution of practice roles.

Individuals involved in practice-related decision making should review these documents.

Further reading

ASHP long-range vision for the pharmacy work force in hospitals and health systems (2007) *Am J Health Syst Pharm* **64**:1320–1330.

A vision for pharmacy's future roles, responsibilities, and manpower needs. American College of Clinical Pharmacy (2000). *Pharmacotherapy* **20**:991–1022.

1 Bond CA, Raehl CL (2007). Clinical pharmacy services, pharmacy staffing and hospital mortality rates. *Pharmacotherapy* **27**(4):481–493.

2 Bond CA, Raehl CL, Franke T (1999). Clinical pharmacy services, pharmacist staffing, and drug costs in United States hospitals. *Pharmacotherapy* **19**(12):1354–1362.

3 Bond CA, Raehl CL, Pitterle ME, et al. (1999). Health care professional staffing, hospital characteristics, and hospital mortality rates. *Pharmacotherapy* **19**(2):130–138.

Medication therapy management

Medication therapy management (MTM) services are patient-focused services aimed at improving therapeutic outcomes. MTM is independent of, but may occur with, the provision of a medication product. MTM encompasses a range of activities and responsibilities within the scope of pharmacy practice.

MTM services are individualized for each patient and may include the following:

- Performing or obtaining necessary assessments of the patient's health status.
- Formulating a medication treatment plan.
- Selecting, initiating, modifying, or administering medication therapy.
- Monitoring and evaluating the patient's response to therapy, including safety and effectiveness.
- Performing a comprehensive medication review to identify, resolve, and prevent medication-related problems, including adverse effects.
- Documenting the care delivered and communicating essential information to the patient's PCP.
- Providing verbal education and training designed to enhance patient understanding and appropriate use of medications.
- Providing information, support services, and resources designed to enhance patient adherence with therapeutic regimens.
- Coordinating and integrating MTM services within the broader health care–management services being provided to the patient.

MTM service programs provide the following:

- Patient-specific and individualized services provided directly by a pharmacist to the patient. Services are separate from population-focused quality-assurance measures for medication use.
- Face-to-face interaction between the patient and pharmacist is the preferred method of delivery. MTM program structure should support establishment and maintenance of the patient–pharmacist relationship.
- Opportunities for pharmacists or other health-care providers to identify patients who should receive services.
- Payment for MTM services consistent with contemporary provider payment rates that are based on time, clinical intensity, and resources required to provide services.
- Processes to improve continuity of care, outcomes, and outcome measures.

In some situations, MTM services may be provided to the caregiver or other persons involved in the care of the patient.

Core elements of MTM

The five core elements of the MTM pharmacy practice service model are:

- Medication therapy review.
- Personal medication record.
- Medication-related action plan.
- Intervention and/or referral.
- Documentation and follow-up.

Credentialing

Credentialing is an essential step in delivering MTM services and is being required by many payers. Advanced credentialing programs provide practice recognition among peers, patients, and other health-care providers and certify that the pharmacist possesses the specialized experience and skills to provide the highest level of professional services. Opportunities for credentialing are as follows:

- Board of Pharmaceutical Specialties recognizes specialties in nuclear pharmacy, nutrition support pharmacy, oncology pharmacy, pharmacotherapy (with added qualifications in cardiology and infectious diseases), and psychiatric pharmacy (http://www.bpsweb.org/Home.html)
- Certified Diabetes Educator (http://www.ncbde.org/)
- Certified Asthma Educator (http://www.naecb.org/)
- Certified Geriatric Pharmacist (http://www.ccgp.org/)
- Certified Anticoagulation Care Provider (http://www.ncbap.org/index.aspx)
- Council on Credentialing in Pharmacy (http://pharmacycredentialing.org/ccp/index.htm)

Further reading

American Pharmacists Association and National Association of Chain Drug Stores Foundation (2008). Medication therapy management in pharmacy practice: core elements of an MTM service model (version 2.0). *J Am Pharm Assoc* **48**(3):341–353.

Chapter 13

Medication management

Brian Baird
Katharine A. Sheldon

Medication management

Medication management consists of two main components:

- The clinically skilled use of medications to cost-effectively improve patient's lives, and
- The safe, secure, and efficient handling and storage of medicines.

Department capabilities

Hospitals are complex, challenging systems. In order to function effectively as this critical component of the patient-care system, the department must be able to perform the following missions:[1]

- Maintain security and accountability for all medications stored in the facility.
- Ensure pharmacist review of new medication orders, and periodically review existing orders.
- Efficiently deliver drugs in a manner adaptable to rapid changes in patient condition and location.
- Operate clinical programs that ensure patients receive quality pharmaceutical care.
- Maintain a supply of formulary-approved medications, and conscientiously review, add, and remove drugs from this formulary as warranted.
- Distribute drug information to other members of the health-care team.
- Educate and maintain the competency of the pharmacy staff.

Required systems and processes

Hospital pharmacies should have the following systems in place to ensure effective medication management:[2]

- Secure drug storage and monitoring of drug disposition
  - Drugs must be protected at all times from unauthorized access, including patient and visitor access. All medication storage rooms must be locked. Areas to which drugs are delivered and deliveries themselves must be secure, as required by the Joint Commission.
  - Individual state law and the Drug Enforcement Agency (DEA) regulate controlled substances; refer to specific laws for details.
  - In hospitals without 24/7 pharmacist presence, the pharmacy must be locked. Non-pharmacists are not allowed access.[2]
- Distribution systems able to react to sudden changes in patient location and condition, while remaining cost-efficient. Tube systems, couriers, and robotic deliveries may be used in different combinations to fulfill this purpose.
- 24/7 pharmacist availability. Many hospitals do not have pharmacists on-site 24/7. When the pharmacy is closed, services may be provided by other methods. Some of the more common methods include the following, and a hospital may be served by a combination of these systems:
  - Automated dispensing cabinets or machines that allow nursing access to additional medications during hours the pharmacy is closed.
  - On-call services by a pharmacist who is able to answer questions or report to the pharmacy if needed.
  - Retrospective review of medication orders begun when a pharmacist was not present.

 - Telepharmacy services, including scanning or faxing of new paper orders for review by a pharmacist in another location. Many hospitals may pool together to use these services from a single pharmacist.
- A pharmacy and therapeutics committee (or equivalent). The committee should be able to effectively do the following:
  - Review new drugs and new indications, and determine whether certain medications should be used by the hospital or not (added to the formulary or not).
  - Review usage of already-approved medications and determine whether usage is appropriate, and take action when inappropriate.
  - Approve new policies relating to use of medications and the pharmacy department in general.
- Clinical programs tailored to generate the best outcomes for patients
  - Service lines offered by each hospital vary, and involvement by pharmacists should be aligned according to the services present.
  - Research evaluating clinical services associated with positive outcomes provides a general guide to where emphasis in clinical programs should be placed to achieve these outcomes.[3]
- Effective processes for managing medication errors, also known as adverse drug reactions. The pharmacy department should be able to
  - Effectively work with other departments on errors that involve multiple departments.
  - Track errors and identify trends in order to change systems that are systematically generating errors.
  - Report certain drug reactions to their manufacturers and governmental agencies (e.g., MedWatch) in charge of aggregating such data from many sites.
- Drug information systems that can readily disseminate both urgent and routine information to members of the pharmacy department and to other health-care providers in the institution
- Education plans for the pharmacy staff, including routine assessments of skills and updates on areas particular to the institution. A year's list of topics is a good framework. Education may be developed internally or purchased, and several forms are available, including Web-based and paper. Common approaches include the following:
  - High-risk service lines of the hospital, such as pediatrics, should trigger routine competencies specific to these patient populations.
  - Other routine topics of education and competency assessment include aseptic technique and calculations.[3]

1 American Society of Health-System Pharmacists (US). Best Practices for Hospital and Health-System Pharmacy 2007–2008. www.ashp.org/Import/PRACTICEANDPOLICY/PolicyPositions GuidelinesBestPractices.aspx

2 American Society of Health-System Pharmacists (US). Assuring Continuous Compliance with Joint Commission Standards: A Pharmacy Guide 2008. www.ashp.org/s_ashp/sec_detail.asp?CID=1472&DID=7488

3 Bond CA, Raehl CL, Patry R (2004). Evidence-based core clinical pharmacy services in United States hospitals in 2020: services and staffing. *Pharmacotherapy* **24**(4):427–440.

Evaluating new drugs

This section is intended to help practitioners evaluate a product approved for use by the Food and Drug Agency (FDA). For information on how the FDA approves drugs, see U.S. Drug Approval Process, p. 278.

New drugs are approved and appear on the market constantly, and health-care professionals are bombarded with promotional materials from the pharmaceutical industry. Because the pharmaceutical industry's business is to sell drugs, promotional materials should be reviewed with caution.

The FDA approves drugs for use in the United States. However, simply because a drug has received regulatory approval does not necessarily indicate that the drug is a clinically significant advance. Because the FDA places the emphasis of its evaluation on safety and efficacy, not therapeutic value, many drugs are similar to existing products. Assessments of the value of new drugs in Canada, France, and the United States have shown that, at best, only one-third offer some additional clinical benefit and as few as 3% are major therapeutic advances.[1]

Premarketing trials are often placebo-controlled and so do not typically compare the drug to an established "reference" treatment. Even if the trial does compare the new drug with a reference treatment, the trial might be too small or short to provide certain meaningful data. In particular, rare adverse drug reactions (ADRs) or differences in response in subgroups of patients are unlikely to be identified from smaller trials.[2]

Much of the data presented by the pharmaceutical industry relies on surrogate markers rather than patient outcomes. These two types of data can be substantially different in their real-life meaning. For example, cyclo-oxygenase 2 (COX-2) NSAIDs cause fewer endoscopically detected ulcers than standard NSAIDs; however, many of these ulcers are not clinically significant and would spontaneously heal. A better evaluation would be to determine the difference between COX-2 NSAIDs and standard NSAIDs in causing symptomatic or bleeding ulcers, because this outcome would be more meaningful.

The STEPS acronym is a useful tool for evaluating new drugs:[3]

- ***Safety***. Evaluate the safety of the new drug with that of a standard reference preparation, ideally using comparison studies that reflect the real-life situation. Pharmaceutical companies often highlight differences in ADRs that are relatively trivial or rare. Check especially for ADRs that would place the patient at particular risk:
  - Liver, kidney, or bone-marrow toxicity
  - Cardiovascular events, such as myocardial infarction (MI), stroke
  - CNS events, such as seizure
  - Significant skin or hypersensitivity reactions, such as anaphylaxis or toxic epidermal necrolysis
  - GI bleeding
  - Congenital abnormalities

Compare the frequency of these events within the context of the significance of the disease. A 5% risk of hepatotoxicity for a drug that treats a life-threatening disease is more acceptable than the same risk when treating a self-limiting disease.

- ***Tolerability***. Are side effects likely to affect adherence? Evaluate dropout rates in clinical trials; if there is a high dropout rate due to more ADRs than with the reference drug, this makes the new drug of less therapeutic value. If patients won't take the drug, it won't work.
- ***Effectiveness***. Compare the new drug to a reference drug in a head-to-head trial. Ask if this new drug works as well as or better than the reference drug. The number needed to treat (NNT) is the simplest way to assess therapeutic value (see Chapter 8, p. 152). If the new drug's NNT is the same as or lower than the reference drug's, it is worth considering.
- ***Price***. Consider purchase price primarily, and fairly compare products over a similar time span. For example, if the new drug is only given 1 week out of 4, ensure that cost is compared to 4 weeks of comparator's therapy. Also, check for additional costs associated with the new drug vs. those of the reference. These costs could include
  - Administration cost, such as IV sets and tubing
  - Monitoring costs, such as lab work and patient visits
  - Additional time or travel if a patient has more office visits
- ***Simplicity***. Is it easy for the patient to use the drug? Review the following attributes, and consider any additional ones:
  - Doses per day, and number of tablets per dose
  - Injectable vs. oral administration
  - Easy-to-use dispensing device, if applicable (inhaler, injector, etc.)
  - Special storage requirements, such as refrigeration

After considering these criteria, the drug should be discussed and the action taken. This is often the role of the Pharmacy and Therapeutics Committee at the hospital in question, a committee required by the Joint Commission. Whoever reviews the drug for use must decide if it will not be used or kept on hand (non-formulary drug), if it will be kept on hand for use (formulary drug), or on some restriction representing a middle point. Restrictions may be placed on drugs so that only certain areas or prescribers may use them, although this entails additional work for the pharmacy department. Following are some examples of such restrictions:

- Monitored use: no restrictions on use, but approval has conditional review of usage or some other quality assurance plan
- Restricted to a certain area or prescribers, or for certain conditions

Either of these conditions may also feature a time limit, stating that the drug will be removed from the formulary after a specified period of time if some defined conditions are not met.[4]

1 Howland R (2006). A look back at the pharmaceuticals market 2005: deregulation continues. Prescrire International **15**(82):75–79.

2 Howland RH (2008). How are drugs approved? Part 3. The stages of drug development. *Psychosoc Nurs Ment Health Serv* **46**(3):17–202.

3 Preskorn SH (1994). Antidepressant drug selection: criteria and options. *J Clin Psychiatry* **55**(Suppl A):6–24, 98–100.

4 American Society of Health-System Pharmacists (US). Best Practices for Hospital and Health-System Pharmacy 2007–2008. www.ashp.org/Import/PRACTICEANDPOLICY/PolicyPositionsGuidelinesBestPractices.aspx

How to write a protocol

Protocols, particularly medication protocols, are documents that specify all of the critical parts of a certain kind of therapy. Generally, protocols are used when the treatment is somewhat complex and is expected to be used repeatedly. Protocols of this kind help to ensure that drugs are used safely, cost-effectively, and in a standardized manner within the hospital setting. Examples of such protocols include the following:

- Treatment of stroke, including thrombolytic therapy
- Heparin infusions, including dose adjustments for PTT results
- Initiating and monitoring dofetilide (Tikosyn)

The need for a drug protocol is usually brought to light by a complicated procedure or practice that would benefit from having the existing practice reviewed and written out. Protocols may consist of drugs only, a diagnosis whose treatment consists partly of medication therapy, or other combinations. It is important that a pharmacy representative be able to review such protocols before they are published and used, as no other member of the health-care team provides the same perspective.[1]

Stages of protocol development

Identification of need

A new or existing practice is recognized as being cumbersome, unsafe, or otherwise in need of revision.

For example, a new use for a drug is developed that requires compounding in a specific way, additional monitoring, and adjunctive medication therapy. It has begun use with these orders written in longhand, but the inconsistency of this practice and increased likelihood of error make clear the need for a prewritten protocol.

Assignment of responsibility

A leader should be identified for the project. Although a group may be responsible for the final form, projects such as this typically require a leader who is responsible for moving the work along.

Gathering evidence and best practices

The leader and group obtain other, similar protocols and enquire about their strengths and weaknesses. Other departments that will be affected by the protocol or whose work contributes to the project should be contacted with questions, although they may not need to sit on the committee. Literature searches are made to collect current evidence and best practices. These data should be reviewed and vetted, and the most useful results distributed to those working on the project, if applicable.

Draft compilation

After reviewing the available evidence, the leader or committee drafts a protocol. The protocol should be reviewed and revised by the committee or its writer until no great flaws remain. At times, substantive decisions must be delayed until the protocol can be reviewed by the next committee. Or, committee members from the next committee may be asked their opinion so that the protocol-drafting group can deliver a better result. After the draft has been rewritten and edited, the protocol is submitted to the appropriate hospital committee. After this committee's review, the protocol should assume a final or near-final form.

Education and rollout

The completed protocol is often submitted to an education department to gain their expertise in training staff members. The date to begin using the protocol may also be set according to the time it will take for staff to be educated. It is important to remember that implementation of a protocol may need to be delayed after its approval if staff education is required. Staff members should be allowed to have the opportunity to familiarize themselves with a protocol before being expected to act on it.

It is imperative that pharmacists be able to review a protocol during its development. The protocol should be reviewed with great scrutiny because it will be used many times. A protocol containing drugs or focused on drug therapy should be reviewed for the following details:

- Generic and trade names for each drug, with emphasis on the generic name
- Correct route, dose, and frequency for each medication
- Indication for each PRN medication
- Frequency of administration
- Dilution instructions for each drip present
- All ambiguous statements clarified
- Contraindications or reasons not to use drugs prominently placed

Limitations

A protocol may not be made to deal with every eventuality. Rather, a well-designed protocol will succinctly provide a framework for dealing with a particular set of circumstances. Patients will inevitably fall outside of these circumstances; thus a protocol should be developed with these limitations in mind so it does not become inappropriately complex.[2]

1 Fugate S, Chappe J (2008). Standardizing the management of heparin-induced thrombocytopenia. *Am J Health Syst Pharm* **65**(4):334–339.

2 American Society of Health-System Pharmacists (US). Best Practices for Hospital and Health-System Pharmacy 2007–2008. www.ashp.org/Import/PRACTICEANDPOLICY/PolicyPositionsGuidelinesBestPractices.aspx

U.S. drug approval process

All products legally called "drugs" in the United States have been approved by the Food and Drug Administration (FDA), based in Rockville, Maryland. The FDA consists of nine divisions; the divisions primarily concerned with approval of new drugs are the Center for Drug Evaluation and Research (CDER), and the Center for Biologics Evaluation and Research (CBER). The CDER reviews most drugs and the CBER reviews vaccines. The other types of therapies (such as gene therapy) assigned to the CBER have so far yielded few products that have required review or are currently being marketed.

Regardless of the reviewing center, the research and approval process proceeds in a general pattern. A new compound is "sponsored," generally by a pharmaceutical company, through the approval process. The process may be voluntarily halted at any point by the sponsor of the product or by the FDA when a safety problem is detected.

Below is a typical pattern of approval. It assumes each step is completed successfully.[1]

- A company identifies a potentially useful compound. The company performs animal or other testing that indicates that the product may be useful in humans.
- The company may patent the compound early in this process, usually when the compound begins to show promise. This patent gives the company the exclusive right to perform research with the compound and market it, if the FDA later allows.
- The company files an "Investigational New Drug Application" (IND) with the FDA, which is an application to study the drug in humans.
- The FDA reviews the IND. Usually, the decision for IND approval or rejection is returned within 60 days.
- The investigating company must get approval from an institutional review board (IRB), which oversees studies as they progress. The IRB may be local to an institution or be a national company that provides IRB services. The IRB is a multidisciplinary group including physicians; its purpose is to review studies and ensure the safety of patients enrolled in trials that will be performed in its area of responsibility. Among other responsibilities, the IRB must strive to ensure that only quality studies are approved, that patients' confidentiality is respected, and that patients receive informed consent so that they may decide whether they wish to participate or not.
- *Phase I studies*, usually enrolling 20–80 healthy volunteers, are used to determine a profile of pharmacokinetic properties, overall effects, and the toxicities of the product.
- In *phase II studies* the drug is used in patients with the targeted disease. These studies are bigger than phase I trials and usually contain a few dozen to 300 people. This larger number of subjects and use of the drug in a population with a disease better establish the drug's profile. This additional data guides later decisions regarding which dose and schedule to use, and well as other important decisions.

1 J Howland RH (2008). How are drugs approved? Part 3. The stages of drug development. *Psychosoc Nurs Ment Health Serv* **46**(3):17–202.

- In *phase III studies* data obtained from previous trials are used to estimate the dose, schedule, etc. and to determine what form of the drug to use. Also, efficacy data from the phase II trials guide the size and statistical-power needed for phase III trials. Phase III trials may range in size from 100 to several thousand patients, depending on the drug in question.
- When the sponsoring company thinks that its evidence is sufficient, it engages the FDA during a pre–New Drug Application (NDA) time period. The FDA and the company address any necessary data that are not available.
- The company submits a completed NDA to the FDA.
- The FDA reviews the drug by means of a specialist system, with a committee composed of experts from a particular field responsible for reviewing the drugs fitting their field. Examples of such committees are the Oncologic Drugs Advisory Committee and the Gastrointestinal Drugs Advisory Committee.
- The FDA advisory committee meets to discuss whether to approve the drug for use and any additional restrictions that may be imposed. The actions of the committee are considered "advice" or "recommendations" only, and are then submitted to an FDA executive panel.
- The executive committee acts on the advisory committee's recommendation. Usually the advice is taken; however, the executive committee reserves the right to act independently.
- The FDA sends the sponsoring company a "complete response" letter, which details any additional steps that must be taken before or after drug approval.

The manufacturing facility for the drug is also inspected during the drug approval process. This occurs regardless of whether the facility is within the United States. Also, a product used during clinical trials may have been manufactured on a small scale, in a laboratory setting. Therefore, the manufacturing facility may be unfamiliar with the needed processes. The drug can be produced prior to the FDA's approval; however, it may not be shipped from the manufacturing facility until after approval.

Development time needed for each step varies from drug to drug, but generally the total amount of time needed for the entire process from beginning to end is several years.

Companies may pay the FDA a user fee to speed up the review process. This logic behind the fee is that a company wishing to have a drug reviewed with priority uses more of the FDA's resources, so they should pay additional fees so that the FDA can hire more reviewers. This program has been in existence for over 10 years, and most companies that think a drug has the potential to make a substantial profit will make use of this program to move the drug to the U.S. market more quickly.[1]

As a condition of approval, the drug may be required to go through additional *phase IV safety trials*. These trials investigate data that the FDA thinks need greater study, generally safety data. Often, large trials are used to detect subtle or rare safety problems that occur too infrequently to be detected by smaller trials. If these or other conditions attached to the drug's approval are not carried out, the FDA may remove the drug from the market.[2]

There are some additional corporate dynamics inherent to this process, such as company mergers and acquisitions. A company may purchase another company in order to take over the rights of a promising compound, or a small company may engage with a larger company in a licensing risk–profit sharing arrangement to gain resources needed to complete development.

1 Shulman SR, Kaitin KI (1996). The Prescription Drug User Fee Act of 1992. A 5-year experiment for industry and the FDA. *Pharacoeconomics* **9**(2):121–133.

2 U.S. Food and Drug Administration. Managing the risks from medical product use. Available at: www.fda.gov/oc/tfrm/Part4.html

Pharmacy and therapeutics committees

Each hospital has a pharmacy and therapeutics (P&T) committee or an equivalent. The P&T committee is generally responsible for pharmacy-related policies and procedures and drug formulary decisions (See references, p. 283).[1]

Membership

A P&T committee should consist of a multidisciplinary group of practitioners, including representatives from the following disciplines:

- Medical staff: internal medicine, anesthesia, and other physicians from areas of the hospital that have high medication use or high patient load. Typically, the chair of the committee is a physician.
- Director of pharmacy, other pharmacy representatives as appropriate
- Nursing: chief nursing officer or representatives
- Administration
- Education, usually nursing education[2]

Other attendees are invited as needed, on a standing or ad hoc basis. Often, if a new drug that impacts a particular specialty is being added to the formulary, that specialty will send a member to the meeting at which the agent will be reviewed. Also, if an important medication-use evaluation is to be presented, members of the groups who use the medication may be invited to comment on it.

The P&T committee should have rules stating who the voting members are. Some committees only allow physicians to vote; others have voting rights for various members. The committee should meet at least quarterly, although monthly meetings allow more timely actions.

Agenda and duties

Generally, the director of pharmacy will set the agenda for the meeting in conjunction with the chair of the committee. The agenda and items to be reviewed are often sent to members several days prior to the meeting for review.

A primary focus of the committee is to add or remove drugs to and from the hospital formulary. The members of the committee must ensure that new drugs are safe and necessary, have an acceptable evidence base, and are cost-effective. Typically, a drug monograph is presented to provide committee members with unbiased information; see Evaluating New Drugs (p. 274).

In addition to adding or removing drugs from the hospital's formulary, the P&T committee usually has a role in the following areas:

- Review of medication-use evaluation results and recommending changes based on them
- Updating and maintaining policies and procedures relevant to the department of pharmacy or specific to medications
- Analyzing adverse drug reactions and medication errors, and making recommendations based on them
- Reviewing medication expenditures

Actions

The actions of the P&T committee must be codified into minutes that are reviewed and approved as determined by the hospital's committee structure. These minutes should then be published to all affected hospital departments in a summarized form.

Actions passed at a P&T committee meeting are assigned to a group for implementation. Typically, progress of implementation, if applicable, is reported at the following P&T committee meeting.[3]

1 American Society of Health-System Pharmacists (US). Best Practices for Hospital and Health-System Pharmacy 2007–2008. www.ashp.org/Import/PRACTICEANDPOLICY/PolicyPositions GuidelinesBestPractices.aspx

2 American Society of Health-System Pharmacists (US). ASHP Guidelines on the Pharmacy and Therapeutics Committee and the Formulary System. www.ashp.org.

3 Tyler LS, Cole SW, May JR, et al. (2008). ASHP guidelines on the pharmacy and therapeutics committee and the formulary system. *Am J Health Syst Pharm* **65**(13):1272–1283.

Clinical pathways and collaborative practice arrangements

In an effort to raise health-care quality, methods of planning and managing a patient's hospital stay have been developed. One of these methods, the clinical pathway, has become popular in many U.S. hospitals. The clinical pathway is also variously known as a care plan or care map, depending on the institution or region.

Fundamentally, use of a clinical pathway involves selecting a discrete medical condition, such as coronary artery bypass or carotid endarterectomy, and exhaustively listing all of the components of care that should occur for the patient. Such components may be such things as addition or removal of medications, changes in dressing types, and dietary advancement, among others. These changes are listed in a temporal sequence so that the plan is followed in a logical order.

For example, a clinical pathway for carotid artery surgery (carotid endarterectomy) may include all of the tests needed prior to the surgery, the dietary restrictions beforehand, and suggestions for medications. Provision of information to the patient and family may be included in the plan so that this is not overlooked. After the surgery, the care plan should carefully incorporate all relevant aspects of care, including typical medications, vital signs, follow-up imaging or Doppler examinations, dietary advancement, and discharge planning.

Development

There are several approaches to the development of a clinical pathway. Since many specific types of surgery have clinical similarities across hospitals in the United States, products have been developed that outline clinical pathways for these common procedures. Also, clinical pathways are often adapted from other hospitals in a health-care system and then adopted for use locally. Finally, care plans may be developed in their entirety on-site.

No matter which approach is taken, it is crucial to consider the parties who will be affected by the clinical pathway when it is implemented. Primarily, having multidisciplinary involvement during development promotes a system-wide view of the processes. This method is less likely to overlook important parts of the process, which can happen when a department is performing an important function but is not represented during development of the clinical pathway. In addition, not including important contributors leads to a greater likelihood of rejection of the clinical pathway by those not included in its development.

Each clinical plan should incorporate relevant guidelines and thus lead to evidence-based practice, because guidelines are based on evidence. Updates to clinical pathways should be made routinely when new guidelines are published or when significant changes in the standards of care emerge.[1]

Value

The ultimate purpose of the clinical pathway is to provide better care to the patient. Like the guidelines they are based on, clinical pathways have been shown to improve outcomes. Patient outcomes will vary by the object of the pathway, the difference between the standard of care and the level of care brought to pass by the clinical pathway, and the rigidity with which the clinical pathway is adhered to.

Additionally, cost benefits have been a driving factor in the adoption of clinical pathways. The use of pathways has been shown to decrease costs, primarily by decreasing length of stay. This decrease in length of stay is mostly attributable to the standardization of care brought about by the pathway and by better planning procedures resulting from the clearly listed goals of therapy in the pathway. Again, these improvements vary according to the subject of the pathway.

Other, more intangible benefits may also be realized from the use of clinical pathways. Their development and maintenance tend to bring together multidisciplinary groups of practitioners, often leading to an increase in morale and more engagement by members of the group. Patients like early discharge; however, patients also appreciate knowing which steps are before them in the care process, as these stages can be related directly from the clinical pathway.

Collaborative practice agreements

It is possible to establish formal arrangements between pharmacists and prescribers (generally physicians) that allow pharmacists to manage patients within a certain, predesignated scope of care. The exact legal ramifications of this type of practice vary from state to state and may change with legislation.

Collaborative practice agreements, also known as pharmacist-based disease-state management and collaborative practice arrangements, begin under various circumstances. Often, they evolve from a close physician–pharmacist relationship in which the realization is made that the pharmacist, if given a protocol or certain amount of authority with which to practice, could work apart from the physician and consult the physician only when the occasion required. Typically the care area is specialized in nature and the scope of practice is intentionally limited.[2]

A policy or legal agreement is needed for the pharmacist, so that the limits of their practice are defined. This agreement is essentially a delegation of authority by the prescriber. The details of such an agreement vary by state and by how much delegation a physician wishes to provide, as well as how much authority the pharmacist is willing to accept. In a practice with multiple physicians, some physicians may choose to participate in the agreement, whereas others may not. The pharmacist would then have

1 Bohmer R (1998). Critical pathways at Massachusetts General Hospital. *J Vasc Surg* **28**:373–377.

2 Ferro LA, Marcrom RE, Garrelts L, et al. (1998). Collaborative practice agreements between pharmacists and physicians. *J Am Pharm Assoc* **38**:655–664.

authority under the agreement only with patients of the physicians who are participating in the agreement.[3]

Some research has shown that patients receiving care under collaborative practice arrangements have better outcomes than those of control groups. The two main goals of such an arrangement are the improvement of patient care and the transfer of a limited scope of care to pharmacists. This delegation can free physicians' time for more complex patients and lead to better overall care.[4]

3 Harris IM, Baker E, Berry T, et al. (2008). Developing a business-practice model for pharmacy services in ambulatory settings. *Pharmacotherapy* **28**(2):7e-34e.

4 Leal S, Soto M (2008). Chronic kidney disease risk reduction in a Hispanic population through pharmacist-based disease-state management. *Adv Chron Kidney Dis* **15**(2):162–167.

Electronic prescribing

Since the advent of the Internet and World Wide Web, interest in electronic prescribing has increased exponentially. Although some closed systems, such as the Veterans Administration (VA) system, have already employed electronic prescribing on a long-term basis, it is a new development for general practice.

Currently, over 100 electronic prescribing systems are available commercially and over 35 million electronic prescriptions were processed in 2007. This figure was expected to triple for 2008, and the overall growth of electronic prescribing remains strong.[1]

Additionally, in 2008, the U.S. Congress passed legislation tying physician Medicare reimbursement incentives to electronic prescribing, which should spur even greater adoption of this technology. Electronic prescribing is also referred to as "Computerized Prescriber Order Entry."

A variety of system types are available, which gives those considering purchase of these systems several choices based on features and cost. Some of the major features include the following:

- Electronic prescribing only, or a full electronic medical-records system that includes electronic prescribing as a component
- Inpatient and outpatient systems
- Handheld vs. desktop functionality
- Availability of refill records
- Formulary decision support from regional insurance companies[2]

It should be noted that both prescribers and pharmacies must possess systems for the electronic functions to work. However, many systems are able to print prescriptions on demand when it is determined that electronic prescribing cannot proceed.

The impetus for electronic prescribing is multifaceted. The main advantages are noted below:

- Prescriptions are legible.
- Prescriptions are typically not lost.
- With faster transmission, prescriptions can be readied sooner at the pharmacy.
- Supports decision making when prescribing (can flag errors)
- Improved safety for patients with drug allergies
- Accessibility of information between primary care and specialist care
- Drug-usage reports for individual patients
- Improved use of patient and staff time
- Better audit trails
- Improved patient compliance with protocols
- The pharmacy as early identification of new scripts for screening and supply.[3]

Electronic prescribing systems are often intelligent and flag areas of drug interaction, incorrect dosing, other prescribing errors, additional information required for safe drug administration, and formulary issues. These systems require input and maintenance by pharmacy and information technology teams.[4]

Pharmacy and prescriber staff using an electronic prescribing system require training in its use before working with the system. These systems have various levels of security, depending on the role of the professional in the use of the system. It is essential that there is good security for any electronic prescribing system, with frequent backup, and a system must be in place in case of system failure.[5]

1 American Society of Health-System Pharmacists (US). Best Practices for Hospital and Health-System Pharmacy 2007–2008. www.ashp.org/Import/PRACTICEANDPOLICY/PolicyPositionsGuidelinesBestPractices.aspx

2 Gray MD, Felkey BG (2004). Computerized prescriber order-entry systems: evaluation, selection, and implementation. *Am J Health Syst Pharm* **61**(2):190–197.

3 Donyai P, O'Grady K, Jacklin A, Barber N, Franklin BD (2008). The effects of electronic prescribing on the quality of prescribing. *Br J Clin Pharmacol* **65**(2):230–237.

4 Bobb A, Gleason K, Husch M, Feinglass J, et al. (2004). The epidemiology of prescribing errors: the potential impact of computerized prescriber order entry. *Arch Intern Med* **164**(7):785–792.

5 Jayawardena S, Eisdorfer J, Indulkar S, et al. (2007). Prescription errors and the impact of computerized prescription order entry system in a community-based hospital. *Am J Ther* **14**(4):336–340.

Incident reporting

Each hospital pharmacy should have a policy in place for the reporting of incidents. This is typically an electronic system that allows entries to be made from any computer terminal and collected centrally by those who are tasked with monitoring the incidents. Good systems allow users to input incident information anonymously.[1]

An *incident* is usually defined as an event or circumstance that could have, or did, lead to unintended or unexpected harm, loss, or damage. Incidents might involve actual or potential injury, damage, loss, allergic reaction, violence, abuse, falls and other accidents, and hospital-acquired infections. Such a policy should apply to all hospital staff and is generally taught during orientation.[2]

- An incident-reporting program should identify, assess, and manage risks that could compromise or threaten the quality of patient services or staff working in a safe environment, as part of the overall management of risk. It is a confidential process, and all staff should complete the appropriate documentation if involved in or aware of an incident.
- Incidents need to be reported to ensure that the hospital can analyze the data for trends, causes, and costs. Action plans may then be developed to mitigate future similar incidents.[3]
- Reporting of incidents allows staff to have input into changing practices and procedures. Incident reporting must follow a "no-blame" or "non-punitive" culture in which the reporter of the incident is not punished.
- Medication incidents must be reported through this mechanism to ensure that there can be a review of trends, analysis of failures, arrangements for improvements, and follow-up audits.
- The type of incident that a pharmacist can report includes medication errors and failure of a system or process that affects patient care.
- In addition to reporting an incident, a pharmacist or their supervisor may also deal with an incident by communicating with the relevant members of staff involved.[4]

1. Dixon JF (2002). Going paperless with custom-built Web-based patient occurrence reporting. *Jt Comm J Qual Improv* **28**(7):387–395.

2. Tamuz M, Thomas EJ, Franchois KE (2004). Defining and classifying medical error: lessons for patient safety reporting systems. *Qual Saf Health Care* **13**(1):13–20.

3. Pronovost PJ, Thompson DA, Holzmueller CG, et al. (2006). Toward learning from patient safety reporting systems. *J Crit Care* **21**(4):30–315.

4. Crone KG, Muraski MB, Skeel JD, Love-Gregory L, et al. (2006). Between a rock and a hard place: disclosing medical errors. *Clin Chem* **52**(9):1809–1814.

Pharmaceutical sales representatives

Pharmaceutical sales representatives, also known as "drug reps," provide information to health-care practitioners about their company's products, but their primary function is to promote and sell them. The background of pharmaceutical sales representatives is generally not medical, although a few nurses and pharmacists serve as these representatives. Often, they have a business, biology, or similar Bachelor's degree.

These salespeople are generally assigned a territory, consisting of certain physician offices, hospitals, and/or pharmacies in a certain area. Areas vary widely according to the drug being marketed.

The representative will be instructed on the sales approach for their drug or drugs, and will then work within their area, promoting the product in various ways. Part of the duty is simply to ensure the drug is easily remembered when it may be prescribed. Fulfilling this role consists of brief office visits, visits to pharmacies to promote stocking of the drug, and provision of promotional materials.

Additional duties include educating prescribers and pharmacists on the characteristics of the drug, being present at seminars and conferences, and organizing speaker presentations on the drug or its disease states. The estimated expenditures for promotion of new drugs to U.S. physicians ranges from $27.7 to $57.5 billion per year as of 2006.[1]

Representatives should not be confused with medical science liaisons (MSLs), who are licensed medical professionals such as pharmacists, nurses, and physicians. These individuals generally carry no overt marketing materials with them and are able to discuss off-label uses, upcoming trial results, and other data that are off-limits to pharmaceutical representatives.

A few guidelines regarding pharmaceutical representatives are noted below:

- Medical representatives should provide their service according to the Pharmaceutical Research and Manufacturers of America (PhRMA) Code on Interactions with Healthcare Professionals. The newest and most restrictive version of the code went into effect in January 2009. The specifics of this code may be found on the phrma.org Web site.[2]
- In addition to the PhRMA code, most hospitals have a local policy for dealing with pharmaceutical representatives. Occasionally this policy is combined with a policy dealing with other vendors, such as those marketing devices, bandages, etc.
- Many hospitals do not allow pharmaceutical representatives to leave samples, or have specific procedures for the samples. Check for such a policy before accepting samples from pharmaceutical representatives.
- The best practice for pharmaceutical-representative visits is to restrict them to appointments only when meeting with a member of the pharmacy staff. Additionally, some hospital policies restrict the grades of staff that are allowed to meet with medical representatives.[3]

- Pharmaceutical representatives are not allowed to promote medications for indications that are not FDA approved or off-label, and should not answer questions that relate to these situations. Generally, representatives may note questions of this type and refer them to their medical information office for that office to provide written answers.[4]

Finally, pharmaceutical representatives typically have access to wholesaler buying data and will know when a physician or hospital is using a product on the basis of these data. However, these data are limited solely to units purchased; they do not reveal the prescriber or provide other useful information. For outpatient use of drugs, this information is often available at the prescriber level unless a prescriber has opted out of this program.[5]

1 Gagnon MA, Lexchin K (2005). The cost of pushing pills: a new estimate of pharmaceutical promotion expenditures in the United States. *PLoS Med* **5**(1):e1

2 Pharmaceutical Research and Manufacturers of America. Guidelines for Interactions with Healthcare Professionals. www.phrma.org/files/PhRMA%20Marketing%20Code%202008.pdf

3 Institute of Safe Medical Practices. Safety Alert! May 22, 2008. www.ismp.org/newsletters/ acutecare/articles/20080522.asp

4 Hatton RC, Chavez ML, Jackson E, et al. (2008). Pharmacists and industry: guidelines for ethical interactions. *Pharmacotherapy* **28**(3):410–420.

5 American Medical Association: Physician Data Restriction Program. www.ama-assn.org/ama/ pub/category/12054.html.

Confidentiality

Pharmacists and pharmacy staff are expected to maintain the confidentiality of any patient or customer they have contact with during the course of their professional duties. The Health Information Portability and Protection Act (HIPAA) codified this expectation and set rules for the protection of patient's confidentiality.[1] Information that should remain confidential includes the following:

- Patient's past, present, or future condition and health, including mental health
- The provision of health care to the individual, including medications
- Past, present, or future health-care payments[2]

De-identification

It should be noted that there are few restrictions on the use or disclosure of de-identified health information. There are two ways to de-identify information, but the most common method applicable to pharmacists is to remove identifiers of the individual and their personal contacts if any are included. Identifiers include, but are not limited to

- Names
- Social Security numbers
- Specific geographic descriptions such as address
- Birthdates, admission or discharge dates, and age for patients over 89 years of age
- Pictures of the entire face
- Phone numbers
- E-mail addresses
- Health plan beneficiary numbers[3]

To avoid unintentional disclosures, it is important to develop good habits when dealing with patient information:

- Discussing a patient with colleagues is often necessary for patient care or training purposes, but be cautious about revealing names or other patient identifiers. Reveal only information that is necessary.
- Do not discuss patients in public areas such as elevators or hallways.
- If talking about work to family or friends, only talk about patients in general terms without specific, identifying details.
- Ensure that written information such as patient medication profiles and prescriptions are not left where other patients or the public can see it.
- If discussing medication with a patient, try to do this in a reasonably private area. If hospital patients have visitors, ask if the patient would like you to return when they have gone.
- Ensure that computer systems have strong passwords, and always log off at the end of a session.[2]

Disclosure of information

In some situations, pharmacists might have to disclose confidential information outside of the scope of patient care. The HIPAA also provides guidance for when these disclosures might be necessary:

- If required by law, court order, or statute
- For a minor
- If necessary to prevent serious injury or damage to the health of the patient, a third party, or the public health[3]

1 Health Insurance Reform: Security Standards. 45 C.F.R. Parts 160, 162, and 164. February 20, 2003.

2 HIPAA Administrative Simplification. 45 C.F.R. Parts 160, 162, and 164. February 16, 2006.

3 Health Insurance Reform: Security Standards. 45 C.F.R. Part 164.514(a)(c). February 20, 2003.

Conflicts of interest

A conflict of interest exists when a pharmacist has a professional interest competing with a personal interest. The primary interest of a pharmacist should always be one of patient welfare if the pharmacist has a clinical practice; some pharmacists may have a primary interest of research or some other field. The conflicting, secondary interest generally is one involving some sort of personal or financial gain for the pharmacist. Examples of relationships that may be perceived as conflicts of interest include the following:

- Ownership of mutual funds that invest in a specific area of business, such as certain biotech funds
- Ownership of individual stock or options in pharmaceutical companies
- Gifts from pharmaceutical representatives, including invitations to social events or entertainment
- Honoraria or contract employment by industry
- Review of a manuscript for a product in whose company the pharmacist has a financial interest[1]

Importantly, a conflict of interest may exist only as perception of patients or colleagues; the person thought to have the conflict may have a neutral or negative view of the situation that leads to this perception. For example, a pharmacist holding stock in a pharmaceutical company may have a negative opinion about that company due to stock losses; however, the holding of the stock may still be perceived as a conflict of interest by patients or colleagues.[1]

Disclosure

Pharmacists may be required to disclose conflicts of interest in certain circumstances. Some reasons for this include formulary decision-making responsibilities, publication of research, and service on investigational review boards. A disclosure allows the group to evaluate the reason for the conflict of interest and determine how it should be dealt with. Depending on the circumstance, abstention from voting, simple notation, or other actions may be appropriate.[2]

It is important to realize that disclosure does not absolve the pharmacist from conflict of interest. Disclosure is helpful in that it reveals to others what possible conflicts exist for the one who discloses; it does not remove the conflicts.

1 Hatton RC, Chavez ML, Jackson E, et al. (2008). Pharmacists and industry: guidelines for ethical interactions. *Pharmacotherapy* **28**(3):410–420.

2 American Society of Health-System Pharmacists (US). Best Practices for Hospital and Health-System Pharmacy 2007–2008. www.ashp.org/Import/PRACTICEANDPOLICY/PolicyPositions GuidelinesBestPractices.aspx

Disposal of medicines

Pharmaceutical waste can be generated through a variety of processes in hospitals, including but not limited to intravenous (IV) preparation, general compounding, spills, partially used vials, syringes and IVs, unused preparations, patients' personal medications, and outdated medications.[1] Appropriate pharmaceutical-waste management is a new challenge facing hospitals and other health-care facilities.[1] Each hospital should have policies and procedures in place that adhere to pharmaceutical-waste regulations established by national and state regulatory organizations.

Medicines supplied by the hospital department

All out-of-date medicines and any drugs no longer required for a specific patient are usually returned to the pharmacy, whose staff will either return the medication into stock or arrange for destruction (as appropriate). Hospital-specific procedures for return of medication into stock and destruction of medication should be in place.

Transportation of returns to pharmacy

- By dedicated pharmacy box or return bin: unused or expired products
- By pneumatic tube systems or dumb waiters: unused or expired products
- By unit or department personnel: controlled substances

Medicines brought into hospital by patients

Many times a patient will bring his or her medicine into the hospital. In most situations, these medications will either be sent home or stored in a secure location during the patient's stay. If the patient cannot arrange for home medications to be returned home, the hospital will store them in a secure location. Most pharmacies will destroy a patient's home medications if they are not retrieved within a specified time frame by the patient (e.g., 30 days after patient discharge).

Disposal of medicines

Many pharmacies use reverse distributors to dispose of expired pharmaceuticals. These reverse distributors ship all expired drugs back to the manufacturer for credit, and any items that do not meet the manufacturers' return policy becomes waste at the reverse distributor, who will then destroy the medications.[2]

When disposing of partially used vials, IV admixtures, or broken materials, most pharmacies and nursing units use biohazardous sharps containers.[2] Many pharmacies have used the drain to dispose of pharmaceuticals, although that practice is beginning to diminish because of environmental concerns.[2]

Federal regulations such as the Resource Conservation and Recovery Act (RCRA) in addition to state regulations have increased the complexity of hazardous pharmaceutical-waste management. It is important to check with federal and state regulators to make sure all pharmaceuticals are being disposed of properly.

Disposal and destruction of controlled substances by the pharmacy

Typically the pharmacy will use a reverse distributor to dispose of and destroy controlled substances. The reverse distributor must be registered with the Drug Enforcement Agency (DEA); it is the pharmacy's responsibility to verify that the reverse distributor is DEA registered.[3]

When the pharmacy transfers Schedule II controlled substances to a reverse distributor for destruction, the distributor must issue an Official Order Form (DEA Form-222) to the pharmacy. When the pharmacy transfers Schedule III-V controlled substances to a reverse distributor for destruction, the pharmacy must document in writing the drug name, dosage form, strength, quantity, and date transferred.

The reverse distributor who will destroy the controlled substances is responsible for submitting a DEA Form-41 to the DEA when the drugs have been destroyed. The DEA Form-41 should not be used when transferring the controlled substances between the pharmacy and reverse distributor responsible for disposing of the drugs.[3]

When a reverse distributor is not used, controlled substances must be destroyed so that they are beyond reclamation, and two licensed healthcare professionals must document the destruction.[1]

Records of destruction

In some cases state law may be more stringent about record-keeping requirements than federal law; in those cases, the state law must be complied with in addition to federal law.

According to federal law, the records involving the transfer or destruction of medications must be kept readily available for 2 years from the date of disposal for inspection and copying by the DEA.[4]

Records of controlled substances listed in Schedules I and II must be maintained separately from all other records. Records of controlled substances listed in Schedules III, IV, and V must be maintained either separately from all other records or in such form that the information required is readily retrievable from the ordinary business records.[4]

Disposal of medicines at home

Recent environmental studies have shown that flushing expired or unused medications can have an adverse impact on the environment. Patients should be counseled on how to properly dispose of their medications at home.

1 Hospitals for a Healthy Environment (2008). Managing pharmaceutical waste: a 10-step blueprint for health care facilities in the United States. August 2008. Available at: www.hercenter.org/hazmet/tenstepblueprint.pdf

2 Smith C (2002). Managing pharmaceutical waste—what pharmacists should know. *J Pharm Soc Wisc* Nov/Dec;17–22.

3 *The Pharmacist's Manual*, a summary of the DEA disposal requirements. www.deadiversion.usdoj.gov/pubs/manuals/pharm2/index.htm/

4 Code of Federal Regulations. Section 1304: Records and Reports of Registrants. http://www.deadiversion.usdoj.gov/21cfr/cfr/2104cfrt.htm

The American Pharmacists Association has developed guidance on proper disposal at home: 1) do not flush unused medications down the toilet or sink unless the label specifically states to do so and 2) when discarding unused medications, protect children and pets by crushing solid medications or dissolve in water and mix with kitty litter or solid kitchen substance (e.g., coffee grounds), then place in a sealed plastic bag. It is important to remind patients to remove and destroy all identifying personal information from the medication container prior to disposal.[5]

Many states and communities offer programs that allow the public to bring unused drugs to a central location for proper disposal. Check for approved state and local collection programs to direct patients to the best option for proper disposal of their unused or expired medications.

5 American Pharmacists Association (2008). APhA Provides Guidance on Proper Medication Disposal Use with Respect and Discard with Care. www.pharmacist.com

Chapter 14
Research

Michelle W. McCarthy
Nathan Powell

Audit and research

Research on humans should be subject to ethical committee review. Sometimes, there is a blurred distinction between audit or quality-assurance activities and research. Pharmacists need to consider projects carefully and ensure that they comply with local requirements. The following discussion helps to distinguish research from audit and quality assurance.

Audit (which might not need to go to IRB review)

- Measures the process and outcome of care
- Is not randomized
- Is usually initiated and conducted by those providing the clinical service
- Involves review of recorded data by those entitled to have access to such data
- Analysis is not performed with the intent to publish or present.

Research (should go to IRB review if it involves patients or volunteers)

- Randomized studies
- Data collection if outside personnel can access sensitive information about patients
- Interventions involving contact with patients by a health professional previously unknown to them
- Questionnaires asking for personal data or sensitive sociodemographic details
- If there is an intention to publish or present data as research
- If pharmaceutical data are collected (other than post-marketing surveillance)
- If patients or volunteers have any procedure additional to normal medical care
- If patient samples of any sort are taken additional to normal medical care

Writing a research proposal

Structure of a research proposal

- Title of project
- Purpose of the project
- Background of project
- Central research question(s)
- Research design
- Data analysis
- Timetable
- Research staff required
- Resources required
- Proposed budget
- References

Title of project

- Descriptive
- Clear
- Succinct
- Use recognizable key words
- Comprehendible (to nonspecialists)
- Should not imply an expected outcome

Examples

- "A randomized controlled trial of amitriptyline in chronic pain."
- "A descriptive study of the needs of patients on an orthopedic surgery unit."

Purpose of the project

- Why undertake the project?
- Who will benefit?
- Academic potential or contribution?
- Clinical potential or contribution?
- Patient potential or contribution?
- What gaps are likely to be filled?

Background of project

- Literature review
- Critical appraisal of literature and evidence
- Establish scientific adequacy of evidence
- Establish clinical and social adequacy of evidence
- Identify positive evidence and the potential to support, replicate, or challenge it
- Identify negative evidence and the potential to support, replicate, or challenge it
- Identify uncertain evidence and the potential to clarify, support, or reject it
- Identify lack of evidence and the potential to remedy this
- Justify research questions

Research questions

- Clear
- Specific
- Distinctive
- Comprehendible (to self and others)
- Answerable
- Feasible (scientifically and financially)

Research design

- Type of design
- Randomized controlled trial
- Matched comparison
- Cohort study
- Single case study
- Descriptive, ethnographic
- Sampling frame
- Sample selection criteria
- Baseline and follow-up strategy
- Measures and data to be collected (methods, outcome, satisfaction, costs)
- Access to data arrangements
- Ethical considerations (research often requires approval from an IRB or equivalent body (see Chapter 7, Institutional Review Boards, p. 122).

Data analysis

- How data will be stored?
- Manually and computerized
- Coded
- Entered
- Confidentiality and anonymity
- How data will be retrieved from computer?
- How data will be manipulated?
- Descriptive versus inductive
- Univariate, bivariate, or multivariate analysis

- Tests of significance
- Qualitative data handling
- Which statistical or epidemiological package? (e.g., SPSS)
- Data-presentation strategy
- Report-writing strategy (e.g., report, journal publications, book, meeting presentation or poster)

Timetable
- Preparation time
- Start baseline data collection
- Follow-up data collection
- End-of-data collection
- Data-retrieval time
- Data analysis
- Report preparation, writing and dissemination
- Do not underestimate the time involved—be realistic and keep to the schedule.

Research staff required
- Self
- Research assistants
- Interviewers
- Secretarial, administrative support
- Data entry, data retrieval, and handling staff
- Consultants (statistician, specialist advice, support)

Resources required
- Staff
- Accommodation (office space and storage space)
- Equipment
  - Computer hardware and software
  - Telephones, fax, e-mail
  - Furniture, filing cabinets, storage
  - Audio- and video-recording machinery
  - Specialist, technical equipment
- Laboratory time and access
- Books, journals, and library services
- Printing and stationery
- Postage
- Travel—both staff and reimbursement for participants in the study
- Overhead (staff and agency).

References

Provide supporting references in a standard format, according to Uniform Requirements or *American Medical Association Manual of Style* (see Chapter 14, p. 309)

Reference management software

Reference management software allows users to create personal database files so that references can be quickly stored, retrieved, and inserted into word-processing programs.

- Add references manually or by importing them directly from databases and publisher Web sites.
- Abstracts, tags, and other attachments such as pdf files can be downloaded and linked to specific references.
- Organize references by folder, author, or key word.
- Notes on each reference can be kept within the database and searched easily, allowing researchers to quickly find the information they need.

One of the most useful features of reference management software is the integration with word processors and the ability to forget about formatting in-text citations or bibliographies so that the writer can fully concentrate on content.

- The program will add the reference or a placeholder in the document and then create in-text citations or a bibliography based on the format the user chooses.
- Most programs come with hundreds of predefined output styles and users can add their own.
- As an example, it takes seconds to convert the in-text citations and bibliography of an entire document from the style required for *Pharmacotherapy* to the style required for *Annals of Pharmacotherapy*.

References can be exported in formatted bibliographies and some software programs even allow electronic sharing of references for seamless collaboration between researchers.

It is important that users become familiar with the range of products available. Some of the most popular programs for users in the sciences and health-care professions are Reference Manager®, ProCite®, EndNote®, and RefWorks®. Some are Web-based applications, meaning the reference database is accessible from any computer that has access to the Internet. Other programs store the reference databases on the user's computer or on a portable storage device and are available whether Internet access is available or not.

Most reference manager software products offer a trial period. It is recommended that prospective buyers define their own needs and find a product that is best suited for them.

Preparation of materials for publication

There are a variety of styles used to cite publications in the medical literature. Editors of several medical journals have established guidelines for the format of manuscripts submitted to their journals. This group, known as, the International Committee of Medical Journal Editors (ICMJE), has broadened its focus beyond manuscript and reference formatting to include ethical principles related to publication in biomedical journals. Many journals now follow ICMJE's *Uniform Requirements for Manuscripts Submitted to Biomedical Journals.*

Review of the Uniform Requirements is beyond the scope of this book. Those preparing materials for publication should review the following:

- *Uniform Requirements for Manuscripts Submitted to Biomedical Journals: Writing and Editing for Biomedical Publication.* October 2008. Available at: www.icmje.org/
- Patrias K. *Citing Medicine: The NLM Style Guide for Authors, Editors, and Publishers*, 2nd ed. Bethesda, MD: National Library of Medicine, 2007. Available at: www.nlm.nih.gov/citingmedicine
- Iverson C, Christiansen S, Flanagin A, et al. *AMA Manual of Style: A Guide for Authors and Editors*, 10th ed. New York: Oxford University Press, 2007.

Additionally, it is important to review and follow the "Information for Authors" for the journal to which the manuscript will be submitted.

Chapter 15
Therapy-related issues

Allergy and immunology

Lynn Limon

Cardiology

William D. Cahoon, Jr.
Frank A. Fulco
Donna M. White
Whitney D. Raper

Critical care

David Volles

Electrolyte disorders

Lena M. Maynor
Trisha N. Branan
Tina M. Grof
Amber G. Ormsby
Kelly L. Branham
Jessica L. Johnson
Shelby Raynor

Endocrinology

Donna M. White
Julie J. Kelsey
Nicole L. Metzger

Gastroenterology

Nancy S. Yunker
Jason C. Gallagher

Infectious diseases

Jason C. Gallagher
Patricia Pecora Fulco
Michelle W. McCarthy

Neurology

Kathleen A. Bledsoe

Oncology

Nikki M. Yost
Kathlene DeGregory
Mika Raye Kessans

Pain

Laura Morgan

Psychiatry

Ericka L. Breden

Pulmonary

Stacey Baker Pattie
Shelby Raynor
Chrissie V. Shirley
Jessica L. Johnson
Donna M. White

Transplant

Nathan Powell
Leah W. Paige

Toxicology

S. Rutherfoord Rose

Allergic rhinitis

Allergic rhinitis (AR) is caused by exposure to inhaled antigens that results in inflammation of nasal membranes. Diseases to rule out are infectious rhinitis, rhinitis medicamentosa, and hormonal rhinitis, as well as idiopathic and anatomic causes.

Nasal symptoms
- Excess mucus production
- Sneezing
- Congestion
- Nasal pruritus
- Rhinorrhea

Ocular symptoms
- Lacrimation
- Pruritus
- Edema

Constitutional symptoms
- Fatigue
- Malaise
- Headache

The process of sensitization and allergic response involves immunoglobulin E (IgE) antibodies, which line mucous membranes. After the initial allergen contact, IgE production increases and IgE then binds to the surface of mast cells. Upon re-exposure, allergen molecules bind and cross-link IgE on the mast cells of the nose and throat. Symptoms emerge after mast cell degranulation.

Immediate (or early-phase) response generates histamine, cytokines, kinins, proteases, interleukins, leukotrienes, and prostaglandins, triggering sneezing, itching, and rhinorhhea. Congestion is a late-phase response.

Types of allergic rhinitis
- Seasonal allergic rhinitis (SAR)
- Perennial allergic rhinitis (PAR)
- Mixed SAR/PAR

In those with SAR, nasal and ocular symptoms, such as tearing and conjunctivitis, occur during well-defined seasons, predominately in the spring (tree pollen, grass pollen) and autumn (ragweed pollen). Mowing of lawns in the spring and summer and raking of leaves in the autumn release outdoor mold spores into the air.

Symptoms from PAR persist most of the year because of allergy of antigens present year-round. These are due primarily to indoor allergens, such as house dust mites, animal dander, cockroaches, and indoor mold spores.

Treatment
- Allergen avoidance
- Allergen-specific immunotherapy
- Medications

Allergen avoidance and immunotherapy are the first and last treatments, respectively, for AR.

- Avoiding or at least minimizing exposure to environmental triggers is the most effective way to control symptoms. Indoor allergen avoidance includes controlling for dust mites, animal dander, insects, and indoor molds. Pollens and molds should be avoided outdoors and minimized inside by closing windows and using air conditioners.
- Immunotherapy consists of subcutaneous (SC) injections of identified allergens (for a duration of 3 to 5 years); tolerance gradually develops and patients have fewer AR symptoms.

The traditional SAR and PAR classifications are not helpful for specific selection of drug treatment. Instead, symptom assessment by 1) intermittent vs. persistent and 2) mild, moderate, or severe are now being used.

Intermittent is defined as occurring ≤4 days per week and ≤4 weeks in duration. *Persistent* symptoms continue for >4 days per week and >4 weeks in duration. *Mild* symptoms do not interfere with sleep, work, or school activities, whereas *moderate to severe* symptoms do interfere with these activities.

A stepwise approach is recommended, with an oral H1 antihistamine or an intranasal H1 antihistamine, a nasal chromone, or nasal saline for mild, intermittent symptoms. With moderate to severe intermittent symptoms, nasal corticosteroids are added to those options. In contrast, for moderate to severe persistent symptoms, nasal corticosteroids are the drugs of choice.

Antihistamines

First-generation oral H1 antihistamines include diphenhydramine, chlorpheniramine, brompheneramine, and hydroxyzine. While effective in controlling rhinnorhea, sneezing, and pruritus, the adverse effect of sedation is nearly universal. Even bedtime administration results in substantial residual daytime sedation. These agents are also poorly selective and agonize muscarinic receptors, resulting in other anticholinergic effects. These agents are not recommended for rhinitis treatment.

The second-generation oral H1 antihistamines are more selective and have anti-inflammatory properties. Overall, they are less sedating and have a faster onset, minimal CNS penetration, and a longer duration of action compared to the first-generation agents. Table 15.1 summarizes comparative dosing regimens for these agents.

Azelastine (1–2 sprays/nostril, bid) and olopatadine (2 sprays nostril, bid) are nasal antihistamines with a faster onset than that of their oral counterparts.

Nasal corticosteroids (see Table 15.2)

Nasal corticosteroids are effective in relieving both early- and late-phase symptoms in the nose, including congestion, itching, rhinnorhea, and sneezing. This class of agents is considered the most effective therapy for AR when taken consistently, although maximum efficacy may require at least 2 weeks of use. Unlike oral agents, nasal corticosteroids do not affect the hypothalamic–pituitary–adrenal (HPA) axis. Patients may prefer one product over another because of taste, smell, and aftertaste, as well as drug dripping down the throat.

Table 15.1 Second-generation oral H1 antihistamines

Rx/OTC	Generic name	Brand name	Dosage
OTC	Cetirizine	Zyrtec, generic	10 mg qd
Rx	Desloratadine	Clarinex	5 mg qd
Rx	Fexofenadine Immediate release Sustained release	Allegra, generic	60 mg bid 180 mg qd
Rx	Levocetirizine	Xyzal	5 mg qd
OTC	Loratadine	Claritin, generic	10 mg qd

Table 15.2 Corticosteroid nasal sprays

Generic name	Brand name	Daily dose/nostril
Beclomethasone	Beconase AQ	1–2 sprays bid
Budesonide	Rhinocort AQ	2 sprays qd
Ciclesonide	Omnaris	2 sprays qd
Flunisolide	Nasarel (generic)	2 sprays bid
Fluticasone propionate	Flonase (generics)	2 sprays qd
Fluticasone furoate	Veramyst	2 sprays qd
Mometasone	Nasonex	2 sprays qd
Triamcinolone	Nasocort AQ	2 sprays qd

Decongestants

Decongestants (nasal, oral, ocular) are considered adjunctive therapy. Nasal formulations are more effective; however, rebound congestion will occur within 3–5 days, limiting duration of use. Tissue hypertrophy and tachyphylaxis are also a risk.

Patients with hypertension, hyperthyroidism, benign prostatic hyperplasia, and glaucoma are not good candidates for oral decongestants. Table 15.3 lists these agents, showing their duration of effect.

Table 15.3 Decongestants

Dosage form	Duration of activity (hours)
Topical (nasal or ophthalmic)	
Phenylephrine	4
Naphazoline	4–6
Tetrahydrozoline	4–6
Oxymetazoline	12
Xylometazoline	10
Oral	
Ephedrine	4
Phenylephrine	4
Pseudoephedrine immediate release	4–6
Pseudoephedrine sustained release	12

Other agents

Montelukast
- Oral leukotriene modifer
- Useful for those with concomitant asthma
- Usual dose: 10 mg daily

Cromolyn
- Mast-cell stabilizer nasal spray (see Table 15.4)
- Works best when used around the clock
- Available over the counter (OTC)
- Drawback is the qid administration schedule

Ipratropium
- Anticholinergic nasal spray (see Table 15.4)
- Excellent for treating rhinorrhea
- Use 2 to 4 times daily

Table 15.4 Nasal spray administration

Clear nasal passages
Shake bottle
Tilt head forward
With bottle in right hand, place nozzle in left nostril away from nasal septum
Inhale and actuate bottle at the same time
Hold breath 5–10 seconds
Exhale slowly
Repeat steps, using left hand to spray right nostril
Don't blow nose for at least 1 minute
Close bottle and store as directed

Further reading

The most recent guidelines for the management of AR are from the World Health Organization's workshop for Allergic Rhinitis and Its Impact on Asthma (ARIA). An update to a 1999 publication was released in 2007 and is available at http://www.whiar.org

Dermatological drug reactions

Dermatological drug reactions occur via nonimmunological or immunological mechanisms. With nonimmunological reactions, cutaneous effects result from a variety of factors, including cumulative toxicity, overdose, drug–drug interactions, and metabolic alterations.

With immunological reactions, drugs or their metabolites act as haptens, binding covalently with peptides, becoming immunogenic. They can be characterized according to the Gell and Coombs classification of hypersensitivity, types I–IV.

Gell Coombs classification

Type I reaction

- IgE mediated
- Uticaria
- Angioedema
- Symptoms occur after 1–2 hours (with oral medications)

Type II reaction

- IgG or IgM mediated
- Antibiotic-induced hemolytic anemia and thrombocytopenia
- Autoimmune bullous disease (i.e., drug-induced pemphigus)

Type III reaction

- Circulating soluble complexes of drug antigens and specific IgG or IgM antibodies deposit in tissue
- Antibiotic-associated serum sickness

Type IV reaction

- Delayed-type hypersensitivity reactions mediated by T lymphocytes that recognize antigens
- Contact dermatitis
- Exanthematous drug eruptions
- Fixed drug eruptions
- Stevens–Johnson syndrome (SJS)
- Toxic epidermal necrolysis (TEN)

Diagnosis

- Chronology of drug administration
- Patient age and hormonal status
- Accurate description of primary skin lesions
- Suspect medications known to cause dermatological reactions
- Discontinue suspected drug(s)

Exanthematous drug eruptions

- Most common type of cutaneous drug reaction
- Maculopapular rash, similar to measles, distributed on trunk or pressure areas, often symmetrical
- Begins 7–14 days after initiation of therapy
- Typically resolves in 1–2 weeks without sequelae
- Most frequently associated with penicillin family

- Differential diagnosis is a viral exanthema
- Symptomatic treatment with oral antihistamines and topical corticosteroids

Fixed drug eruptions

- Second most common type of cutaneous drug reaction
- Erythematous or hyperpigmented round or local lesion, up to 20 cm in diameter
- Appears on face, lips, hands, feet, genitalia
- Color varies: red, red-brown, gray, blue, violaceous
- Begins 7–14 days after initiation of therapy
- Upon rechallenge, lesion appears in identical place
- Sulfonamides, NSAIDs, tetracyclines, barbiturates, carbamazepine
- Differential diagnosis is an insect bite
- Asymptomatic; treatment is discontinuation of drug
- Hyperpigmentation can persist for weeks to months after resolution of the eruption

Urticaria

- Acute urticaria is eruption of edematous papules and plaques.
- Lesions appear within minutes to days; abate in less than 24 hours
- >6 weeks in duration is chronic urticaria
- Etiology
  - Penicillins, cephalosporins, sulfonamides, tetracyclines
  - Interaction between infectious agent and medication (i.e., Epstein–Barr virus and amoxicillin)
- Anaphylactoid reactions
  - Mimic type I reactions
  - Caused by histamine release from mast cells
  - Aspirin, NSAIDs, morphine, codeine, quinine, radiological contrast media
- May progress to angioedema and/or anaphylaxis

Drug-mediated photosensitive drug eruption

- Occurs only on sun-exposed skin
- Begins as exaggerated sunburn, progresses to papules, vesicle formation, edema in minutes to hours
- Localized eruption suggests reaction to topical agent; widespread eruption suggests reaction to systemic photosensitizing agent
- Discontinue agent; symptomatic treatment is with corticosteroids
- Phototoxic drug reaction
  - Absorption of UV radiation, releasing energy damaging to epidermal cells
  - Thiazide diuretics, furosemide, diltiazem, sulfonamides, psoralens, fluoroquinolones, tetracyclines
- Photoallergic drug reaction
  - Absorption of UV radiation causes drug to bind as hapten to native protein on epidermal cells
  - Creates antigen that sensitizes nearby lymphocytes
  - Dapsone, quinidine, phenothiazines

Drug-induced pseudoporphyria

- Fragile blisters develop in sun-exposed areas that resemble porphyria lesions.
- Dorsum of the hands, forearms, ears, face
- Naproxen, other NSAIDs, tetracyclines
- Does not produce hypertrichosis and dyschromia, as with porphyria

TEN, SJS, and erythema multiforme

Anticonvulsants, sulfonamides, allopurinol, NSAIDs, and dapsone can cause all three syndromes.

TEN

- Influenza symptoms prodrome lasting up to 14 days
- Epidermal–dermal bonding is disrupted
- Widespread, full-thickness epidermal necrosis in >30% of body surface area
- 40% mortality
- Skin sloughing more treatable than surfaces lined with mucosa (conjunctiva, gastrointestinal tract)
- Medical emergency; patients should be managed in burn units
- Treatment is fluid replacement, nutritional supplementation, sterile technique, and wound care.
- Use of corticosteroids is controversial.

SJS

- Characterized by widespread erythematous or purpuric macules and targetoid lesions
- Rate of epidermal detachment is <10%
- 5% mortality
- Treatment is fluid replacement, nutritional supplementation, sterile technique, and wound care.

Erythema multiforme

- Characterized by targetoid lesions, with or without blisters
- Most cases secondary to prior herpes virus infection
- Low morbidity and mortality
- May be the same disease process as SJS

Drug hypersensitivity syndrome

- Dermatological manifestation along with internal-organ toxicity
- Triad of fever, skin eruption, and internal organ involvement
- Begins 1–6 weeks after initiation of therapy
- Prodrome mimics viral upper respiratory tract infection
- May result in exanthematous eruptions, erythroderma, SJS, or TEN
- Internal-organ damage may include lymphadenopathy, hepatitis, nephritis, or pneumonitis.

Hyperpigmentation

- Caused by medication or disturbances in melanin production
- Oral contraceptives, antimalarial agents, phenothiazines, tetracyclines, amiodarone

Drug desensitization

Desensitization is the process of decreasing a patient's sensitivity to an allergen. In most cases, an alternative agent should be used that doesn't cross react with the drug to which the patient is sensitive. This can be of the same drug class but with a different side chain.

Desensitization involves introducing minute amounts of the drug and then slowly increasing the dose (usually by doubling) every 15–20 minutes until a full therapeutic dose is achieved. The potential for a reaction is lessened when the oral route is used. Drug desensitization is accomplished over hours, as compared to the methods used for allergy shots (i.e., allergy to pollen, dust), which are much slower, usually needing months to complete the process.

During the procedure the appearance of mild skin reactions such as pruritus or urticaria is common. The sensitized state lasts only as long as the drug is given. Once it is stopped, the patient becomes sensitive again in 8–48 hours and must be desensitized again. A low dose of the agent may be given daily if it is anticipated that the drug will be given again.

Common examples of drugs for which desensitization has been successful include antimicrobial agents, aspirin, insulin, and cancer agents. All doses, whether oral or parenteral, should be prepared under controlled conditions, preferably in the hospital pharmacy.

The following precautions should be observed during desensitization:

- The patient must give written consent.
- Any other drugs know to exacerbate allergic reactions should be discontinued.
- The procedure must be performed in a controlled setting.
- Emergency drugs and someone to administer them must be present throughout the procedure.
- Intravenous access is obtained before the procedure begins.
- Prophylaxis (antihistamines, corticosteroids) is not advised, as this may mask a reaction.
- Monitoring before each dose and at every interval includes:
- Temperature, blood pressure, pulse, respiratory rate
- Observation and direct questioning regarding signs and symptoms of allergic reactions (skin flushing, rash, itching, wheeze, shortness of breath, tingling of lips or tongue)
- The patient should be observed for at least 1 hour following the final dose of the desensitization schedule.

Rheumatoid arthritis

Rheumatoid arthritis (RA) is the most common systemic inflammatory disease that causes chronic pain, stiffness, swelling, and limitation in the motion and function of multiple, and usually symmetrical, joints. The small joints in the hands and feet are most commonly affected. Inflammation may develop extra-articularly, causing vasculitis, eye inflammation, neurological dysfunction, cardiopulmonary disease, lymphadenopathy, and splenomegaly.

RA is three times more common in women than in men. While it is still unclear why RA occurs, a genetic predisposition and exposure to unknown environmental factors may be responsible. Chronic inflammation of synovial tissue results in proliferation that produces erosions of bone and cartilage. Better understanding of the complex immunological factors involved in this disease have led to newer, very effective disease-modifying pharmacological agents.

Signs, symptoms, and laboratory findings

- Morning stiffness
- Rheumatoid nodules
- Energy loss
- Low-grade fevers
- Appetite loss
- Dry mouth, dry eyes (Sjogren's syndrome)
- Normocytic, normochromic anemia
- Thrombocytosis
- Elevated erythrocyte sedimentation rate (ESR)
  - Elevated with other inflammatory diseases
- Elevated C-reactive protein (CRP)
- Rheumatoid factor (RF)
  - Present in 60%–70% of RA patients
  - Large interpatient variability
- Antinucelar antibodies (ANA)
- Turbid synovial fluid
- Radiological findings
  - Periarticular osteoporosis
  - Erosions
  - Used periodically to monitor disease progression

Treatment

Cartilage damage and bony erosions may occur within the first 2 years of RA. The early use of disease-modifying drugs and the continuing availability of newer biological agents has dramatically improved the outcomes of most RA patients.

Treatment requires a wide-ranging plan to support patients medically, socially, and emotionally. Options include medications, reduction of joint stress, physical and occupational therapy, and surgical intervention.

Goals of therapy

- Achieve lowest possible level of RA disease activity, with remission if possible
- Minimization of joint damage
- Enhance physical function
- Improve quality of life

Pharmacological therapy

Nonsteroidal anti-inflammatory agents (NSAIDs), corticosteroids, and disease-modifying antirheumatic drugs (DMARDs) are the three general classes of drugs commonly used in the treatment of RA. In general, NSAIDs and corticosteroids act more quickly than DMARDs, which take weeks or months to demonstrate a clinical effect.

NSAIDs

- Reduce stiffness by decreasing acute inflammation
- Provide analgesia
- High end of dosage range
- Trial period should be weeks to 1 month
- Seldom used as monotherapy

Corticosteroids

- Control symptoms before onset of action of DMARDs
- Local injections in joints and soft tissue used to control local inflammation
- Provide DMARD action but adverse events (e.g., osteoporosis, infection) preclude long-term chronic use
- Pulse therapy used for acute flares

The 2008 guidelines from the American College of Rheumatology include recommendations for the use of nonbiological and biological DMARDs. Not included in this updated list of medications are familiar agents historically used for RA treatment—gold, cyclophosphamide, D-penicillamine, azathioprine, cyclosporine, and tacrolimus. One of the newer biological DMARDs, anakinra, is also not included in their recommendations.

DMARDs—nonbiological

- *Methotrexate:* 7.5 mg PO once weekly or 2.5 mg PO every 12 hours for 3 doses once weekly (maximum dose 20 mg weekly)
- *Leflunomide:* 100 mg PO daily for 3 days then 20 mg PO daily (may reduce maintenance dose to 10 mg PO daily if side effects)
- *Hydroxychloroquine:* 400–600 mg PO daily for 4–12 weeks, then 200–400 mg PO daily
- *Minocycline:* 100 mg PO twice daily
- *Sulfasalazine:* 0.5–1 g PO daily (or in divided dose of twice daily), then 1 g PO twice daily (maximum dose 3 g daily)
- Double- and triple-agent combinations

DMARDs—biological

Anti-tumor necrosis factor (TNF) agents

- *Adalimumab* (for moderate to severe RA and receiving other DMARDs): 40 mg SC every other week; dose may be increased to 40 mg SC weekly if not receiving concomitant methotrexate
- *Etanercept:* 50 mg SC weekly
- *Infliximab:* 3 mg/kg IV infusion at weeks 0, 2, 6, then every 8 weeks (in combination with methotrexate); may increase to 10 mg/kg every 8 weeks or 3 mg/kg every 4 weeks if incomplete responses

T-cell costimulatory blocking agents

- *Abatacept:* 500 mg IV infusion (<60 kg), 750 mg IV (60–100 kg), 100 mg (>100 kg) at weeks 2 and 4 after the initial dose, then every 4 weeks

B-cell deleting agents

- *Rituxumab:* 1000 mg IV infusion for 2 doses (separated by a 2 week interval). Use in combination with methotrexate

All of the biologics require careful monitoring and have the potential for serious adverse effects. Refer to individual package inserts for this information.

Further reading

Recent guidelines on the use of DMARDs for the management of RA are:

Saag KG, Teng GG, Patkar NM, et al. (2008). American College of Rheumatology 2008 recommendations for the use of nonbiologic and biologic disease-modifying antirheumatic drugs in rheumatoid arthritis. *Arthritis Rheum* **59**:762–784. Also available at: www.rheumatology.org/practice/#guidelines

Systemic lupus erythematosus and other collagen-vascular diseases

Collagen-vascular diseases are a heterogenous group of diseases that have an immune-mediated pathogenesis and varied clinical manifestations. Systemic lupus erythematosus (SLE) is the most well known. Other commonly seen collagen-vascular diseases include systemic sclerosis, polymyositis/dermatositis, polymyalgia rheumatica/giant cell arteritis, and drug-induced vasculitis. Drug-induced lupus erythematosus is related to these diseases.

Systemic lupus erythematosus

SLE is a disease most commonly observed in young women who are African American, Hispanic, Native American, or Asian. The etiology of abnormal autoantibody production with formation of immune complexes is largely unknown. Inflammatory reactions leading to tissue damage result from defective clearance of the immune complexes.

Clinical presentation

Each patient presents differently, although most initially complain of arthritis and arthralgia. A butterfly rash on the face is also initially present in approximately 50% of newly diagnosed patients.

Common signs and symptoms

- Arthritis, arthralgia
- Fatigue, fever, weight loss
- Butterfly rash, photosensitivity, Raynaud's phenomenon, discoid lesions
- Psychosis, seizures
- Pleuritis
- Pericarditis, myocarditis, heart murmur, hypertension
- Nephritis
- Nausea, abdominal pain, bowel hemorrhage
- Anemia, leukopenia, thrombocytopenia
- Lymphadenopathy

Treatment goals

- Management of symptoms and induction of remission
- Maintenance of remission for as long as possible between flares

Nonpharmacological therapy

- Balanced routine of rest and exercise to help counter fatigue
- Limited exposure to sunlight

Pharmacological therapy

NSAIDs are used initially to manage fever, arthritis, and serositis. NSAIDs may affect renal function by decreasing blood flow and glomerular filtration. This can be mistakenly attributed to the effects of lupus nephritis.

Of note, NSAID-associated hepatotoxicity is observed more often in SLE patients than in the normal population, and there is an association in those with SLE between aseptic meningitis and NSAID use.

Antimalarials are useful for SLE-associated cutaneous problems, arthralgia, pleuritis, pericardial inflammation, fatigue, and leucopenia. Hydroxychloroquine (used most often) and chloroquine both need at least 3 months to achieve effectiveness. Dose and duration are based on tolerability and toxicity, particularly to the retina.

Corticosteroids are not used in patients with mild disease. However, as SLE progresses, or in those with lupus nephritis, CNS disease, pneumonitis, polyserositis, vasculitis, and/or thrombocytopenia, corticosteroids are indicated. The lowest dose possible to manage symptoms is used, ranging from prednisone 10–20 mg/day to 1–3 mg/kg/day. High-dose pulse therapy with parenteral methylprednisolone followed by prednisone tapered back down to maintenance doses is used for patients who have life-threatening SLE manifestations.

The cytotoxic immunosuppressant agent cyclophosphamide, in combination with prednisone, is an established treatment for SLE, particularly in those with lupus nephritis. Clinical trial data support this combination as it preserves renal function and decreases the risk of developing end-stage renal failure. Cyclophosphamide is dosed at 1–3 mg/kg orally and 0.5–1.0 g/m^2 for intravenous (IV) administration (used concomitantly with mesna to prevent hemorrhagic cystitis). A common regimen is every month for 6 months, then every 3 months of either 2 years or for 1 year after the nephritis is in remission.

Azathioprine may be used as a steroid-sparing agent.

Newer therapies include mycophenolate and rituxumab; many other biological agents are being investigated on the basis of better understanding of the immunological basis of SLE.

Drug-induced lupus erythematosus

Drug-induced lupus erythematosus can develop months to years after exposure to a drug. The most commonly implicated drugs are hydralazine, procainamide, quinidine, isoniazid, diltiazem, and minocycline. An extensive list of drugs associated with drug-induced lupus is available at www.Emedicine.com/DERM/topic107htm

Differential diagnosis of idiopathic SLE and drug-induced lupus is

- Exposure to a suspected drug
- No prior history of idiopathic SLE
- Development of antinuclear antibodies (ANAs)
- At least one clinical feature of SLE
- Rapid decline of ANAs and symptomatic improvement when drug is discontinued

Systemic sclerosis

Clinical manifestations

- Sclerosis of the skin
- Raynaud's phenomenon
- Dyspepsia
- Constipation
- Diarrhea
- Steatorrhea
- Esophageal dysmotility

Treatment

- D-penicillamine
- Angiotensin-converting enzyme (ACE) inhibitors
- Calcium channel blockers

Polymyositis (PM) and dermatomyositis (DM)

Clinical manifestations

- Inflammation of skeletal muscle (PM) and skin (DM)
- Muscle weakness
- Arthritis
- Raynaud's phenomenon

Treatment

- Physical therapy
- Prednisone (muscle weakness is also a potential adverse effect of long-term corticosteroid therapy)
- Azathioprine for prednisone resistance
- Immunosuppressant

Polymyalgia rheumatica and giant cell arteritis

Approximately 15% of patients with polymyalgia rheumatica develop giant cell arteritis (GCA) and approximately 50% of patients with GCA have associated polymyalgia rheumatica.

Clinical manifestations

- Proximal myalgia of the hip and shoulder girdles with accompanying morning stiffness that lasts >1 hour
- Low-grade fever
- Weight loss
- Malaise
- Fatigue
- Depression

Treatment

Corticosteroids induce a complete or near-complete remission.

Drug-induced vasculitis

Clinical manifestations

- Rash
- Glomerulonephritis
- Hepatitis
- Fatigue
- Myalgias
- Arthralgias
- Fever

Treatment

- Discontinue drug
- Corticosteroids and/or immunosuppressive therapy if symptoms continue

Angina

Angina pectoris is the clinical manifestation of transient myocardial ischemia caused by an imbalance of myocardial oxygen supply and demand. Angina often manifests as chest discomfort described as pressure, tightness, heaviness, squeezing, or burning, though pain may radiate to the arms, neck, or jaw. Patients may also experience atypical signs of angina, such as shortness of breath, nausea/vomiting, or lightheadedness.

Types of angina (Table 15.5)

- Chronic stable angina
- Unstable angina
- Variant (Prinzmetal's) angina

Risk factors

- Cigarette smoking
- Diabetes
- Hypercholesterolemia
- Hypertension
- Sedentary lifestyle
- Family history of premature heart disease

Goals of therapy

- Relief of symptoms
- Prevention or slowing of disease progression
- Prevention of cardiac events
- Improved survival

Table 15.5 Types of angina

	Chronic stable angina	Unstable angina	Variant (Prinzmetal's) angina
Predictable?	Yes	No	No
Relieved by rest?	Yes	No	No
Relieved by SL NTG?	Yes	Variable	Yes
Fixed coronary stenosis?	Yes	No	Variable
Evolving coronary stenosis?	No	Yes	No
Coronary vasospasm?	No	No	Yes

NTG, nitroglycerin.

Acute angina therapy

- Sublingual (SL) NTG 0.4 mg every 5 minutes for a maximum of 3 doses in 15 minutes
- Translingual [spray] NTG 0.4 mg every 5 minutes for a maximum of 3 doses in 15 minutes

Avoid nitrates if patient has used sildenafil (Viagra®) in the previous 24 hours or tadalafil (Cialis®) or vardenafil (Levitra®) in the previous 5 days.

Patients should be instructed to sit or lie down when taking NTG because of the risk of hypotension. If symptoms have not improved within 5 minutes of the first dose of NTG, patients should seek emergency medical care.

Continuing treatment

Chronic stable angina

Antiplatelets

- Aspirin 75–162 mg should be started and continued indefinitely in all patients without contraindications.
- Clopidogrel 75 mg daily should be used as an alternative in patients with contraindications to aspirin.

Angiotensin-converting enzyme (ACE) inhibitors

- ACE inhibitors should be started and continued indefinitely in patients with left ventricular ejection fraction (LVEF) $<$40%, or those with diabetes, hypertension, or chronic kidney disease.
- Angiotensin receptor blockers (ARB) should be used in patients with indications for, but who are intolerant of, ACE inhibitors.

Anti-anginals (see Table 15.6)

All anti-anginals—nitrates, calcium-channel blockers, beta-blockers—prolong exercise tolerance prior to the onset of angina and/or ischemia. It is reasonable to start therapy with any of the three classes of anti-anginals, though combinations may be necessary to adequately control anginal symptoms. Caution is advised with the combination of beta-blockers and non-dihydropyridine calcium-channel blockers (e.g. diltiazem, verapamil).

Ranolazine

Ranolazine, which was FDA approved in 2006, provides anti-anginal effects without affecting hemodynamic parameters (e.g., BP, heart rate). Ranolazine should be reserved for patients on optimal doses of other anti-anginals, or for patients who cannot tolerate anti-anginal dose increases because of hemodynamic limitations (e.g., hypotension, bradycardia).

Risk factor management

Risk factor reduction is central to achieving the goals of anginal therapy. Slowing progression and reducing cardiovascular events and mortality can be achieved by managing risk factors:

- Smoking cessation
- Blood pressure management (BP $<$140/90 mmHg, or $<$130/80 mmHg in those with diabetes or chronic kidney disease)
- Diabetes management (near-normal hemoglobin A1c [HbA1c])

Table 15.6 Dosing regimens for anti-anginals in chronic stable angina

Drug	Class	Dose range
Isosorbide mononitrate	Nitrate	Regular release: 5–20 mg twice daily Extended release: 60–240 mg once daily
Isosorbide dinitrate	Nitrate	5–80 mg twice to 3 times daily
NTG patch	Nitrate	0.2–0.8 mg/hr worn for 12 hours
Atenolol	Beta-blocker	50–200 mg/day
Metoprolol	Beta-blocker	50–200 mg twice daily
Amlodipine	Ca-channel blocker	5–10 mg/day
Nifedipine	Ca-channel blocker	30–90 mg/day
Diltiazem	Ca-channel blocker	Immediate release: 30–90 mg 4 times daily Delayed release: 120–320 mg daily
Verapamil	Ca-channel blocker	Immediate release: 80–160 mg 3 times daily Delayed release: 120–480 mg daily

- Lipid management (LDL <100 mg/dL, with optional goal of <70 mg/dL)
- Encourage physical activity (30–60 minutes, 7 days per week)
- Weight reduction

Variant (Prinzmetal's) angina

Medical therapy of variant angina consists of risk factor management (as with chronic stable angina) and pharmacological therapy with vasodilators. Calcium-channel blockers and nitrates are first-line therapy, as they are effective vasodilators of the coronary vasculature.

Further reading

The American College of Cardiology (ACC) and American Heart Association (AHA) have produced joint guideline statements on the management of chronic stable angina. The 2007 focused guideline update is available at: http://circ.ahajournals.org/cgi/reprint/CIRCULATIONAHA.107.187930

Unstable angina and non-ST elevation myocardial infarction

Unstable angina (UA) and non-ST elevation myocardial infarction (NSTEMI) are manifestations of progressive ischemic heart disease caused by plaque rupture and coronary thrombosis. UA and NSTEMI compromise blood flow and, therefore, oxygen supply to areas of the myocardium, thereby producing ischemia.

Signs and symptoms

Unlike chronic stable angina, UA and NSTEMI are characterized by less predictable and inconsistent chest pain that is more frequent and less responsive to sublingual (SL) NTG, and not relieved by rest (angina at rest >20 minutes). Angina associated with UA and NSTEMI is often characterized as chest discomfort or pressure that may radiate to the shoulders, arms, neck, or jaw.

Some patients, often the elderly, diabetics, or women, may present with atypical signs and symptoms of UA and NSTEMI:

- Shortness of breath
- Sweating
- Nausea/vomiting
- Palpitations
- Syncope

Diagnosis

The diagnosis of UA or NSTEMI is based on several factors:

- Patient history
- Physical exam
- Electrocardiogram (ECG)
- ST-segment depression (2 or more contiguous leads)
- T-wave inversion
- Biochemical (cardiac) markers (i.e., troponin, creatine kinase-MB)

UA and NSTEMI are often indistinguishable at initial presentation and are considered part of the same clinical syndrome. NSTEMI may be distinguished from UA solely by the presence of positive biochemical markers.

Goals of therapy

- Immediate relief of ischemia
- Prevention of serious adverse outcomes (i.e., death or re-infarction)

Risk stratification

Early risk stratification is useful in identifying high-risk patients who may benefit from more aggressive therapy. One risk stratification tool, the TIMI risk stratification score, identifies seven independent variables associated with patient outcome following UA or NSTEMI[1]:

- Age ≥65 years
- Presence of at least three coronary heart disease risk factors

1. Antman EM, Cohen M, Bernink PJ, et al. (2000). The TIMI risk score for unstable angina/non-ST elevation MI: a method for prognostication and therapeutic decision making. *JAMA* **284**:835–842.

- Prior coronary stenosis ≥50%
- Presence of ST-segment deviation on ECG
- At least two anginal episodes in previous 24 hours
- Elevated serum cardiac markers
- Use of aspirin in the past 7 days

Patients receive one point for each independent risk factor present. Patients with 0–2 points are considered low risk, 3–4 points are intermediate risk, and 5–7 points are at high risk for recurrent ischemia, recurrent myocardial infarction, and all-cause mortality.

Initial therapy

Initial management of UA or NSTEMI should consist of morphine, oxygen, nitrates, aspirin, and a beta-blocker (Table 15.7).

Morphine

In theory, morphine may be beneficial for reducing ischemia by reducing the oxygen demand associated with pain and anxiety. Morphine, however, has not been demonstrated to improve cardiovascular outcomes following UA and NSTEMI. Despite the lack of outcomes data, morphine remains a standard of care due to its analgesic and anxiolytic properties.

Oxygen

Oxygen should be administered to all UA and NSTEMI patients with arterial oxygen saturations <90%. Increasing arterial oxygen supply may serve to lessen ischemia.

Nitrates

Nitrates have the beneficial effects of reducing myocardial oxygen demand while improving oxygen supply. Though not shown to reduce mortality or to improve other cardiovascular outcomes, nitrates are beneficial in attenuating ischemia and alleviating patients' symptoms.

Table 15.7 Dosing regimens for initial therapy in UA and NSTEMI

Drug	Dose	Notes
Morphine	2–4 mg every 5–15 minutes as needed	Monitor blood pressure
Oxygen	Inhaled oxygen to maintain saturation >90%	Supplemental oxygen may be given to all UA/NSTEMI patients
Nitrates	SL NTG: 0.4 mg every 5 minutes IV NTG: 10 mcg/min	SL: may give up to 3 doses IV: titrate every 3–5 minutes
Aspirin	162–325 mg orally or chewed	Chewing achieves high blood concentrations more rapidly
Beta-blocker	PO: Metoprolol 25 mg IV: Metoprolol 5 mg	IV administration reserved for tachycardia or hypertension

Aspirin

Aspirin, an antiplatelet agent, is the only initial therapy with proven mortality and cardiovascular benefits. Aspirin diminishes platelet aggregation, a key step in thrombus formation, thereby limiting the degree of arterial occlusion.

Beta-blockers

Beta-blockers reduce myocardial oxygen demand by competitively inhibiting the sympathetic nervous system's effects on heart rate and myocardial contractility. Beta-blockers, administered orally, should be given early in the course of care. IV administration may be considered in limited situations, including ongoing angina with associated hypertension or tachycardia.

Anticoagulant therapy (Table 15.8)

Heparin

Heparin, an anti-thrombin agent, is the historic gold standard for anticoagulation in UA and NSTEMI. While enoxaparin has more predictable effects and requires less monitoring, heparin does not require renal dose adjustment. Heparin is a first-line agent for either invasive or conservative management of UA and NSTEMI.

Low-molecular-weight heparin (LMWH)

Enoxaparin, a low-molecular weight heparin, has demonstrated superiority when directly compared with unfractionated heparin. Enoxaparin also has the added benefits of a more predictable response while not requiring laboratory monitoring. Like heparin, LMWH is a first-line agent for either invasive or conservative management of UA and NSTEMI.

Bivalirudin

Bivalirudin, an IV direct thrombin inhibitor, has recently been added to the list of anticoagulants available for UA and NSTEMI management. On the basis of the ACUITY study, which showed similar rates of ischemia and bleeding to those with heparin, bivalirudin is now a first-line

Table 15.8 Dosing regimens for anticoagulants in UA and NSTEMI

Drug	Dose	Notes
Heparin	Bolus: 60 mg/kg Infusion: 12 mg/kg/hr	No renal dose adjustment required
Enoxaparin	Bolus: 30 mg IV Maintenance: 1 mg/kg every 12 hours	Renal dose adjustment required
Bivalirudin	Bolus: 0.1 mg/kg Infusion: 0.25 mg/kg/hr	Contraindicated: CrCl <30 mL/min
Fondaparinux	2.5 mg SC once daily	Renal dose adjustment required

alternative to heparin or LMWH in patients undergoing invasive management.[2] Bivalirudin also provides a non-heparin alternative in patients with a history of heparin-induced thrombocytopenia (HIT) undergoing UA or NSTEMI management.

Fondaparinux

Like bivalirudin, fondaparinux is a recent addition to the list of anticoagulants available for UA and NSTEMI management. Fondaparinux, a subcutaneous factor Xa inhbitor, demonstrated a reduction in major bleeding while maintaining a similar risk reduction to that with enoxaparin.[3] Fondaparinux is a first-line alternative to heparin or LMWH in patients undergoing either invasive or conservative management. Fondaparinux may be the agent of choice for conservative management of patients with a high risk of bleeding.

Antiplatelet therapy

Aspirin

Aspirin is an antiplatelet agent with proven mortality and cardiovascular outcomes benefits. Aspirin should be administered as soon as possible after presentation and continued indefinitely. In patients with a previous history of gastrointestinal (GI) bleeding, proton pump inhibitors (PPIs) may be given concurrently to prevent recurrent GI bleeding.

Thienopyridines

Ticlopidine and clopidogrel are adenosine diphosphate (ADP) inhibitors that have antiplatelet activity. Ticlopidine has an increased risk of causing myelotoxicity, thus clopidogrel is used over ticlopidine in patients intolerant of or allergic to aspirin.

Clopidogrel should also be given with aspirin in certain clinical situations. For example, patients being treated with an initial conservative strategy should receive aspirin and clopidogrel. For patients undergoing an invasive management strategy, either clopidogrel or a glycoprotein IIb–IIIa inhibitor should be given in addition to aspirin before angiography. Clopidogrel should be held for 5–7 days prior to CABG.

Glycoprotein IIb–IIIa inhibitors (Table 15.9)

Glycoprotein IIb–IIIa inhibitors inhibit platelet aggregation by blocking the final common platelet receptor. For invasive management, glycoprotein IIb–IIIa inhibitors have proven benefits and may be given in addition to aspirin before angiography. In conservative management, however, glycoprotein IIb–IIIa inhibitors should be limited to patients with high-risk features, including recurrent ischemia, continued cardiac biomarker elevation, hemodynamic instability, and TIMI risk score >4.

The optimal timing of administration of these agents has yet to be clearly defined. In certain circumstances, such as patients with high-risk features, the combination of aspirin, clopidogrel, and glycoprotein IIb–IIIa inhibitors may be considered when benefits outweigh risk of bleeding.

2 Stone GW, McLaurin BT, Cox DA, et al. (2006). Bivalirudin for patients with acute coronary syndromes. *N Engl J Med* **355**:2203–2216.

3 Yusuf S, Mehta SR, Chrolavicius S, et al. (2006). Comparison of enoxaparin and fondaparinux in acute coronary syndromes. *N Engl J Med* **354**:1464–1476.

Table 15.9 Dosing regimens for glycoprotein IIb–IIIa inhibitors in UA and NSTEMI

Drug	Dose	Renal adjustment	Reversible
Abciximab	Bolus: 0.25 mg/kg Infusion: 10 mcg/min	No	No
Eptifibatide	Bolus: 180 mcg/kg Infusion: 2 mcg/kg/min	Yes	Yes
Tirofiban	First 30 minutes: 0.4 mcg/kg/min Continued dose: 0.1 mcg/kg/min	Yes	Yes

Invasive vs. conservative management

Two management strategies, invasive and conservative, exist for UA and NSTEMI management. Invasive management typically consists of diagnostic angiography within the first 4–24 hours of admission, with percutaneous coronary intervention (PCI) or coronary artery bypass grafting (CABG) as indicated. Patients treated with invasive management are also, however, treated with the previously mentioned UA/NSTEMI medications (i.e., anticoagulants, antiplatelets, and anti-ischemics).

In the conservative management strategy, diagnostic angiography is used only in those who fail medical therapy (i.e., refractory angina) or in those with evidence of ongoing ischemia, such as a positive stress test.

The decision to follow an invasive or conservative management strategy is at the discretion of the individual patient and/or treating physician. However, the conservative strategy is generally reserved for patients with a low-risk score in the absence of high-risk features.

Invasive management, by contrast, is preferred for patients with recurrent angina, elevated cardiac markers, hemodynamic instability, sustained ventricular tachycardia, PCI within the previous 6 months, prior CABG, or reduced LVEF.

Continuing treatment

The goals of continued treatment following UA or NSTEMI are to moderate and control risk factors, reduce recurrence of ischemia, and improve survival. Several medication classes have been identified that address these goals and should be a routine component of post-UA/NSTEMI care.

Statins

Statins have proven benefits, including primary and secondary prevention of coronary heart disease, for patients post-UA/NSTEMI. These benefits, however, extend beyond lipid lowering. Pleiotropic effects, including plaque stabilization, decreased inflammation, and decreased thrombogenicity, have been demonstrated and are thought to contribute to the morbidity and mortality benefits of statin therapy.

Antiplatelet therapy

Aspirin 75–162 mg should be prescribed and continued indefinitely in patients recovering from UA or NSTEMI. Higher initial doses (aspirin 162–325 mg) should be considered in patients who are revascularized (i.e., undergo catheterization with intervention).

Clopidogrel 75 mg daily should be prescribed for at least 1 month and ideally up to 1 year in all post-UA/NSTEMI patients. Patients who receive bare metal stents (BMS) should be prescribed clopidogrel for at least 1 month, whereas those who receive drug-eluting stents (DES) should continue clopidogrel for at least 1 year.

ACE inhibitors

ACE inhibitors have proven beneficial effects after acute ST-elevation MI; however, less data is available regarding their efficacy post-UA/NSTEMI. ACE inhibitors are indicated in patients recovering from UA or NSTEMI with heart failure, low ejection fraction (i.e., EF $<$40%), hypertension, or diabetes, unless contraindicated.

Aldosterone antagonists

Aldosterone antagonists (i.e., spironolactone and eplerenone) are relatively new additions to the continuing treatment of post-UA/NSTEMI patients. Aldosterone antagonists have proven mortality benefits in select patient populations. Patients post-UA/NSTEMI on concomitant ACE inhibitor therapy and with low ejection fractions (EF $<$40%), a serum potassium $<$5 mEq/L, and serum creatinine $<$2.5 mg/dL are candidates for aldosterone antagonist therapy.

Life-threatening hyperkalemia, though rare, can occur with aldosterone antagonist use; therefore, serum potassium levels should be closely monitored.

Beta-blockers

Beta-blockers are indicated for all post-UA/NSTEMI patients without contraindications and should be continued indefinitely. The benefits of beta-blockers include reduced myocardial oxygen demand, improvement of ischemic symptoms, decreased cardiac remodeling and subsequent improvements in LV function, and a reduction in morbidity and mortality.

Caution is advised in patients with a history of asthma, current heart failure symptoms, or hemodynamic compromise (hypotension or bradycardia).

Further reading

The American College of Cardiology (ACC) and American Heart Association (AHA) have produced joint guideline statements on the management of UA/NSTEMI. The 2007 guideline update is available at: http://www.circ.ahajournals.org/cgi/reprint/102/10/1193

ST-elevation myocardial infarction

ST-elevation myocardial infarction (STEMI) is the most severe form of the acute coronary syndromes (ACS) (which includes UA, NSTEMI, and STEMI). STEMI occurs when a fibrin-rich occlusion leads to complete blockage of a coronary artery. This blockage, in turn, results in myocardial ischemia and may result in irreversible damage to the myocardium.

Signs and symptoms

Patients with STEMI may present with "typical" angina, consisting of chest pain, pressure, or tightness, that is not relieved by rest or sublingual nitroglycerin. Certain populations, however, may present with atypical signs or symptoms of STEMI, which include dyspnea, diaphoresis, nausea and vomiting, and syncope. Patient populations more likely to present with atypical signs and symptoms include the following:

- Elderly
- Diabetics
- Females
- Non-white race
- Prior heart failure

Diagnosis

Prompt diagnosis and subsequent treatment are vital in the management of STEMI. Patients presenting with signs or symptoms concerning for ACS should undergo evaluation encompassing the following:

- Patient history
- Physical exam
- Electrocardiogram (ECG)
  - ST-segment elevation (2 or more contiguous leads)
  - T-wave inversion
- Biochemical (cardiac) markers (i.e., troponin, creatine kinase-MB)

Time delays in the elevation of cardiac makers limit their usefulness in the early diagnosis of STEMI. For this reason, the diagnosis of STEMI relies primarily on ECG findings and patient symptoms.

Goals of therapy

- Relief of ischemic pain
- Prompt reperfusion of infarct-related artery
- Reduce morbidity and mortality
- Prevent or slow progression of coronary heart disease
- Manage patient-related risk factors

Risk stratification

Like UA and NSTEMI, risk stratification can help guide early management of STEMI. Similar to the UA/NSTEMI risk stratification tool, the TIMI risk score for STEMI evaluates independent variables associated with patient outcome[1]:

- Age
- History of diabetes, hypertension, or angina
- Systolic blood pressure <100 mmHg

- Heart rate >100 beats/min
- Killip class II–IV
- Weight <67 kg
- Anterior ST-elevation or left bundle branch block (LBBB)
- Time to reperfusion >4 hours

Patients with higher TIMI risk scores have higher rates of in-hospital mortality following STEMI.[1]

Reperfusion

The primary goal of acute STEMI care is to reperfuse (or open) the infarct-related artery as soon as possible. Reperfusion of arteries can be achieved by one of two methods: pharmacological fibrinolysis or primary percutaneous coronary intervention (PCI) (via cardiac catheterization).

When both treatment options are readily available, primary PCI is the preferred method of reperfusion as it demonstrates enhanced survival and decreased intracranial hemorrhage when directly compared with fibrinolysis. If, however, there is a delay (>90 minutes) to primary PCI or if primary PCI is unavailable, fibrinolysis should be initiated.

Primary PCI

Primary PCI, when performed within an appropriate time frame, has demonstrated superior outcomes to those with fibrinolysis. Adjunctive therapy with an anticoagulant, antiplatelet agent, and beta-blocker should be given at the time of PCI.

Fibrinolysis

Fibrinolytic agents (see Table 15.10) decrease mortality in acute STEMI and, due to widespread availability, remain an important option in reperfusion. Fibrinolytics (or thrombolytics) activate the conversion of plasminogen to the clot-lysing enzyme plasmin.

Absolute contraindications to fibrinolysis

- Any prior intracerebral hemorrhage
- Known structural cerebrovascular lesion
- Known malignant intracranial neoplasm
- Ischemic stroke within past 3 months
- Suspected aortic dissection
- Active bleeding or bleeding diathesis
- Significant closed head or facial trauma in past 3 months

Adjunctive anticoagulation (see Table 15.11)

Adjunctive anticoagulation should be provided for all STEMI patients undergoing reperfusion. Primary anticoagulation options include heparin and low-molecular-weight heparin (LMWH). Bivalirudin can be used as an alternative agent in patients with known heparin-induced thrombocytopenia (HIT) who are treated with streptokinase.

1 Morrow DA, Antman EM, Parsons L, et al. (2001). Application of the TIMI risk score for ST-elevation MI in the National Registry of Myocardial Infarction 3. *JAMA* 286(11):1356–1359.

Table 15.10 Dosing regimens for preferred fibrinolytics in STEMI

Drug	Dose	Advantages	Limitations
Streptokinase	1.5 million units over 30–60 minutes	Less expensive	Less effective
Alteplase	Bolus: 15 mg 0.75 mg/kg over 30 minutes 0.5 mg/kg over 60 minutes	Better outcomes	Administration Cost
Tenecteplase	Bolus over 5–10 minutes based on body weight	Administration	Cost
Reteplase	10 units over 10 minutes Repeat bolus after 30 minutes	Administration	Cost

Table 15.11 Dosing regimens for anticoagulation in STEMI

Drug	Dose	Notes
Heparin	Bolus: 60 units/kg intravenous Infusion: 12 units/kg/hr	No renal dose adjustment required
Enoxaparin	Bolus: 30 mg intravenous Maintenance: 1 mg/kg every 12 hours, subcutaneous	Renal dose adjustment required Patients >75 years of age: omit bolus, decrease dose to 0.75 mg/kg
Bivalirudin	Bolus: 0.25 mg/kg Maintenance: 0.5 mg/kg/hr for first 12 hours, then 0.25 mg/kg/hr for next 36 hours	Renal dose adjustment required

Adapted from American College of Rheumatology Subcommittee on Osteoarthrits Guidelines. Recommendations for the medical management of osteoarthritis of the hip and knee. Arthritis Rheum 2000; 43:1905–1915, with permission of John Wiley & Sons, Inc.

Initial therapy

In addition to reperfusion, initial management of STEMI, like that of UA and NSTEMI, should consist of morphine, oxygen, nitrates, antiplatelet agents, and a beta-blocker (see Table 15.12).

Morphine

Pain may often be severe with acute STEMI, resulting in increased sympathetic activity. Morphine may be beneficial for reducing ischemia by

Table 15.12 Dosing regimens for initial therapy in STEMI

Drug	Dose	Notes
Morphine	2–4 mg every 5–15 minutes as needed	Monitor blood pressure
Oxygen	Inhaled oxygen to maintain saturation >90%	Supplemental oxygen may be given to all STEMI patients
Nitrates	SL NTG: 0.4 mg every 5 minutes	SL: may give up to 3 doses
	IV NTG: 10 mcg/min	IV: titrate every 3–5 minutes
Aspirin	162–325 mg orally or chewed	Chewing achieves high blood concentrations more rapidly
Beta-blocker	PO: Metoprolol 25 mg IV: Metoprolol 5 mg	IV administration reserved for tachycardia or hypertension

reducing the oxygen demand associated with pain and anxiety. Morphine, however, has not been demonstrated to improve cardiovascular outcomes following STEMI. Despite the lack of outcomes data, morphine remains a standard of care due to its analgesic and anxiolytic properties.

Oxygen

Oxygen should be administered to all STEMI patients with arterial oxygen saturations <90%. Increasing arterial oxygen supply may serve to lessen ischemia.

Nitrates

Nitrates have the beneficial effects of reducing myocardial oxygen demand while improving oxygen supply. Though not shown to provide significant mortality benefit, nitrates are beneficial in attenuating ischemia and alleviating patients' symptoms.

Antiplatelet therapy

The antiplatelet agents aspirin and clopidogrel have proven mortality and cardiovascular benefits. These agents diminish platelet aggregation, a key step in thrombus formation, thereby limiting the degree of arterial occlusion. Dual antiplatelet therapy with aspirin and clopidogrel is recommended in all STEMI patients regardless of whether they receive reperfusion therapy.

Beta-blockers

Beta-blockers reduce myocardial oxygen demand by competitively inhibiting the sympathetic nervous system's effects on heart rate and myocardial contractility. Beta-blockers, administered orally, should be given early in the course of care. IV administration may be considered in limited situations, such as ongoing angina with associated hypertension or tachycardia.

Continuing treatment

The goals of continued treatment following STEMI are to moderate and control risk factors, reduce recurrence of ischemia, and improve survival. Several medication classes have been identified that address these goals and should be initiated and continued indefinitely following STEMI.

Statins

Statins have proven benefits, including primary and secondary prevention of coronary heart disease, for patients post-STEMI. These benefits extend beyond lipid lowering. Pleiotropic effects, including plaque stabilization, decreased inflammation, and decreased thrombogenicity, have been demonstrated and are thought to contribute to the morbidity and mortality benefits of statin therapy.

Antiplatelet therapy

Aspirin 75–162 mg should be prescribed and continued indefinitely in patients recovering from STEMI. Higher initial doses (aspirin 162–325 mg) should be considered in patients who are revascularized (i.e., undergo catheterization with intervention).

Clopidogrel 75 mg daily should be prescribed for at least 1 month and ideally up to 1 year in all post-STEMI patients. Patients who receive bare metal stents (BMS) should be prescribed clopidogrel for at least 1 month, while those who receive drug-eluting stents (DES) should continue clopidogrel for at least 1 year.

ACE inhibitors

ACE inhibitors have proven beneficial effects after acute ST-elevation MI. ACE inhibitors are indicated in patients recovering from UA/NSTEMI with heart failure, low ejection fraction (EF <40%), hypertension, or diabetes, unless contraindicated.

Aldosterone antagonists

Aldosterone antagonists (e.g., spironolactone and epleronone) are relatively new additions to the continuing treatment of post-STEMI patients. Aldosterone antagonists have proven mortality benefits in select patient populations. Patients post-STEMI on concomitant ACE inhibitor therapy with low ejection fractions (EF <40%), serum potassium <5 mEq/L, and serum creatinine <2.5 mg/dL are candidates for aldosterone antagonist therapy.

Life-threatening hyperkalemia, though rare, can occur and serum potassium levels should be closely monitored.

Beta-blockers

Beta-blockers are indicated for all post-STEMI patients without contraindications. The benefits of beta-blockers include reduced myocardial oxygen demand, improvement of ischemic symptoms, decreased cardiac remodeling and subsequent improvements in LV function, and a reduction in morbidity and mortality.

Caution is advised in patients with a history of asthma, current heart failure symptoms, or hemodynamic compromise (hypotension or bradycardia).

Risk factor modification

Risk factor modification is an important component of continued treatment following STEMI. In addition to proper medical therapy, risk factor modification provides secondary prevention of cardiovascular disease and improves mortality. Risk factor modification should include:

- Smoking cessation
- Diabetes management (A1c goal <7%)
- Hypertension management (goal BP <140/90; <130/80 in diabetics)
- Cardiac rehabilitation
- Dietary modification

Further reading

The American College of Cardiology (ACC) and American Heart Association (AHA) have produced joint guideline statements on the management of STEMI. The 2007 focused guideline update is available at: http://circ.ahajournals.org/cgi/reprint/CIRCULATIONAHA.107.188209

Tolerance to nitrate therapy

Tolerance develops rapidly to forms of nitrate administration delivering continuous, stable concentrations of the drug (e.g., NTG patch, isosorbide dinitrate dosed 3 to 4 times daily). This is of particular importance in patients receiving extended courses of nitrates, such as those with chronic stable angina.

Mechanisms of nitrate tolerance are incompletely understood. Proposed mechanisms include impaired nitroglycerin bioconversion to nitric oxide, decreased vascular responsiveness to nitric oxide–mediated vasodilation, and neurohormonal activation leading to vasoconstriction.

Practical management of nitrate tolerance is to prevent its development by allowing a nitrate-free interval. The optimal duration of nitrate-free interval is unknown, though a 10- to 12-hour off period has been recommended. The timing of nitrate administration should allow for this nitrate-free interval.

Nitrate-free interval dosing strategies

- Isosorbide dinitrate dosed at 8 AM, 1 PM, and 6 PM
- Isosorbide mononitrate dosed at 8 AM
- NTG patch applied at 8 AM, removed at 8 PM

It should be noted that patients with a low ischemic threshold may develop rebound ischemia during the nitrate-free interval. Isosorbide mononitrate has not been reported to cause rebound ischemia and may be useful in patients with a very low ischemic threshold.

Acute decompensated heart failure

Acute decompensated heart failure (ADHF) is a clinical syndrome characterized by dyspnea and respiratory distress often secondary to left ventricular (LV) systolic or diastolic dysfunction. LV dysfunction may cause a reduction in cardiac output and elevations in cardiac filling and pulmonary pressures that can lead to pulmonary fluid accumulation (cardiogenic pulmonary edema). Clinical manifestations of ADHF include dyspnea, tachypnea, decreased organ perfusion, and hypo- or hyper- tension.

Goals of therapy

- Hemodynamic stability
- Proper oxygenation/ventilation
- Relief of symptoms
- Reduced morbidity (e.g., rehospitalization)
- Reduced short-term mortality

Nonpharmacological interventions

Although ADHF is often the result of worsening disease processes, medication and dietary noncompliance are important factors that can contribute to decompensation. Non-drug interventions have a significant impact on achieving goals of therapy.

- Sodium-restricted diet (goal <2 g sodium/day)
- Fluid restriction (goal <2 L/day)
- Supplemental oxygen (maintain oxygen saturation >90%)
- Patient education

Pharmacological treatment

Medical therapy for ADHF should be individualized on a patient-specific basis and is guided by both clinical signs and symptoms and hemodynamic parameters.

Diuretics

Given the pathophysiology of ADHF, patients are often volume overloaded, though on rare occasions pulmonary edema can occur in the absence of significant volume overload (e.g., aortic or mitral insufficiency). Regardless of etiology, patients with ADHF benefit from improved oxygenation and symptom relief secondary to diuresis.

Loop diuretics (e.g., furosemide, bumetanide, torsemide) are the diuretics of choice with patient-specific IV dosing (see Table 15.13). Patients with previous loop diuretic use often require higher initial doses that are at least equivalent to their home maintenance doses (e.g., furosemide 120 mg IV for a patient who takes 120 mg orally daily).

Strategies for patients with inadequate initial diuretic response

- Doubling IV dose until adequate diuresis occurs
- Addition of thiazide diuretic (e.g., hydrochlorothiazide, metolazone)
- Continuous IV infusion of loop diuretic

Vasodilators (see Table 15.14)

IV vasodilators decrease cardiac filling and pulmonary pressures that can decrease pulmonary edema and reduce patient symptoms. Vasodilators

Table 15.13 Common diuretic doses for ADHF

Loop diuretics	Initial dose	Maximum dose	Continuous infusion
Furosemide	20–40 mg IV	200 mg single IV dose	10–40 mg/hr
Bumetanide	0.5–1 mg IV	10 mg/day	0.5–2 mg/hr
Torsemide	10–20 mg IV	200 mg single IV dose	5–20 mg/hr
Thiazide diuretics	**Initial dose**	**Maximum dose**	**Comments**
Metolazone	2.5 mg	20 mg/day	Intermittent dosing; give prior to loop diuretic
Hydrochlorothiazide	25 mg	100 mg/day	Give prior to loop diuretic

Table 15.14 Vasodilators for ADHF

Inotrope	Class of agent	Dose	Comments
Nitroglycerin	Nitrate	5–10 mcg/min	Tolerance develops within 24–48 hours
Nitroprusside	Vasodilator	0.25–0.5 mcg/kg/min	Monitor for signs of cyanide toxicity
Nesiritide	Human B-type natriuretic peptide	2 mcg/kg (bolus); 0.01 mcg/kg/min	Caution with prolonged infusion (>48 hours)

are often given to patients with concomitant ischemic disease or those with inadequate response to diuretic therapy.

Caution should be used when using these in patients with hypotension, and use should generally be avoided with SBP <90 mmHg.

Nitroglycerin

IV nitroglycerin is a commonly used potent vasodilator and, while effective, requires frequent dose titration. Doses up to 160 mcg/min may be required. Nitrate tolerance develops quickly with continuous infusions (24–48 hours).

Nitroprusside

Nitroprusside, which produces both arterial and venous dilation, is reserved for specific clinical situations in ADHF (e.g., hypertensive emergency, aortic or mitral regurgitation). Metabolites of nitroprusside can accumulate and produce cyanide toxicity.

Nesiritide

Nesiritide is a recombinant form of human B-type natriuretic peptide (BNP) that acts as a vasodilator. Clinical trials of nesiritide in ADHF have demonstrated improved hemodynamic parameters and a reduction of patient symptoms. Post-marketing analyses have raised concerns of increased mortality and renal impairment.

Inotropes (see Table 15.15)

Patients with signs or symptoms of low cardiac output (e.g., cool extremities, decreased urine output, etc.) or poor organ perfusion may benefit from IV inotropes. Inotropes improve cardiac output, increase systemic perfusion, and decrease symptoms.

Despite these benefits even short-term IV inotrope therapy has been associated with increased mortality. Therefore, use of IV inotropes should be reserved for symptomatic patients with severe hemodynamic compromise (e.g., low cardiac output, hypotension) and to improve end-organ function.

Table 15.15 Inotropic agents for ADHF

Inotrope	Class of agent	Dose range	Comments
Dobutamine	Beta-receptor agonist	2.5–20 mcg/kg/min	Avoid concomitant beta-blockers
Milrinone	Phosphodiesterase Enzyme Inhibitor	0.25–0.75 mcg/kg/min	Avoid if SBP <90 mmHg

Further reading

Guideline statements specific to ADHF are limited to a brief section of the 2006 Heart Failure Society of America (HFSA) Comprehensive Heart Failure Practice Guideline, available at: http://www.hfsa.org/hf_guidelines.asp.

The European Society of Cardiology, however, has published guideline statements specific to acute heart failure. Available at: http://www.escardio.org/NR/rdonlyres/CBA6844E-56D7-43B4-B0FB-6A4FAF0C0E98/0/guidelines_AHF_FT_2005.pdf

Chronic heart failure

Chronic heart failure (CHF) is a clinical syndrome in which the heart is unable to pump blood at a rate sufficient to meet the body's metabolic demand. CHF is the result of a structural or functional disorder that impairs the ventricle's ability to fill with or eject blood. The New York Heart Association (NYHA) has classified the stages of CHF (Table 15.16).

Signs and symptoms

Clinically, patients can range from being asymptomatic with structural changes that predispose patients to CHF to having continual symptoms with end-stage disease. Symptoms vary with etiology and classification of CHF but classically include one or more of the following:

- Dyspnea
- Orthopnea
- Peripheral edema
- Fatigue
- Persistent cough
- Early satiety and/or nausea

Goals of therapy

- Improve symptoms
- Slow or reverse deterioration of myocardial function
- Improve quality of life
- Reduce mortality

Nonpharmacological interventions

Non-drug interventions can have a significant impact on CHF management. These interventions can improve patients' functional capacity, improve quality of life, and decrease mortality.

- Sodium-restricted diet (goal <2 g sodium/day)
- Fluid restriction (goal <2 L/day)
- Smoking cessation
- Restriction of alcohol consumption
- Monitoring daily weight
- Physical activity as tolerated
- Patient education
- Participation in cardiac rehabilitation program

Pharmacological treatment

Multiple drugs and drug classes are commonly used in the management of CHF (see Table 15.17). Each of these interventions, with the exception of diuretics and digoxin, has shown mortality benefit in patients with CHF secondary to systolic dysfunction.

Angiotensin-converting enzyme (ACE) inhibitors

Evidence supports the routine use of ACE inhibitors in patients with left ventricular dysfunction (EF <40%) regardless of whether they are symptomatic (see Table 15.18). These agents moderate activation of the renin–angiotensin aldosterone system (RAAS) and angiotensin II production, which produces

Table 15.16 NYHA classification of CHF

Class	Patient symptoms
I	No limitation of physical activity. Ordinary activity does not cause undue fatigue, palpitation, or dyspnea.
II	Slight limitation of physical activity. Comfortable at rest, but ordinary physical activity results in fatigue, palpitation, or dyspnea.
III	Marked limitation of physical activity. Comfortable at rest, but less than ordinary activity causes fatigue, palpitation, or dyspnea.
IV	Unable to carry out any physical activity without discomfort. Symptoms of cardiac insufficiency at rest. If any physical activity is undertaken, discomfort is increased.

Table 15.17 Drug indications by NYHA classification

Drug intervention	NYHA Class I	NYHA Class II	NYHA Class III	NYHA Class IV
ACE inhibitors	Yes	Yes	Yes	Yes
ARBs*	Yes	Yes	Yes	Yes
Aldosterone antagonists	No	No	Yes	Yes
Beta-blockers	Consider	Yes	Yes	Yes
Digoxin†	No	Consider	Consider	Consider
Diuretics	No	Yes	Yes	Yes
Isosorbide dintrate/hydralazine‡	No	No	Yes	Yes

* As alternative in patients unable to tolerate ACE inhibitor therapy.

† Consider for symptom relief in patients on optimized medical regimen.

‡ Indicated for NYHA class III and IV heart failure in African Americans.

Crouch MA. *Contemporary Management of Heart Failure. Clinical Consult 2002; Supplement 1* (Vol. 17). Reprinted with permission of the American Society of Consultant Pharmacists, Alexandria, Virginia.

Table 15.18 Common doses of ACE inhibitors for CHF

ACE inhibitor	Initial dose	Target dose
Captopril	6.25–12.5 mg 3 times daily	50 mg 3 times daily
Enalapril	2.5 mg once or twice daily	10–20 mg twice daily
Fosinopril	10 mg daily	40 mg daily
Lisinopril	2.5–5 mg daily	20–40 mg daily
Quinapril	5 mg once or twice daily	20 mg twice daily

vasodilation and a reduction in sodium and water retention. ACE inhibitors have proven beneficial in reducing hospital readmission and mortality and slowing disease progression.

Angiotensin receptor blockers (ARBs)

Like ACE inhibitors, ARBs moderate the RAAS and produce vasodilation and a reduction in sodium and water retention (see Table 15.19). ARBs have proven efficacious as alternatives in patients who are unable to tolerate ACE inhibitors because of adverse effects (e.g. cough).

The clinical effects of ARBs are similar to ACE inhibitors in regard to hospital readmission, mortality, and disease progression. Though controversial, the addition of an ARB to ACE inhibitor therapy may be considered in patients who remain symptomatic on conventional therapy.

Aldosterone antagonists (see Table 15.20)

Neurohormonal activation of the RAAS leads to an increase in aldosterone production, which results in sodium and water retention and ventricular remodeling. Aldosterone antagonists directly compete with aldosterone for binding sites and have proven morbidity and mortality benefits in patients with NYHA Class III and IV heart failure.

Hyperkalemia is a major adverse effect of aldosterone antagonists and precaution is advised in patients with baseline renal insufficiency (serum creatinine >2.0 mg/dL in females, >2.5 mg/dL in males) or those with concomitant ACE inhibitor or ARB therapy. Aldosterone antagonists should not be administered in patients with a history of severe hyperkalemia or with a current serum potassium >5 mEq/L.

Beta-blockers (see Table 15.21)

Prolonged activation of the sympathetic nervous system has numerous deleterious effects including vasoconstriction, myocardial ischemia,

Table 15.19 Common doses of ARBs for CHF

ARB	Initial dose	Target dose	Comments
Valsartan	20–40 mg twice daily	160 mg twice daily	May cause dizziness
Candesartan	4–8 mg once daily	32 mg once daily	Contraindicated in severe hepatic disease

Table 15.20 Common aldosterone antagonist doses for CHF

Aldosterone Antagonist	Initial dose	Maximum dose	Comments
Spironolactone	12.5–25 mg once daily	50 mg daily	Consider dose reduction with hyperkalemia
Eplerenone	25 mg daily	50 mg daily	Useful alternative for patients unable to tolerate spironolactone

Table 15.21 Common beta-blocker doses for CHF

Beta-blocker	Initial dose	Target dose	Comments
Metoprolol tartrate	6.25 mg twice daily	50–100 mg twice daily	Regular-release formulation
Metoprolol succinate	12.5–25 mg daily	200 mg daily	Extended-release formulation
Carvedilol	3.125 mg twice daily	25–50 mg twice daily	Contraindicated in severe hepatic disease
Bisoprolol	1.25 mg once daily	5–10 mg once daily	Titrate dose slowly in renal impairment

ventricular remodeling, and reduced responsiveness to beta-agonists (decreased contractile function). Beta-blockers moderate these deleterious effects and have been shown to slow disease progression, improve functional status, and prolong survival.

Patients may experience worsened symptoms for the first 4–10 weeks of therapy before any improvement is noted.

Digoxin

Digoxin promotes an increase in intracellular calcium concentration, which improves myocyte contractility and LV systolic function. Digoxin, used anecdotally for heart failure for over 200 years, has not been shown to improve mortality. It does, however, reduce hospitalization rates from heart failure and provide symptomatic benefit.

Digoxin should be reserved for patients with symptomatic heart failure despite optimal medical therapy or for rate control in patients with concomitant atrial fibrillation. Digoxin levels should be maintained between 0.5 ng/mL and 0.8 ng/mL, as higher levels are associated with increased toxicity and no evidence of increased efficacy.

Diuretics

Like digoxin, diuretics have not been shown to improve mortality but are instead used for symptom relief. Diuretics (and salt restriction) are recommended for symptomatic patients with decreased ejection fraction and signs or symptoms of edema.

Loop diuretics (e.g., furosemide, bumetanide, torsemide) are the diuretics of choice with patient-specific dosing (see Table 15.22).

Isosorbide dinitrate/hydralazine (see Table 15.23)

The combination of isosorbide dinitrate and hydralazine demonstrated modest benefits in reducing heart failure–associated mortality when compared with placebo. The use of this combination of agents has not become an accepted standard of care, as ACE inhibitors, when directly compared, showed a more significant mortality benefit. Further, compliance with

Table 15.22 Common diuretic doses for CHF

Loop diuretic	Initial dose	Incremental dose increase	Typical dosing interval
Furosemide	20–80 mg/dose	20–40 mg/dose	Daily or twice daily
Bumetanide	0.5–1 mg/dose	0.5–1 mg/dose	Daily or twice daily
Torsemide	10–20 mg/dose	10–20 mg/dose	Daily

Table 15.23 Isosorbide dinitrate and hydralazine doses for CHF

Agent	Initial dose	Target dose	Comments
Isosorbide dinitrate	10 mg 3 times daily	120–160 mg daily in 3–4 divided doses	Dose limited by headache
Hydralazine	10–25 mg 3–4 times daily	225–300 mg daily in 3–4 divided doses	Requires close blood pressure monitoring

isosorbide dinitrate and hydralazine is historically low because of pill burden (3–4 times daily) and adverse effects (e.g., headache).

African Americans with NYHA Class III or IV heart failure may gain the most benefit from this combination of agents, as a recent study has demonstrated.[1] The addition of isosorbide dinitrate and hydralazine to standard of care (including ACE inhibitors) resulted in significant mortality improvement in this patient population. Questions remain about the utility of isosorbide dinitrate and hydralazine in other heart-failure patient populations.

1 A-HeFT Investigators (2004). Combination of isosorbide dinitrate and hydralazine in blacks with heart failure. *N Eng J Med* **351**(20):2049–2057.

Further reading

Several CHF guideline statements have been published by a number of committees and professional societies. These guidelines cover a range of topics from diagnosis to palliative management of end-stage disease.

American College of Cardiology/American Heart Association (ACC/AHA): http://circ.ahajournals.org/cgi/reprint/112/12/e154

European Society of Cardiology (ESC): http://www.escardio.org/NR/rdonlyres/8A2848B4-5DEB-41B9-9A0A-5B5A90494B64/0/guidelines_CHF_FT_2005.pdf

Heart Failure Society of America (HFSA): http://www.hfsa.org/hf_guidelines.asp

Acute cardiogenic pulmonary edema

Pulmonary edema is the extravasation of fluid from the pulmonary vasculature into the interstitial space of the lungs. Two distinct types of pulmonary edema, cardiogenic and noncardiogenic, may occur, which present with similar clinical manifestations.

Prompt diagnosis of the underlying cause is necessary as this is a medical emergency requiring urgent treatment. The focus of this section is on the treatment of cardiogenic pulmonary edema.

Cardiogenic pulmonary edema is caused by a rapid increase in pulmonary hydrostatic pressure leading to fluid extravasation into the lungs. This pulmonary edema leads to symptoms of dyspnea, tachypnea, and hypoxemia. Common causes of cardiogenic pulmonary edema are

- Myocardial ischemia/infarction
- Exacerbation of heart failure
- Dysfunction of mitral or aortic valve
- Severe systemic hypertension
- Acute tachycardia or bradycardia

Nonpharmacological interventions

Oxygen

Oxygen should be administered with the goal of decreasing hypoxia while maintaining oxygen saturations >90%. If hypoxia persists despite attempts at oxygenation, ventilatory support may be required.

Noninvasive positive pressure ventilation

Two forms of noninvasive positive pressure ventilation, continuous positive airway pressure (CPAP) and bilevel positive airway pressure (BiPAP), are used in treating cardiogenic pulmonary edema. Either form decreases patient work of breathing and improves patient comfort by maintaining alveolar patency and improving gas exchange.

Mechanical ventilation

Mechanical ventilation provides airway support and promotes optimal oxygenation and ventilation. Mechanical ventilation is usually reserved for patients with ongoing hypoxia despite optimal oxygenation, failed noninvasive positive pressure ventilation, worsening clinical appearance, and cardiogenic shock.

Assisted circulation

Assisted circulation provided by the placement of an intra-aortic balloon pump (IABP) is used in patients with ongoing cardiogenic shock. IABP provides temporary blood pressure support and improves cardiac output while patients are awaiting more definitive therapies.

Pharmacological treatment

Loop diuretics

Intravenous loop diuretics are the cornerstone of cardiogenic pulmonary edema therapy as they decrease preload and pulmonary pressure by providing diuresis and direct venodilation. Patients with pre-existing diuretic therapy or those with impaired renal function often require larger doses with dose determinations made on an individual-patient basis.

Nitroglycerin

Nitroglycerin, administered in sublingual, intravenous, or transdermal form, produces effective and rapid preload reduction resulting in significant symptomatic improvement. Nitroglycerin is rapidly titratable while possessing a short half-life that allows for discontinuation if hypotension occurs.

Nesiritide

Nesiritide is a recombinant form of human B-type natriuretic peptide (BNP) that produces reduced pulmonary pressures, increased stroke volume, and increased cardiac output. Nesiritide is currently indicated for acute decompensated heart failure, though it may play a role in select patients with cardiogenic pulmonary edema. Nesiritide should be reserved for those patients in whom nitroglycerin is contraindicated (e.g., current sildenafil use) or when prolonged nitroglycerin use is expected, because nitrate tolerance limits its effectiveness.

Angiotensin-converting enzyme (ACE) inhibitors

ACE inhibitors produce several beneficial effects in cardiogenic pulmonary edema. ACE inhibitors decrease systemic vascular resistance (afterload) and improve renal perfusion, which may improve cardiac output and increase the effectiveness of diuretics, respectively. Caution is advised when using ACE inhibitors in hypotensive patients.

Inotropes

Inotropic agents (e.g., dobutamine, milrinone) improve cardiac output in patients with cardiogenic pulmonary edema and concomitant depressed myocardial function. These agents also, however, cause tachycardia, induce dysrhythmias, increase myocardial oxygen demand, and increase myocardial ischemia. Inotropic agents are thus reserved for cardiogenic pulmonary edema patients who are hypotensive and cannot tolerate previously mentioned preload- and afterload-reducing therapy.

Morphine

Morphine is an historical component of cardiogenic pulmonary edema therapy as it is thought to produce preload reduction, though there is no available evidence to support this theory. Any hemodynamic benefits are likely related to reduced anxiety and subsequent reductions in myocardial oxygen demand.

Cardiopulmonary resuscitation in adults

Cardiopulmonary resuscitation (CPR) is an organized sequence of assessments and interventions used to manage the patient experiencing cardiac arrest. The management of cardiopulmonary arrest is commonly divided into two categories: basic life support (BLS) and advanced cardiovascular life support (ACLS).

Epidemiology

Sudden cardiac arrest (SCA) is a leading cause of death in the United States and Canada. Estimates suggest approximately 330,000 people in the United States die annually in the out-of-hospital and emergency department settings from coronary heart disease. Incidence of SCA in North America is approximately 0.55 per 1000 population.

The most common cause of SCA results from the pulseless cardiac-arrest rhythms ventricular fibrillation (VF) and ventricular tachycardia (VT), which will be highlighted in this chapter.

Basic life support

BLS is the first-responder phase of the chain of survival and may be carried out by anyone who has taken a basic first-aid course. It includes recognizing signs of SCA, heart attack, stroke, and foreign-body airway obstruction as well as administering CPR and defibrillation with an automated external defibrillator (AED).

Once the scene of an in-hospital arrest is deemed safe, the first responder should do the following:

- Assess the patient and check for response to confirm an arrest has occurred.
- Once arrest is suspected, ask a bystander to activate the emergency medical response system and to bring an AED, if available.
- Open airway and check breathing using head tilt–chin lift maneuver—if there is no head or neck trauma—then look, listen, and feel for breathing.
- If the patient is not breathing, give 2 rescue breaths, each over 1 second, to produce chest rise.
- Check for pulse, taking no longer than 10 seconds.
- If no pulse is detected, give cycles of 30 chest compressions and 2 breaths. If advanced airway is in place during two-person CPR, ventilate at 8–10 breaths per minute without interruptions during chest compressions. The rescuer should compress the lower half of the sternum 1 1/2 to 2 inches at a rate of approximately 100 compressions per minute until an AED arrives, emergency medical response providers take over, or the victim starts to move.
- If an AED is available, check for shockable rhythm—one that responds to defibrillation.
- If shockable, provide 1 shock then resume CPR for 5 cycles (approximately 2 minutes).

- If not shockable, resume CPR for 5 cycles, checking rhythm every 5 cycles until emergency medical response providers take over or victim starts to move.

Advanced cardiovascular life support

ACLS is an extension of BLS and generally begins with the arrival of the emergency response team. It is important to recognize that common ACLS therapies including advanced airways and pharmacological support of circulation have not been shown to increase rates of survival to hospital discharge. Basic CPR and early defibrillation are the only interventions proven to benefit survival in cardiac arrest. However, medications do have a role and should always be considered.

Once on the scene of a pulseless arrest, check for the following:

- BLS is maintained
- The patient's airway is secured and oxygen administered
- IV access is obtained (in hospital, blood is taken for urgent blood-gas analysis and determination of electrolyte levels). CPR should not be interrupted to obtain access.
- Cardiac monitor or defibrillator is attached to allow diagnosis of the arrhythmia.
- Rhythm is assessed to determine if it is a shockable rhythm. The most common shockable rhythms that lead to SCA are ventricular fibrillation (VF) and pulseless ventricular tachycardia (VT).
- If shockable, give a single shock followed by immediate resumption of CPR (30 compressions to 2 ventilations). Complete 5 cycles of CPR before reassessing rhythm or feeling for a pulse. The recommended initial energy for biphasic defibrillators is device-specific, typically between 120 and 200 joules (J). Give second and subsequent shocks at the same or higher doses. The recommended energy when using monophasic defibrillators is 360 J for initial and subsequent shocks.
- If VF or VT persists after 1 or 2 shocks plus CPR, give a vasopressor (epinephrine 1 mg IV/intraosseous [IO]) every 3–5 minutes; one dose of vasopressin 40 units IV/IO may replace either the first or second dose of epinephrine).
- If shockable rhythm persists after 2 or 3 shocks plus CPR and administration of a vasopressor, consider antiarrhythmic therapy such as amiodarone 300 mg IV/IO. An additional dose of 150 mg of amiodarone may be administered if return of spontaneous circulation is not achieved with continued CPR. Lidocaine (1–1.5 mg/kg IV/IO first dose, then 0.5–0.75 mg/kg IV/IO, up to a maximum 3 doses or 3 mg/kg) may be considered as an alternative. Consider IV magnesium if the rhythm is identified as torsades de pointes.

Additional rhythms that may cause pulseless arrest include asystole and pulseless electrical activity (PEA). *Asystole* is the absence of any heart rhythm. *PEA* is the presence of organized electrical activity that fails to result in mechanical contraction of the heart. These are considered non-shockable rhythms, as they cannot be corrected using defibrillation.

Administration of a vasopressor (epinephrine or vasopressin) may be considered. For asystole or slow PEA, administration of atropine may be considered (1 mg IV/IO repeat every 3–5 minutes up to 3 doses).

Drug administration

Medication administration during ACLS should be given as soon as possible following rhythm check without interruption in CPR.

For IV administration, a flush of 20 mL of sodium chloride 0.9% solution should be administered after each drug dose to enhance its passage from the peripheral to the central circulation. Alternatively, the dose can be given in tandem with a fast-flowing IV fluid. Elevation of the extremity for 10–20 seconds may facilitate drug delivery to the central circulation.

- Epinephrine is administered at a dose of 1 mg IV/IO (10 mL of 1:10000 prefilled syringe) every 3–5 minutes during cardiac arrest.
- Vasopressin is administered at a dose of 40 units IV/IO. It may replace either the first or second dose of epinephrine in VF and pulseless VT arrest.
- Atropine is often used in the management of asystole, PEA, and bradycardia to block excessive vagal activity that might be contributing to a decline in heart rate. For asystole and PEA, the recommended dose is 1 mg IV, which may be repeated every 3–5 minutes up to a maximum total dose of 3 mg.
- Amiodarone is the antiarrhythmic of choice in resistant VF or pulseless VT. A dose of 300 mg in 20 mL dextrose 5% in water is given as a slow bolus over a period of at least 3 minutes. Because amiodarone is incompatible with normal saline, bags of dextrose 5% in water should be available to enable prompt preparation and for flushing after dose(s). A repeat bolus of 150 mg may be administered if return of spontaneous circulation is not achieved. If rhythm is restored, an infusion of 1 mg/min for 6 hours and then 0.5 mg/min for 6 hours may be used.
- Lidocaine should be considered an alternative to amiodarone in the management of VF and pulseless VT. The recommended dose is 1–1.5 mg/kg IV. Additional doses of 0.5– 0.75 mg/kg IV push may be considered at 5- to 10-minute intervals up to a maximum of 3 mg /kg.
- Magnesium is the agent of choice in cardiac arrest associated with torsades de pointes, a type of arrhythmia that is often drug induced. It is commonly administered as magnesium sulfate at a dose of 1–2 g diluted in 10 mL D5W IV/IO push, typically over 5–20 minutes.
- Atropine, epinephrine, lidocaine, naloxone, and vasopressin may be administered via an endotracheal tube if alternative access cannot be established. Give 2 to 2.5 times the IV dose diluted in 5–10 mL of water or 0.9% sodium chloride followed by five ventilations to assist absorption.

Further reading

2005 American Heart Association Guidelines for Cardiopulmonary Resuscitation and Emergency Cardiovascular Care, Part 4: Adult Basic Life Support. *Circulation* **112**(Suppl . IV): IV-19–IV-34.

2005 American Heart Association Guidelines for Cardiopulmonary Resuscitation and Emergency Cardiovascular Care, Part 7: Advanced Cardiovascular Life Support. *Circulation* **112**(Suppl. IV): IV-51–IV-88.

Hypertension

Hypertension (HTN) is characterized by elevated arterial BP. High BP increases the risk of stroke, MI, angina, renal failure, heart failure, or other vascular complications. High BP is one of many risk factors for cardiovascular disease (CVD).

Epidemiology

- CVD risk doubles for each increment of 20/10 mmHg over 115/75 mmHg.
- In persons >50 years old, SBP >140 mmHg is a more important CVD risk factor than diastolic BP.
- Normotensive individuals at age 55 have a 90% lifetime risk for hypertension development.
- A 5 mmHg drop in systolic BP results in a 14% reduction in stroke, 9% reduction in coronary heart disease, and 7% reduction in all-cause mortality.

Diagnosis

High BP is diagnosed after at least two elevated BP checks on separate occasions, based on values in Table 15.24.

Causes

The following are identifiable causes of hypertension and resistant hypertension:

- Sleep apnea
- Chronic kidney disease
- Primary aldosteronism
- Pheochromocytoma
- Thyroid or parathyroid disease
- Coarctation of the aorta
- Excessive sodium intake
- Nonadherence to antihypertensive drug therapy

Table 15.24 BP classification

Classification	Systolic/ diastolic BP (mm Hg)
Normal	<120/80 mm Hg
Pre-hypertension	120–139 or 80–89 mmHg
Stage 1 hypertension	140–159 or 90–99 mmHg
Stage 2 hypertension	≥160 or ≥100 mmHg

Data from: The Seventh Report of the Joint National Committee on Prevention, Detection, Evaluation, and Treatment of High Blood Pressure—Complete Report. http://www.nhlbi.nih.gov/guidelines/hypertension/jnc7full.htm

Drugs

- NSAIDs (including cyclooxygenase-2 inhibitors)
- Corticosteroids
- Oral contraceptives
- Sympathomimetics (decongestants or anorexics)
- Excessive licorice (in some chewing tobacco)
- Cyclosporin and tacrolimus
- Illicit drugs such as cocaine or amphetamines
- Erythropoietin
- Some antidepressants (venlafaxine)

Treatment

Nonpharmacological therapy

- Lifestyle modifications to reduce both BP and cardiovascular risk should be introduced in all patients with hypertension and for prevention of hypertension.
- Some patients may only require lifestyle modifications.
- Two lifestyle modifications can be equivalent to one drug therapy in treating hypertension (see Table 15.25).

Table 15.25 Impact of lifestyle modifications

Modificationt	Recommendation	~SBP Reduction
Weight reduction	Maintain normal body weight	5–20 mmHg/10kg
Healthy eating plan	Eat a diet rich in fruits, vegetables, lean meats, low-fat dairy products; limit high-fat snacks, desserts	8–14 mmHg
Sodium reduction	Limit sodium intake to ≤2.4 g/day	2–8 mmHg
Physical activity on most days of the week	30 minutes of aerobic exercise, e.g., walking	4–9 mmHg
Limit alcohol* consumption	Men ≤2 drinks/day; Women ≤1 day;	2–4 mmHg

*Alcoholic drink = one 12 ounce beer, one 5 ounce glass of wine, or 1.5 ounces of 80 proof liquor

Data from The Seventh Report of the Joint National Committee on Prevention, Detection, Evaluation, and Treatment of High Blood Pressure—Complete Report. http://www.nhlbi.nih.gov/guidelines/hypertension/jnc7full.htm

Pharmacological treatment

- Antihypertensive therapy is associated with a 40% reduction in stroke; a ≥50% reduction in heart failure, and a 20%–25% reduction in myocardial infarction.
- If BP is ≥160/100 mmHg or 20/10 mmHg higher than goal, two agents should be initiated.
- Most hypertensive patients will require ≥2 agents to control BP.
- Thiazide diuretics should be used in most patients initially or in combination with other agents for compelling indications (see Table 15.26).
- The major objective is to achieve satisfactory BP control and prevent end-organ damage while avoiding adverse effects.
- Begin with monotherapy, unless BP is ≥160/100 mmHg or when BP is 20/10 mmHg above the goal BP for a compelling indication.
- The major classes of drugs used to treat hypertension are
  - Diuretics
  - Beta-blockers (BB)
  - Angiotensin-converting enzyme inhibitors (ACEI)
  - Calcium-channel blockers (CCB)
  - Angiotensin receptor blockers (ARB)
  - Aldosterone antagonists (AldoAnt)

The compelling indications for which specific drugs are indicated are provided in Table 15.27.

Diuretics

- Excellent choice in African Americans and for isolated systolic HTN
- Diuretics useful in all patient populations
- Thiazide diuretics
  - May cause hypokalemia, hyponatremia, hypomagnesemia, hyperuricemia (avoid in gout), hypercalcemia (good choice in osteoporosis)
  - Interact with lithium (↑ levels)
  - NSAIDs can negate effects
- Loop diuretics
  - Same as thiazides except hypocalcemia
- Potassium-sparing diuretic
  - Use with caution with K supplements, ACEI, ARB, renin inhibitor

Selective aldosterone receptor antagonists

- Spironolactone and eplerenone
- Patients should be monitored for hyperkalemia, hyponatremia
- May increase triglycerides or cholesterol
- Drug interactions possible with eplerenone due to metabolism by CYP3A4

Beta-blockers

- Grouped based on cardioselectivity
  - Cardioselective (e.g., atenolol)
  - Non-cardioselective (e.g., propanolol)
  - Selectivity can be lost at high doses
- Metoprolol best choice in renal dysfunction

Table 15.26 Management of blood pressure in adults (≥18 years old)

BP classification SBP/DBP (mmHg)	Without compelling indication	With compelling indication
Pre-hypertension	No drug therapy	Drug(s) for compelling indications
Stage 1 HTN	Thiazide for most	Drug(s) for compelling indications
Stage 2 HTN	Thiazide plus other drug; usually BB, CCB, ACEI, or ARB	Drug(s) for compelling indication plus other antihypertensives as needed

Data from The Seventh Report of the Joint National Committee on Prevention, Detection, Evaluation, and Treatment of High Blood Pressure—Complete Report. http://www.nhlbi.nih.gov/guidelines/hypertension/jnc7full.htm

Table 15.27 Drug recommendations for compelling indications

Compelling indication	Recommended drug
Heart failure	Diuretic, BB, ACEI, ARB, AldoAnt
Postmyocardial infarction	BB, ACEI, AldoAnt
High coronary disease risk	Diuretic, BB, ACEI, CCB
Diabetes	Diuretic, BB, ACEI, ARB, CCB
Chronic kidney disease	ACEI, ARB
Recurrent stroke prevention	Diuretic, ACEI

Data from The Seventh Report of the Joint National Committee on Prevention, Detection, Evaluation, and Treatment of High Blood Pressure—Complete Report. http://www.nhlbi.nih.gov/guidelines/hypertension/jnc7full.htm

- Avoid coadministration with non-dihydropyridine CCB due to increased risk of third-degree heart block
- Rebound hypertension can occur with abrupt withdrawal at high doses; dosage should be tapered
- Monitor when used with other drugs that can alter conduction (digoxin, amiodarone, etc.)

Angiotension-converting enzyme inhibitors

- Multiple agents on U.S. market
- Patients should be monitored for hyperkalemia.
- Cough is a problematic adverse effect that may result in discontinuation.
- Angioedema is a rare, but life-threatening adverse effect.
- May increase lithium levels
- NSAIDs may decrease effectiveness.

- A 30%–35% increase in serum creatinine from baseline is permissible in patients with renal insufficiency.
- Patients should be advised to have adequate fluid intake.
- Excellent choice in patients with renal failure, to further protect kidneys and decrease proteinuria
- Avoid in pregnancy

Calcium-channel blockers

Non-dihydropyridine

- Decrease heart rate by decreasing SA and AV nodal conduction
- If possible, avoid in combination with beta-blockers or other drugs that can potentiate decrease in heart rate, because of increased risk of second- or third-degree heart block
- Can be useful in decreasing proteinuria (patients who can't tolerate ACE inhibitor or ARB or for additional effect)

Dihydropyridine

- Causes dose-dependent peripheral edema
- Excellent choice in isolated systolic HTN

Angiotension receptor blockers

- Monitor for hyperkalemia
- May be useful in patients who have experienced ACEI-induced cough
- Beneficial effects in heart failure
- Avoid in pregnancy

Renin inhibitors

- Monitor for hyperkalemia (infrequent alone, but increased risk in renal patients and in combination therapy with other agents that increase potassium)
- May be alternative use for ACEI-induced cough; incidence is 30%–50% less than with ACEI
- Avoid in pregnancy

α_1-adrenergic blockers

- With first dose hypotension often occurs
- Take at bedtime
- Beer's list drug (doxazosin only, see Medicines for Elderly People, Chapter 10, p. 213)
- Beneficial choice in patients with benign prostatic hypertrophy

In the ALLHAT Trial, the alpha-blocker arm of the trial was terminated early because of a 25% increased risk of combined cardiovascular disease, including death from coronary heart disease and doubling in the risk of heart failure, compared to the risk with diuretic chlorthalidone.

Centrally acting α_2-agonists

- Not first line
- Can cause drowsiness, dry mouth, bradycardia
- Beer's list drug
- Rebound hypertension if clonidine is withdrawn abruptly.
- Methyldopa: drug of choice in pregnancy

Peripheral-acting adrenergic antagonists

- Postural hypotension, sedation, diarrhea, confusion, and peripheral edema are possible side effects
- Avoid use in patients with depression or heart failure and with monamine oxidase inhibitors
- Seldom used

Direct vasodilators

- Possible side effects: headache, edema, reflex tachycardia, orthostatic hypotension, flushing, lupus syndrome associated with hydralazine
- Patients often unable to tolerate side effects
- Used in difficult to control hypertension (resistant hypertension)

Target BP

- Target BP is <140/90 mmHg, but some patients, especially the elderly, might not achieve or tolerate these levels.
- Target BP for diabetes or chronic kidney disease is <130/80.
- Some suggest a goal BP of 125/75 mmHg in patients with proteinuria >1 g/day.[1]

Further reading

The ALLHAT Officers and Coordinators for the ALLHAT Collaborative Research Group (2000). Major cardiovascular events in hypertensive patients randomized to doxazosin vs chlorthalidone: the Antihypertensive and lipid-Lowering Treatment to Prevent Heart Attack Trial (ALLHAT). *JAMA* **283**:1967–1975.

The Seventh Report of the Joint National Committee on Prevention, Detection, Evaluation, and Treatment of High Blood Pressure (2003). *JAMA* **289**:2560–2571. Available at: http://www.nhlbi.nih.gov/guidelines/hypertension/jnc7full.pdf

1 Levey A.S. Nondiabetic Kidney Disease (2002). *N Engl J Med* **347**:1505–1511.

Understanding anticoagulation

Anticoagulation therapy becomes necessary in patients who have a type of blood clot referred to as a venous thromboembolism or VTE. Even patients who do not have a VTE, but who have risk factors for VTE may require anticoagulation as a preventive measure.

Vascular damage, venous stasis, and hypercoagulability are the three primary mechanisms by which clotting risk becomes elevated. Hospitalized patients often have more than one of these mechanisms at work. For example, surgery or trauma may result in vascular damage. Damage to valves within the cardiovascular system and physical immobility result in venous stasis.

Hypercoagulability has many etiologies, including hereditary clotting factor disorders, or pathologies such as sepsis or hyperhomocysteinemia. These risk factors are frequently associated with hospitalization, putting this patient population at risk.

Regulation of coagulation

When functioning normally, clotting of the blood occurs by way of 12 plasma proteins called coagulation factors that are produced in the liver. They circulate continuously through the bloodstream in their inactive form, and each is referred to by its corresponding roman numeral (I–XII). They can become activated by several stimuli. Usually, vascular endothelial damage is the inciting trigger.

Once activation occurs, some of the coagulation factors begin to activate others enzymatically, resulting in the subsequent activation of more and more clotting factors until a clot made out of fibrin is formed. Activation of clotting factor II, also called thrombin, facilitates the formation of fibrin, the main structural component of a clot.

Other proteins circulate through the bloodstream to keep the clotting cascade under control by balancing clotting factor initiated coagulation with anticoagulation. Such endogenous anticoagulation-inducing proteins include antithrombin, protein C, and protein S.

Measuring the degree of anticoagulation

Laboratory assays

Activated partial thromboplastin time (aPTT)

- Quantifies unfractionated heparin-related anticoagulation
- Each commercially available aPTT reagent is uniquely responsive to heparin, so each institution should establish a therapeutic range for VTE treatment based on the reagent used.
- Institution-specific therapeutic range for VTE treatment = aPTT that correlates with heparin concentration of 0.3–0.7 anti-factor Xa units/mL
- aPTT should be checked at baseline and 6 hours after initiating VTE treatment, anytime the dose has been changed, and as needed to remain in the therapeutic range during VTE treatment, which is usually daily.
- (aPTT monitoring is not usually necessary for VTE prophylaxis.)

Anti-factor Xa

- Quantifies low-molecular-weight heparin (LMWH)-related anticoagulation
- Therapeutic range for VTE treatment = 0.5–1 anti-factor Xa units/mL if dosed every 12 hours, or if larger doses are given once every 24 hours, 1–2 anti-factor Xa units/mL is acceptable
- Anti-factor Xa does not need to be monitored routinely in patients using LMWH for VTE prophylaxis or treatment, unless they meet the following criteria:
  - Weight >150 kg
  - Renal insufficiency
  - Pregnancy
  - Neonates
- A peak anti-factor Xa level should be checked 4 hours after the third dose is administered.

International normalized ratio (INR)

- Quantifies vitamin K antagonist–related anticoagulation
- Measures ratio of patient's prothrombin time (PT) to a standard control PT
- Therapeutic range is determined by indication for therapy
- Usual therapeutic INR range for treatment of VTE = 2–3

Factors that may potentiate anticoagulation and increase bleeding risk

- Thrombocytopenia
- Platelet dysfunction
- Aspirin/NSAIDs
- SSRIs

Reversing excessive anticoagulation

Patients who experience major bleeding should receive intravenous protamine as an antidote to UFH or LMWH therapy.

- 1 mg of protamine should be administered for every 1 mg of LMWH (maximum of 50 mg)
- 1 mg of protamine should be administered for every 100 units of UFH (maximum of 50 mg)
- No antidotes are available to reverse anticoagulation from
  - Factor Xa inhibitors
  - Direct thrombin inhibitors

Reversal of excessive anticoagulation with the vitamin K antagonist warfarin is usually accomplished by holding warfarin doses and administering oral vitamin K if necessary (see Adjusting Therapy, p. 385).

Coagulation cascade

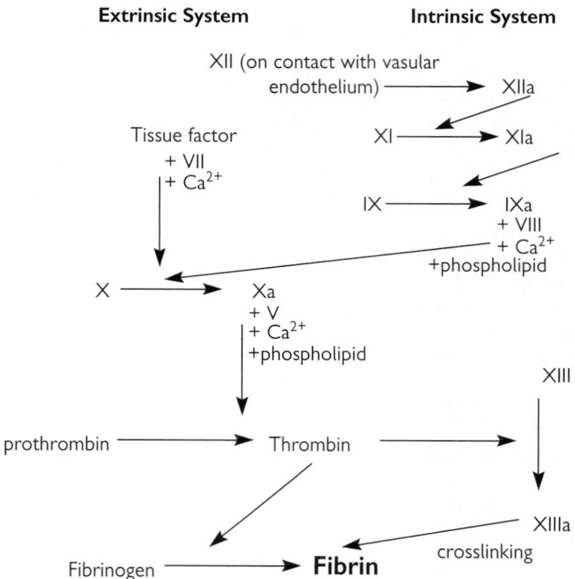

Figure 15.1 The intrinsic and extrinsic pathways of blood coagulation. From Longmore M, Wilkinson IB, Rajagopalan S (2004). *Oxford Handbook of Clinical Medicine*, 6th ed. Oxford: Oxford University Press. By permission of Oxford University Press.

Anticoagulation therapy

Anticoagulation therapies target different aspects of the clotting cascade to counter clot formation. Some inhibit clotting factors, while others enhance endogenous anticoagulation mechanisms. There are four main categories of anticoagulation therapy: antithrombin potency enhancers, factor Xa inhibitors, direct thrombin inhibitors, and vitamin K antagonists.

Commonly used pharmacologic agents in each class include the following:

- Antithrombin efficacy enhancers
- Unfractionated heparin (UFH)
- Low-molecular-weight heparin (LMWH)
  - Enoxaparin, Dalteparin, Tinzaparin
- Factor Xa inhibitors
  - LMWH
  - Fondaparinux
- Vitamin K antagonists (affecting factors II, VII, IX, and X and proteins C and S)
  - Warfarin
- Direct thrombin inhibitors
  - Argatroban, Bivalrudin, Lepirudin

Clinical use of anticoagulants

Prevention of venous thromboembolism

Venous thromboembolism (VTE) describes two major contributors to morbidity and mortality during hospitalization: deep vein thrombosis (DVT) and pulmonary embolism (PE). The benefits of VTE prevention far outweigh the danger, cost, and long-term sequelae associated with clot development and treatment. VTE often prolongs hospital stay and increases readmission rates, as history of VTE is the most significant predictor of a subsequent VTE.

Populations requiring prophylaxis

All inpatients should be screened for VTE prophylaxis indications because hospitalization for medical illness correlates with an eight-fold increase in the risk of VTE over that of healthy individuals. A patient's risk of developing a VTE during hospitalization ranges from 10% to 80%, with spinal cord injury, major trauma, and cancer patients being at the highest end of the risk stratification.

Although uncomplicated general medicine patients have the smallest risk of VTE (10%–20%), they comprise the majority of hospitals' censuses, making them responsible for 70%–80% of the overall incidence of VTE. Thus, all patients should be screened for risk factors that warrant VTE prophylaxis, particularly those who are unable to ambulate early in their hospitalization.

The 2008 American College of Chest Physicians (ACCP) VTE prophylaxis guidelines identify several high-risk populations that are targeted for preventive therapy (see Table 15.28).

Venous thromboembolism prophylaxis

Both pharmacological and nonpharmacological modalities of VTE prophylaxis are available. Non-drug devices may be used as a means of mechanical VTE prophylaxis. Pharmacological measures include drug therapies that produce anticoagulation.

In patients who would likely incur more risk than benefit from pharmacological anticoagulation, mechanical prophylaxis is preferable, although it is generally not as effective as drug therapy. The primary use of nonpharmacological or mechanical prophylaxis is in patients with a very high risk of bleeding.

Some patients may not require either prophylaxis modality. If patients are young and do not have risk factors for clotting or risk factors for falling, frequent ambulation while in the hospital often eliminates the need for either pharmacological or nonpharmacological therapy.

Pharmacological prophylaxis

- UFH is an appropriate, cost-effective agent for VTE prophylaxis, but LMWHs are increasingly replacing UFH in prophylaxis in certain patient populations.
  - Both UFH and LMWH are associated with a risk of heparin-induced thrombocytopenia (HIT) (see Chapter 15, p. 382).
  - Risk of HIT is lower with LMWH than with UFH.

Table 15.28 Risk factors for VTE

Acute medical illness*	Malignant cancer
Advanced age	Myeloproliferative disease
Burns*	Nephrotic syndrome
Cancer*	Obesity
Central-vein catheter placement	Oral contraceptive therapy
Critical illness*	Pregnancy
Venous compression	Respiratory failure
Heart failure	Lower-extremity trauma
History of VTE	Spinal cord injury*
Immobility	Surgery*
Inflammatory bowel syndrome	Thrombophilia
Long-distance travel	Trauma*
Erythropoiesis-stimulating agents	SERM therapy

* Highest risk. Data from: Geerts WH, Bergqvist D, Pineo GF, et al. (2008). Prevention of venous thromboembolism: American College of Chest Physicians Evidence-Based Clinical Practice Guidelines (8th ed.). Chest 133(6):381s–453s.

  - Avoid UFH and LMWH in patients with a history of HIT.
  - Direct thrombin inhibitors may be used in the treatment of HIT.
- LMWH is recommended over UFH for VTE prevention in patients who have undergone total hip replacement (THR) or total knee replacement (TKR).
  - Fondaparinux and warfarin are suitable alternatives to UFH or LMWH in THR, TKR, and hip fracture surgery.
- Although aspirin is effective in prevention of cardiovascular events, it is a weak inhibitor of venous thrombosis. Aspirin is not recommended as a sole means of prophylaxis in patients with VTE risk factors.

Commonly used prophylaxis regimens

- UFH: 5000 units subcutaneously (SC) every 8 hours
- LMWH: All LMWH regimens require renal adjustment
  - Enoxaparin 40 mg SC daily (for most medical indications)
  - Enoxaparin 30 mg SC every12 hours (some orthopedic surgeries)
    - —Patients with CrCl <30 should receive 30 mg SC daily
    - —CrCl <20–25 mL/min: use UFH instead of enoxaparin
- Dalteparin 5000 international units SC daily.
    - —Dosing is weight-based; consult package insert for dosing recommendations
- Fondaparinux: 2.5 mg SC daily (may be safer in patients with a history of HIT, but there is still a risk)
  - Fondaparinux is renally cleared and is contraindicated in patients with CrCl <30 mL/min and inpatients undergoing hemodialysis.

Duration of pharmacological therapy

VTE prophylaxis should continue until a patient is fully ambulatory or being discharged from the hospital. In particularly high-risk surgeries, including hip and knee arthroplasty and oncology surgery, post-hospitalization prophylaxis for 10–35 days should be strongly considered, based on patient risk factors.

High-risk gynecology-oncology surgery patients and trauma patients with major mobility impairments should receive consideration for post-hospitalization anticoagulation as well.

Some contraindications to pharmacological anticoagulation therapy

- Active bleeding
- Hemophilia
- Malignant hypertension
- Severe thrombocytopenia (platelets <20,000)
- Some high-risk surgeries

Anticoagulation agents should only be used with extreme caution in the time period surrounding insertion or removal of a spinal needle or epidural catheter as well as with deep peripheral nerve blockade procedures. Patients can develop severe complications, including permanent paralysis, if an epidural hematoma forms.

Nonpharmacological prophylaxis

Mechanical prophylaxis

The three primary types of mechanical prophylaxis are:

- Graduated compression stockings
- Intermittent pneumatic compression devices
- Venous foot pumps

Mechanical VTE prophylaxis is not as effective as pharmacological therapy, and although DVT incidence may decrease, the incidence of PE is not reduced with mechanical prophylaxis. When contraindications to pharmacological therapy are present, however, mechanical prophylaxis is often the only means of reducing the risk of VTE by preventing venous stasis in immobilized patients.

Mechanical prophylaxis can be used in conjunction with pharmacological anticoagulation therapy in patient populations with very high VTE risk for additive protection.

Treatment of deep vein thrombosis

The goal of DVT treatment is to prevent thrombus extension, PE, post-thrombotic syndrome, and recurrent VTE. Diagnosis of DVT is made by ultrasound or venography.

The treatment of choice for acute DVT is LMWH initiated simultaneously with an oral vitamin K antagonist (usually warfarin 5 mg daily) to provide VTE prophylaxis until the INR is therapeutic for at least 24–48 hours. A regimen of simultaneous warfarin and UFH is equally acceptable to treat DVT, but does not facilitate early hospital discharge like LMWH regimens do.

Any of the following regimens are recommended for 5–7 days (in addition to prolonged warfarin therapy):

- Enoxaparin 1 mg/kg SC every 12 hours
- Enoxaparin 1.5 mg/kg SC daily
- Dalteparin 200 international units (IU)/kg SC daily
  - If patient weighs between 139 and 180 kg, dose should be split into100 IU/kg SC every 12 hours
  - If used for >1 month, 150 IU/kg daily should be used.
- Tinzaparin 175 IU/kg SC daily (dosing is weight-based; consult package insert for recommendations)
- Fondaparinux 7.5 mg SC daily (dosing is weight-based; consult package insert for recommendations)

All LMWH requires dose adjustment in renal dysfunction. Factor Xa monitoring should be used in renal dysfunction and patients with body weight <50 kg or >150 kg.

LMWH should be changed to UFH when CrCl <20–25 mL/min, and in patients getting hemodialysis.

Fondaparinux is contraindicated with CrCl <30 mL/min.

UFH day 1 dosing recommendations (below) must be titrated to institution-specific therapeutic aPTT, or to 1.5- to 2.5-fold prolongation of patient's baseline aPTT.

- 80 unit/kg IV bolus + 18 units/kg/hr continuous infusion
- Platelets should be checked at baseline and at least three times a week to monitor for HIT.

LMWH or UFH and warfarin are initiated simultaneously because warfarin therapy may not yield a therapeutic INR (2–3 for DVT treatment) for a few days, and patients can be in a hypercoagulable state during this time. The duration of warfarin therapy differs according to diagnosis (see Table 15.29).

Table 15.29 Duration of warfarin anticoagulation at INR 2–3 following DVT

Diagnosis	Duration
First DVT with a reversible risk factor	3 months
First DVT of unknown cause	3 months (consider lifelong)
Second or subsequent DVTs	Lifelong
DVT in a cancer patient (warfarin not started until after 3–6 months LMWH)	Lifelong or while cancer is active

*Lifelong therapy is reserved for patients with low bleeding risk, and risk vs. benefit of anticoagulation should be evaluated periodically.

Data from Hirsh J, Hylek E, et al. (2008). Pharmacology and management of the vitamin K antagonists: American College of Chest Physicians Evidence-Based Clinical Practice Guidelines (8th ed.). *Chest* **133**(6):160s–198s.

Daily monitoring of INR is required to titrate to a therapeutic level, and the INR should be stable for at least 24–48 hours before LMWH is discontinued, which is usually 5–7 days after LMWH therapy initiation.

All patients treated for DVT should be ambulatory as early as possible and use graduated compression stockings to limit the incidence and severity of the post-thrombotic syndrome.

Treatment of pulmonary embolism

PE without hemodynamic compromise

The primary treatment for PE without hemodynamic compromise is supportive medical care, including oxygen, analgesia, and anticoagulation. LMWH and warfarin should be initiated simultaneously, and therapy should be overlapped for at least 5 days and until the INR is stable within the therapeutic range (2–3).

PE with hemodynamic compromise

Patients with major PE generally have persistent tachycardia, hypotension, right heart failure, and/or severe hypoxemia. These patients require supportive medical treatment with high-flow oxygen. Severe chest pain may also require analgesia.

For anticoagulation:

- LMWH therapy is preferred over UFH for PE treatment, except in the case of massive PE or a PE that will be treated with fibrinolytic therapy.
- UFH is still commonly used. In the acute stages of a major thromboembolic episode, heparin resistance is common. Since it can suddenly reverse, it is very important to monitor the aPTT closely in acute treatment of a clot.
- When UFH is used, aPTT should be checked every 6 hours and the UFH dose should be adjusted if the aPTT is not within the therapeutic range. Most institutions have specific heparin protocols.
- Warfarin should be initiated within 48 hours. The target INR range is is the same for PE as it is for DVT treatment (2–3). The indication-based duration of warfarin therapy in PE is the same as for DVT.

Heparin-induced thrombocytopenia (HIT)

HIT is a severe, immune-mediated activation of platelets that causes hypercoagulability. Patients who develop HIT are at increased risk for thrombotic complications. Diagnosis of HIT is made when any of the following occur in the presence of HIT antibodies, as determined by the serotonin release assay and the heparin-platelet factor 4 assay:

- An unexplained fall in platelet count of ≥50% from baseline
- Otherwise unexplained thrombosis within the first 5–14 days following initiation of heparin therapy
- Necrotizing skin lesions at heparin injection sites
- Acute systemic (anaphylactoid) reactions that occur after IV heparin administration.

Even if a patient does not have an active thrombosis or definitive diagnosis of HIT, if it is strongly suspected, anticoagulation with the following non-heparin products is recommended

- Argatroban: initial infusion of 2 mcg/kg/min in non-critically ill patients with normal hepatic function. Initial doses of 1 mcg/kg/min should be considered in critically ill patients. In patients with AST or ALT >3 times the upper limit of normal, initial doses of 0.5 mcg/kg/min should be used.
- Lepirudin: bolus dose followed by 0.15 mg/kg/hr (up to 110 kg) infusion, with dose adjustment based on renal function and aPTT monitoring
- Bivalirudin and danaparoid are also recommended in the *Chest* guidelines.
- Initiation of warfarin therapy is appropriate once the platelet count has stabilized. Warfarin should be overlapped with the non-heparin anticoagulant until an appropriate INR level is reached after a minimum of 5 days of overlapping therapy.
- Fondaparinux is an alternative bridging agent in patients being transitioned from non-heparin anticoagulant therapy to warfarin, but is not FDA approved for this indication. This option should not be used in patients with renal impairment.

Further reading

Ansell J, Hirsh J, Hylek E, et al. (2008). Pharmacology and management of the vitamin K antagonists: American College of Chest Physicians Evidence-Based Clinical Practice Guidelines (8th ed.). *Chest* **133**:160s–198s.

Geerts WH, Bergqvist D, Pineo GF, et al. (2008). Prevention of venous thromboembolism: American College of Chest Physicians Evidence-Based Clinical Practice Guidelines (8th ed.). *Chest* **133**:381s–453s.

Hirsh J, Bauer KA, Donati MB, et al. (2008). Parenteral anticoagulants: American College of Chest Physicians (8th ed.). *Chest* **133**:141s–159s.

Kearon C, Kahn SR, Giancarlo A, et al. (2008). Antithrombotic therapy for venous thromboembolic disease: American College of Chest Physicians Evidence-Based Clinical Practice Guidelines (8th ed.). *Chest* **133**:454s–545s.

Warfarin dosing

Initial dosing

- Patients are generally started on 5 mg of warfarin daily.
- Lower (≤5 mg daily) initial doses are usually recommended, especially in patients with:
  - Older age (>60 years old)
  - Malnourishment
  - Debilitation
  - Liver disease
  - Heart failure
  - Bleeding risk (e.g., recent major surgery, history of bleeding).
  - Some concomitant drug therapies (e.g., amiodarone) may warrant empirically starting at lower warfarin doses.
  - Patients with recent heart valve replacement surgery should be started on a daily warfarin dose of 2–3 mg.

When warfarin therapy is being initiated and rapid anticoagulation is required (e.g., when actively treating a thromboembolism or a patient with a high risk of clot formation), UFH should be overlapped with the first 4–5 days of warfarin therapy or until a therapeutic INR has been maintained for two measurements (taken 24 hours apart).

Maintenance dose

The maintenance dose of warfarin is unique for each patient, depending on the indication and the target INR (see Table 15.30).

A maintenance dose can be established by carefully titrating the warfarin dose until the INR is within the indicated therapeutic range.

Table 15.30 INR targets for anticoagulation therapy

Indication	Target INR (range)
Antiphospholipid antibody syndrome (lupus anticoagulant)	2.5 (2.A0–3.0)
Atrial fibrillation or atrial flutter	2.5 (2.0–3.0)
Deep vein thrombosis treatment	2.5 (2.0–3.0)
Pulmonary embolism treatment	2.5 (2.0–3.0)
Bioprosthetic valve (aortic or mitral position)	2.5 (2.0–3.0)
St. Jude bileaflet mechanical valve (aortic position)	2.5 (2.0–3.0)
St. Jude bileaflet mechanical valve (mitral position)	3.0 (2.5–3.5)
Mechanical heart valve	3.0 (2.5–3.5)
Recurrence of DVT or PE (with therapeutic INR)	3.0 (2.5–3.5)

Data from Hirsh J, Hylek E, et al. (2008). Pharmacology and management of the vitamin K antagonists: American College of Chest Physicians Evidence-Based Clinical Practice Guidelines (8th ed.). *Chest* 133(6):160s–198s.

- INR should be checked within 48 hours of initiating therapy and at least 2 times during the first week of therapy.
- INR should be checked weekly for 2 weeks, then every 2 weeks, and then monthly, depending on the patient's stability within the therapeutic INR range.

Adjusting therapy

- INR should be monitored monthly once a patient's INR has become stabilized.
- Any change to warfarin therapy requires follow-up monitoring within 2 weeks.
- INRs deviating very slightly from the therapeutic goal may be managed by increased monitoring frequency without dose adjustments when a modifiable cause of deviation may be identified and corrected.
- The total weekly warfarin dose may be changed by 5%–20% (usually 10%) at a time to help achieve a therapeutic INR when a dose change needs to be made.
- Generally, trends should guide warfarin dose adjustments.
- When an INR is higher than the goal INR, as long as there is no evidence of active bleeding, hold one or more doses of warfarin to reduce the INR, and monitor the patient more frequently. Consideration should also be given to reducing the total weekly dose.
  - Once INR exceeds 5.0–9.0 (without active bleeding), all of the above INR reducing measures should be taken, and treatment with 1–5 mg of oral vitamin K should be considered.
- Any incidence of significant, active bleeding should be referred immediately for inpatient evaluation, as this may warrant treatment with slow infusions of IV vitamin K, fresh frozen plasma, or recombinant factor VIIa.

Monitoring therapy

Modifiable causes of INR fluctuation include the following:

- Nonadherence—missed doses or doses taken at the wrong time
- Changes in kinetic parameters— weight change and fluid shifts
- Diseases—infections, liver disease, renal impairment, and GI or absorption disturbances
- Changes in social behavior—excessive alcohol consumption
- Vitamin K content of diet—daily low-dose oral vitamin K therapy (100–200 mcg) may be used to help stabilize labile INRs
- Stress
- Genetics—patients with variant genotypes of CYP2C9 and vitamin K epoxide reductase complex subunit 1 (VKORC-1) may require lower warfarin doses.
- Drug interactions, including over-the-counter medicines and herbal supplements (see Table 15.31)

Duration of therapy

While some patients require life-long anticoagulation therapy, many indications for anticoagulation require only 3–12 months of therapy.

Table 15.31 Drug interactions with warfarin

Drugs and herbal supplements that potentiate anticoagulation	Drugs and herbal supplements that reduce anticoagulation
Alcohol (with liver disease)	Carbamazepine
Amiodarone	Cholestyramine
Cimetidine	Etodolac
Ciprofloxacin	Griseofulvin
Citalopram	Mercaptopurine
Clofibrate	Mesalamine
Diltiazem	Nafcillin
Erythromycin	Phenobarbital
Fenofibrate	Ribavirin
Fluconazole	Rifampin
Gemfibrozil	Sucralfate
Ginkgo biloba	Trazodone
Isoniazid	
Metronidazole	
Omeprazole	
Piroxicam	
Propafenone	
Propranolol	
Sertraline	
Sulfinpyrazone	
Sulfamethoxazole-trimethoprim	
Voriconazole	
Zileuton	

Data from Holbrook AM, Pereira JA, Labiris R, et al. (2005). Systematic overview of warfarin and its drug and food interactions. *Arch Intern Med* **165**:1095–1106.

Counseling patients treated with warfarin

After the decision had been made to initiate therapy, patients should be educated about the dynamics of warfarin therapy and the associated risks. In addition to verbal counseling, patients should also be provided written information.

Educational materials and verbal teaching should include:

- The reason that anticoagulation is required for the patient
- How warfarin works—a patient-specific discussion with varying complexity, based on the patient's education and cognitive ability
- Dose—how much, how often, and the indication-specific duration of therapy
- The importance of adherence (see Chapter 1, Adherence)
- The importance of taking warfarin at the same time each day. (Usually, evening dosing is best because it allows at least 12 hours between dose administration and INR checking.)
- What to do when a dose is missed
- Signs of clotting and bleeding, and when it is appropriate to seek emergency medical attention (see Tables 15.32 and 15.33)
- The need for frequent INR monitoring through blood testing
- Meaning and interpretation of INR
- Patients should know their specific INR goal and range.
- Importance of reminding health-care professionals (dentists, pharmacists, and physicians) about warfarin treatment
- Avoidance of drug interactions (see Table 15.31), including over-the-counter medicines (especially aspirin-containing products) and herbal preparations
- Maintaining limited, consistent alcohol intake
- Importance of maintaining consistent dietary vitamin K intake (completely eliminating it from the diet is not required); see Table 15.34)
- Using contraception when appropriate, since warfarin is pregnancy category X
- Taking precautions to avoid injury that could lead to bleeding (avoiding contact sports, using sharp objects carefully, not walking barefoot outdoors, and avoiding electric razors)
- Purchasing an anticoagulation ID card or medical ID bracelet

Patients should know that INR monitoring is necessary for the entire duration of warfarin therapy. All patients taking warfarin should be connected with an anticoagulation clinic or have access to INR monitoring services of some kind.

Patients should be aware that any time they are hospitalized, have changes to their medications, or undergo surgery or other invasive procedures the INR should be monitored more closely. Specific guidelines are available and should be used to guide warfarin therapy discontinuation before surgical procedures for prevention of intraoperative bleeding.

Table 15.32 Signs of bleeding

Normal signs of anticoagulation-related bleeding	Signs of anticoagulation-related bleeding requiring immediate medical attention
Bleeding gums	Severe headache (hemorrhagic stroke)
Cuts may bleed longer T	Severe stomach pain (GI bleed)
Easy bruising	Uncontrollable bleeding of any kind
Minor nosebleeds	Vomiting blood, bloody stools, or severe stomach pain.
Minimal, hemorrhoid-related bleeding from lower GI tract	

Table 15.33 Signs of clotting requiring immediate medical attention

- Acute shortness of breath, wheezing or crackles in the lungs, unexplained rapid breathing, or chest wall tenderness (pulmonary embolism)
- One-sided weakness or slurred speech (ischemic stroke)
- Intense chest pain or pressure (myocardial infarction)
- One-sided redness or swelling of an extremity that is often painful (deep vein thrombosis)

Table 15.34 Foods with high vitamin K content

Asparagus	Lettuce
Avocado	Olive oil
Broccoli	Peas
Brussels sprouts	Pistachio nuts
Cabbage	Soybean products
Collard greens	Spinach
Green onions	Vegetable oils

Data from Brown C (2006). *An Overview of Traditional Anticoagulants*. U.S. Pharmacist.

Outpatient anticoagulation management

Anticoagulation management may be provided by pharmacists in the outpatient setting. Anticoagulation clinics provide ongoing monitoring of the PT/INR. This service is critical because warfarin has a narrow therapeutic index, with a relatively small margin between safety and toxicity. The goal of any anticoagulation clinic is to provide intensive follow-up and maintain the PT/INR within the target therapeutic range for each patient.

Each outpatient anticoagulation clinic will have institution-specific protocols and guidelines to direct warfarin dose adjustments, determine the INR range at which point-of-care testing needs to be verified with laboratory results (point-of-care devices often have reduced accuracy at higher INRs) and many other clinical practices. Anticoagulation clinics often incorporate the following services into each visit:

- Review of the current dose and INR goals
- INR testing—point-of-care testing or through a laboratory
- Adherence and consistency assessment (number of missed doses)
- Re-education and assessment of signs of bleeding or clotting
- Lifestyle assessment
  - Dietary changes (especially vitamin K content)
  - Alcohol use
- Medication history and drug-interaction screening (including herbals and over-the-counter medications)
- Making appropriate dose adjustments when necessary
- Inquiry about upcoming dental or surgical procedures
- Referring patients for escalation of care when appropriate
- Clearly educating patients about dose changes and how they should be executed
- Ensuring that patients will receive timely follow-up
- Ensuring that patients have medication refills when needed
- Documenting that all the services listed above have been provided
- Maintaining communication with patients for rescheduling any missed appointments

Home-based services

When patients are home bound, qualified home health nurses may be able to help manage anticoagulation therapy.

Future of services

With the growth of technology, anticoagulation management is undergoing change, with an increasing number of patients testing their own INR at home, and adjusting their warfarin dose in coordination with a pharmacist by telephone. Computer programs have been shown to be effective in making warfarin-dosing recommendations, based on dose-to-INR correlation trends.

Additionally, the growth of pharmacogenomics (see Chapter 10. Pharmacogenomics, p. 238) is making it possible to predict how patients will respond to medication therapy on the basis of genetic makeup. Tests to determine which patients will be at a higher bleeding risk and will require lower doses of warfarin therapy based on CYP2C9 and VKORC1 genotype are already available.

Clinical trials have been conducted to determine if genotyping patients and then empirically reducing starting warfarin doses in patients with variant genotypes will help reduce the incidence of bleeding or unnecessarily high INRs. Results of these trials are conflicting.

Further reading

Ansell J, Hirsh J, Hylek E, et al. (2008). Pharmacology and management of the vitamin K antagonists: American College of Chest Physicians Evidence-Based Clinical Practice Guidelines (8th ed.). *Chest* **133**(6):160s–198s.

Dager W (2003). Initiating warfarin therapy. *Ann Pharmacother* **37**(6):905–908.

Kearon C, Kahn SR, Giancarlo A, et al. (2008). Antithrombotic therapy for venous thromboembolic disease: American College of Chest Physicians Evidence-Based Clinical Practice Guidelines (8th ed.). *Chest* **133**(6):454s–545s.

Hyperlipidemia

Coronary heart disease (CHD) is the leading cause of morality in the United States. Hyperlipidemia is a major cause of atherosclerosis and often results in CHD. Hyperlipidemia is preventable; however, patients often do not meet established lipid goals. The National Cholesterol Education Program (NCEP) Expert Panel on Detection, Evaluation, and Treatment of High Blood Cholesterol in Adults has developed guidelines for cholesterol management.

To prevent coronary events, patients must be assessed for risk. Along with low-density lipid (LDL) cholesterol, risk determinants include presence or absence of CHD, other atherosclerotic diseases (e.g., peripheral arterial disease, abdominal aortic aneurysm, and symptomatic carotid artery disease), and major risk factors other than LDL (see Table 15.35).

Risk categories

- *Very high risk:* CHD plus either multiple major risk factors (diabetes), severe and poorly controlled risk factors (continued cigarette smoking), multiple risk factors of the metabolic syndrome (high triglycerides [TG] ≥200 mg/dL plus non–high-density lipids [HDL] ≥130 mg/dL with HDL <40 mg/dL), or acute coronary syndrome
- *High risk:* CHD or CHD risk equivalents >20% chance of CHD within 10 years
- *Moderately high risk:* ≥2 risk factors; 10%–20% chance of CHD in 10 years
- *Moderate risk:* ≥2 risk factors; <10% chance of CHD in 10 years
- *Low risk:* 0–1 risk factors, 10-year risk assessment not assigned

Risk equivalents

- Clinical manifestations of noncoronary forms of atherosclerotic disease (peripheral artery disease, abdominal aortic aneurysm, and carotid artery disease [transient ischemic attacks or stroke of carotid origin >50% obstruction of carotid artery])
- Diabetes
- ≥2 risk factors

Treatment of elevated LDL includes therapeutic lifestyle changes and drug therapy. Table 15.36 details the primary LDL goal for each risk category and when to initiate these two interventions.

Pharmacological treatment

HMG CoA reductase inhibitors

- Atorvastatin, fluvastatin, lovastatin, pravastatin, rosuvastatin, simvastatin
- LDL reduction: 18%–63%
- HDL increase: 5%–15%
- Triglyceride reduction: 7%–30%
  - Dose: see Table 15.37
  - It is estimated that for every doubling of a statin dose, LDL is lowered by approximately 6%.

Table 15.35 Major risk factors that impact LDL goals

- Cigarette smoking
- Hypertension (BP ≥140/90 or on antihypertensive medication)
- Low HDL cholesterol (<40 mg/dL)
- Family history of premature CHD (CHD in female first-degree relative <65 years old and CHD in male first-degree relative <55 years old)
- Age (men ≥45 years; women ≥55 years)

Data from ATP III Update 2004: Implications of Recent Clinical Trials for the ATP III Guidelines. http://www.nhlbi.nih.gov/guidelines/cholesterol/atp3upd04.htm

Table 15.36 Risk categories and LDL lipid goals

Risk category	Primary LDL goal (mg/dL)	LDL level (mg/dL) for initiating therapeutic lifestyle changes*	LDL level (mg/dL) for considering drug treatment
Very high risk	<70	>100	>100
High risk	<100	≥100	≥100
Moderately high risk	<130 optional goal <100	≥130	≥130 (100–129 drug therapy optional)
Moderate risk	<130	≥130	≥160
Low risk	<160	≥160	≥190

*Therapeutic lifestyle changes: saturated fat intake <7% of calories; cholesterol intake <200 mg/day; increasing soluble fiber (20–25 g/day); and plant stanols/sterols (2 g/day) as options to enhance LDL lowering, Weight management and increased physical activity also reduce risk.

Data from ATP III Update 2004: Implications of Recent Clinical Trials for the ATP III Guidelines. http://www.nhlbi.nih.gov/guidelines/cholesterol/atp3upd04.htm

Table 15.37 Usual statin dose for reducing LDL 30%–40%

Drug and dose	LDL reduction (%)
Atorvastatin 10 mg	39
Fluvastatin 80 mg	36
Lovastatin 40 mg	34
Pravastatin 40 mg	40
Rosuvastatin 5–10 mg	39–45
Simvastatin 20–40 mg	38–50

Data from ATP III Update 2004: Implications of Recent Clinical Trials for the ATP III Guidelines. http://www.nhlbi.nih.gov/guidelines/cholesterol/atp3upd04.htm

- Statins are generally well tolerated; there is a risk of myopathy or increased LFTs (stop if >3× upper limits of normal [ULN])
- May interact with other drugs metabolized by cytochrome P-450 isoenzymes
- Check creatinine kinase (CK) level if renal decline, or complaints of myopathy. Discontinue statin if CK> 10× ULN
- Consider other drugs in combination with statins when LDL remains 30 mg/dL above goal and TG are >200 mg/dL or if elevated TG or low HDL

Bile acid sequestrants

- Cholestyramine, colestipol, colesevelam
- LDL reduction: 15%–30%
- HDL increase: 3%–5%
- TG reduction: no change or increase; therefore, contraindicated when TG >400 mg/dL
  - Dose: cholestyramine 4–16 g/day, colestipol 5–20 g/day, colsevelam 2.6–3.8 g/day
  - Adverse effects include GI distress, constipation, decreased absorption of other medications
  - May have patient adherence issues due to granule formulation (cholestyramine, colestipol)

Nicotinic acid

- Nicotinc acid immediate release (Niacin), nicotinic acid extended release (Niaspan)
- LDL reduction: 5%–25%
- HDL increase: 15%–35%
- TG reduction: 20%–50%
  - Dose: nicotinc acid immediate release 1.5–3 g/day (titrate dose), nicotinic acid extended release 1–2 g/day
  - Adverse effects include flushing, hyperglycemia, hyperuricemia, hepatotoxicity
  - Flushing can be minimized with use of extended-release formulation, starting with 500 mg and titrating up slowly. Flushing is also reduced when given with a non-fatty meal and with 325 mg aspirin or 200 mg ibuprofen given 30 minutes prior to dose.

Fibrates

- Gemfibrozil, fenofibrate
- LDL reduction: 5%–20%
- HDL increase: 10%–20%
- TG reduction: 20%–50%
- Dose: gemfibrozil 600 mg/day (divided bid), fenofibrate 200 mg/day
- Adverse effects include dyspepsia, myopathy, gallstones
- Fenofibrate is renally cleared; therefore, a serum creatinine should be drawn prior to therapy (start lowest dose for serum creatinine <50 mL/min)
- Check LFTs and discontinue if >3× ULN

Intestinal cholesterol absorption inhibitor

- Ezetimibe
- LDL reduction: 15%–20%
- HDL increase: 3%–5%
- TG reduction: <8%
- Dose: 10 mg/day
- Adverse effects include abdominal pain, myalgia, headache, sinusitis
- Take 2 hours before or after administration of bile acid sequestrant

Omega 3 fatty acids

- Fish oil, flax seed oil, and prescription fish-oil formulation containing 440 mg EPA and 260 mg DHA
- Significantly decrease TG alone and in combination
- Adverse effects include fishy-taste disturbance

Combination therapy (with a statin)

- Drug therapy with non-statins lowers LDL by 5%–30%, depending on the dose; this is equivalent to increasing a statin 2–3 times.
- Combination therapy allows increased focus on non-HDL-cholesterol; non-HDL-cholesterol correlates strongly as a predictor of CVD and mortality, more than LDL cholesterol.
- When combining a statin with a fibrate, fenofibrate is preferred, as there is no inhibition of statin metabolism, <1.0% risk for myopathy. Gemfibrozil should be avoided in combination, if possible, as it shares a second metabolic pathway, glucuronidation, common to statins and increases the risk of myopathy.
- Niacin is often added to a statin if the HDL is low and/or TGs are elevated.

Other considerations

- Treat TGs first if ≥500 mg/dL to avoid possible pancreatitis. If patient has diabetes and hemoglobin A1C is >8%, then blood glucose control is paramount in decreasing TG levels, as diabetes promotes lipogenesis and, subsequently, elevations in TG.
- Dietary fat restriction and simple carbohydrate restriction also help reduce TG.
- Low HDL is considered an independent risk factor for CVD; the Framingham study showed that for every 20 mg/dL reduction in HDL, CHD risk increases by 50%.
- In diabetes, LDL goal is <100 mg; with high risk, <70 mg/dL. The American Diabetes Association recommends a 30%–40% reduction from baseline LDL.

Further reading

Grundy SM, Cleeman JL, Merz CN, et al. (2004). National Heart, Lung, and Blood Institute; American College of Cardiology Foundation; American Heart Association. Implications of recent clinical trials for the National Cholesterol Education Program Adult Treatment Panel III guidelines. *Circulation* **110**:227–239.

Liu J, Sempos CT, Donahue RP, et al. (2006). Non-high-density lipoprotein and very-low-density lipoprotein cholesterol and their risk predictive values in coronary heart disease. *Am J Cardiol* **98**:1363–1368.

Introduction to critical care

Critical care medicine involves caring for patients with extensive monitoring and care needs that can only be provided in an intensive care unit (ICU) setting. This may involve mechanical ventilation for acute respiratory compromise or continuous cardiac monitoring for hemodynamically unstable patients.

Care of these patients involves an array of equipment and devices such as central venous line catheters, arterial lines, endotracheal tubes for mechanical ventilation, renal replacement therapies, and monitors for hemodynamic and respiratory status.

Many hospitals also have intermediate-care or step-down units for patients who do not require the full complement of comprehensive critical care services but still require a certain degree of monitoring or care beyond what can be provided on the general ward.

Critical care team

The practice of critical care has increasingly become more multidisciplinary. In addition to the physician intensivist and critical care–trained nurse, the team may include pharmacists, respiratory therapists, social workers, physical and occupational therapists, and nutrition support specialists. Each member of the team contributes their expertise and knowledge, allowing for well thought-out decisions and treatment plans resulting in better patient outcomes.

In recent years, there has been a tremendous increase in the number and quality of evidenced-based critical care medicine studies advancing the practice of critical care medicine.

Pharmacotherapy in critical care

Critically ill patients often require a broad variety of different medications, including broad-spectrum antibiotics, cardiovascular medications such as vasopressors and antihypertensive agents, fluid replacement, anticoagulants, sedatives, analgesics, and agents to decrease the incidence of gastrointestinal bleeding (H2 blockers and proton pump inhibitors). Patients in the ICU receive nearly twice as many different drugs as other hospitalized patients, which increases the chance for medication errors, drug interactions, and adverse drug events.

Patients in the ICU are also known to have altered medication pharmacokinetics as a result of decreased renal function and liver function, alterations in volume status, and changes in drug protein binding. Alterations in pharmacokinetics and pharmacodynamics may alter the response to various medications, necessitating careful monitoring of clinical outcomes and adverse events.

Scoring systems in critical care

Many scoring systems are used in critical care practice, including systems for severity of illness such as the commonly used APACHE II score. The APACHE II score is based on 12 physiological and biochemical variables. It provides a measure of severity of illness and allows for estimation of the risk of death. The APACHE II score is also used in clinical research to stratify patients according to severity of illness.

The injury severity score (ISS) is commonly used for trauma patients to aid in triage and to allow for comparisons of trauma patients in a hospital over time or between different hospitals. Scoring systems are also used for assessing levels of neurological function and sedation.

Scoring systems for neurological function

- The Glascow Coma Score (GCS) has a scale of 1–15 and uses eye opening, motor response, and verbal response for assessment.
- Ramsay sedation scale
- Richmond Agitation and Sedation Scale (RASS)

Role of the critical care pharmacist

Pharmacists are assuming greater roles and responsibilities in the care of critically ill patients and have become integral members of the ICU multidisciplinary team. Involvement of critical care pharmacists has been shown to decrease drug-related costs, prevent adverse drug events, and reduce patient morbidity in critically ill ICU patients. The Society of Critical Care Medicine (SCCM) as well as other physician and pharmacy organizations have deemed pharmacists an essential component of critical care practice.

Activities of critical care pharmacist

- Make rounds with the critical care multidisciplinary team
- Review profiles and identify drug-related problems
- Teaching role (students and residents)
- Medication reconciliation of patients' medication regimens
- Pharmacokinetic monitoring
- Nutritional support monitoring
- Identify and report adverse drug reactions
- Participate in departmental and institutional quality improvement and protocol and guideline development committees
- Scholarly activity, including conducting of clinical research and submission of manuscripts for publication

Common critical care therapies with pharmacist interventions

- Stress ulcer prophylaxis
- Deep vein thrombosis and pulmonary embolism prophylaxis
- Antibiotic therapy
- Total parenteral nutrition
- Glycemic control
- Sedation, analgesia, and neuromuscular blockade
- Treatment of thromboembolic diseases with anticoagulants
- Renal dysfunction drug-dosing adjustments
- Electrolyte replacement
- Treatment of sepsis
  - Fluid resuscitation
  - Vasopressors
  - Corticosteroids
  - Activated protein C

Importance of communication

Good communication among all members of the critical care team is essential to ensure that all health-care providers are aware and involved in the plan of care. Plans of care are more likely to succeed if those involved in implementing the plan are involved in discussion of the care plan, and this includes the pharmacist.

Pharmacists on the critical care team will need to effectively communicate with the physicians, nurses, and sometimes the patient to gather medication histories when appropriate. There are often many different disciplines and teams involved in the care of the ICU patient, making this communication more challenging.

There also are differences between "open" ICUs, in which a different team other than the critical care team has primary responsibility for the patient, and a "closed" ICU, in which the intensivist and the critical care team has primary responsibility for the patient. In open ICUs it can be difficult to determine which team or member of the team is the appropriate person to address concerns to.

Communication with patients can be difficult because of decreased mental status from sedative medications and the effects of acute critical illness. It is important to realize, however, that patients still may be able to hear conversations among the medical team, despite the appearance of not being able to do so.

Further reading

Boucher BA, Wood GC, Swanson JM (2006). Pharmacokinetic changes in critical illness. *Crit Care Clin* **22**:255–271.

Kane SL, Weber RJ, Dasta JF (2003). The impact of critical care pharmacists on enhancing patient outcomes. *Intensive Care Med* **29**:691–698.

Leape LL, Cullen DJ, Clapp MD, et al. (1999). Pharmacist participation on physician rounds and adverse drug events in the intensive care unit. *JAMA* **282**:267–270.

Maclaren R, Devlin JW, Martin SJ, et al. (2006). Critical care pharmacy services in Unites States hospitals. *Ann Pharmacother* **40**:612–618.

Acid–base disorders

The body produces a large amount of acidic compounds daily, including carbon dioxide (CO_2, converted to carbonic acid when it combines with water) and hydrogen ions from the metabolism of carbohydrates, fats, and proteins. Under normal conditions, the pH is maintained in a narrow range (7.35–7.45) by excretion of CO_2 and hydrogen ions and through buffering with bicarbonate.

The kidneys and lungs maintain acid–base balance. The renal system coordinates bicarbonate and hydrogen ion production and excretion and the lungs regulate the excretion of CO_2.

Increased intake, altered production, or impaired or excessive excretion of acid or base leads to derangements in blood pH. *Acidosis* is characterized by a low pH (<7.35) and may be induced by a low serum bicarbonate (<24 meq/L) or by an elevation in partial pressure of carbon dioxide in arterial blood ($PaCO_2$; >40 mmHg). *Alkalosis* is characterized by an elevated pH (>7.45) and may be induced by an elevated serum bicarbonate (>30 meq/L) or a decrease in $PaCO_2$ (<35 mmHg).

Acid–base balance equation

$$CO_2 + H_2O \leftrightarrow H_2CO_3 \text{ (carbonic acid)} \leftrightarrow H^+ + HCO_3^-$$

Metabolic acid–base disorders

Metabolic acidosis and metabolic alkalosis are common acid–base disorders in the ICU. Metabolic acid–base disorders involve increases or decreases in the serum bicarbonate.

Metabolic acidosis

Metabolic acidosis is associated with a low pH and low serum bicarbonate. Acidosis is the most common metabolic acid–base disorder encountered in the ICU and includes anion gap (AG) and non-AG acidosis.

$$AG = \text{Serum sodium} - (\text{Serum chloride} + \text{Serum bicarbonate})$$

The normal AG is 8–12 mEq/L and an elevation in the AG indicates the presence of an additional pathologic anion. Normal AG acidosis occurs in the setting of bicarbonate loss, but without the presence of an additional pathologic anion.

Causes of increased AG acidosis

- Lactic acidosis
- Toxic ingestions (methanol, propylene glycol)
- Diabetic ketoacidosis
- Rhabdomyolysis
- Renal failure and uremia

Causes of normal AG acidosis

- GI losses of bicarbonate (diarrhea, intestinal fistula output)
- Renal losses of bicarbonate
- Excessive saline administration

Treatment of metabolic acidosis

Treatment of a metabolic acidosis is directed at correcting the underlying cause of the process (e.g., insulin and fluid for diabetic ketoacidosis, dialysis for renal failure, and treatment of sepsis for lactic acidosis). Administration of bicarbonate is controversial as it may actually worsen some clinical parameters. Bicarbonate therapy should be considered for life-threatening acidosis (pH <7.1 and/or sodium bicarbonate <12 meq/L).

Metabolic alkalosis

Metabolic alkalosis is associated with a high pH and elevated serum bicarbonate. Causes of metabolic alkalosis involve loss of H^+ ions in relation to bicarbonate resulting in an elevated serum bicarbonate (>30 meq/L).

Causes of metabolic alkalosis

- Excessive loss of gastric secretions including H^+ (GI tube drainage, vomiting)
- Contraction alkalosis from diuretics
- Excessive sodium bicarbonate or citrate
- Drugs including corticosteroids and laxatives

Treatment of metabolic alkalosis

- Replacement of fluid with saline
- Acetazolamide 500 mg IV or PO q8h until corrected
- Spironolactone for hyperaldosteronism-related alkalsosis

Respiratory acid–base disorders

Respiratory acid–base disorders involve disturbances in the plasma levels of CO_2 measured on arterial blood gas as $PaCO_2$. A normal $PaCO_2$ value for healthy adults is 35–45 mmHg. In respiratory acidosis, lack of adequate alveolar ventilation results in elevated levels of CO_2 (>45 mmHg), which is converted to carbonic acid leading to acidosis.

Hyperventilation leads to decreases in CO_2, leading to respiratory alkalosis. Any condition that results in hyperventilation may lead to respiratory alkalosis.

Mixed acid–base disorders and compensation

Metabolic and respiratory acid–base disorders may occur independently or also very commonly coexist in the same patient. A primary metabolic acid–base disorder will generate a respiratory response to compensate for the acidosis in the body's attempt to maintain a normal pH.

A patient with a metabolic acidosis will have increased respiration rate to get rid of CO_2 as a compensatory mechanism. A patient with a metabolic alkalosis will decrease respiration rate to retain CO_2 and compensate for the alkalosis. The kidneys are also able to compensate for a respiratory acid–base disorder by retention or excretion of bicarbonate.

Further reading

Gunnerson KJ (2005). Clinical review: The meaning of acid–base abnormalities in the intensive care unit part I—epidemiology. *Crit Care* **9**:508–516.

Mechanical ventilation

Mechanical ventilation, also referred to as positive pressure ventilation, involves forcing air into the central airways, which then flows to the alveoli. Mechanical ventilation may be required for patients with acute or chronic respiratory failure. Patients in respiratory failure may either have inadequate oxygenation of blood (passage of oxygen across the alveoli membrane) or difficulty with ventilation (movement of air into and out of lungs) with subsequent increases in CO_2.

Indications for mechanical ventilation

Mechanical ventilation may be indicated for patients with either oxygenation or ventilatory insufficiency. A variety of physical signs and biochemical variables are used to determine when patients may require ventilatory support (respiratory rate, $PaO_{2,}$, CO_2, and pH) Patients with a variety of acute and chronic diseases may require mechanical ventilation.

Noninvasive ventilation

Selected patients might initially be managed with noninvasive techniques, such as a tight-fitting face or nasal mask to augment spontaneous breathing in compliant patients by assisting with the inspiration effort or providing continuous positive airway pressure (CPAP). A nasogastric tube may also be placed to decompress the stomach, which can become inflated through air swallowing.

Invasive ventilation

The more conventional form of mechanical ventilation is through the insertion of a plastic tube (endotracheal tube) into the patient's trachea and connection of the tube to a ventilator device. The process of placing the tube is known as "intubation." The tube may be placed through the upper airway (nasal or oral) or directly into the trachea (tracheotomy).

Drugs used to facilitate intubation

Intubation requires overcoming the body's natural barriers to objects entering the trachea. Insertion of a tube into the trachea is an extremely uncomfortable procedure that produces coughing and agitation. A variety of medications may help to blunt the noxious effects of intubation:

- Bezodiazepines such as lorarepam or midazolam (1–2 mg)
- Propofol (2 mg/kg)
- Thiopental (3–5 mg/kg)
- Etomidate (0.2–0.6 mg/kg)
- Fentanyl (2 mcg/kg)
- Neuromuscular blockers such as rocuronium (1 mg/kg) or succinylcholine (2 mg/kg)
- Lidocaine (1.5–2 mg/kg) or as topical 4% solution

Modes of ventilation

There are a plethora of different types of ventilators with a vast array of different features that provide for numerous ventilator modes and may facilitate improvements in ventilation, oxygenation, and patient comfort.

Volume-limited ventilation

With volume-limited ventilation, inspiration is terminated after the delivery of a preset tidal volume. There are several modes of mechanical ventilation that deliver volume-limited ventilation.

Controlled mechanical ventilation (CMV)

- Ventilator controls the movement of gas through the lungs
- Very high level of support
- Preset number of breaths are delivered to supply all the patient's ventilatory requirements
- Does not take into account any residual breathing effort and does not require patients to initiate any breaths

Assist controlled mechanical ventilation (ACV)

- Ventilator controls movement of gas through the lungs
- Preset number of controlled breaths provided by ventilator
- Patient may trigger additional assisted breaths through initiation of a spontaneous breath
- High level of support that allows additional assisted breaths initiated by the patient

Intermittent mandatory ventilation (IMV)

- Ventilator controls movement of gas through lungs
- Allows for spontaneous patient-initiated breaths in between mandatory breaths
- Allows patients to breath over the ventilator and increase overall minute ventilation rate

Synchronized intermittent mandatory ventilation (SIMV)

- Ventilator controls movement of gas through lungs
- Attempts to synchronize the ventilator breaths with patient-initiated spontaneous breaths
- Attempts to avoid having a mandatory breath occur during a spontaneous breath

Pressure support ventilation (PSV)

- A flow-limited mode of ventilation that adds a preset inspiratory pressure to the ventilator circuit
- The pressure support required is adjusted to ensure adequate tidal volumes
- Augments the flow of gas through the lungs in patients taking spontaneous breaths
- Well suited for weaning patients from mechanical ventilation but not suited to provide full ventilatory support

- More comfortable mode of ventilation
- Pressure support may also be added to other modes of ventilation (ACV with pressure support)

Continuous positive airway pressure (CPAP)

- Ventilator maintains the ventilator circuit pressure at a constant value above the ambient pressure during spontaneous breaths
- No additional pressure is provided and patients must initiate all breaths
- May be useful for sleep-related breathing disorders or for obese patients

Positive end-expiratory pressure (PEEP)

- Pressure applied at the end of the expiration
- Added to other modes of ventilation to prevent the alveoli from collapsing

High-frequency oscillation ventilation (HFOV)

- Employs very high respiratory rates and small tidal volumes
- May be able to achieve adequate gas exchange when conventional ventilator modes fail (severe ARDS)
- Very uncomfortable mode, which may require use of sedation and neuromuscular blockers

Further reading

Slutsky AS (1993). Mechanical ventilation. American College of Chest Physicians' Consensus Conference. *Chest* **104**:1833–1859.

Calfee CS, Matthay MA (2005). Recent advances in mechanical ventilation. *Am J Med* **118**:584–591.

Motility stimulants

The provision of early enteral feeding is an important goal in critically ill patients and has several advantages over parenteral feeding. Several factors contribute to impaired gastrointestinal (GI) tract motility in critically ill patients, leading to poor absorption of enteral feeds and oral medications.

Factors contributing to GI dysmotility

- Surgery
- Intestinal inflammation due to trauma or intestinal manipulation
- Medications, including opioids and anticholinergic agents
- Diabetes
- Dehydration
- Electrolyte disorder (hypokalemia, hypomagnesemia)
- Hemodynamic distrubance

Impaired GI motility may include delayed gastric emptying (gastroparesis) or ileus (often postoperative ileus), a generalized GI tract dysmotility in which the normal propulsive activity of the intestines is disrupted. Postoperative ileus is usually short-lived and self-limiting. Prolonged ileus, however, may result in pain, discomfort, and decreased mobility and cause delays in oral feeding, resulting in compromised nutrition.

Markers such as bowel sounds, gastric residual volume on aspiration, and patient tolerance of tube feedings are used to assess gut motility. Neither bowel sounds nor gastric residual volume are particularly reliable for determining gut motility. There is controversy about the upper limit of acceptable gastric residual volume (>300 mL is commonly used limit).

Several medications have been used to treat impaired GI motility in critically ill patients. Unfortunately, only very weak evidence exists to suggest that these agents have much of an effect on GI motility.

Metoclopramide

- Widely used agent for promoting gut motility and advancing feeding tubes
- Dopamine antagonist in the stomach and small bowel
- Increases lower esophageal sphincter pressure
- Very limited data to suggest efficacy for gastroparesis or ileus
- Usual dose is 10 mg 3–4 times daily (IV or oral)
- Associated with extrapyramidal symptoms and depression

Erythromycin

- Macrolide antibiotic used to promote GI motility
- Limited data suggesting utility in critically ill patients
- Motilin receptor agonist
- Stimulates fundic contractility and induces gastric contractions
- Widely variable doses used: 70–250 mg IV three times daily
- Smaller doses appear more effective (70–125 mg three times daily)
- Toxicity may include QT-interval prolongation, nausea, vomiting, ototoxicity pseudomembranous colitis
- Concern for development of antibiotic resistance

Alvimopan

- Oral peripherally acting mu-opioid antagonist
- Minimal crossing of blood–brain barrier (doesn't reverse analgesia)
- Usual dose is 12 mg before surgery followed by 12 mg twice daily for up to 7 days (not to exceed 15 doses)
- Appears to hasten postoperative GI recovery after bowel surgery
- Most common side effects include low blood calcium levels, anemia, and GI problems (constipation, heartburn, flatulence)
- Concern for risk of MI (no causal relationship determined)
- Very limited FDA approval (small or larger bowel resection surgery)
- Use is restricted to indication and for inpatients only
- Only available to hospitals enrolled in special registration program to ensure appropriate education (E.A.S.E. program)

Methynaltrexone

- Peripherally acting mu-opioid antagonist
- FDA approved only for constipation associated with chronic opioid use
- Decreases the constipating effect of chronic opioids
- Dose is weight based (0.15 mg/kg) SC every other day
- 8 mg SC for weight of 38–62 kg, 12 mg SC for 62–114 kg
- Common side effects include GI effects and dizziness
- Controlled trial found no benefit for postoperative ileus

Neostigmine

- Acetylcholinesterase inhibitor
- Stimulates acetylcholine release within the gut wall
- Useful for colonic pseudo-obstruction (Ogilvie's syndrome)
- Usual dose is 2 mg slow IV push
- Concern for severe bradycardia requires monitoring
- Also given as continuous infusion to lessen risk of bradycardia (2 mg in 50 mL normal saline given over 24 hours)

Further reading

Camilleri M (2007). Diabetic gastroparesis. *N Engl J Med* **356**:820–829.

Traut U, Brugger L, Kunz R, et al. (2008). Systemic prokinetic pharmacologic treatment for postoperative adynamic ileus following abdominal surgery in adults. *Cochrane Database Syst Rev* **1**:CD004930.

Renal-replacement therapy

Acute renal failure is a common feature of critical illness and is associated with high mortality. Renal function recovers in the majority of patients who survive, although a proportion of these patients go on to require chronic renal support. During the period of time it takes for the kidneys to recover, renal-replacement therapy in the form of intermittent hemodialysis or continuous renal replacement is required to undertake some of the functions that the healthy kidneys would normally perform.

In the hemodynamically unstable critically ill patient, continuous forms of renal replacement are preferred because of the large fluid shifts leading to hypotension with standard hemodialysis.

Indications for renal replacement therapies

- Fluid excess (pulmonary edema)
- Hyperkalemia
- Metabolic acidosis
- Clearance of dialyzable drugs or nephrotoxins
- Uremic symptoms

Terminology

Confusion often arises over the various techniques used for renal-replacement therapy. Abbreviations add to the confusion, but there are basically two main renal replacement modes, with a hybrid of the two also being commonly employed. Blood follows a pressure gradient that is either generated by taking blood from an artery and returning it to a vein (arteriovenous; AV) or taking blood from a vein and using the machine to generate the pressure gradient required before returning the blood to a vein (venovenous; VV).

Putting the various abbreviations together with the form of renal replacement gives the appropriate abbreviation for the technique (e.g., continuous venovenous hemodiafiltration [CVVHDF]). In critically ill patients, continuous replacement therapies are used until the patient is hemodynamically stable and able to tolerate intermittent dialysis.

Hemodialysis (HD)

Intermittant HD is not normally used in critical care, but may be used when a patient already has chronic renal failure and is hemodynamically stable. Blood is pushed through thousands of small tubes made of a semi-permeable membrane (see Fig. 15.2). Clearance of small, water-soluble molecules occurs by diffusion through a semi-permeable membrane into dialysis fluid that bathes the tubes. Water can also be drawn off by altering the concentration of glucose in the dialysis fluid.

Clean fluid can be infused back into the patient if required, although this is unusual for this form of renal replacement.

Hemofiltration (HF)

In HF, blood passes through thousands of small tubes made of a membrane full of small holes (typically 20,000 Da in diameter). A pressure gradient pushes the patient's plasma through the holes (filtration) and the eluent is discarded (Fig. 15.3). Clean fluid is infused back into the patient.

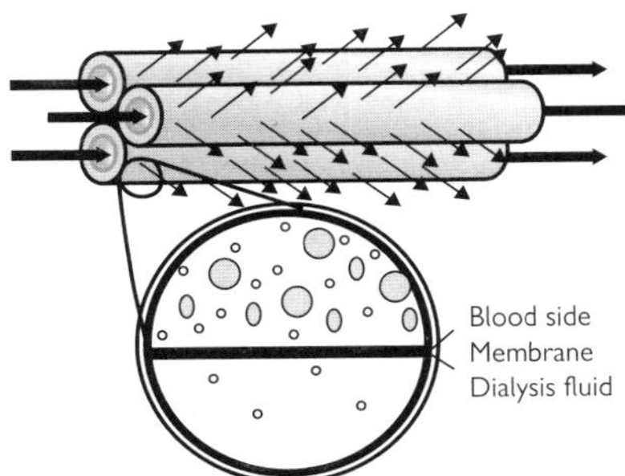

Figure 15.2 Hemodialysis.

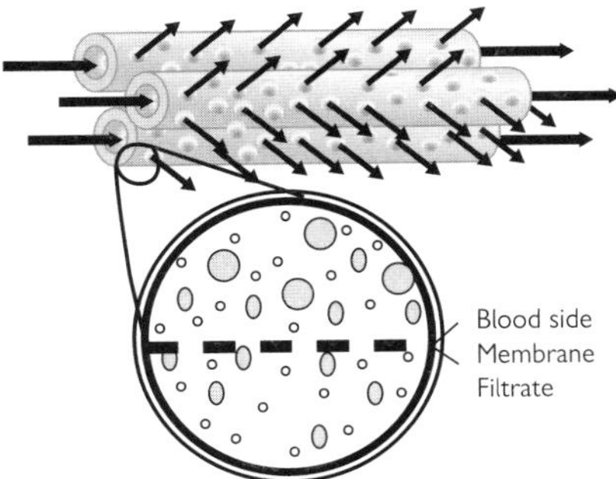

Figure 15.3 Hemofiltration.

Hemodiafiltration (HDF)

HDF is a hybrid form of filtration that adds a dialysis element to hemofiltration by allowing dialysis fluid to be added to the eluent generated from the filter, thus diluting it and causing an additional diffusion process to occur.

Slow extended daily dialysis (SLEDD)

This has been developed more recently to combine the advantages of HD and continuous renal replacement therapies.

Membrane filters

Membranes are usually hollow fiber polyacrylonitrile, polyamide, or polysulphone.

Buffer and replacement fluid

Whichever technique is employed, vast quantities of fluid are required for the process to take place. One of the many small molecules cleared is bicarbonate. Bicarbonate is central to the acid–base balance of the human body. Acid–base status is monitored closely during renal replacement and bicarbonate is administered to establish appropriate acid–base balance,

A buffered balanced solution is used, with lactate or bicarbonate as a buffer. Fluid removal is adjusted to achieve the desired fluid balance.

Anticoagulation of the circuit

The passage of blood through the extracorporeal circuit activates clotting pathways (see Fig. 15.4). The resulting coagulation clogs the filter circuit, reducing its efficiency and ultimately destroying its patency.

Anticoagulants are employed to maintain circuit patency, unless the patient is particularly coagulopathic.

Heparin

Heparin has long been used to maintain filter patency through its inhibitory effects on the enzyme cascade. It can be infused into the circuit or the patient, to maintain an aPTT of 1.5–2 times normal. Heparin is poorly cleared by renal-replacement therapy.

Prostacyclin

Prostaglandins produced by the endothelial lining of the vasculature inhibit the effect of thromboxane on platelet activation. This activity is lost in an extracorporeal circuit. Prostacyclin is used as an anticoagulant and is infused into the circuit at 2–10 nanograms/kg/min.

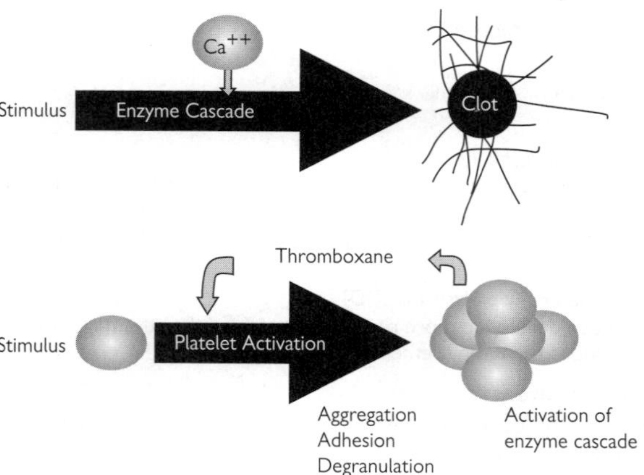

Figure 15.4 Activation of clotting cascade.

Citrate

Citrate has been used to bind up ionized calcium in the circuit, thus inhibiting several calcium-dependant steps in the clotting cascade and inhibiting calcium influx into platelets, preventing platelet activation. Large quantities of citrate are needed, and this results in a large solute load and metabolic alkalosis.

Pharmacist issues with renal replacement

- Evaluate all medications for dosing adjustment
- CVVHF or CVVHD removes more drug than HD
- Dose after HD for drugs removed by HD
- Monitor for electrolyte disturbances
- Adjust electrolytes in total parenteral nutrition
- Identify acid–base disturbances
- Minimize extra fluid when appropriate
- Be aware of drug–membrane interactions (avoid ACE inhibitors with CVVHDF)

Further reading

Kellum JA, Mehta R, Angus DC, Palevsky P, Ronco C, for the ADQI workgroup (2002). The First International Consensus Conference on Continuous Renal Replacement Therapy. *Kidney Int* **62**:1855–1863.

Heintz BH, Matzke GR, Dager WE (2009). Antimicrobially dosing concepts and recommendations for critically ill adult patients receiving continuous renal replacement therapy or intermittent hemodialysis. *Pharmacotherapy* **29**(5):562–577.

Sedation, paralysis, delirium

Patient discomfort and distress is common in the ICU setting and may result from being intubated or undergoing painful procedures, or from the difficulty communicating with caregivers. Patient distress may result in undesirable physiological consequences such as increases in cortisol, catecholamines, prostaglandins, and free fatty acids, subsequently leading to organ ischemia and fluid and electrolyte disturbances.

Pain, anxiety, and delirium are common causes of distress in ICU patients. These conditions should be monitored for and treated to enhance patient comfort and avoid undesirable physiological consequences. Pain is commonly treated with opioid narcotics such as fentanyl, morphine, or hydromorphone in the ICU.

Anxiety

Anxiety is a sustained state of apprehension and autonomic arousal in response to real or perceived threats. In the ICU, loss of control, difficulty communicating, and fear of suffering and of death contributes to anxiety.

Sedative medications used to treat ICU anxiety include benzodiazepines (midazolam and lorazepam), propofol, and dexmedetomidine. Intermittent PRN bolus doses of benzodiazepines are usual first-line agents for sedation. Patients requiring frequent doses may require a continuous infusion, although continuous infusions should be used cautiously to avoid oversedation.

Midazolam

- Benzodiazepine acts on the GABA receptor
- Lacks analgesic activity
- Anticonvulsive activity
- Produces amnesia
- Rapid onset and short duration with a single dose
- Useful for acute agitation due to rapid onset
- Metabolized in the liver
- Active metabolites may accumulate with prolonged infusion
- Caution with using a continuous infusion longer than 48 hours
- Tolerance develops, requiring higher doses over time
- Usual dose is 2–5 mg IV PRN or infusion initiated at 2 mg/hr

Lorazepam

- Benzodiazepine acts on the GABA receptor
- Lacks analgesic activity
- Anticonvulsive activity
- Slow onset (less useful for acute agitation)
- Metabolized by glucuronidation
- No active metabolites, less risk for infusion to accumulate
- Long half-life of 12–15 hours makes titration of infusion difficult
- Usual dose is 1–4 mg IV or PO PRN or infusion initiated at 1 mg/hr
- Higher infusion rates associated with propylene glycol toxicity

Propofol

- General anesthetic agent
- Sedative and hypnotic properties
- Lacks analgesic properties
- Highly lipophilic
- Very rapid onset and short duration after discontinuation
- Metabolized in liver to inactive metabolites
- Available in a lipid emulsion vehicle (1.1 kcal/mL)
- Prolonged use may cause hypertriglyceridemia
- Tachyphylaxis may occur but is variable
- Very high doses associated with lactic acidosis and cardiac arrest
- Requires a dedicated IV line because of infection risk
- Tubing changed every 12 hours for infusion
- Anticonvulsive properties
- Side effects include bradycardia and hypotension
- Usual dose is 5–10 mcg/kg/min titrated to desired sedation

Dexmedetomidine

- Selective, centrally acting α_2-agonist
- Analgesic properties in addition to sedation
- Approved for use <24 hours
- Synergistic with opioids (may lessen opioid use)
- Minimal respiratory depression
- Patients more easily aroused
- Side effects include bradycardia and hypotension
- Usual dose is 0.2–0.7 mcg/kg/hr continuous infusion

Sedation scales and daily interruption of infusions

Sedation goals for ICU patients should be set each day on the basis of available validated sedation scales, such as the Richmond Agitation Sedation Scale (RASS) or the Ramsay Scale. Use of sedation scales assists with the titration of medication to the lowest effective dose, minimizing oversedation.

To avoid excessive sedation, use of intermittent bolus doses rather than continuous infusions should be considered. If continuous infusions must be used, a daily interruption of the infusion may decrease the incidence of excessive sedation and decrease the duration of mechanical ventilation. Patients must be observed for withdrawal symptoms as sedation is reduced, since benzodiazepines may produce a withdrawal reaction upon abrupt discontinuation.

Paralysis

Neuromuscular blocking agents may be used in the ICU to facilitate intubation or facilitate mechanical ventilation when analgesia and sedation alone do not permit adequate mechanical ventilation. Modern ICU practice and improvements in ventilators have dramatically decreased the need for paralysis. The continued need for paralysis should be reassessed frequently, as long-term use of neuromuscular blocking agents is associated with myopathy and long-term weakness. Patients should always receive appropriate sedation when receiving paralytic agents.

Cisatracurium

- Nondepolarizing neuromuscular blocker
- Eliminated through Hoffman degradation
- Does not rely on kidneys or liver for elimination
- Usual bolus dose is 0.15–0.2 mg/kg
- Continuous infusion rate of 3 mcg/kg/min

Pancuronium

- Nondepolarizing neuromuscular blocker
- Eliminated via the kidneys (avoid in renal failure)
- Side effects include tachycardia and prolonged weakness
- Avoid in patients with ischemia heart disease
- Usual dose 0.05–0.1 mg/kg bolus dose
- Intermittent dose every 30–60 minutes as needed

Vecuronium

- Nondepolarizing neuromuscular blocker
- Eliminated via liver (avoid in hepatic failure)
- Associated with prolonged weakness
- Usual bolus dose is 0.1 mg/kg
- Continuous infusion rate of 0.8 mcg/kg/min

Delirium

Delirium is a neurological syndrome characterized by impairment of consciousness and cognitive function that fluctuates in severity. It is an acute change in cognitive function affecting attention, arousal, orientation, or perception. Delirium is associated with greater length of stay, higher mortality, and risk for permanent cognitive disability.

Any potential causes such as drugs or other medical conditions causing delirium should first be addressed. Traditional antipsychotic medications such as haloperidol as well as newer atypical antipsychotic medications including quetiapine, risperidone, and olanzapine have been used for ICU delirium. Scheduled regimens are more effective than PRN.

Further reading

Jacobi J, Fraser GL, Coursin DB, et al. (2002) Practice guidelines for the sustained use of sedatives and analgesics in the critically ill adult. *Crit Care Med* **30**:119–141.

Kress JP, Pohlman AS, O'Connor MF, Hall JB (2000). Daily interruption of sedative infusions in critically ill patients undergoing mechanical ventilation. *N Engl J Med* **342**:1471–1477.

Stress-ulcer prophylaxis

Endoscopic evidence of mucosal damage is evident in most ICU patients (75%–100%) within a day or two of ICU admission, although in most cases the damage is superficial and heals quickly. Clinically overt bleeding (hematemesis, gross blood, or "coffee grounds" in nasogastric [NG] aspirate, or melena) occurs in 5%–25% of critically ill patients.

The incidence of clinically important bleeding, defined as clinically overt bleeding complicated by hemodynamic instability or a dramatic decrease in hemoglobin requiring a transfusion, is much lower, with an incidence of 2%–6% in patients not receiving prophylaxis, according to clinical data through 1999.

Prospective studies since 1999 indicate that the risk for clinically important bleeding has decreased dramatically (incidence of 0.1%–4%) as a result of advances in ICU care. These include optimization of hemodynamic status and improvements in tissue oxygenation, reducing underlying gut ischemia.

Pathophysiology

It is thought that mucosal damage is brought about by a number of factors, such as disturbances in mucosal blood flow caused by cardiovascular instability and hypoperfusion, leading to a relative mucosal ischemia. Splanchnic hypoperfusion specifically is a major factor in the development of stress-related mucosal damage.

The presence of elevated gastric luminal pH and altered mucosal protective mechanisms contribute to mucosal stress ulceration. At pH <4, the proteolytic enzyme pepsin destroys clots forming on damaged gastric mucosa, increasing the probability of bleeding and the extent of gastric damage.

Risk factors

A number of risk factors have been identified as causing stress ulceration. The two most important ones are mechanical ventilation for >48 hours and coagulopathy have both identified as independent risk factors for bleeding. Following is a list of all risk factors for stress ulceration:

- >48 hours of mechanical ventilation*
- Coagulopathy*
- Acute renal failure
- Acute liver failure
- Sepsis
- Hypotension
- Severe head injury
- History of GI bleeding
- Burns covering >35% of body surface area
- Major surgery
- Medications including corticosteroids or NSAIDs

* Identified as an independent risk factor for bleeding

Goals of stress-ulcer prophylaxis therapy

An increase in the gastric pH to >4 is thought to be sufficient to prevent superficial stress ulceration, which may progress to a more serious and difficult-to-treat pathological state. The aim of stress-ulcer prophylaxis therapy is to prevent further attack on the already injured mucosa by decreasing gastric acidity and/or preventing proteolytic enzymes from attacking unprotected gastric mucosa.

Medications used for stress-ulcer prophylaxis

Several drugs have been used to prevent stress-related mucosal bleeding, including histamine (H2) antagonists, proton pump inhibitors (PPIs), sucralfate, and antacids.

Their use has been assessed in several large randomized, placebo-controlled studies, with conflicting results arising from each. The therapy of choice has changed a number of times over the years. Generally, H2 antagonists and PPIs are most commonly used because of the dosing issues and questionable efficacy with antacids and sucralfate.

H2 antagonists are commonly used first-line agents:

- Famotidine 20 mg IV or PO twice daily
- Ranitidine 50 mg IV three times daily
- Tolerance to H2 antagonists occurs within 72 hours
- Generally safe and well tolerated
- Central nervous system (CNS) side effects including confusion and delirium have been observed
- Rare cases of thrombocytopenia

PPI use is growing because of concerns and adverse effects associated with H2 antagonists (i.e., CNS side effects, thrombocytopenia, and development of tolerance), although there is no definitive study identifying PPI as first-line therapy. PPI drugs inhibit the final step in acid production (i.e., transport of H^+ by the proton pump). Once-daily injections of esomeprazole or pantoprazole have been used.

Extemporaneously prepared enteral formulations of omeprazole, lansoprazole, and pantoprazole (prepared by mixing PPI in sodium bicarconate) have been used for administration down various GI tubes (NG tubes or feeding tubes). Quick-dissolving formulations of lansoprazole have also been used, including administration down gastric tubes:

- Esomeprazole 40 mg IV or PO once daily
- Pantoprazole 40 mg IV or PO once daily
- Omeprazole 40 mg PO once daily
- Lansoprazole 30 mg PO once daily
- Generally safe and well tolerated
- Reports of abdominal pain, diarrhea, and nausea
- Intravenous PPIs including esomeprazole, pantoprazole, and lansoprazole are also used to prevent rebleed after a GI bleed.
  - Esomeprazole and pantoprazole: loading dose of 80 mg followed by continuous infusion of 8 mg/hr for 72 hours
  - Lansoprazole: loading dose of 60 mg followed by continuous infusion of 6 mg/hr for 72 hours

Unwanted effects of stress-ulcer prophylaxis

Stress-ulcer prophylaxis therapy has not been shown to reduce mortality and may be associated with negative consequences, especially if continued in patients without risk factors for stress-related mucosal disease.

One study found an increased incidence of nosocomial pneumonia with H2 antagonists; however, this remains controversial, as a meta-analysis did not find a significant increase in the risk of pneumonia with H2 antagonists.

The incidence of *Clostidium difficile* is greater in patients who take acid suppressants (higher for PPIs than with H2 antagonists).

It is appropriate to cease stress-ulcer prophylaxis when the risk factors for GI ulceration no longer apply (i.e., mechanical ventilation, coagulopathy) and/or when nasogastric feeding is established.

Unfortunately, it is common for patients to continue on stress-ulcer prophylaxis when it is not indicated even through to discharge from the ICU and the hospital. This is an area where pharmacists can play a large role in eliminating unnecessary PPI and H2-antagonist therapy.

Further reading

American Society of Health-System Pharmacists (1999). Therapeutic guidelines on stress ulcer prophylaxis. *Am J Health Syst Pharm* **56**:347–379.

Vasoactive drugs

Vasoactive drugs include both vasopressors and inotropes. Certain agents may act as both vasopressor and inotrope, depending on the dose (infusion rate).

- *Vasopressors* induce vasoconstriction, resulting in elevations in blood pressure (mean arterial blood pressure [MAP]).
- *Inotropes* increase contractility, increasing the force of contraction of the heart and resulting in higher cardiac output.
- *Chronotropic agents* affect the heart rate.

Receptors activity

- Alpha-adrenergic (α_1) receptors are located in vascular walls and induce vasoconstriction when activated, which results in elevated MAP.
- Beta-adrenergic (β_1) receptors are located mostly in the heart and cause increases in inotropic and chronotropic activity. β_2 receptors are located on blood vessels and induce vasodilation when activated.
- Dopamine (D_1) receptors are located in splanchnic, renal, coronary, and cerebral vascular beds and activation of these receptors leads to vasodilation, increasing perfusion to area.

Use of vasoactive drugs

- Hypotension from hypovolemia, heart failure, or septic shock
- Pressors indicated for decrease in systolic blood pressure (BP) of >30 mmHg from baseline or a >60 mmHg decrease in MAP
- Vasoactive agents should only be used after the patient has been adequately fluid resuscitated.
- Charts of receptor activity are available; however, it is important to recognize different activities predominate at different infusion rates.
- Vasoactive drugs should be titrated to appropriate MAP and cardiac output (CO) goals in addition to evidence of end-organ perfusion.
- Vasoactive drugs are usually given via central line, when possible (low-dose dopamine may be given peripherally).

Dopamine (α_1^{++}, β_1^{++}, β_2^{++}, D_1^{+++}, D_2^{+++})

Dose range effects (dosing range 1–30 mcg/kg/min)

- Low doses (<3 mcg/kg/min):
  - Predominant D_1-receptor stimulation leads to ↑ renal, mesenteric, and coronary perfusion. Increases urine output.
- Medium doses (3–6 mcg/kg/min):
  - Predominant β_1-adrenoceptor stimulation leads to an increase in heart rate, stroke volume, and cardiac output.
- Large doses (>6 mcg/kg/min):
  - α_1-adrenoceptor stimulation predominates, leading to vasoconstriction, which increases systemic vascular resistance and increases BP.

Uses

Dopamine is used to treat cardiogenic shock or as a second-line agent for septic shock. In general, dopamine should not be used as a renoprotective agent, as it has not been proven to prevent acute renal failure or reduce the need for renal-replacement therapies, although it may result in higher urine output.

Dobutamine (α_1^+, β_1^{++}, β_2^+)

Dose range effects (dosing range 2–20 mcg/kg/min)

- Usual dose (2.5–10 mcg/kg/min):
  - Predominant β_1-adrenoceptor stimulation leads to ↑ CO.

Uses

Dobutamine is used for cardiogenic shock.

Other effects

BP can fall in hypovolemic patients.

Epinephrine (α_1^{+++}, β_1^{+++}, β_2^{++})

Dose range effects (dosing range 0.01–0.4 mcg/kg/min)

- Low doses (<0.01 mcg/kg /min):
  - Predominant β_2 stimulation leads to dilatation of skeletal vasculature, resulting in a reduction in BP.
- Medium doses (0.04–0.1 mcg/kg/min):
  - Predominant β_1 stimulation leads to an increase in heart rate, stroke volume, and CO.
- Large doses (0.1–0.3 mcg/kg/min):
  - α1-stimulation predominates, leading to vasoconstriction with increased systemic vascular resistance and increased BP.
- Larger doses (>0.3 mcg/kg/min):
  - Increased α_1 adrenoceptor stimulation causes decreased renal blood flow and decreased splanchnic vascular bed perfusion. GI motility and pyloric tone are also decreased.

Uses

Epinephrine is used to treat anaphylactic shock and severe congestive cardiac failure and as a second-line agent for septic shock.

Other effects

Infusions of epinephrine can lead to arrhythmias, hyperglycemia, and metabolic acidosis. There is a risk of mesenteric ischemia at higher doses.

Norepinephrine (Levarterenol) (α_1^{+++}, β_1^{++})

Dose range effects (dosing range 0.5–30 mcg/min)

- Low doses (<2 mcg/min):
  - Predominant β_1-adrenoceptor stimulation leads to an increase in heart rate, stroke volume, and CO.
- Higher doses (>4 mcg/min):
  - Predominant α_1-adrenoceptor stimulation leads to vasoconstriction. Baroreceptor-mediated bradycardia is possible; however, this is offset by the chronotropic effect and heart rate usually remains unchanged or only slightly decreased.

Uses

Norepinephrine is the drug of choice for septic shock and is used to increase MAP in severe head injury.

Other effects

Infusion of norepinephrine can lead to arrhythmias, hyperglycemia, and metabolic acidosis. It is not useful for cardiogenic shock, due to increased afterload.

Phenylephrine (α_1^{+++})

Dose range effects (dosing range 10–360 mcg/min)

- Usual maintenance dose (40–100 mcg/min):
  - Pure α_1-adrenoceptor stimulation leads to vasoconstriction, which increases MAP. Minimal effects on inotropy or chronotropy

Uses

Phenylephrine is used for patients with hypotension and a low systemic vascular resistance. It is used commonly for anesthesia-induced hypotension and as a second-line agent in severe sepsis. It may also be added to other vasoactive drug regimens.

Other effects

Reflex bradycardia, metabolic acidosis, and decreased renal perfusion leading to lower urine output can occur.

Milrinone

Pharmacology

This agent inhibits phosphodiesterase, causing an intracellular excess of cAMP and consequent calcium ion influx. This in turn causes increased myocardial contractility and smooth-muscle relaxation and results in inotropic activity with significant vasodilation and hypotension.

Dose

- Usual maintenance dose: 0.375–0.75 mcg/kg/min

Uses

Milrinone is used for cardiac failure. It is associated with a lower incidence of cardiac arrhythmias than that with other inotropic agents.

Other effects

Hypotension is caused by vasodilatation.

Vasopressin

Pharmacology

Vasopressin is an antidiuretic hormone analogue that binds to V_1 receptors, resulting in vasoconstriction. Vasopressin also increases responsiveness of the vasculature to catecholamines.

Dose

- Usual maintenance dose: 0.02–0.04 units/min (not titrated)

Uses

Vasopressin is a second-line agent for septic shock not responsive to other vasopressors. It may allow for reduction in doses of other vasopressors, improving renal blood flow and urine output.

Other effects

There is a concern for vasoconstriction of coronary arteries and mesentery vasculature potentially resulting in ischemic complications.

Further reading

Hollenberg SM, Ahrens TS, Annane D, et al. (2004). Practice parameters for hemodynamic support of sepsis in adult patients: 2004 update. *Crit Care Med* **32**:1928–1948.

Wound care

The skin is the largest organ of the body. Its function is to serve as a protective barrier against the environment. Wounds represent a major cause of morbidity and impaired quality of life, consuming substantial health-care resources.

- 1.25 million people in the United States have burns every year
- 6.5 million people in the United States have chronic skin ulcers
  - Pressure ulcers
  - Venous stasis
  - Diabetes mellitus
- Breaching the skin barrier exposes underlying tissue to the following:
  - Mechanical damage
  - Dehydration
  - Microbial invasion
  - Temperature variations

Classification of wounds

Various classifications of wounds have been developed. For the purposes of wound care, the following descriptions are useful because they correspond to dressing choice. Some wounds may demonstrate more than one of the following features.

Epithelializing or granulating: A clean, red, or pink wound. Usually shallow with minimal exudates. This represents a well-healing wound.

Sloughy: Yellow slough covers all or part of wound. This may be a dry or wet wound.

Necrotic: Dead tissue creates a black, dry, leathery eschar.

Infected: Yellow or greenish in color with possible surrounding cellulitus of unbroken skin. The wound may also have an offensive odor.

Exuding: Any of the above wounds (except necrotic) may produce exudates to varying degrees. High levels of exudates can lead to maceration of surrounding skin.

Cavity: The wound forms a shallow or deep cavity. Sinuses are narrow cavities that can extend to some depth, including tracking to bone or between two wounds.

Malodorous: Fungating tumors and infected and necrotic wounds may have an offensive odor.

Factors promoting wound healing

- Moist but not excessively wet
- Adequate warmth
- Adequate oxygen
- Good nutrition and appropriate protein intake
- Relatively free of contamination (including slough and necrotic tissue)

Patient factors inhibiting wound healing

- Poor perfusion (peripheral vascular disease)
- Older age

- Concurrent diseases (diabetes, cancer, anemia)
- Drugs (steroids, cytotoxic drugs)
- Smoking
- Immobility

Wound dressings

As wounds heal, the type of dressing appropriate to the wound can change. Slough and necrotic tissue are effectively foreign bodies that inhibit wound healing and should be removed. After removal the underlying tissue should be granulating.

The wound care plan should be reviewed on a regular basis. Frequency of dressing changes depends on the severity and nature of the wound. An infected or exudating wound may require daily dressing changes whereas a well-healing, granulating wound may only require a dressing change every few days.

Characteristics of ideal wound dressing

- Maintain moist environment
- Manage excessive exudates
- Allow oxygenation
- Provide barrier to microorganisms
- Maintain a warm environment
- Should not shed particles or fibers
- Decrease or eliminate odor
- Acceptable to patient
- Cost effective

Types of wound dressings

Wound-care dressings provide active wound management by interacting with the wound surface. The type of dressing should be matched to the wound.

- Primary dressing—applied directly to wound surface
- Secondary dressing—placed over the primary dressing
- Alginate dressing—used for exuding, sloughy, or cavity wound
- Foam dressing—exuding or highly exuding wounds
- Films and membranes—shallow, granulating wounds
- Hydrocolloid—shallow would with light edudates
- Hydrogels—dry, sloughy wound
- Paraffin gauze—granulating wound

Topical antimicrobials

These agents are usually not recommended because of the potential for increased resistance and local sensitivity reactions. There is little evidence that topical antimicrobials work, and infection should be treated with systemic antibiotics. However, topical antimicrobials may be indicated in certain situations:

- Povidone iodine preparations for wounds infected with microorganisms
- Silver sulfadiazine for burn wounds to treat *Pseudomonas* spp.

Vacuum-assisted closure (VAC)

VAC therapy is a form of wound care in which negative pressure is applied to a porous dressing, which is placed in the wound cavity or over a flap or graft. VAC helps to remove excess exudates and mechanically draws the edges of the wound inward, promoting healing. It is suitable for any chronic open wound or acute and traumatic surgical wounds. VAC should not be used for infected wounds.

Further reading

Singer AJ, Clark RAF (1999). Cutaneous wound healing. *N Engl J Med* **341**:738–746.
www.worldwidewounds.com

Management of calcium imbalance

Normal range: 8.6–10.2 mg/dL

Hypocalcemia

Causes of hypocalcemia

- Malabsorption, inadequate intake, vitamin D deficiency
- Hypoalbuminemia
- Hyperphosphatemia
- Hypomagnesemia
- Pancreatitis
- Hypoparathyroidism

Complications of hypocalcemia

- Dysrhythmias
- Muscle cramping
- Paresthesias
- Seizures
- Stridor
- Tetany

Nonpharmacological treatment

- Treat underlying disorder

Pharmacological treatment

Mild hypocalcemia (7.6–8.5 mg/dL), asymptomatic

- Most commonly related to hypoalbuminemia; therefore, correct for hypoalbuminemia (if Ca "normal" when corrected, treatment is unnecessary):

$$Ca_{corrected} = [(4\text{-}Alb_{measured}) \times (0.8)] + Ca_{measured}$$

- Evaluate ionized calcium levels when albumin <2.0 g/dL.
- Acute mild, asymptomatic hypocalcemia may not require treatment.
  - If treatment is desired, 1000–2000 mg calcium gluconate IV infusion
  - Dilute in 100 mL D5W or NS and infuse over 30–60 minutes
- Chronic mild, asymptomatic hypocalcemia may be treated with oral supplementation (e.g., calcium carbonate, calcitriol, vitamin D replacement).

Severe hypocalcemia (<7.6 mg/dL), symptomatic

- 1000 mg calcium chloride slow IV push over 10 minutes or 3000 mg calcium gluconate slow IV push over 10 minutes (see Table 15.38)
- May repeat as necessary
- Refractory hypocalcemia may require a continuous calcium infusion.
  - Calcium chloride maximum concentration 20 mg/mL; maximum infusion rate 100 mg/min (0.8–1.5 mEq/min)
  - Calcium chloride maximum concentration 50 mg/mL; maximum infusion rate 300 mg/min (0.8–1.5 mEq/min)
  - Rapid infusions may cause hypotension and cardiac arrhythmias.
  - Hypomagnesemia may cause refractory hypocalcemia.
- For severe hyperkalemia with ECG changes, calcium chloride 1000 mg IV push over 2–5 minutes (central line preferred)

Important considerations

- Serum calcium levels must be corrected for hypoalbuminemia.
- Ionized Ca^+, which will provide an accurate assessment of calcium stores independent of serum albumin, may be preferred in symptomatic hypocalcemia.
- Ionized Ca^+ normal range: 1.12–1.30 mmol/L

Monitoring

- Serum calcium every 4–6 hours until corrected
- Serum magnesium if hypomagnesemia suspected

Hypercalcemia

Causes of hypercalcemia

- Hyperparathyroidism
- Hyperthyroidism
- Malignancy
- Renal dysfunction
- Medications (e.g., thiazide diuretics, lithium, vitamin D)

Complications

- Lethargy
- Psychosis
- Coma
- Polydipsia/polyuria
- Anorexia (nausea/vomiting)
- Soft tissue calcification

Nonpharmacological treatment

- Treat underlying disorder

Pharmacological treatment (see Hypercalcemia unit, p. 644)

Table 15.38 Characteristics of IV calcium preparations

Preparation	Supplied as	Elemental calcium content per 1 g (100 mL)	Administration
Calcium chloride	Injection solution (10%) 100 mg/mL	13.6 mEq	Central line preferred. May cause severe extravasation
Calcium gluconate	Injection solution (10%) 100 mg/mL	4.65 mEq	Preferred for peripheral administration

Management of magnesium imbalance

Normal range: 1.5–2.4 mg/dL

Hypomagnesemia

Causes of hypomagnesemia

- Malnutrition
- Burns
- Trauma
- Alcoholism
- Medications (e.g., amphotericin B, cisplatin, cyclosporine, loop diuretics)

Complications of hypomagnesemia

- Hypokalemia
- Hypocalcemia
- Tetany
- Seizure
- Arrhythmias
- Cardiac arrest

Treatment

Oral magnesium replacement (see Table 15.39)

- Slow onset of action
- GI intolerance
- Utility in acute hypomagnesemia may be limited
- Useful for maintenance

Mild to moderate hypomagnesemia (1.0–1.5 mg/dL)

- 1000–4000 mg magnesium sulfate IV infusion
- May be appropriate to reduce dose by 50% in renal dysfunction
- Dilute in D5W or NS to a 20% concentration
- Up to 50% of IV magnesium sulfate is eliminated renally, therefore administer at a maximum rate of 1000 mg/hr

Severe hypomagnesemia (<1.0 mg/dL)

- 4000–8000 mg magnesium sulfate IV infusion
- Dilute in D5W or NS to a 20% concentration
- Up to 50% of IV magnesium sulfate is eliminated renally, therefore administer at a maximum rate of 1000 mg/hr
- May be appropriate to reduce dose by 50% in renal dysfunction
- 1000–2000 mg magnesium sulfate IV push over 5 minutes for torsades de pointes

Monitoring

- Daily serum magnesium until normalized

Hypermagnesemia

Causes of hypermagnesemia

- Renal insufficiency
- Hypothyroidism
- Medications (e.g., lithium)

Complications of hypermagnesemia

- Hypotension
- Bradycardia
- Confusion
- Respiratory depression
- Coma

Nonpharmacological treatment

- Treat underlying disorder
- External cardiac pacing (symptomatic)
- Mechanical ventilation (symptomatic)
- Dialysis (use only in emergent situations, unless patient is already on dialysis)

Pharmacological treatment

- 1000 mg calcium gluconate slow IV push over 10 minutes
- Hydration with normal saline (200 mL/hr)
  - Add calcium gluconate 1000 mg to each liter of fluid
- Loop diuretics (e.g., furosemide 40 mg IV push) to maintain urine output

Monitoring

- Serum magnesium every 2 hours until normalized and patient is asymptomatic

Table 15.39 Selected oral preparations

Preparation	Elemental magnesium/tablet (mg)
Magnesium oxide tablet (400 mg)	242
Magnesium gluconate tablet (500 mg)	27
Magnesium chloride tablet, controlled release (64 mg)	64

Management of phosphate imbalance

Normal range: 2.7–4.5 mg/dL

Hypophosphatemia

Causes of hypophosphatemia

- Malnutrition
- Increased urine excretion of phosphorus
- Hyperparathyroidism
- Refeeding syndrome
- Medications

Complications of hypophosphatemia

- Myalgias
- Peripheral neuropathy
- Paralysis
- Rhabdomyolysis
- Seizures
- Acute respiratory failure

Treatment (see Table 15.40)

Mild, asymptomatic hypophosphatemia (2.3–2.7 mg/dL)

- Oral phosphate repletion may be adequate if absorption from GI tract is normal.
- GI tract absorption may be unpredictable.
- Oral phosphorus preparations may cause diarrhea.
- Can be given as IV infusion if oral phosphorus cannot be tolerated (0.08–0.16 mmol/kg phosphorus IV infusion)

Moderate hypophosphatemia (1.5–2.2 mg/dL), symptomatic

- 0.16–0.32 mmol/kg phosphorus as IV infusion
- IV preparations available as potassium phosphate or sodium phosphate
- Dilute in D5W or NS to maximum concentration of 0.12 mmol/mL
- Infuse total dose over 4–6 hours to avoid infusion related reactions

Severe hypophosphatemia (<1.5 mg/dL)

- 0.32–0.64 mmol/kg as IV infusion

Monitoring

- Repeat serum phosphorus level 2–4 hours after phosphorus administration.

Hyperphosphatemia

Causes of hyperphosphatemia

- Renal insufficiency
- Acidosis
- Hypoparathryoidism
- Tumor lysis syndrome
- Medications (e.g., phosphate supplements, bisphosphonates)

Complications of hypophosphatemia
- Calcium/phosphate complex formation and deposit in muscle
- Tetany
- Mortality

Nonpharmacological treatment
- Treat underlying condition
- Dialysis (use only in emergent situations, unless patient is already on dialysis)

Pharmacological treatment
- Phosphate binders
- Calcium carbonate: 1250 mg PO tid with each meal
- Calcium acetate: 667–1334 mg PO tid with each meal
- Sevelamer: 800–1600 mg PO tid with each meal
- Aluminum-based products are not usually recommended because of aluminum toxicity.

Monitoring
- Serum phosphorus levels until normal
- Serum calcium levels

Table 15.40 Select phosphate-containing preparations

Oral preparations	Phosphorus content	Potassium content	Sodium content
Potassium and sodium phosphate powder (Neutra Phos®)	8 mmol/packet	7.1 mEq/packet	7.1 mEq/packet
IV preparations			
Potassium phosphate	3 mmol/mL	4.4 mEq/mL	0
Sodium phosphate	3 mmol/mL	0	4 mEq/mL

Management of potassium imbalance

Normal range: 3.5–5.0 mEq/L

Hypokalemia

Causes of hypokalemia

- Excessive loss through GI tract or kidney
- Hypomagnesemia
- Intracellular shift
- Medications (e.g., diuretics)

Complications of hypokalemia

- Nausea and vomiting
- Weakness and fatigue
- Constipation
- Paralysis
- Respiratory failure
- Arrhythmias
- Sudden death

Risks associated with IV potassium

- Rapid administration of IV potassium or administration of concentrated IV potassium can result in hyperkalemia, leading to paralysis, respiratory failure, arrhythmias, and asystole.
- Potassium should NOT be administered undiluted or IV push
- Peripheral administration of potassium may lead to burning and phlebitis. Therefore, less concentrated solutions should be used peripherally.

Safety measures for IV potassium

In 2002, the Joint Commission (JCAHO) included the removal of concentrated potassium from general patient care areas in their National Patient Safety Goals (NPSG), which has resulted in a decrease in medication errors related to accidental administration of concentrated potassium. This has been retired as a NPSG; however, it is still included as a Medication Management standard by JCAHO.[1]

Other safety measures include the following:

- Warning labels for concentrated potassium stored in specialized patient-care areas
- Including desired concentration and rate of infusion in physician orders
- Use of standardized concentrations and premixed solutions

Treatment

Mild to moderate hypokalemia (2.5–3.4 mEq/L)

- Oral potassium repletion is preferred for patients who are asymptomatic.
- Serum potassium decreases 0.3 mmol for each 100 mmol decrease in total body stores. Therefore, for each 0.1 mEq/L increase in serum potassium desired, ~10 mEq potassium is required.

1 FAQs for the 2008 National Patient Safety Goals (2008) Accessed July 9, 2008, from: http://www.joint comission.org

- Potassium chloride is the most commonly used agent for repletion.
- 20–40 mEq potassium chloride IV infusion if the patient cannot tolerate oral potassium or the GI tract is nonfunctional

Severe hypokalemia (<2.5 mEq/L), symptomatic

- 40–80 mEq potassium chloride IV infusion (see Table 15.41)
- Solutions containing dextrose may cause intracellular potassium shift; therefore, dilute in non-dextrose containing solution.
- Maximum concentration 80 mEq/L for peripheral line, 120 mEq/L for central line
- Maximum rate of administration: 10 mEq/hr without cardiac monitoring
- Administration rates >20 mEq/hr rarely necessary

Monitoring

- Serum potassium level every 1–6 hours if severe or symptomatic or if IV treatment ongoing
- Serum magnesium may be indicated if hypokalemia is resistant to treatment.
- Cardiac monitoring if rate of administration >10 mEq/hr

Hyperkalemia

Causes of hyperkalemia

- Renal insufficiency
- Increased oral intake (salt substitutes)
- Acidosis
- Adrenal insufficiency
- Medications (e.g., ACE inhibitors, ARBs, potassium-sparing diuretics, NSAIDs, K^+ supplements)

Complications

- ECG changes (peaked T waves, QRS widening, loss of p-wave)
- Nausea and vomiting
- Muscle weakness
- Cramping
- Paralysis

Table 15.41 Selected premixed potassium-containing preparations

Diluent	Number of mEq in diluent
D5W	20, 30, 40 mEq/1000 mL
D5W and LR	20, 30, 40 mEq/1000 mL
D5W and 1/2 NS	10 mEq/500 mL; 10, 20, 30, 40 mEq/1000 mL
D5W and NS	20, 40 mEq/1000 mL
1/2 NS	20, 40 mEq/1000 mL
NS	20, 40 mEq/1000 mL
SWFI	10, 20 mEq/50 mL; 10, 20, 30, 40 mEq/100 mL

Nonpharmacological treatment

- Treat underlying disorder
- Dialysis (use only in emergent situations, unless patient is already on dialysis)

Pharmacological treatment

Mild or moderate hyperkalemia (5.5–6.9 mEq/L), asymptomatic

- Sodium polystyrene (exchange capacity: approximately 1 g of resin binds 1 mEq of potassium)
- Dose (adults): 15 g, may repeat every 6 hours
- Rectal (retention enema 30–60 minutes): 30–50 g, may repeat every 6 hours
- Effect within 60 minutes

Severe hyperkalemia (>7.0 mEq/L) or symptomatic

- Protect the heart (effect within 1–2 minutes)
- 1000 mg calcium chloride slow IV push over 10 minutes or 3000 mg calcium gluconate slow IV push over 10 minutes
- Repeat every 10 minutes until ECG changes resolve
- Shift K^+ intracellularly (effect within 30 minutes)
- 50 mL of dextrose 50% IV push over 3–5 minutes; regular insulin 10 units IV push
- 50 mL of 8.4% sodium bicarbonate slow IV push over 3–5 minutes
- 20 mg albuterol (nebulized), may repeat every 10 minutes
- Bind potassium (effect within 60 minutes)
- Sodium polystyrene (see above for dosing)

Monitoring

- Serum potassium every 1–2 hours until normal and patient is asymptomatic

Management of sodium imbalance

Normal range: 135–145 mEq/L

Hyponatremia

Causes of hyponatremia (see Table 15.42)

- Typically a manifestation of water imbalance
- Total body sodium can be decreased, normal, or increased.
- Multiple medications cause syndrome of inappropriate antidiuretic hormone (SIADH; e.g., selective serotonin reuptake inhibitors [SSRIs], tricyclic antidepressants [TCAs], venlafaxine, desmopressin, carbamazepine, NSAIDs, antipsychotics, cyclophosphamide)

Complications of hyponatremia

- Headache
- Lethargy
- Nausea
- Vomiting
- Muscle weakness
- Seizures
- Severity of complications depends on the acuity of decreased sodium concentration

Pharmacologic treatment

Mild to moderate hyponatremia (121–134 mEq/L), asymptomatic

- Asymptomatic or chronic hyponatremia should be corrected at a rate ≤0.5 mEq/L/hr with a maximum change in 24 hours of 8–12 mEq/L.
- Fluid restriction is usually effective in mild, asymptomatic patients.
- Demeclocycline 900–1200 mg PO daily in 3 divided doses. May take 7–10 days for therapeutic effect

Severe hyponatremia (<120 mEq/L) or symptomatic

- For symptomatic hyponatremia with serum Na^+ >120 mEq/L, 0.9% sodium chloride may be an appropriate replacement fluid.
- For acute hyponatremia associated with seizures or coma, serum sodium correction rate 1–2 mEq/L/hr with 3% sodium chloride until symptoms resolve
  - Once symptoms have resolved, increase serum sodium at a rate of ≤0.5 mEq/L/hr with a maximum change in 24 hours of 8–12 mEq/L
- Estimate the amount of sodium required to correct serum Na^+ using the following equation:

$$Na^+ \text{ Deficit (mEq)} = \text{Total body water} \times (140 - Na^+_{measured})$$

- Total body water (TBW) = Body weight (kg) x 0.6 for males (or x 0.5 for females)
- ~1/3 Na^+ deficit can be replaced during the first 12 hours of treatment, provided the rate of replacement does not exceed 0.5 mEq/L/hr.
- The remaining 2/3 should be replaced gradually over several days.
- To estimate the expected change in serum Na^+ after 1 L of 3% sodium chloride:

$$\text{Change in serum } Na^+ \text{ (mEq)} = (512 \text{ mEq/L} - Na^+_{measured}) / \text{TBW} + 1$$

- To estimate the expected change in serum Na^+ after 1 L of 0.9% sodium chloride:

  Change in serum Na^+ (mEq) = $(154 \text{ mEq/L} - Na^+_{measured}) / \text{TBW} + 1$

- The rate of fluid administration depends on the desired rate of serum Na^+ concentration change.
- Conivaptan, a vasopressin antagonist, may have some utility.
  - 20 mg IV over 30 minutes, followed by 20 mg continuous IV infusion over 24 hours. May be administered for additional 1–2 days, total duration not to exceed 4 days
- Contraindicated in hypovolemic hyponatremia

Important considerations

- Overly aggressive replacement of sodium (>12 mEq in 24 hours) may be associated with central pontine myelinolysis, which can result in severe, irreversible neurological impairment.
- Serum Na^+ should be corrected in the setting of hyperglycemia using the following equation:

  $Na^+_{corrected} = Na^+_{measured} + 1.6\ [(\text{serum glucose} - 100)/100]$

Monitoring

- Serum sodium every 2–4 hours until patient is asymptomatic, then every 4–8 hours until corrected
- Signs of neurological complications

Hypernatremia

Causes of hypernatremia (see Table 15.42)

- Typically a manifestation of water deficit
- Total body sodium can be decreased, normal, or increased.

Table 15.42 Causes of sodium imbalance

	Hyponatremia	
Hypovolemic	**Euvolemic**	**Hypervolemic**
Excessive diuresis Adrenal insufficiency Cerebral salt wasting Blood loss GI losses	SIADH Adrenal insufficiency Hypothyroidism	Congestive heart failure Cirrhosis Nephrotic syndrome
	Hypernatremia	
Hypovolemic	**Euvolemic**	**Hypervolemic**
GI losses Burns Osmotic diuresis	Diabetes insipidus	Hypertonic saline infusion Hyperaldosteronism

Complications of hypernatremia

- Restlessness
- Irritability
- Lethargy
- Hyperreflexia
- Intracranial bleeding
- Seizures
- Coma

Pharmacological treatment

Mild hypernatremia (146–154 mEq/L), asymptomatic

- Asymptomatic or chronic hypernatremia should be corrected at a rate of ≤0.5 mEq/L/hr with a maximum change in 24 hours of 8–12 mEq/L
- Removal of any agents contributing to TBW loss and increasing fluid intake may be adequate to reverse mild, asymptomatic hypernatremia.

Severe hypernatremia (>155 mEq/L) or symptomatic

- For severe, acute hypernatremia, correction should occur ≤1–2 mEq/L/hr to avoid cerebral edema.
- For severe, chronic hypernatremia, correction should occur ≤0.5 mEq/L/hr to avoid cerebral edema, herniation, or death.
- Risk of cerebral edema, herniation, and death is greater in chronic hypernatremia.
- Estimate the amount of water required to correct serum Na^+ using the following equation:

$$\text{Water deficit (L)} = \text{TBW} \times [(\text{Na}^+_{\text{measured}}/140) - 1]$$

- 1/2 water deficit can be replaced during the first 24 hours of treatment, provided the rate of replacement does not exceed 0.5 mEq/L/hr.
- The remaining 1/2 should be replaced gradually over 2–3 days.
- To estimate the expected change in serum Na^+ after 1 L of 5% dextrose solution:

$$\text{Change in serum Na}^+ \text{ (mEq)} = (0 \text{ mEq/L} - \text{Na}^+_{\text{measured}})/\ \text{TBW} + 1$$

- To estimate the expected change in serum Na^+ after 1 L of 0.45% sodium chloride:

$$\text{Change in serum Na}^+ \text{ (mEq)} = (77 \text{ mEq/L} - \text{Na}^+_{\text{measured}})/\ \text{TBW} + 1$$

- The rate of fluid administration depends on the desired rate of serum Na^+ concentration change.

Monitoring

- Serum sodium every 2–4 hours until patient asymptomatic, then every 4–8 hours until corrected
- Signs of neurological complications

Prescribing intravenous fluids

Prescribing intravenous fluids

Reasons for IV fluid treatment

- Maintain fluid balance (euvolemia)
- Correct dehydration (hypovolemia)
- Fluid resuscitation (e.g., acute sepsis)

Maintenance IV fluids (see Table 15.43)

- To maintain euvolemia, total daily intake should equal total daily output.
- Normal daily adult requirement for overall intake is 30 mL/kg.
- Selection of maintenance fluid should incorporate electrolyte (i.e., sodium and potassium) needs.
  - The Dietary Reference Intake[1] (DRI) for Na^+ 1.2 g/day ~56.2 mEq Na^+ and upper limit for daily Na^+ intake 2.3 g/day ~99.5 mEq Na^+
  - Fluid containing sodium chloride can provide daily sodium needs. Serum Na^+ should also be used to guide sodium content of selected IV fluid.
  - The DRI for K^+ 4.7 g/day ~120 mEq K^+
  - Potassium is sometimes added to IV fluid to maintain body potassium stores. Serum potassium should be used to guide the decision to add potassium to IV fluid.
- For example, for a 70 kg man, 0.45% sodium chloride infused at 85 mL/hr over 24 hours would provide 29 mL/kg intake, 157 mEq Na^+, and 1020 mL free water.
- In hospitalized patients who are able to tolerate oral intake, IV fluids may not be necessary to maintain fluid balance.

Table 15.43 Characteristics of select IV fluids

Solution	Tonicity	Sodium content (mEq/L)	Dextrose content (g/L)	Considerations
0.9% sodium chloride	Isotonic	154	0	Can cause hypernatremia if used for maintenance for extended period
5% dextrose/ 0.45% sodium chloride	Hypotonic	77	50	Useful for maintenance fluid or mildly dehydrated patients
5% dextrose	Hypotonic	0	50	Not useful for intravascular volume expansion

IV fluids for dehydration

- IV fluids may be necessary to replace fluid from acute volume loss (see Table 15.43).
  - Acute blood loss
  - Vomiting
  - Diarrhea
- The initial goal of therapy is for total daily intake to exceed total daily output until euvolemia is achieved.
  - Monitoring should include strict ins/outs, taking insensible losses into consideration, and daily weight checks.
- Selection of IV fluid should be based on the type of volume loss.
  - Gastrointestinal fluids tend to have relatively high sodium content.
  - Severe diarrhea may result in hyponatremia and hypokalemia.

Other considerations

- Patients who are hypernatremic may benefit from fluids that contain at least some free water, i.e., hypotonic fluids
- When hyponatremia is present, serum osmolality is less than normal; therefore, IV fluid normally considered isotonic will actually be hypertonic relative to the serum and will have the effect of drawing free water into the vasculature.
- Patients with congestive heart failure and kidney dysfunction are at increased risk of volume overload. Therefore, monitoring of daily ins/outs and daily weights is extremely important in these patients.

Fluid resuscitation in sepsis

- IV fluids are used in sepsis to assist in achieving hemodynamic stability.
- Some controversy exists regarding the optimal type of fluid that should be administered in acute sepsis.

Crystalloid solutions

- Crystalloids are solutions made of small organic molecules and inorganic ions in water that are capable of passing through semi-permeable membranes (e.g., 0.9% sodium chloride and 5% dextrose/0.45% sodium chloride solutions).
- Because a relatively small percentage of crystalloids remain in the vasculature, large volumes of crystalloids may be required to maintain hemodynamic stability in sepsis.
- Crystalloid solutions are substantially less expensive than colloids.
- When crystalloids are used in treating sepsis, 0.9% sodium chloride is generally the agent of choice.

Colloid solutions

- Colloids are solutions with greater osmolality than that of serum. They cannot cross semi-permeable membranes (e.g., albumin).
- Colloids increase oncotic pressure in the vasculature and draw water into the intravascular space.
- Colloids are sometimes referred to as "volume expanders."

- Colloids require significantly less volume to achieve goals of therapy, but are expensive.
- Albumin-containing solutions are the most commonly used colloid in sepsis.

Surviving Sepsis Campaign Guidelines 2008[2]

- Albumin has been shown to be as effective as 0.9% sodium chloride for fluid resuscitation in sepsis.
- Current guidelines recommend the use of either crystalloid or colloid for fluid resuscitation.
- An initial fluid challenge of at least 1000 mL of crystalloid or 300–500 mL of colloid over 30 minutes should be administered.
- Increased volumes or more rapid infusion may be necessary depending on hemodynamic status.
- Many patients will need aggressive fluid resuscitation for the first 24 hours of treatment (see Table 15.44).

Table 15.44 Goals of fluid resuscitation in sepsis

Parameter	Goal
Central venous pressure (CVP)	≥8 mmHg (12 mmHg if mechanically ventilated)
Mean arterial pressure (MAP)	≥65 mmHg
Urine output	≥0.5 ml/kg.hr

1 Standing Committee on the Scientific Evaluation of Dietary Reference Intakes, Food and Nutrition Board, National Academy of Sciences (2004). Dietary reference intakes for water, potassium, sodium, chloride, and sulfate. Washington, DC: National Academy Press, accessed July 7, 2008, from: www.nap.edu

2 Dellinger RP, Levy MM, Carlet JM, et al. (2008) Surviving Sepsis Campaign: international guidelines for management of severe sepsis and septic shock: 2008. *Crit Care Med* **36**:296–327.

Fluid balance

- Total body water (TBW) accounts for ~50% lean body weight (LBW) in adult females and ~60% LBW in adult males.
- TBW is compartmentalized in the body as either intracellular fluid (ICF) or extracellular fluid (ECF).

Intracellular fluid

- Fluid contained within cells; rich in potassium, magnesium, and protein
- ICF makes up 2/3 TBW

Extracellular fluid

- Fluid contained outside of cells, i.e., intravascular and interstitial space
- Rich in sodium, chloride, and bicarbonate
- ECF makes up 1/3 TBW

Osmolality

- Osmotic pressure created by nonpermeable solutes, referred to as *effective osmoles*, results in movement of water across the membrane in the direction of increased numbers of solute molecules.
- Effective osmoles in ECF consist primarily of sodium, chloride, and bicarbonate.
- In the ICF, effective osmoles consist primarily of potassium and phosphates.
- Water moves freely across membranes to maintain osmotic equilibrium between the ECF and ICF.
- Normal plasma osmolality is 275–290 mosmol/kg

$$\text{Serum osmolality} = (2 \times Na^+) + (\text{glucose}/18) + (\text{BUN}/2.8)$$

Tonicity

- Effective osmolality is referred to as *tonicity*.
- IV fluids may be isotonic, hypertonic, or hypotonic relative to their osmolality compared with serum osmolality.
- Distribution of IV fluids in the body depends on tonicity (see Table 15.45).
  - Isotonic fluids have the same tonicity as serum and will distribute to intravascular and interstitial space.
  - Hypotonic fluids have less tonicity than serum, resulting in distribution intracellularly.
  - Hypertonic fluids have greater tonicity than serum and will remain mostly in the vasculature.

Maintenance of fluid balance

- Maintenance of fluid balance in the body requires that volume lost on a daily basis be replaced; "water in" must equal "water out" (see Table 15.46).
- When water intake does not equal output, patients may develop hypernatremia or hyponatremia.

Table 15.45 Distribution of commonly used IV fluids

Solution	Osmolality (msomol/L)	% Intracellular	% Intravascular	% Interstitial
0.9% sodium chloride	304	0	25	75
0.45% sodium chloride	154	37	15.75	47.25
5% dextrose/ 0.45% sodium chloride	154*	33.3	16.7	50
5% dextrose	0*	66.7	8.3	25
3% sodium chloride	1027	0	75	25

*For 5% dextrose, actual osmolality is 277 mosmol/L; however, dextrose is rapidly metabolized and has no effect on serum osmolality under normal circumstances.

Table 15.46 Potential sources of water intake and output

Intake	Output
Oral intake	Urine
IV medications and fluids	Stool
Parenteral nutrition	Insensible loss (skin/respiratory)
Water flushes for feeding tubes	Emesis
	Surgical drains

Practical issues concerning parenteral nutrition

The identification and selection of patients who require parenteral nutrition (PN), and the subsequent provision and monitoring of this treatment, consists of a number of overlapping phases.

If there is concern about a patient's nutrition, the patient should be referred to the nutrition support team for a full assessment.

Initiation of parenteral nutrition

Once referred to the nutrition support team, the patient will be formally assessed, and if appropriate, line access will be planned. For short-term PN (7–10 days), this will usually be a peripherally inserted venous catheter (PICC), and a tunneled central line will be used if the anticipated duration of PN is longer or if peripheral access is limited.

Before initiating PN, baseline biochemistry should be checked and fluid and electrolyte abnormalities corrected (see Table 15.47). In those at risk of developing refeeding syndrome, additional IV vitamins may be needed.

Early monitoring phase

During the first week of PN (and subsequently if the patient is unstable with respect to fluid and electrolyte or metabolic issues) the patient is monitored intensely. This consists of a minimum set of mandatory assessments and appropriate blood and other laboratory tests. The aim is to optimize nutritional support while remaining aware of the other therapeutic strategies in the patient's overall care plan.

It may be necessary to modify either nutritional support or the overall patient care plan to obtain the best patient outcomes.

Stable patient phase

After the patient is stabilized on PN, a less intensive monitoring process is required.

Reintroduction of diet

At a certain point, diet or enteral feed is usually introduced in a transitional manner. Collaboration with the nutrition support team is essential and, if appropriate, reduction or cessation of PN is recommended.

Cessation of parenteral nutrition

PN is usually stopped when oral nutritional intake is deemed adequate for the individual patient. As a general rule of thumb, cessation of PN is determined on the basis of a variety of factors and is a multidisciplinary decision.

IV access

Peripheral cannulae (Venflons) should not routinely be used for the administration of PN and should only be used in the short term for the administration of peripheral-formulated PN.

PICC lines are usually used for medium duration and then switched to long-term venous access (2–6 months).

Tunneled, cuffed central venous catheters (CVCs) are inserted via the subclavian (or jugular) vein for long-term feeding.

A dedicated single-lumen line is the safest route for PN administration. There is a greater risk of infection the more times a line is manipulated. Obviously, aseptic technique should be used. Nothing else should be given through this lumen, nor should blood be sampled from the line under normal circumstances (it might be appropriate for blood sampling in patients receiving parenteral nutrition at home).

If a multilumen line must be used for clinical reasons, one lumen should be dedicated for PN use only. Again, ideally, nothing else should be given through this lumen, nor should blood be sampled from it.

Prescribing PN

Patients' nutritional requirements are based on standard dietetic equations. A regimen close to a patient's requirements should be provided in a formulation prepared to minimize risk.

Nitrogen

Protein in parenteral nutrition is provided in the form of amino acids. Individual nitrogen requirements are calculated.

Carbohydrate and lipid

The energy in parenteral nutrition is generally described as non-protein calories (i.e., the figure excludes the energy provided from amino acids).

Total energy intake is best given as a mixture of glucose and lipid, usually in a ratio of 60:40. This might be varied if clinically important glucose intolerance develops or there is a requirement for lipid-free PN.

Volume

In general, PN should provide all fluid volume requirements, including losses from wounds, drains, stomas, and fistulae, etc. However, if these losses are large or highly variable, they should be replaced and managed separately.

Electrolytes

These are modified according to clinical requirements and with particular regard to extrarenal losses.

Electrolytes should be reviewed daily and modified as necessary. Monitoring of urinary electrolyte losses is useful.

Vitamins, minerals, and trace elements

These are added routinely on a daily basis. Extra zinc or selenium may be required in patients with large GI losses. Patients on long-term PN should undergo routine micronutrient screening (see Table 15.47).

Other medications

In general, drug additions should not be made to the PN on grounds of stability, unless stability work is undertaken. Certain drug additions are known to lead to incompatibility, e.g., heparin.

Recommended monitoring and care

- Daily weight (before starting PN and daily thereafter)
- Take temperature and BP reading every 4–6 hours (observe for clinical evidence of infection, and general well-being)

Table 15.47 Suggested monitoring guide (refer to local guidelines)

	Baseline	New patient or unstable	Stable patient
Blood biochemistry			
Urea and creatinine	Yes	Daily	Three times weekly
Sodium	Yes	Daily	Three times weekly
K^+	Yes	Daily	Three times weekly
Bicarbonate	Yes	Daily	Three times weekly
Chloride	Yes	Daily	Three times weekly
LFTs: bilirubin	Yes	Daily	Three times weekly
Alk phos	Yes	Daily	Three times weekly
AST or ALT	Yes	Daily	Three times weekly
Albumin	Yes	Daily	Three times weekly
Calcium	Yes	Daily	Three times weekly
Magnesium	Yes	Daily	Three times weekly
Phosphate	Yes	Daily	Three times weekly
Zinc	Yes	Weekly	Every 2 weeks
Copper	Yes	Monthly	Every 3 months
CRP	Yes	Three times weekly	Three times weekly
Full blood count	Yes	Three times weekly	Weekly
Coagulation			
aPTT	Yes	Weekly	Weekly
INR	Yes	Weekly	Weekly
Lipids			
Cholesterol	Yes	Weekly	Weekly
Triglycerides	Yes	Weekly	Weekly

Alk phos, alkaline phosphatase; ALT, alanine aminotransferase; aPTT, activated partial prothrombin time; AST, asparate aminotransferase; CRP, C-reactive protein; INR, international normalized ratio; LFTs, liver function tests.

- Accurate fluid-balance chart and summary (to maintain accurate fluid balance and homeostasis). Bag change should be undertaken at the same time of day.
- Capillary blood glucose monitoring q6h during the first 24 hours, then twice or once daily when the patient is stable (generally, the glucose target should be 72–180 mg/dL [4–10 mmols/L]). Return to capillary blood glucose monitoring every 6 hours when the patient is being weaned off PN.
- Daily assessment for CVC or PICC site infection or leakage. Change dressing for CVCs at least every 72 hours and more frequently if loose, soiled, or wet. Change PICC dressings weekly.
- 24-hour urine collections for nitrogen balance and electrolytes should be undertaken according to local practice.

Storage of PN on ward

PN bags not yet connected to the patient must be stored in a refrigerator (between 35.6° and 46.4°F [2–8°C]). Bags stored in a drug refrigerator must be kept away from freezer compartments to prevent ice crystal formation in the parenteral nutrition.

Bags that have been refrigerated should be removed at least 1–2 hours before being hung and infused so that the solution can reach room temperature. Bags connected to the patient should be protected from light with protective covers.

Normal nutritional requirements

The Harris–Benedict equation is commonly used to calculate basal energy expenditure (BEE) in kilocalories (kcal) per day.

It is always best to be cautious by starting low and titrating up (depending on tolerance and clinical response). Use actual body weight if the patient is less than their ideal body weight (IBW). Use an adjusted body weight if the patient is >140% of their IBW because fat is not as metabolically active as muscle. Adjusted body weight can be calculated by IBW + [(Actual body weight – IBW) x 0.4].

Macronutrients

Calories

- Most patients should receive 25–35 kcal/kg/day.

Harris–Benedict equation (BEE)

BW = body weight in kg, Ht = height in cm, age = age in years

Men: BEE = 66 + (13.7 x BW) + (5 x Ht) – (6.8 x age)

Women: BEE = 655 + (9 x BW) + (1.7 x Ht) – (4.7 x age)

Stress factors

- Low stress: 1.2
- Moderate stress: 1.2–1.3
- Severe stress: 1.3–1.5
- Burns: up to 2 (depends on surface area of body burned)

Total caloric requirement equals the BEE multiplied by the stress factor.

Composition of parenteral nutrition regimens

- If possible, a patient-specific nutrition regimen should be developed to deliver a balance of glucose, protein, and lipids to provide the total calculated caloric need.
- *Protein:* most patients should receive between 0.2 and 2.5 g/kg/day of protein, depending on their level of stress and renal function.
  - 1 g protein = 4 kcal
- *Lipids:* limit to 25%–40% of total calories
  - Fat = 9 kcal/g, 10% lipid = 1.1 kcal/mL, 20% lipid = 2 kcal/mL
  - Keep serum triglycerides <350 mg/dL
- *Glucose:* minimum of 100 g/day, usually the remainder of the caloric intake after protein and lipids are calculated
  - IV dextrose = 3.4 kcal/g

Nitrogen

- Normal nitrogen requirements are 0.14–0.2 g/kg body weight
- Requirements in catabolic patients can be in the range of 0.2–0.3 g/kg body weight
- Nonrenal nitrogen losses should be taken into consideration, e.g., with wound, fistula, or burn losses

Electrolytes

- Sodium (normal range 1–2 mEq/kg)
  - Sensitive to hemodilutional effects; actual low sodium level is usually only a result of excessive losses, and a moderately low level is unlikely to be clinically significant
- Potassium (normal range 1–2 mEq/kg)
  - Affected by renal function, drugs, or excessive losses
- Calcium (normal range 10–15 mEq)
  - Minimal supplementation generally adequate in short term
- Magnesium (normal range 10–15 mEq)
  - Renally conserved, minimal amounts generally suffice
- Phosphorus (normal range 20–40 mmol)
  - Influenced by renal function, refeeding syndrome, and onset of sepsis

Trace elements and vitamins

Commercial multivitamin and mineral preparations are suitable for most short- to medium-term patients. For long-term patients, requirements are dictated by monitoring.

Specific clinical conditions affecting parenteral nutrition requirements and provision

Refeeding syndrome

- Start with low calories/day (max. 20 kcal/kg/day).
- Monitor and supplement potassium, magnesium, and phosphorus as required.
- Ensure adequate vitamin supply, especially thiamine.

Acute renal failure

- Consider fluid, potassium, and phosphorus restriction.

Chronic renal failure

- Influenced by dialysis status
- Consider need for protein, potassium, and phosphate restriction.

Acute liver failure

- Use dry body weight (especially if ascites is present) to calculate requirements.
- Patients may require sodium and fluid restriction. Protein restriction is not necessary.
- Provision of nutrition usually outweighs risks of abnormal LFTs.

Congestive cardiac failure

- Consider need for sodium and fluid restriction.

Nutritional support in adults

Parenteral support

Poor nutritional status is a major determinant of morbidity (as a consequence of depressed cell-mediated immunity and wound healing) and mortality.

The decision to provide nutritional support must be made thorough clinical patient assessment. Parenteral nutritional support is the least preferred method of providing nutritional support and should be reserved for patients in whom it is the only viable option to provide the necessary substrates for metabolism.

Appropriate indications for parenteral nutrition

- Inability to provide sufficient nutrients enterally
- Short bowel syndrome
- Severe malabsorption/steatorrhea
- High-output enterocutaneous fistula
- Prolonged paralytic ileus
- Severe pancreatitis
- Multiple injuries involving the viscera
- Intractable vomiting or diarrhea
- Persistent GI hemorrhage
- Lack of enteral access
- Malnourished patients in whom the use of the intestine is not anticipated for >7 days after major abdominal surgery
- Conditions severely affecting the GI tract, such as severe mucositis following systemic chemotherapy

Guide to calculating parenteral nutritional requirements in adults

Nutritional assessment

Patient assessment is necessary to determine nutritional needs and to predict any metabolic changes that may occur. A number of techniques are available to assess nutritional status. Some factors to consider are weight loss in the previous 6 months; recent dietary intake compared to usual intake; presence of anorexia, nausea, vomiting, or diarrhea for >2 weeks; functional capacity; metabolic demands of underlying conditions; and physical exam.

Common criteria used to define malnutrition are recent weight loss, body mass index (BMI) changes, and ideal body weight (IBW).

Identifying high-risk patients

- Unintentional weight loss: 5%–10% is clinically significant
- Poor oral intake
- Underlying conditions: take edema, ascites, or dehydration into consideration

$$\text{BMI} = \frac{\text{Weight (kg)}}{\text{Height (m)}^2}$$

BMI categories
- Underweight: <18.5
- Healthy: 18.5–24.9
- Overweight: 25–29.9
- Unhealthy: >30

BMI is a useful measure that has a low correlation with height, but a higher correlation with independent measures of body fat for adults. A BMI of 14–15 is associated with mortality.

The only clinical method to assess nutritional status that has been validated is the Subjective Global Assessment (SGA). Data from the patient's history and physical examination are subjectively weighted to classify the patient as well nourished, moderately malnourished, or severely malnourished.

IBW
- Requires patient's height to calculate
- Men: 50 kg + 2.3 kg for every inch over 60 inches
- Women: 45.5 kg + 2.3 kg for every inch over 60 inches

Children's parenteral nutrition regimens

Parenteral nutrition in children

Parenteral nutrition has been used successfully in pediatric patients since 1944. It is a means to provide the necessary calories, protein, and fat to sustain life until enteral nutrition is indicated. Patients may only require short-term (<2 weeks) parenteral nutrition given the following clinical situations: major intestinal surgery, chemotherapy, severe acute pancreatitis, trauma, burns, sepsis, or low birth weight. Others will need long-term parenteral nutrition in the event of prolonged episodes of intestinal failure.

There are two techniques used to provide nutrients to patients: peripherally and centrally. An infusion of a more concentrated solution requires a central line. This reduces the risk of thrombophlebitis, which can occur when a concentrated solution is given through a peripheral line. The peripheral line is used for less concentrated solutions.

Nutritional requirements (see Tables 15.48, 15.49, 15.50, 15.51, and 15.52)

Fluid requirements depend on the patient's size, abnormal losses (e.g., diarrhea, fever), surgical procedures, and disease states. The requirements of fluid to body weight are much greater in very small children

Table 15.48 Estimated average requirements for fluid, calories, protein, and fat

Age	Fluid (mL/kg/day)	Calories (kcal/kg/day)	Protein (g/kg/day)	Fat (g/kg/day)
Preterm infant	100–200	90–110	2.5–3.5	3
Term infant to 1 year	95–120	90–100	2.0–2.5	3
1–10 years	75–100	50–90	1.5–2.0	1–2
>10 years	50–75	40–50	1.0–1.3	1–2

Table 15.49 Normal baseline electrolyte requirements

Electrolytes	Daily requirements (mg)	
	Neonates	Infants & children
Sodium	120	200–500
Potassium	500	700–2000
Calcium	400	600–800
Magnesium	40	60–170
Phosphate	300	500–800
Chloride	180	300–750

Table 15.50 Normal requirements for trace elements

Element (mg)	Preterm	Infant	Children
Zinc	5	5	10
Copper	0.4–0.6	0.5–1	1–3
Selenium	10	15	20–30
Manganese	0.3–0.6	0.6–1	1–1.5
Iron	6	10	10

Table 15.51 Normal requirements for water-soluble vitamins

Vitamin	Preterm	Infant	Children
B_1 (mg)	0.3	0.4	0.7–1
B_2 (mg)	0.4	0.5	0.8–1.2
B_6 (mg)	0.3	0.6	1–1.7
B_{12} (mcg)	0.3	0.5	0.7–1.4
C (mg)	30	35	40–45
Biotin (mcg)	10	15	20
Folate (mcg)	25	35	50–100
Niacin (mg)	5	6	9–13

Table 15.52 Requirements for fat-soluble vitamins

Vitamin	Preterm	Infant	Children
A (mcg)	375	375	400–700
D (IU)	*	400	400
E (mg)	3	4	6–7
K (mcg)	5	10	15–30

*American Academy or Pediatrics 2008 Guidelines did not report

than in older children and adults. Infants have a much larger body surface area relative to weight than do older patients. Fluid maintenance is often dependent on body weight:

- <10 kg: 100 mL/kg/day
- 11–20 kg: 1000 mL plus 50 mL/kg for each kg above 10 kg
- >20 kg: 1500 mL plus 20 mL/kg for each kg above 20 kg

Infants are more susceptible to insensible water losses due to evaporation from bilirubin lights and radiant warmers. Infants also dissipate more heat per kilogram. Patients with high urinary outputs, increased ileostomy or gastrostomy tube outputs, diarrhea, and vomiting should have replacement fluids for these excessive losses, in addition to their maintenance fluid requirements.

The patient's weight and assessment of intake and output can be used to estimate hydration status. It is important that patients receiving parenteral nutrition be weighed regularly (initially daily, then twice to three times weekly with growth plotted when their condition stabilizes) and have their fluid balance monitored.

Carbohydrate

Glucose (in the form of dextrose monohydrate), which provides 3.4 kcal/g of dextrose, is the carbohydrate of choice in parenteral nutrition. Dextrose infusions are introduced in a stepwise manner to prevent hyperosmolality and hyperinsulinemia.

Neonates, extreme low–birth weight (ELBW) infants (<1000 g body weight) in particular, may not tolerate large amounts of dextrose initially because of insulin resistance. Initial infusions of >8.6 g/kg/day may lead to hyperglycemia and serum hyperosmolality, resulting in osmotic diuresis. For this reason, dextrose is introduced at 5 g/kg/day with a gradual increase of 3 g/kg/day, while monitoring serum glucose.

Older infants and children are able to tolerate higher amounts of dextrose and are initiated at 10 g/kg/day, and can withstand a more rapid increase per day (ranging from 5 to 30 g/kg/day).

The concentration of dextrose that can be infused depends on the type of line access available. The dextrose concentration in parenteral nutrition infused peripherally is limited to 12.5%. If central access is available, 20%–30% glucose can be infused. Infusion of parenteral nutrition with dextrose concentrations >20% has been associated with cardiac arrhythmias.

Lipids

Fat is an important parenteral substrate because it is a concentrated source of calories in an isotonic medium, which makes it useful for peripheral administration. It is a useful substitute for carbohydrate if dextrose calories are limited because of glucose intolerance.

Lipid emulsions are available in a 10% solution (1.1 kcal/mL) or 20% solution (2 kcal/mL). They are composed of triglycerides stabilized with egg phospholipids and isotonically balanced with glycerol.

Essential fatty acid deficiency can develop in the premature newborn during the first week of life on lipid-free regimens. The amount of lipid required to prevent fatty acid deficiency is 0.5–1 g/kg/day. Initiation of lipids should not exceed 1 g/kg/day (0.5 g/kg/day in neonates); however, the amount used for non-glucose caloric needs often requires 3–4 g/kg/day. In lipid doses >4 g/kg/day there is an increased risk for fat overload syndrome, characterized by jaundice, fever, leukocytosis, coagulopathy, seizures, and shock.

Serum triglycerides should be monitored to assess tolerance. Triglycerides should be drawn 4–8 hours after completion of the infusion. If the serum triglyceride level is >150 mg/dL, the lipid infusion rate should be reduced.

Protein

Nitrogen retention refers to the body's ability to hold onto its critical nitrogen for natural body processes to take place. Nitrogen is needed for growth, the formation of new tissues (e.g., wound healing), and the synthesis of plasma proteins, enzymes, and blood cells.

Requirements vary according to age, nutritional status, and disease state. Infants and children experiencing periods of growth have higher nitrogen requirements than those of adults. Low–birth weight (LBW) infants have relatively high total amino acid requirements to support maintenance, growth, and developmental needs.

In term infants requiring parenteral nutrition, amino acid intake (2.0–2.5 g/kg/day of protein) results in nitrogen retention comparable to that of the healthy enteral-fed infant. Premature infants require 2.5–3.5 g/kg/day of protein to promote nitrogen retention.

Choice of amino acid solution

The proteins of the human body are manufactured from 20 different amino acids; of these, there are eight essential amino acids. Premature infants and children are unable to synthesize or metabolize some of the amino acids that are "nonessential" for adults.

The use of amino acid solutions designed for adults have resulted in abnormal plasma amino acid profiles in infants. Infants fed with adult amino acid solutions have been shown to develop high concentrations of phenylalanine and tyrosine and low levels of taurine. The amino acid preparations available for pediatrics (TrophAmine® and Aminosyn PF®) yield a plasma amino acid pattern resembling that seen in breast-fed infants.

Administration of nutrition

- The aqueous phase runs over a period of 24 hours and the solution is filtered using a 0.2-micron filter.
- Lipids normally run over a period of 12–24 hours and are filtered with a 1.2-micron filter, although some centers prefer not to use filters.
- The weight used for calculation is usually the actual weight of the child. In some cases of LBW infants, birth weight will be used because of fluctuations in the first days of life.

Complications

Catheter related

Complications can occur from central catheter insertion (e.g., malposition, hemorrhage, pneumothorax, air embolism, or nerve injury) or may occur subsequently (e.g., infection, occlusion, or thromboembolism). The major catheter-related complication is infection. This is due to the catheter, which provides direct access to the central circulation. It is reported that close to 50% of catheters will lead to infection.

Metabolic related

Metabolic complications consist of hyperglycemia, hypoglycemia, azotemia, electrolyte disorders, acid–base disorders, etc. These complications often resolve by adjusting the additives in the parenteral nutrition.

Parenteral nutrition–associated cholestasis

Cholestasis is more likely to develop in LBW infants. The exact etiology is unknown; however, it seems to be multifactorial (e.g., absence of enteral feeding, calorie overload, amino acids and fasting). If the parenteral nutrition is withdrawn, liver dysfunction should reverse; however, cirrhosis has been associated with fibrosis and death.

If parenteral nutrition cannot be discontinued, then other options for administering parenteral nutrition should be employed (e.g., nutrition can be turned off for part of the day, excessive calories decreased to maintain normal growth and metabolism, minimal enteral feeding initiated to stimulate the gut when possible).

Monitoring of children receiving parenteral nutrition in the hospital

Clinical and laboratory monitoring, observations, and assessment of growth are required. Growth is evaluated by accurate measurement of weight and height as well as by development assessment. These measures are plotted over time. Fluid balance, temperature, and bowel movements need to be assessed daily.

Laboratory monitoring

- Initial assessment: daily for first 3–4 days, then twice weekly, dependent on the patient's clinical status
- Complete blood count
- Basic metabolic panel
- Calcium, magnesium, phosphate, bilirubin, ALP, AST, ALT, blood glucose, albumin, triglycerides, and cholesterol

Enteral feeding

Types of tube feeding

Enteral feeding should be considered in patients with a functioning gastrointestinal (GI) tract who are unable to meet nutrition requirements with ordinary diet, food fortification, or oral nutritional supplements. Enteral nutrition is contraindicated in patients with intestinal obstruction, paralytic ileus, GI ischemia, intractable diarrhea, and diffuse peritonitis.

Enteral-access device selection is based on several patient-specific factors, including GI anatomy, gastric emptying, duration of tube placement, and aspiration potential. Postpyloric feeding is indicated if there is gastric outflow obstruction or severe pancreatitis, or if the patient is at risk for aspiration with intragastric feeding.

Intragastric feeding

- Nasogastric (NG)
- Orogastric (OG)
- Percutaneous endoscopic gastrostomy (PEG)

Post-pyloric feeding

- Nasoduodenal
- Nasojejunal
- Percutaneous endoscopic gastrojejunostomy (PEG-J)
- Percutaneous endoscopic jejunostomy (PEJ)
- Surgically placed jejunostomy

Feeding tube–specific issues

Site of delivery

- Gastric tubes end in the stomach, whereas duodenal and jejunal tubes end in the duodenum and jejunum, respectively.
- Enteral tubes should be flushed with 20–30 mL of warm water every 4 hours with continuous feeds, and before and after intermittent feedings and medication administration.
- Do not use acidic solutions; proteins precipitate and may clog the tube (see Chapter 10, p. 230)

Differences between tubes

- Fine-bore—soft, smooth, very flexible, increased patient comfort, decreased nasal irritation
- Large-bore nasogastric—decompression and gastric drainage
- Number of lumens
- Rate of flow
- Length

Tube complications

- Removal by patient
- Incorrect positioning of tube
- Mechanical complications (blockage)
- Nasal tubes—nasopharyngeal ulceration, nasal septum necrosis, bacterial sinusitis
- Enterostomies—perforation, hemorrhage, wound infection, bowel obstruction and necrosis

Categories of feeds

Polymeric feeds

Polymeric feeds contain whole protein, carbohydrate, and triglycerides and can be used as a sole source of nutrition for those patients without any special nutrient requirements. The standard caloric density is 1–2 kcal/mL and 35–60 g/L of protein.

Formulas may be supplemented with fiber, which can help improve bowel function, if problematic. Polymeric feeds are viscous and may require the use of large-bore feeding tubes and an infusion pump.

Monomeric (elemental) feeds

Monomeric feeds contain free amino acids, glucose or maltodextran, and a very low fat content. The standard caloric density is approximately 1 kcal/mL with 40–50 g/L of protein. They are used in situations of malabsorption, such as fistula and pancreatitis.

Disease-specific feeds and modular supplements

Certain clinical conditions should be considered when determining enteral nutrition needs, such as those with organ dysfunction, inflammatory bowel disease, pancreatitis, and diabetes, among others. For example, patients with renal insufficiency should receive feeds that are calorie dense, low in protein, and contain modified electrolytes, whereas dialysis patients should receive higher amounts of protein.

Modular supplements are single nutrient components, such as protein, carbohydrates, and fat, used in patients suffering from malabsorption and hypoproteinemia. They are not nutritionally complete and thus should be given with a complete formula.

Administration of tube feeds

For intragastric feeds, continuous tube feeds are the most frequent method used in hospitals and nursing homes and are given over 16–24 hours per day, resulting in fewer instances of diarrhea and vomiting. Postpyloric feeding is generally performed by continuous infusion because it is deemed more physiological.

Alternatively, feeds may be administered via intermittent boluses of 240–480 mL by syringe over a period of 20–40 minutes 4 to 8 times daily, although complications such as aspiration and delayed gastric transit times have been reported more frequently with this approach. Intermittent tube feeds are also used in the instance of pertinent drug–food interactions, as seen with phenytoin administration.

Complications from feeds

Diarrhea

Diarrhea is the most common complication associated with enteral nutrition, occurring in 21%–72% of patients. Severe diarrhea can cause life-threatening electrolyte changes and hypovolemia.

Diarrhea typically becomes worse with the use of laxative-containing and prokinetic medications (see Critical Care section, p. 396). Concomitant use of these medications needs to be rationalized, and antidiarrheal medications, such as loperamide, and fiber may be of use.

Potential underlying disease states, including *Clostridium difficile*, should be considered. If diarrhea persists after treatment, consider switching to the postpyloric route.

Constipation

Constipation is usually a result of a combination of inadequate fluid, dehydration, immobility, and medications. If functional pathology is excluded, management is with laxatives and suppositories.

Vomiting, aspiration, or reflux

Aspiration is one of the most serious complications of enteral nutrition, which can lead to pneumonia and death in critically ill patients. While both nasogastric and postpyloric feeding can increase the risk of aspiration, many associate less aspiration risk with postpyloric feeds; however, evidence is lacking.

Aspiration risk factors include vomiting and excessive gastric residuals of >200 mL.

Metabolic complications

Refeeding syndrome

Refeeding syndrome occurs more frequently with parenteral nutrition; however, it can still occur with enteral nutrition and oral feeding. Patients at greatest risk for refeeding syndrome are those who have not received nutrition for long periods of time and have adapted to using free fatty acids and ketones as a primary energy source.

When enteral nutrition is started in these patients, the presence of excess carbohydrate stimulates insulin release. This leads to intracellular shifts of phosphate, magnesium, and potassium that can lead to cardiac arrhythmias or neurological events.

Emaciated patients must have their tube feedings introduced gradually and serum electrolytes should be closely monitored and replaced daily.

Vitamin and trace-element deficiencies

The incidence of vitamin and trace-element deficiencies is rare, since commercially available feeds are nutritionally complete. Patients being fed over extended periods should be monitored periodically for appropriate vitamin and trace-element levels.

Hyperglycemia

Hyperglycemia is a common adverse event that occurs with enteral feeds secondary to carbohydrate administration. In critically ill patients, it is important that blood glucose be monitored and controlled, as studies have shown that tight glycemic control improves mortality rates.

Intravenous therapy at home

As defined by the American Society of Health-System Pharmacists, *home care* is the provision of specialized, complex pharmaceutical services and clinical assessment and monitoring to patients in their homes. Home intravenous (IV) therapy encompasses a variety of therapeutic modalities for the treatment of many different disease states or conditions.

A safe and effective home IV therapy regimen requires a multidisciplinary approach among a variety of health-care providers, including physicians, nurses, and pharmacists.

IV therapies

- Antimicrobial agents
- Parenteral antimicrobial therapy in the home care setting represents a multibillion-dollar-a-year industry provided to 1 in 1000 Americans on an annual basis.
- Chemotherapy
- Total parenteral nutrition
- Pain management
- Hydration
- Immune globulins
- Immunosuppressant agents
- Growth hormone

Initiation of home IV therapy

Factors influencing the choice of drug delivery method

- Drug stability
- Dose frequency and duration
- Rate and volume of infusion
- Type of vascular access device
- Age of patient
- Functional limitations of patient and caregiver
- Reimbursement

Preadmission assessment

- Patient, family, and caregiver agreement with provision of home IV therapy
- Review of patient's past medical history and medication profile
- Nutritional assessment
- Assessment of patient's home environment
- Availability of psychosocial and family support
- Ongoing prescriber involvement in assessment and treatment of patient
- Establishment of a prognosis with clearly defined outcome goals
- Appropriate indication, dosage, route, and method of medication administration
- Appropriate laboratory tests for monitoring therapy

Role of the physician

- Preadmission assessment
- Establish diagnosis

- Select therapy
- Establish appropriate monitoring parameters
- Ongoing assessment of patient's clinical response to therapy
- Monitor patient for signs of toxicity or adverse drug effects
- Management of vascular access problems
- Coordinate multidisciplinary team efforts
- Approve any changes in therapy
- Provide education and training to patient and family: information on risk of infection, complications, treatment plans, potential problems, communication, and expected outcomes

Role of the nurse

- Preadmission assessment
- Assess patient's functional limitations, cognitive and technical skills
- Administer medication
- Routine maintenance and care of vascular access device
- Ongoing assessment of patient's clinical response to therapy
- Monitor patient for signs of toxicity or adverse drug effects
- Provide education and training to patient and family: information on risk of infection, complications, treatment plans, potential problems, communication, and expected outcomes
- Interdisciplinary communication and coordination of care

Role of the pharmacist

- Preadmission assessment
- Acquire, store, compound, dispense, and deliver medication
- Assess medication storage and stability requirements
- Monitor pharmacokinetics
- Monitor patient for signs of toxicity or adverse drug effects
- Monitor patient for potential drug interactions
- Consult with physician on dose recommendations
- Provide patient education regarding IV medications
- Interdisciplinary communication

Role of the patient and caregiver

- Adherence to therapy
- Care of vascular access device, including flushes
- Change injection caps, IV tubing, and bags
- Change dressings

With careful collaboration between members of a multidisciplinary team and the patient, home IV therapy allows for successful medication administration with minimal interruption in a patient's daily life.

Further reading

American Society of Health-System Pharmacists (2000). ASHP guidelines on the pharmacist's role in home care. *Am J Health Syst Pharm* **57**:1252–1257.

Oseland S, Querciagrossa AJ (2003). Collaboration of nursing and pharmacy in home infusion therapy. *Home Healthc Nurse* **21**:818–824.

Tice AD, Rehn SJ, Dalovisio JR, et al. (2004). Practice guidelines for outpatient parenteral antimicrobial therapy. *Clin Infect Dis* **38**:1651–1672.

Sodium content of parenteral drugs

A number of parenteral formulations contain a significant amount of sodium ions (see Table 15.53). This sodium load is unlikely to be important in most patients but could be clinically significant for some patient groups, e.g., neonates and patients with significant liver impairment.

Table 15.53 is not exhaustive but lists the sodium content of more frequently used drugs or drugs in which the sodium level is especially high. The absence of a drug from the table does not necessarily mean that it has low sodium content (check additional sources).

If a drug is reconstituted or infused with sodium chloride 0.9% solution, this further increases the sodium load.

Note that some oral preparations, especially soluble tablets, might have high sodium levels.

Table 15.53 Summary of product characteristics

Name	Vial/ ampule size	Sodium content per vial (mEq)
Acetazolamide	500 mg	2.05
Acetylcysteine	6 g	38.3
Acyclovir	500 mg	2.1
Ampicillin	1 g	2.9
Amphotericin lipid complex	100 mg	3.3
Amphotericin liposomal	50 mg	0.5
Cefotaxime	1 g	2.2
Ceftazidime	1 g	2.3
Ceftriaxone	1 g	3.6
Cefuroxime powder	1 g	2.4
Cefuroxime premix	750 mg	4.8
Cefuroxime premix	1.5 g	9.7
Chloramphenicol	1 g	2.25
Chlorothiaide	500 mg	2.5
Ciprofloxacin	200 mg	15.4
Dalteparin	10,000 IU/mL	0.16
Dantrolene	20 mg	0.08
Desmopressin	4 mcg	0.16
Diazoxide	1.5 g	74
Ertapenem	1 g	6
Esomeprazole	20 mg	0.93

Table 15.53 *(Contd.)*

Name	Vial/ ampule size	Sodium content per vial (mEq)
Famotidine premix	20 mg	7.8
Fluconazole	200 mg	16
Foscarnet	6 g	93.6
TFurosemide	20 mg	0.324
Ganciclovir	500 mg	2
Granisetron	1 mg	0.39
Heparin	10,000 IU/mL	0.8
Hetastarch 6%	500 mL	77
Hydrocortisone sodium succinate	1 g	20.7
Imipenem-Cilastatin	500 mg	1.6
Levofloxacin	500 mg	15.4
Levothyroxine	200 mcg	1.6
Meropenem	1 g	3.92
Metoclopramide	10 mg	0.29
Metronidazole	500 mg	14
Midazolam	1 mg/mL	0.14
Nafcillin	1 g	2.9
Nitroprusside	50 mg	0.34
Pantoprazole	40 mg	0.9
Penicillin G potassium	1,000,000 IU/50 mL	1.7
Penicillin G sodium	1,000,000 IU/50 mL	1.68
Pamidronate dry powder	30 mg	0.2
	90 mg	0.3
Pamidronate solution	30 mg	1.1
	60 mg	1.1
	90 mg	1.1
Phenytoin	250 mg	2
Piperacillin	2 g	3.7
Piperacillin + tazobactam powder	2.25 g	4.69
	3.375 g	7.04
	4.5 g	9.39
Piperacillin + tazobactam premix	2.25 g	5.7
	3.375 g	8.6
	4.5 g	11.4

Table 15.53 (*Contd.*)

Name	Vial/ampule size	Sodium content per vial (mEq)
Rifampin	600 mg	0.65
Sodium bicarbonate	4.2% (10 mL)	5
	5% (500 mL)	297.5
	7.4% (50 mL)	44.6
	8.4% (50 mL)	50
Sodium chloride	0.9% (100 mL)	15.65
Terbutaline	1 mg	0.3
Thiopental	1 g	4.9
Ticarcillin	1 g	4.75
Ticarcillin + clavulanic acid	3.1 g	14.3
Valproate	500 mg	3.01
Verapamil	5 mg	0.74

Further reading

Contact the manufacturer for additional information on sodium content.
Medical References. University of Maryland. Available at: http://www.umm.edu/medref/
Trissel L (2007). *Handbook on Injectable Drugs*, 14th ed. Bethesda MD: American Society of Health-System Pharmacists.

Diabetes mellitus

Diabetes mellitus (DM) affects approximately 7.8% of the U.S. population. In 2007, the Center for Disease Control and Prevention (CDC) reported that 23.6 million people in the United States have diabetes. Of these, 5.7 million remain undiagnosed. Another 57 million people have prediabetes.

Type 2 diabetes accounts for 90%–95% of all diabetes and is a result of insulin resistance and pancreatic beta-cell dysfunction. Type 1 diabetes results from an absolute insulin deficiency secondary to autoimmune dysfunction.

Diabetes is the leading cause of kidney failure and the leading cause of blindness in 20- to 74-year-olds. Among diabetics, the risks for stroke, heart disease, and death from heart disease are 2 to 4 times higher than those of the nondiabetic population. Diabetes accounts for more than 60% of all nontraumatic lower limb amputations.

Diabetes is both a deadly and costly disease that continues to reach epidemic proportions. The CDC estimates that in 2007 the total cost from diabetes was $174 billion dollars.

While insulin is used in type 1 diabetes, oral therapy is used alone and in combination with insulin to treat type 2 diabetes.

Diagnosis

Diabetes is diagnosed when:

- Symptoms of diabetes (polydipsia, polyuria, unexplained weight loss) PLUS
- Plasma glucose 200 mg/dL or more, taken at any time of the day

OR

- Fasting plasma glucose 126 mg/dL or more*

OR

- 2 hour postprandial glucose 200 mg/dL or more after 75 g glucose load*

Management

The management of diabetes involves lifestyle and pharmacological therapy. Pharmacological therapy includes insulin and oral hypoglycemics or antihyperglycemics. Medical nutritional therapy and exercise remain the cornerstones for treatment of diabetes.

When HbA1C or blood glucose goals are not met by monotherapy, combination therapy is more effective than switching to another monotherapy. Switching or replacing drug therapy is not recommended.

Combination therapy allows for greater glucose-lowering, addressing both major physiological defects of type 2 diabetes: insulin secretory failure and insulin resistance. It is important to keep in mind the % degree of HbA1C-lowering achievable from monotherapy, combination, and triple therapy when making decisions to help patients reach HbA1C goals.

Hemoglobin A1C approximate lowering (not including insulin):

- Monotherapy lowers A1C from ~0.6% to 2.5%
- Combination therapy ~2%
- Triple therapy ~2% to 2.5%

*must be repeated on 2 different days.

Hemoglobin A1C lowering from insulin:

- No ceiling, but limited by hypoglylcemia
- Hemoglobin A1C >8.5%–9% on monotherapy or double therapy may indicate frank insulin loss and the need for insulin

Insulin

Insulin is necessary for type 1 diabetics and in type 2 diabetics who are inadequately controlled or during periods of stress. Insulin is also used in gestational diabetics inadequately controlled by diet and exercise.

There are various types of insulin based on onset and duration of action (see Table 15.54) as well as premixed combination products (see Table 15.55).

- NPH can be mixed with rapid- or short-acting insulins only.
- Insulin glargine and detemir may not be mixed with any other insulins.

Table 15.54 Insulin types: human and insulin analogs

Insulin	Onset	Peak	Duration
Rapid-acting analogs Lispro, aspart, glulisine	10–15 minutes	1–2 hours	3–5 hours
Short-acting human regular	30–60 minutes	2–4 hours	5–8 hours
Intermediate-acting human NPH	2–4 hours	4–10 hours	10–16 hours
Long-acting analogs Detemir * Glargine*	3–8 hour 2–4 hours	None None	~24 hours Up to 24 hours

* 2 or more injections may be required in some patients.

Table 15.55 Premixed insulins

Insulin	Onset	Peak	Duration
70/30 (70% NPH/30% regular	0.5–1 hour	2–10 hours	10–18 hours
50/50 (50% NPH/50% regular)	0.5–1 hour	2–10 hours	10–18 hours
Humalog 70/25 (75% lispro protamine + 25% lispro)	~15 minutes	1–3 hours	10–16 hours
Humalog 50/50 (50% lispro protamine + 50% lispro)	~15 minutes	1–3 hours	10–16 hours
Novolog 70/30 (70% aspart protamine + 30% aspart)	~15 minutes	1–3 hours	10–16 hours

- Insulin is only stable for 28 days once opened (with the exception of detemir; stable for 42 days) and may be stored in or out of the refrigerator. Unopened refrigerated insulin is stable through the manufacturer's expiration date.
- The goal of any insulin regimen or combination is to target control, avoid hypoglycemia, and be acceptable to the patient.
- Consider insulin therapy when HbA1C >8% and the patient is already on combination or triple therapy and exhibits hyperglycemia. Oral agents should not be discontinued.
- Consider insulin therapy if HbA1C >10% at any time; insulin can be discontinued or modified once hyperglycemic symptoms have subsided.
- Although premixed insulin offers the advantage of decreased injections, it is difficult to adjust either insulin component successfully.
- Insulin dosage may be adjusted every 3–7 days on the basis of patient's self-monitoring of blood glucose.
- Generally, fasting blood glucose is targeted first with long-acting or basal insulin for control, then post-meal glucoses are targeted with meal-coverage insulin.

U-500 insulin (regular concentrated insulin)

- U-500 regular insulin is reserved generally for patients taking more than 200 units per day and >100 units per injection.
- U-500 insulin activity is similar to that of NPH insulin and is generally dosed before breakfast and before dinner, but can be increased to 3 or 4 times daily as doses increase.
- U-500 insulin characteristics:
  - Onset: 1–2 hours
  - Peak: 4–8 hours
  - Duration: 10–20 hours
- Use with caution, as U-500 insulin is 5 times more potent than U-100 insulin.

Insulin pens

- Insulin pens offer flexibility in patient schedules as they are more discrete and may offer an alternative to those who fear injections or have dexterity or visual impairments.
- Pens are either disposable or have replaceable cartridges.
- Pens generally hold either 150 or 300 units of insulin and come in boxes of 5.
- Insulin pen stability must be verified with the manufacturer as stability varies from 10 to 42 days.

Oral agents

Second-generation sulfonylureas

- Mechanism: stimulate insulin release from binding to sulfonlyurea β-cell site
- Targets postprandial glucose
- Place in therapy: monotherapy, combination therapy, can be first line

- Reduction in HbA1c: 0.9&–2.5%
- Glipizide: 5 mg daily to 40 mg daily in 2 divided doses; XL 10–20 mg daily
- Glyburide: 1.25 mg daily to 20 mg daily. Doses >10 mg/day should be divided and given twice per day.
- Glimepiride: 1–8 mg daily
- Give regular-release glipizide before meals in divided doses and XL daily
- Risks: hypoglycemia, weight gain
- No additional benefit at doses >50% of maximum dose

Biguanides

- Mechanism: decreases hepatic glucose production
- Targets fasting blood glucose
- Place in therapy: considered first line, monotherapy, combination therapy
- Reduction in HbA1c: 1%–1.3%
- Metformin immediate release: 500 mg twice daily or 850 mg daily, up to 2550 mg in 3 divided doses
- Metformin extended release (XR): 500–2000 mg daily
- Increase dose by 500 mg/day weekly
- Maximum effective dose is 2000 mg/day
- Lactic acidosis rare (<0.3%, but 50% fatal)
- Contraindicated with serum creatinine ≥1.5 mg/dL in men and 1.4 mg/dL in women
- Regular release should be discontinued just before (if morning surgery, then PM before; if PM surgery, then morning of) surgery or diagnostic tests requiring radiocontrast; XR stop the night before and restart either form 48 hours after renal function is normal
- Use with caution in patients >80 years (should have normal renal clearance) and in those with hepatic dysfunction, alcoholism, unstable congestive heart failure (CHF), or dehydration.
- GI side effects (nausea, vomiting, diarrhea) occur in up to 50% of patients; can give with food; start low and go slow
- Improved lipid profile; weight neutral or weight loss
- Decreased macrovascular events

Meglitinides

- Mechanism: stimulates insulin release from binding to sulfonlyurea β-cell site
- Targets postprandial glucose; short acting
- Place in therapy: monotherapy or combination therapy
- Reduction in HbA1C: 0.6%–0.8%
- Repaglinide: 1.5 mg to 16 mg daily in 3 divided doses 15–30 minutes before meals.
- Nateglinide: 180 mg daily to 360 mg daily in 3 divided doses 15–30 minutes before meals
- Risks: hypoglycemia; weight gain
- The need for frequent dosing may adversely affect compliance.

Thiazolidinedione

- Mechanism: activates PPAR-γ, increasing peripheral insulin sensitivity in skeletal muscle cells
- Targets fasting blood glucose.
- Place in therapy: considered second line, but could be monotherapy in patients with lower hemoglobin A1C (6.5%–8%) range, combination therapy
- Reduction in HbA1C: 1.5%–1.6%
- Pioglitazone: 15–45 mg daily
- Rosiglitazone: 2 mg twice daily to 4 mg twice daily or 4 mg daily to 8 mg daily
- Edema and weight gain occur more in combination with insulin.
- Contraindicated in NYHA Class III and IV heart failure; do not use in patients with underlying liver dysfunction (baseline ALT ≥2.5 ULN). If ALT is ≥3× ULN at any time, must discontinue use
- An increase in bone fracture rates has been reported in women.
- Delayed onset of action, may be 6–8 weeks (or as much as 12 weeks)
- Pioglitazone may have positive effects on lipids (↑ HDL, ↓TG)
- Recent meta-analysis with rosiglitazone suggests increased risk of MI compared to those taking control. ADA no longer recommends rosiglitazone.

α-glucosidase inhibitor

- Mechanism: slows carbohydrate absorption in gut
- Targets postprandial glucose
- Place in therapy: monotherapy or combination therapy
- Reduction in HbA1C: 0.6%–1.3%
- Acarbose: 150–300 mg in 3 divided doses with meals
- Miglitol: 150–300 mg in 3 divided doses with meals
- Must take with carbohydrate-containing meal
- Decreases postprandial glucose; must be taken with first bite of food
- Start low and go slow to avoid GI intolerance.
- If hypoglycemia occurs (risk if on insulin or sulfonylurea too), must treat with glucose, not sucrose

Dipeptidyl peptidase inhibitor (DPP IV)

- Mechanism: slows inactivation of incretin hormones, GLP-1 and GLP, suppressing glucagon secretion and increasing glucose-dependent insulin release
- Targets postprandial blood glucose
- Place in therapy: monotherapy or combination therapy
- Reduction in HbA1C: 0.8%
- Sitagliptin: 100 mg daily
- Dosage adjustment necessary in renal dysfunction
- Creatinine clearance: 30–50 mL/min = 50 mg daily
- Creatinine clearance <30 mL/min = 25 mg daily
- Increases satiety
- Delays gastric emptying
- Weight neutral

Combination oral hypoglycemics

- Place in therapy: second line, convenience; improved adherence
- Combinations in varying strengths are available for the following:
  - Glyburide/metformin
  - Glipizide/metformin
  - Pioglitazone/glimepiride
  - Pioglitazone/metformin
  - Rosiglitazone/glimepiride
  - Rosiglitazone/metformin
  - Sitagliptin/metformin

Newer antidiabetic treatments

Pramlintide (Symlin®)

- Injectable amylin analog
- Mechanism: suppresses glucagon release; slows gastric emptying; enhances satiety
- Place in therapy: adjunct therapy for patients taking mealtime insulin and have not achieved glucose goals
- Reduction in HbA1C: 0.43%–0.56%
- Type 1 DM dose: 15 mcg tid before meals; titrate up to 60 mcg tid
- Type 2 DM dose: 60 mcg tid before meals; titrate to 120 mcg tid
- Requires reduction in preprandial insulin, including rapid, short, or fix-mixed insulin by 50% initially to avoid hypoglycemia
- Common side effects include nausea and vomiting (dose related)
- Contraindicated in hypoglycemic unawareness and in gastroparesis

Exenatide (Byetta®) injectable

- Glucagon-like peptide-1 (GLP-1) incretin mimetics; mimics incretin hormone
- Mechanism: stimulates insulin secretion in response to glucose load, inhibits release of glucagon following a meal; increases satiety; slows absorption of nutrients through delayed gastric emptying
- Place in therapy: adjunct therapy for use in combination with sulfonylureas, metformin, or a combination of these
- Reduction in HbA1C: 0.8%–0.9%
- Type 2 DM dose: 5 mcg bid within 60 minutes of a meal; dosage can be increased to 10 mcg bid if tolerated
- Common side effects include nausea and vomiting (dose related)
- Recent reports of possible exenatide pancreatitis have arisen. Its use is currently not recommended in patients with a history of pancreatitis

Blood glucose monitoring and control

Monitoring

The place of blood glucose monitoring is well recognized in patients with diabetes who require insulin treatment. There is now a wide range of meters available, in addition to lancet devices. It is important to be familiar with a range of machines. Most companies provide meters at low cost directly to patients and many insurance companies will cover the cost of a meter.

Recent developments have decreased the volume of blood required and decreased the speed of analysis to only a few seconds. Some meters have data download features providing charts, averages, and graphs and can estimate average levels according to chosen parameters.

Many meters offer alternative testing site options such as the forearm or the calf. Alternate site testing is subject to variabilities and should be discussed with a diabetes educator or provider.

Monitoring of patients with type 2 DM continues to be controversial; however, there are good reasons for regular, but less frequent, monitoring, and it should be encouraged. It is useful to monitor for lifestyle changes such as increased exercise, change of diet, identifying and managing hypoglycemia, and other influencing factors (stress or illness).

Alternate checking around different meal times or at bedtime may add important information for patients who continue to have controlled fasting blood glucoses, but an elevated hemoglobin A1C.

Control

The American Diabetes Association (ADA) recommends daily checking in type 2 diabetics on insulin and checking 3 to 4 times daily for type 1 diabetics and pregnant women taking insulin. It is important to recognize that the frequency and timing of blood glucose monitoring should be dictated by the patient and should be sufficient to reach blood glucose goals.

The ADA and the American Academy of Clinical Endocrinologists (AACE) have developed treatment target goals for diabetic patients (see Table 15.56).

Table 15.56 Treatment target goals for diabetic patients

Parameter	ADA	AACE
Hemoglobin A1c	<7%	<6.5%
Pre-meal blood glucose	70–130 mg/dL*	<110 mg/dL*
2-hour postprandial blood glucose	<180 mg/dL*	<140 mg/dL*

* Capillary plasma glucose.

Data from American Diabetes Association (2008). Standards of medical care in diabetes. *Diabetes Care* **31**:S12.

AACE Diabetes Mellitus Clinical Practice Guidelines Task Force (2007) AACE Consensus Statement for Glycemic Control. *Endocr Pract* **13**(Suppl 1):5.

Further reading

AACE Diabetes Mellitus Clinical Practice Guidelines Task Force (2007) AACE medical guidelines for clinical practice for the management of diabetes mellitus. *Endocr Pract* **13**(Suppl 1):3–68.

American Diabetes Association (2008) Standards of Medical Care in Diabetes. *Diabetes Care* **31**:S12–S54.

Contraception

Contraception has been an important part of human lives since the early Egyptian days. While methods have changed dramatically over the years, the purpose remains the same: to control fertility.

Most methods used today are female driven and involve hormones. These methods are very effective in preventing pregnancy when taken or used as directed. Barrier methods rely on their availability at the time of intercourse and are more efficacious when used with spermicides.

Factors that need to be considered when selecting a method of contraception include reliability of the patient, age of the patient, medical history, personal history, and reversibility of the agent.

Failure rates for methods include the *perfect rate*, when the method is used perfectly all of the time, and the *typical rate*, which is more consistent with normal use.

Female contraception

Hormonal methods

Oral contraceptive pills

- Combination (21-day, 84-day cycles, continuous)
- Progestin only (28-day cycle, norgestrel, norethindrone)
- Estrogens
  - Ethinyl estradiol, ≤35 mcg is considered low dose
  - Mestranol, ≤35 mcg is considered low dose
- Progestins create the differences between pills, having more androgenic effects, anti-androgenic effects, or progestational effects.
  - Levonorgestrel
  - Norgestrel
  - Norgestimate
  - Desogestrel
  - Norethindrone
  - Norethindrone acetate
  - Drosperinone
  - Ethynodiol diacetate
- Monophasic (same dose every day)
- Triphasic (3 different doses of progestin or estrogen over 21 days)
- The perfect-use failure rates for combined pills and the progestin-only pill are 0.1% and 0.5%, respectively.
- The typical failure rate is 5% for both pill types.
- If one pill is forgotten, take as soon as remembered. If 2 or tablets are missed in the first 2 weeks, 2 tablets should be taken for 2 days with a back-up method for 7 days. If 2 tablets are missed in the third week or more than 2 are missed at any time, a new pack should be started with a back-up method used for 1 week. Condoms along with spermicide are appropriate for a back-up method.

Transdermal

- Ortho Evra contains ethinyl estradiol and norelgestromin, a metabolite of norgestimate.

- The patch is changed weekly for 3 weeks, with the fourth week remaining hormone free.
- The failure rate is 1% for both perfect and typical use.
- Approximately 60% more estrogen is absorbed into the bloodstream than with traditional 35-mcg pills. This places women at higher risk for thrombosis and myocardial infarctions.
- The patch is less effective in women weighing ≥90 kg, and other methods should be considered.
- If a patch change is forgotten in the first week, the woman should change the patch-change day and use a back-up method for the first week of the new cycle. Patch changes forgotten in the second and third week do not need a back-up method as long as the duration was <48 hours. If it was >48 hours, the woman should restart the entire cycle and use a back-up method for the first week.

Transvaginal

- Nuvaring contains ethinyl estradiol and etonorgestrel, a metabolite of desogestrel.
- The ring remains in place for 3 weeks and is removed for the fourth. A new ring is used each month. It can be removed for up to 3 hours.
- Side effects include increased vaginal discharge, irritation, or infection.
- The perfect-use failure rate is <0.3%, and a 2% typical rate.
- The ring can be dislodged with bowel movements.
- If the ring is removed for more than 3 hours, a back-up method should be used for 7 days.

Intrauterine

- Mirena contains levonorgestrel and releases the equivalent of 3 progestin-only pills per week.
- The device may remain in place for 5 years.
- The failure rate is 0.1% for both perfect and typical use.

Injection

- Depo Provera is medroxyprogesterone, which is an intramuscular injection given every 3 months.
- The most common side effect is irregular bleeding, which can last 6–12 months.
- It has been associated with decreased bone mineral density (BMD). Cessation of therapy reverses this effect; however, BMD may not recover to pretreatment levels, especially with long-term therapy.
- The failure rate is 0.3% for both perfect and typical use.

Implantable

- Implanon is a single rod implant that also contains etonorgestrel. It has a 3-year duration.
- It requires a specially trained professional for placement.
- The failure rate is <0.1% for both perfect and typical use.

Contraindications for hormonal methods

- Thromboembolic disorders
- History of cerebral vascular accident
- Coronary artery or ischemic heart disease

- Known or suspected breast cancer
- Known or suspected estrogen-dependent neoplasm
- Benign or malignant liver tumor

Adverse effects of hormonal methods

- Nausea
- Breakthrough bleeding and spotting
- Headaches, including migraines
- Skin changes (chloasma, melasma, rash)
- Breast changes
- Depression
- Fluid retention
- Corneal curvature changes and dry eyes
- Exacerbation of gallbladder disease
- Thrombosis

Nonhormonal methods

Barrier methods

All barrier methods, except the condom and sponge, require fitting and a prescription.

- Female condoms
    - Made of polyurethane
    - Failure rates are 5% for perfect use and 21% for typical use.
- Diaphragm
    - Made of latex
    - Can cause urinary tract infections more often than other methods
    - The perfect-use failure rate is 6% and typical use failure rate is 20%.
- Cervical cap
    - Made of silicone
    - Failure rates depend on parity.
    - —Failure rates for nulliparous women are 9% and 20% for perfect and typical use, respectively.
    - —Failure rates for multiparous women are 26% and 40%.
- Lea's shield
    - Made of silicone
    - Failure rates for typical use are 9% for nulliparous women and 14% for multiparous women.
- Sponge
    - Made of polyurethane
    - Contains non-oxynol-9
    - Should not be used if a woman or her partner is allergic to sulfa drugs
    - Failure rates depend on parity.
    - —Nulliparous women have failure rates of 9% and 16% for perfect and typical use, respectively.
    - —Multiparous women have failure rates of 20% and 32%.

Spermicides

- Nonoxynol-9; the typical failure rate is 6% for perfect use and 26% for typical use.
    - Contraceptive foam
    - Contraceptive film

- Contraceptive suppositories
- Contraceptive gel
- Contraceptive jelly

High doses or prolonged exposure to nonoxynol-9 can increase the incidence of HIV transmission.

Intrauterine device

Copper T can be left in place for up to 10 years. Adverse effects include heavier menstrual periods and increased uterine cramping during menses. Failure rates are 0.6% and 0.8% for perfect and typical use, respectively.

Tubal occlusion

- Surgical methods, both failure rates are 0.5%
- Essure (transcervical sterilization), both failure rates are 0.2%

Male contraception

Condoms

- Failure rates are 3% and 14% for perfect and typical use, respectively.
  - Latex, breakage, or slippage rate 1.6%
  - Non-latex
    —Cannot stretch like latex
    —Higher breakage rate (4%)
    —Slightly higher failure rate
    —Still being studied for efficacy in preventing sexually transmitted diseases (STDs) and HIV
    —Lambskin condoms are only for contraception.

Vasectomy, surgical procedure

- Failure rate for perfect use is 0.1% and for typical use, 0.15%.

Emergency contraception

- Plan B (0.75 mg levonorgestrel tablet x2 doses)
- Yuzpe method (100 mcg ethinyl estradiol and 1 mg norgestrel or equivalent x 2 doses)
- These methods should be used within 72 hours of unprotected intercourse.

Further reading

Hatcher RA, Trussell J, Stewart FH, *et al. (2004). Contraceptive Technology*, 18th ed. New York: Ardent Media.
Planned Parenthood: www.plannedparenthood.org

Menopause

Menopause is the irreversible cessation of the female reproductive cycle and menses that follows a permanent loss of ovarian response to gonadotropins. It occurs spontaneously at the average age of 51; however, smokers will undergo menopause earlier since they metabolize estrogen more quickly.

Approximately 10 years prior to menopause follicular function is less predictable and menopausal symptoms may start to occur. After 1 year of amenorrhea, a woman is considered postmenopausal.

Symptoms

Vasomotor instability

- "Hot flash" or "hot flush"
- Caused by estrogen deficiency
- 75%–85% of women will experience this symptom
- May last for 1–2 years following menopause

Atrophic changes

- Vaginal atrophy
  - Vaginal burning or itching
  - Vaginal bleeding
  - Dyspareunia (painful intercourse)
- Local estrogen therapy is most effective to alleviate vaginal-atrophy symptoms.
- Atrophy of bladder and urethra

Menopausal syndrome

This is usually psychogenic, but consider organic possibilities such as
- Sleep disturbances
- Nocturnal vasomotor symptoms

Symptom management

Lifestyle changes

- Lower core body temperature
  - Dress in layers.
  - Use a fan.
  - Consume cold food and beverages.
- Exercise
- Stop smoking
- Relaxation techniques

Hormone therapy

- Used for the treatment of moderate–severe vasomotor symptoms with lowest dose possible and for treatment of vulvar and vaginal atrophy
- Reduces hot-flush incidence by 70%–90%
- Estrogens should not be used in women with a history of MI, cerebrovascular accident (CVA), or venous thromboembolism (VTE).

Side effects

- Breast tenderness
- Increased breast density
- Bloating
- Headaches
- Increased risk of gallstones
- Bleeding

Other risks

- Endometrial cancer with unopposed estrogen
- Breast cancer (absolute risk is low, estrogen plus progestin appears to increase risk over estrogen alone; consider alternatives in breast cancer survivors)
- Cardiovascular risk—hormone therapy does not increase risks if started close to menopause (within 10 years)
- Thrombosis—risk increases two-fold with hormones, risk is greatest in first year of therapy
- Dementia—initiation in older women seems to increase risk

Nonhormonal therapy

Antidepressants

- Venlafaxine
  - Initial dose: 37.5 mg daily, may increase to 75 mg daily (doses above 75 mg daily have not shown increased efficacy, but had more adverse effects)
  - 61% reduction in hot-flash score vs. 27% for the placebo group
- Paroxetine controlled release (CR)
  - Initial dose: 12.5 mg daily
  - 50%–51% reduction in hot-flash episodes per day vs. 16% reduction with placebo
- Fluoxetine
  - Initial dose: 20 mg daily
  - 50% decrease in hot-flash score compared with 36% for placebo

Gabapentin

- Intial dose 300 mg tid (reduce dose for renal insufficiency)
- 45% reduction in hot-flash frequency vs. 29% for placebo

Clonidine

- Initial dose: 0.05 mg bid or 0.1 mg/day transdermal
- Oral therapy: 37% reduction in hot-flash frequency over placebo (20%)
- Transdermal: 80% reduction in hot-flash frequency (vs. 36% placebo), 73% reduction in severity over 29% with placebo

Methyldopa

- Initial dose: 250 mg bid
- Improvement in frequency (reduction) and visual analog score over placebo

Alternative therapy

- Soy isoflavones have not been shown to be beneficial over placebo in relief of vasomotor symptoms. No safety data exist for use in women with breast cancer.
- Red clover isoflavone (Promensil®) (flavonoids and coumarins) shows a slight reduction in frequency of hot flashes over placebo in some studies. A meta-analysis did not show any benefits of use. Long-term safety data are unavailable.
- In small studies black Cohosh has been shown to be more effective than placebo in women with mild to moderate vasomotor symptoms. Use beyond 6 months has not been studied.

Further reading

Mayoclinic.com: www.mayoclinic.com/health/menopause

National Institutes of Health, Menopausal Hormone Therapy Information: www.nih.gov/PHTindex.htm

North American Menopausal Society (NAMS): www.menopause.org. See their July 2008 position statement.

Obesity

Obesity is a growing health-care issue in developed countries throughout the world. Currently, two-thirds of Americans are classified as overweight or obese. The rate of obesity has increased significantly over the past four decades.

Obesity worsens outcomes, including mortality, in a number of disease states—hypertension, cardiovascular disease, dyslipidemia, type 2 diabetes, osteoarthritis, respiratory conditions, obstructive sleep apnea, and many malignancies (colon, esophageal, breast, uterine, ovarian, kidney, and pancreatic).

Obesity increases the risk of all-cause mortality and is a major cause of preventable death in the United States.

Background

Body mass index (BMI) = Weight (kg)/[Height (meters)]^2

- Normal-weight BMI: 18.5–24.9 kg/m^2
- Overweight BMI: 25–29.9 kg/m^2
- Obese BMI: 30–39.9 kg/m^2
- Extremely obese BMI: > 40 kg/m^2

Patient evaluation

- BMI
- Waist circumference
- Assessment of comorbidities
- Medication review
- Previous weight loss strategies
- Exercise
- Motivation
- Goal is weight loss
- Weight-loss readiness

Weight loss benefits

- Decreased BP, total cholesterol, low-density lipoprotein (LDL), triglycerides, and plasma glucose in patients with type 2 diabetes
- Increased high-density lipoprotein (HDL) and self-esteem

Treatment strategies

Lifestyle modifications

- Dietary changes
  - Involve a dietician to develop a healthy, balanced diet.
  - Weight loss = calories burned > calories ingested.
  - Decreasing total daily caloric intake by 500–1000 kcal results in loss of 1–2 lbs (or approx. 0.5–1 kg) per week.
- Diet options
  - Meal replacements (e.g., SlimFast)
  - Low fat: 7%–30% of total daily kcal
  - Low carbohydrate: <60 g per day (e.g., Adkins, South Beach)

- Low glycemic index: rates foods by how much they increase plasma glucose 2 hours post-consumption
- High protein

Exercise

- Encourage 30 minutes most days of the week
- Results in modest weight reduction without calorie restriction
- Increases HDL
- Decreases blood pressure, triglycerides, and insulin resistance
- Improves body composition (muscle tissue vs. adipose tissue)

Behavioral therapy

- Set weight-loss goals
- Self-monitoring of diet and exercise
- Relapse prevention

Pharmacologic treatment options

Criteria for use

- BMI >30 kg/m^2 or >27 kg/m^2 with existing comorbidities
- Comorbidities: hypertension, dyslipidemia, cardiovascular disease, type 2 diabetes, and obstructive sleep apnea
- Combine with lifestyle modifications

FDA-approved agents for weight loss (see Table 15.57)

- Result in 2%–5% weight loss when combined with lifestyle modifications
- Some abuse potential for diethylpropion and phentermine (Schedule IV)

Herbal products for weight loss

- Multiple products are available: bitter orange, chitosan, chromium, conjugate linoleic acid, fiber, guar gum, green tea, guarana, hoodia, hyroxycitric acid, L-carnitine, natural licorice, usnic acid, white kidney bean extract, willow bark, and yohimbine
- Little scientific evidence to prove efficacy
- Serious safety concerns: elevations in blood pressure, heart rate, and liver failure

Surgical treatment options (see Table 15.58)

Indications

- BMI >40kg/m^2 or >35 kg/m^2 with comorbidities (listed above)
- Failed lifestyle and pharmacological interventions

Table 15.57 FDA-approved agents for weight loss

Generic name	Class	Dose	Mechanism of action	Patient counseling
Diethylpropion	Appetite suppressant	IR: 25 mg tid CR: 75 mg daily	Sympathomimetic	Increases blood pressure and heart rate; insomnia
Phentermine HCl, resin	Appetite suppressant	HCl salt: 18.75–37.5 mg daily Resin: 15–30 mg daily	Sympathomimetic	Increases blood pressure and heart rate; insomnia
Sibutramine	Appetite suppressant	5–15 mg daily	5-HT, NE, DA reuptake inhibitor	Increases blood pressure and heart rate, may interact with other antidepressants
Orlistat	Triglyceride absorption inhibitor	Rx: 120 mg tid OTC: 60 mg tid	Decreases triglyceride absorption by inhibiting triacylglycerol lipase	Omit dose if meal skipped or fat free; flatus, fecal discharge and urgency, and oily stools; consider MVI

CR, controlled release; DA, dopamine; HCl, hydrochloride; IR, immediate release; MVI, multivitamin; NE, norepinephrine, OTC, over-the-counter; Rx, prescription; 5-HT, serotonin.

Data from: Eckel, R (2008). Clinical practice. Nonsurgical management of obesity in adults. N Engl J Med 358(18):1941–1950.

Table 15.58 Surgical treatment options

Procedure	Type	Long-term complications
Adjustable gastric banding	Restrictive	Nausea and vomiting
Gastroplasty	Restrictive	Nausea and vomiting
Vertical restrictive gastrectomy	Restrictive	Nausea and vomiting
Roux-en-Y gastric bypass	Malabsorptive and restrictive	Nausea and vomiting; dumping syndrome; B_{12}, calcium, copper, folate, iron, vitamin E, and thiamine deficiencies
Biliopancreatic diversion with duodenal switch	Malabsorptive	Protein malnutrition, fat-soluble vitamin malabsorption, and magnesium and zinc deficiencies

Data from:

DeMaria EJ (2007). Bariatric surgery for morbid obesity. *N Engl J Med* **356**:2176–2183.

Malone M (2008). Recommended nutritional supplements for bariatric surgery patients. *Ann Pharmacother* **42**:1851–1858.

Griffith DP, Liff DA, Ziegler TR, Esper GJ, Winton EF (2009). Acquired copper deficiency: a potentially serious and preventable complication following gastric bypass surgery. *Obesity* **17**:827–831

Further reading

DeMaria EJ (2007). Bariatric surgery for morbid obesity. *N Engl J Med* **356**:2176–2183.

Eckels RH (2008). Nonsurgical management of obesity in adults. *N Engl J Med* **358**:1941–1950.

National Institutes of Health. Clinical guidelines for the identification, evaluation, and treatment of oberweight and obesity in adults: the evidence report (1998). nhlbi.nih.gov/guidelines/obesity/ob_home.htm

Osteoporosis

At least 10 million people in the United States who are over age 50 have osteoporosis, and another 34 million are at risk. Women are four times more likely than men to have the disease. However, approximately 25% of men over the age of 50 will have a fracture related to osteoporosis.

Once one fracture occurs, the person is at higher risk for another. It is a significant cause of morbidity and mortality, and complications cost more than $20 billion each year.

Bone

Bone types

- Trabecular bone comprises the ends of long bone shafts and vertebrae.
- Cortical bone creates the remaining bone.

Bone remodeling

- Osteoclasts break down bone.
- Osteoblasts create new bone.

Types of osteoporosis

- Type I: loss of estrogen, affects trabecular more then cortical bone
- Type II: aging, affects trabecular and cortical bone the same
- Type III: drug therapy

Risk factors

Nonmodifiable

- Older age
- Female gender
- Asian or Caucasian heritage
- Small frame
- Low BMI
- Menopausal status
- Family history of osteoporosis

Modifiable

- Low activity level
- Estrogen deficiency
- Low testosterone
- Smoking
- Excessive alcohol intake (>7 drinks/week)

Various disease states

- Hyperthryoidism
- Hyperparathyroidism
- Cushing's syndrome
- Multiple myeloma
- Leukemia and lymphoma
- Chronic renal failure
- Gastrectomy
- Hepatobiliary disease
- Pancreatic insufficiency

Various medications

- Corticosteroids
- Heparin
- Anticonvulsant therapy
- Medroxyprogesterone
- GNRH agonists
- Chemotherapy
- Aromatase inhibitors

Diagnosis

- Thorough assessment of risk factors
- Presence of signs and symptoms of osteoporosis (occurrence of fragility fracture)
- Measure of bone mineral density (BMD)
- Dual X-ray absorptiometry (DXA) is the gold-standard test for diagnosing those without an osteoporotic fracture.
  - T-score represents a patient's bone mass in terms of standard deviations from average peak bone mass in normal healthy persons.
    —T-score 0 to −1: within normal range
    —T-score between −1 and −2.5: low bone mass (osteopenia)
    —T-score −2.5 or less: osteoporosis
  - BMD T-scores have traditionally been used to guide treatment.

BMD testing

- All women over 65
- All men over age 70
- Postmenopausal women 60–64 years of age with at least 1 risk factor
- Men 50–70 years of age with at least 1 risk factor
- Men and women over age 50 with a fracture
- Anyone on osteoporosis medications
- BMD testing should not be repeated more frequently than every 2 years.

Nonpharmacologic therapy

- Weight-bearing exercise (e.g., walking, running)
- Fall prevention

Drug therapy

Calcium and vitamin D

- Calcium dose: 1000–1500 mg/day (depending on age and menopausal status)
- Vitamin D dose: 800–1000 IU/day

Bisphosphonates (see Table 15.59)

- First-line therapy for postmenopausal osteoporosis (unless contraindicated, e.g., severe renal insufficiency)
- Inhibit bone resorption.
- Increase BMD at the spine and hip in early and late postmenopausal women
- Reduce risk of fracture at vertebral and nonvertebral sites
- Should be given with calcium and vitamin D supplements

Table 15.59 Bisphosphonates available for treatment and prophylaxis of postmenopausal osteoporosis

Bisphosphonate	Formulation	Treatment dosing	Prophylaxis dosing
Alendronate (Fosamax)*	PO	10 mg once daily 70 mg once weekly	5 mg once daily 35 mg once weekly
Risedronate (Actonel)*	PO	5 mg once daily 35 mg once weekly 75 mg once daily for 2 days, monthly	5 mg once daily 35 mg once weekly 75 mg once daily for 2 days, monthly
Ibandronate (Boniva)*	PO	2.5 mg once daily 150 mg once monthly	2.5 mg once daily 150 mg once monthly
	IV	3 mg IV every 3 months	NA
Zoledronic acid (Reclast)†	IV	5 mg IV every year	NA

*Do not use in patients with CrCl<30 mL/min.

†Do not use in patients with CrCl <35 mL/min.

- Tablets should be taken in the morning with a full glass of water (6–8 ounces) at least 30 minutes before food or liquids. Patients need to remain upright for at least 30–60 minutes after taking oral bisphosphonates.
- Infusions may be preferred for indivduals who are unable to sit upright for 30–60 minuts or have poor adherence.
- Infusions should be given over at least 15 minutes.
- Bisphosphates are not recommended in patients with renal insufficiency (CrCl <30 mL/min [alendronate, risedronate, ibandronate], CrCl <35 mL/min [zoledronic acid]).
- Adverse effects: gastrointestinal events, jaw osteonecrosis

Raloxifene

- Estrogen agonist/antagonist
- Improves BMD in the spine and femoral neck
- Reduces risk of vertebral fracture
- Useful in individuals with low bone mass, younger postmenopausal women with hip fracture risk, or for breast cancer prevention
- Dose for treatment or prophylaxis: 60 mg PO daily
- Should be given with calcium and vitamin D supplementation
- Adverse effects: hot flushes, thromboembolic events, mild cardiac events

Calcitonin

- Inhibits bone resorption
- Helps maintain normal calcium levels in serum and increases mineral stores in bone

- Useful for reduction of vertebral bone pain
- Available in an injectable and intranasal formulations
- Use with caution in those with hypersensitivity to calcitonin-salmon
- Dose for treatment: 100 units IM or SC every other day; 200 units (1 spray) intranasally each day (alternating nostrils)
- Adverse effects: flushing, nausea and vomiting

Teriparatide

- Stimulates bone production
- Increases gastric calcium absorption and renal calcium reabsorption
- Increases BMD in the spine and femoral neck
- Prevents vertebral factures and possibly nonvertebral fractures
- Dose for treatment: 20 mcg SC daily; use >2 years is not recommended
- Concomittant use with bisphosphonates is not recommended.
- Adverse effects: hypotension, hyperuricemia, angina

Hormone therapy

- Increases bone production and decreases resorption
- Decreases incidence of vertebral, nonvertebral, and hip fracture
- Adverse effects: thromboembolic events (i.e., cerebrovascular accident, stroke)

Drug use in special populations

- Low-risk: raloxifene and vitamin D reduce risk for vertebral fracture
- Men: risedronate reduces hip fractures, calcitonin decreases vertebral fractures, teriparitide decreases total fractures and possibly vertebral fractures
- Previous hip fracture: zoledonic acid decreases vertebral and nonvertebral fractures
- Long-term glucocorticoid use: risedronate and alendronate reduce clinical and radiographic fracture rate

Combination therapy

Data are insufficient to support routine use of combination therapy. Various combinations have shown increased BMD over either agent alone; however, efficacy for reducing fractures is unknown.

Further reading

MayoClinic.com: www.mayoclinic.com/health/osteoporosis

National Osteoporosis Foundation: www.nof.org

NIH National Resource Center : www.niams.nih.gov/Health-Info/Bone/

Qaseem A, Snow V, Shekelle P, et al. (2008). Pharmacologic treatment of low bone density or osteoporosis to prevent fractures: A clinical practice guideline from the American College of Physicians. *Ann Intern Med* **149**:404–415.

Thyroid disorders

Thyroid hormones, thyroxine (T4) and triiodothyronine (T3), are responsible for metabolic actions throughout the body. Triiodothyronine is five times more active in the body than T4. Thyroxine is primarily secreted by the thyroid gland, whereas the majority of T3 is produced via peripheral conversion of T4 to T3.

Thyroid disorders affect 5%–15% of the population, with the majority of those being women. The most common disorders in the United States are Hashimoto's disease (hypothyroidism) and Graves' disease (hyperthyroidism). Changes in thyroid function alter metabolic actions throughout the body and manifest as a constellation of systemic symptoms.

Hypothyroidism

Hypothyroidism is decreased thyroid hormone production or secretion.

Etiologies

Primary hypothyroidism

- Hashimoto's disease
- Thyroidectomy
- Thyroid ablation with radioactive iodine
- Irradiation
- Thyroid tumor
- Medications (e.g., amiodarone, interferon, interleukin-2, lithium)

Secondary hypothyroidism

- Pituitary dysfunction
- Hypothalamic dysfunction

Signs and symptoms

See Table 15.60.

Laboratory findings and monitoring

- Thyroid-stimulating hormone (TSH) is the most sensitive
- Check thyroid function tests (TFTs) ≥6 weeks after adjustment to levothyroxine dose or brand
- Check TFTs 6 months after dose stabilization and annually thereafter

Pharmacological treatment strategies

- Levothyroxine (T4) is the drug of choice
    - 1.6 mcg/kg/day
    - Start at 25 mcg/day in the elderly and in patients with cardiovascular disease
- Thyroid hormone USP
- Liothyronine (T3)
- Liotrix (T4:T3)

Drug interactions

- Impaired absorption
- Bivalent and trivalent cations (calcium, magnesium, aluminum, and iron)
- Cholestyramine
- Sucralfate

Table 15.60 Signs and symptoms of hypothyroidism and hyperthyroidism

Hypothyroidism	Hyperthyroidism
Weight gain	Weight loss
Fatigue	Fatigue
Cold intolerance	Heat intolerance
Goiter	Enlarged thyroid
Dry skin	Moist skin
Delayed relaxation phase of reflexes	Brisk reflexes
Constipation	Diarrhea
Difficulty concentrating	Mental disturbances
Depression	Nervousness, anxiety
Menorrhagia	Amenorrhea
Myalgias	Muscle weakness
Bradycardia	Tachycardia
Myxedema	Pretibial myxedema
Other symptoms	
Hoarse voice	Exophthalmopathy
Ataxia	Insomnia
Dyslipidemia	Tremor
Hypothermia	Periorbital edema
	Acropachy

Data from: American Association of Clinical Endocrinologists medical guidelines for clinical practice for the evaluation and treatment of hyperthyroidism and hypothyroidism. (2002). *Endocr Practice* **8**:457–469.

Talbert RL (2005). Thyroid disorders. In: DiPiro JT, Talbert RL, Yee GC. eds. *Pharmacotherapy: A Pathophyisologic Approach*, 6th ed. New York: McGraw-Hill.

- Enzyme induction
- Seizure medications (carbamazepine, phenobarbital, phenytoin)
- Rifampin

Subclinical hypothyroidism

- Mildly increased TSH with normal free T4 and T3
- Common in elderly women
- May require treatment if TSH >10 μLU/mL or TSH between 5 and 10 μLU/mL with concurrent goiter or positive antithyroid antibodies

Myxedema coma

- Life-threatening emergency

Signs and symptoms
- Hypothermia
- Altered mental status

Treatment
- High-dose IV levothyroxine (up to 500 mcg)
- Supportive care

Hyperthyroidism

Hyperthyroidism is increased thyroid hormone production or secretion.

Etiologies

Primary hyperthyroidism
- Graves' disease
- Toxic adenoma
- Toxic multinodular goiter
- Thyroiditis
- Medications (e.g., thyroid hormone, excess iodine, amiodarone)

Secondary hypothyroidism
- Excess TSH production by pituitary

Signs and symptoms (see Table 15.60)

Need at least one of the following to diagnose Graves' disease:
- Hyperthyroidism
- Exophthalmopathy
- Dermopathy (pretibial edema)
- Acropachy (thickening of fingers and toes)

Laboratory findings and monitoring
- TSH is the most sensitive test
- Check TFTs 4–6 weeks after treatment initiation
- Check TFTs every 3–6 months once patient is euthyroid (see Table 15.61)

Pharmacologic treatment strategies (see Table 15.62)

Serious adverse events

Do not challenge with another antithyroid agent.
- Agranulocytosis (absolute granulocyte count <500 cells/m^3)
- Aplastic anemia
- Hepatotoxicity
- Vasculitis

Minor adverse events
- Arthralgias
- Rash
- Fever
- Transient leukopenia (absolute granulocyte count <1500 cells/m^3)

Adjunctive agents
- Nonselective beta-blockers (e.g., propranolol)
- Non-dihydropyridine calcium-channel blockers (diltiazem and verapamil)

Table 15.61 Laboratory findings of hypothyroidism and hyperthyroidism

Laboratory	Hypothyroidism (Hashimoto's disease)	Hyperthyroidism (Graves' disease)
TSH	↑	↓
Free T4	↓	↑
T3	↓	↑
Thyroid autoantibodies (thyroid peroxidase and thyroglobulin)	Positive	Positive
Radioactive iodine uptake	Nondiagnostic	↑

Data from:

Baskin HJ, Cobin RH, Duick DS, et al. (2002). American Association of Clinical Endocrinologists medical guidelines for clinical practice for the evaluation and treatment of hyperthyroidism and hypothyroidism. *Endocr Pract* **8**:457–469.

Pearce EN, Farwell AP, Braverman LE (2003). Thyroiditis. *N Engl J Med* **348**:2646–2655.

Talbert RL (2005). Thyroid disorders.In: DiPiro JT, Talbert RL, Yee GC, eds. *Pharmacotherapy: A Pathophyisologic Approach*, 6th ed. New York: McGraw-Hill.

Table 15.62 Antithyroid agents

Name	Mechanism of action	Dose	T1/2 (hours)	Special considerations
Propylthiouracil	Inhibits organification of iodides and coupling of monoiodotyrosine (MIT) and diiodotyrosine (DIT). Blocks peripheral conversion of T4 to T3	300–600 mg/day; divided every 6–8 hours. Max dose is 1200 mg/day	2.5	Preferred in pregnancy and thyroid storm
Methimazole	Inhibits organification of iodides and coupling of MIT and DIT	5–60 mg/day. Max dose is 120 mg/day	6–9	Crosses placenta and enters breast milk

Data from:

Cooper DS (2005). Antithyroid drugs. *N Engl J Med* **352**:905–917.

Baskin HJ, Cobin RH, Duick DS, et al. (2002). American Association of Clinical Endocrinologists medical guidelines for clinical practice for the evaluation and treatment of hyperthyroidism and hypothyroidism. *Endocr Pract* **8**:457–469.

Talbert RL (2005). Thyroid disorders. In: DiPiro JT, Talbert RL, Yee GC, eds. *Pharmacotherapy: A Pathophyisologic Approach*, 6th ed. New York: McGraw-Hill.

Radioactive iodine (I^{131})

- Treatment of choice for Graves' disease
- Slow onset of action; it does not impact circulating thyroid hormone
- May be used initially combined with antithyroid drugs and adjunct agents
- Contraindications: pregnant or lactating women
- May result in hypothyroidism requiring levothyroxine

Surgical intervention (thyroidectomy)

- Not commonly performed
- May be an option for pediatric patients, patients with large goiters, those who cannot tolerate antithyroid medications, etc.

Subclinical hyperthyroidism

- Decreased TSH (<0.1 μLU/mL) with normal free T4 and T3
- Less common than subclinical hypothyroidism
- May require treatment to avoid progression to hyperthyroidism, development of osteoporosis, or atrial fibrillation

Thyroid storm

- Life-threatening emergency

Signs and symptoms

- High fever (>103°F), tachycardia, tachypnea, hypovolemia, delirium, nausea, vomiting, and diarrhea

Treatment

- Propylthiouracil (PTU)
- Supportive care
- Adjunctive agents (nonselective beta-blockers, steroids)

Further reading

Baskin HJ, Cobin RH, Duick DS, et al. (2002). American Association of Clinical Endocrinologists medical guidelines for clinical practice for the evaluation and treatment of hyperthyroidism and hypothyroidism. *Endocr Pract* **8**:457–469.
Cooper DS (2005). Antithyroid drugs. *N Engl J Med* **352**:905–917.
Pearce EN, Farwell AP, Braverman LE (2003). Thyroiditis. *N Engl J Med* **348**:2646–2655.

Constipation in adults

Description and causes of constipation in adults

Constipation is defined as a symptom-based disorder with unsatisfactory defecation and is characterized by infrequent stools, difficult stool passage, or both.

A person may complain of the following:

- Prolonged time to stool
- Straining
- Sense of difficulty passing stool
- Hard or lumpy stools
- Sense of incomplete evacuation
- Need for manual maneuvers to pass stool

Chronic constipation is defined as the presence of symptoms for at least 3 months. Constipation subgroups include functional constipation (normal transit), slow-transit constipation, and pelvic floor dysfunction.

Causes of constipation include metabolic, endocrine, neurological, muscular, psychological, and gastrointestinal (GI) disorders, e.g., inflammatory bowel disease (IBD), irritable bowel syndrome, and intestinal obstruction.

Patients with alarm symptoms (e.g., hematochezia, weight loss ≥10 pounds, family history of colon cancer, IBD, anemia, positive fecal occult blood test, and acute onset of symptoms in elderly adults) should be evaluated by a physician. One of the most common causes of constipation is a low-residue diet. Constipation is also a side effect of many commonly used drugs.

Some medications commonly causing constipation

- Analgesics (e.g., opioids, NSAIDs)
- Antacids (e.g., aluminum, calcium, and bismuth containing)
- Anticholinergic agents (e.g., tricyclic antidepressants, antihistamines, antipsychotics and antispasmodics, antiparkinsonian agents)
- Antihypertensives (e.g., verapamil, clonidine, beta-blockers, ACE inhibitors)
- Antimotility agents (e.g., diphenoxylate, loperamide)
- Barium
- Iron preparations
- Psychotherapeutic agents (e.g., clozapine, olanzapine, risperidone, and quetiapine)
- Sodium polystyrene sulfonate
- Vinca alkaloids

Changing or stopping these drugs might be all that is required to restore normal bowel function.

Most of the factors predisposing to constipation are potentially magnified or compounded in the older patient. In this group, prolonged constipation can lead to fecal impaction, causing urinary and fecal overflow incontinence. It is an avoidable cause of hospital admission.

Treatment of constipation in adults

Treatment should be initiated when the patient and health-care professional feel the symptoms diminish the patient's quality of life. Especially if ambulatory and otherwise healthy, patients should be encouraged to regulate their bowel activity by attention to diet and exercise. The diet should contain adequate amounts of fiber and fluid. Physical exercise has been shown to decrease intestinal transit time and is believed to stimulate regular bowel movements.

If these measures are ineffective, intermittent or regular use of a laxative may be necessary (see Table 15.63). The duration of treatment with laxatives should be limited to the shortest time possible. The undesirability of long-term laxative use should be explained to the patient.

Diet

The major lifestyle factor leading to constipation is inadequate dietary fiber intake. Dietary fiber consists of plant complex carbohydrates that escape digestion in the small intestine and are only partly broken down by bacterial enzymes in the large intestine. The ingestion of dietary fiber increases stool bulk by increasing both solid residue and stool water content. This results in decreased intestinal transit time and decreased water absorption in the large bowel.

The recommended amount of dietary fiber is 20–35 g/day. The fiber content of the diet should be built up gradually to avoid adverse effects, such as bloating or flatulence.

Patients should be encouraged to choose a wide variety of fiber sources, both insoluble (e.g., whole grain breads, prunes, raisins) and soluble (e.g., beans, oat bran, barley, peas, carrots, citrus fruits, apples), rather than adding a few very high–fiber foods (e.g., unprocessed bran) to the diet. Adequate fluid intake, especially water, is encouraged.

Drug therapy

First-line therapy

If dietary management is not sufficient, oral bulk-forming agents are the laxatives of choice for mildly constipated individuals. Provided good fluid intake is maintained, use the following agents:

- Psyllium increases stool frequency. Side effects include flatulence, abdominal cramping, esophageal and colonic mechanical obstruction, and anaphylactic reactions. It should be separated from other medications by 2 hours.
- While calcium polycarbophil and methylcellulose products are available, insufficient data exist for the guidelines to recommend their use. Some products are sugar free.

Second-line therapy

Osmotic laxatives include PEG 3350, lactulose, and saline preparations. These agents increase stool frequency and stool consistency.

- Lactulose syrup contains the nonabsorbable sugars galactose and lactose but it should be used with caution in patients with diabetes mellitus and is contraindicated in galactosemia. Side effects include nausea, abdominal pain, and flatulence.

Table 15.63 Laxative choice in adults

Constituent(s), form, and preparation	Dose (adult dose, unless otherwise specified)	Time to onset
Note: it is recommended that bulk-forming agents be taken with adequate fluid (at least 8 oz).		
Bulk-forming laxatives		
Psyllium (Metamucil®, Fiberall®)	>12 years old: 2–6 capsules up to three times a day 3.5 g (1 rounded teaspoonful) up to three times daily	12–72 hours
Methylcellulose (Citrucel®)	1 heaping tablespoonful up to three times daily 2–4 caplets up to three times daily	12–72 hours
Calcium Polycarbophil (Fibercon®)	2 tablets up to four times daily	12–72 hours
Osmotic laxatives		
Lactulose syrup	15–30 mL daily, in one or two doses initially	1–2 days
Magnesium hydroxide	Drink a full glass of water following dose. Concentrate: 10–20 mL daily or divided doses Liquid: 30–60 mL daily or divided doses Tablets: 6–8 tablets at bedtime	0.5–6 hours
Polyethylene glycol 3350 powder (MiraLax®)	17 g in 8 oz of water	2–4 days
Phosphate enemas	See product information	2–5 minutes
Stool-softening axatives		
Docusate	100–300 mg daily, in one or divided doses	12–72 hours

Table 15.63 *(Contd.)*

Constituent(s), form, and preparation	Dose (adult dose, unless otherwise specified)	Time to onset
Stimulant laxatives		
Bisacodyl, 5 mg tablets	1–3 tablets daily (up to 6 tablets if complete evacuation is required)	6–12 hours
Bisacodyl, 10 mg suppositories	1 suppository daily (retain for 15–20 minutes)	15–60 minutes
Senna (Senokot®, various)	Tablets: 8.6–34.4 mg sennosides daily	6–12 hours
	Granules: 15–30 mg sennosides daily	
	Concentrate: see product	
Docusate/senna (opioid-induced constipation)	1–4 capsules daily, see product	6–12 hours
Lubricant laxatives		
Glycerol/glycerin suppositories	1 suppository, as required	15–30 minutes
Mineral oil emulsion	10–45 mL at night	6–8 hours
Miscellanous preparations		
Lubiprostone	24 mcg twice daily	1–7 days
Methylnaltrexone	8 mg (for 84 to <136 lb) SC every other day 12 mg (136–251 lb) SC every other day	10 minutes

- PEG solution increases stool frequency and consistency and minimizes straining. Side effects include diarrhea, nausea, abdominal bloating, cramping, and flatulence.
- Saline preparations include magnesium citrate, magnesium hydroxide, sodium phosphate, and sodium biphosphate. Electrolyte disturbances have been reported with these agents. Saline laxatives can interact with some medications and are contraindicated in congestive heart failure. Magnesium salts should be used with caution in patients with impaired renal function, and pregnant women should use only on the advice of their physician.

Other agents include the following:

- Stimulant laxatives—oral senna and bisacodyl. These are used prior to radiological and endoscopic procedures and in the treatment of opioid-induced constipation. Side effects include severe cramping, electrolyte and fluid losses, and malabsorption. Prolonged use of senna is associated with melanosis coli and may turn urine pink to red. Bisacodyl is also associated with metabolic acidosis or alkalosis, hypocalcemia, and tetany. When taken with proton pump inhibitors (PPIs), histamine-2 receptor antagonists (H_2Ras), or antacids, gastric or duodenal irritation may result.
- Lubiprostone improves stool frequency, consistency, and straining. Side effects include nausea, diarrhea, headache, abdominal pain, and flatulence.
- Although stool-softening agents, such as docusate salts, are often used in the treatment of constipation, they have limited effectiveness as monotherapy.

Third-line therapy

If constipation is resistant to first- and second-line measures, re-evaluate the underlying cause(s), including impaction. And, if required, consider the following regimens:

- Glycerin suppository rectally (allow to remain for 15–30 minutes)
- Biscacodyl suppository
- Phosphate enema rectally
- Mineral oil orally. It should not be used in children under the age of 6 and should not be administered to the very old or debilitated due to the risk of aspiration. It can cause a deficiency of fat-soluble vitamins.

Fourth-line therapy

In a minority of patients drug-therapy measures are unsuccessful and manual evacuation, biofeedback, or surgery for functionally significant obstructive defecation may be required.

Opioid-induced constipation

When an opioid is first prescribed a stimulant such as senna should be added as a prophylactic measure. It may be combined with a stool softener.

If the patient is already constipated, considerations can include increasing the dosage of the stimulant or adding an osmotic laxative orally or rectally. For refractory constipation, subcutaneous methylnaltrexone may be considered (see Motility Stimulants, p. 406).

Further reading

Bleser S, Bruton S, Carmichael B (2005). Management of chronic constipation: recommendations from a consensus panel. *J Fam Pract* **54**(8):691–698.

Brandt LJ, Prather CM, Quigley EMM, Schiller LR, Schoenfeld P, Talley NJ (2005). Systematic review on the management of chronic constipation in North America. *Am J Gastroenterol* **100**:(Suppl 1):S5–S21.

Locke GR, Pemberton JH, Phillips SF (2000). American Gastroenerological Association Medical Position Statement: Guidelines on constipation. *Gastroenterology* **119**(6):1761–1778.

Ternent CA, Bastawrous AL, Morin NA, Ellis CN, Hyman NH, Buie D, and the Standards Task Force of the American Society of Colon and Rectal Surgeons (2007). Practice parameters for the evaluation and management of constipation. *Dis Colon Rectum* **50**:2013–2022.

Diarrhea

Description and causes

Diarrhea is a term generally understood to mean an increased frequency or liquidity of bowel movements relative to normal for an individual patient. The normal frequency of bowel movements varies in healthy adults, with a range between two bowel movements a week and three bowel movements a day considered normal.

The mechanisms that result in diarrhea are varied and include secretion or decreased absorption of fluid and electrolytes by cells of the intestinal mucosa and exudation resulting from inflammation of the intestinal mucosa.

Diarrhea is a nonspecific symptom that is a manifestation of a wide range of GI disorders, including inflammatory bowel disease, irritable bowel syndrome, GI malignancy, a variety of malabsorption syndromes, and acute or subacute intestinal bacterial, protozoal, or viral infections.

Diarrhea can be an unwanted effect of enteral nutrition and of almost any drug, particularly those listed below.

Medications commonly causing diarrhea

- Acarbose, miglitol, and metformin
- Alzheimer's disease acetylcholinesterase inhibitors
- Antibiotics: clindamycin, erythromycin, ampicillin, amoxicillin/clavulanate, cefuroxime
- Cholinergic drugs, e.g., bethanechol
- Colchicine
- Cytotoxic agents
- Food, drinks (including alcohol and caffeine), and drug additives
- Laxatives (including surreptitious use)
- Lubiprostone
- Magnesium-containing antacids
- Misoprostol
- NSAIDs
- Orlistat
- Protease inhibitors
- Sorbitol, mannitol, fructose and lactose (lactose intolerance)

All patients presenting with diarrhea should be questioned about the relationship between symptoms and changes in medications or diet. If an underlying cause of diarrhea can be identified, management is directed at that cause rather than at the symptom of diarrhea.

Treatment

Chronic diarrhea

The treatment of chronic diarrhea depends on controlling the underlying disease. Symptomatic management may be used as initial treatment before diagnostic testing, after diagnostic testing has failed to confirm a diagnosis, or when specific treatment of the underlying cause does not cure the problem.

Acute diarrhea

Fluid and electrolyte therapy

Oral replacement solutions are the preferred treatment for mild to moderate diarrhea in children and moderate diarrhea in adults. Even in the presence of diarrhea, water and salt continue to be absorbed by active glucose-enhanced sodium absorption in the small intestine.

Oral replacement solutions are effective if they contain balanced quantities of sodium, potassium, glucose, and water. Glucose is necessary to promote electrolyte absorption. In cases of severe dehydration, intravenous fluids such as lactated ringers should be considered.

Proprietary soft drinks and fruit juices might be inadequate treatment for individuals in whom dehydration poses a significant risk, e.g., the elderly and patients with renal disease.

In adults, an oral rehydration solution should be considered for patients with mild to moderate dehydration, e.g., loss <9% of body weight. Solutions should be made up freshly according to manufacturers' recommendations, refrigerated, and replaced every 24 hours.

Several proprietary rehydration products are available and should be made up according to brand recommendations. The WHO-recommended range of concentrations for rehydration solutions are as follows:

- Sodium: 60–90 mmol/L
- Chloride: 50–80 mmol/L
- Potassium: 15–25 mmol/L
- Citrate: 8–12 mmol/L
- Glucose should at least equal to sodium but not exceed 111 mmol/L.

For adults, encourage 1.5 to 2 times the estimated deficit plus concurrent losses. Generally at least 1/2 of the calculated deficit is replaced in the first 4 hours with the rest given over 20 hours.

Once rehydration is complete, further dehydration is prevented by encouraging the patient to drink normal volumes of an appropriate fluid and by replacing continuing losses with an oral rehydration product.

Drug therapy

Antimotility drugs might be of symptomatic benefit in adults with mild or moderate acute diarrhea. Their most valuable role is in short-term control of symptoms during periods of maximum social inconvenience, e.g., travel and work.

These agents are contraindicated in patients with severe diarrhea, if there is a possibility of invasive organisms, severe inflammatory bowel disease, or dilated or obstructed bowel. Antimotility drugs are also sometimes useful for control of symptoms if treatment of the underlying cause is ineffective or if the cause is unknown.

Antimotility drugs are never indicated for management of acute diarrhea in infants and children.

If an antimotility drug is considered appropriate, it is reasonable to use one of the following regimens:

- Loperamide: 4 mg orally initially, followed by 2 mg orally after each unformed stool (maximum of 16 mg/daily)
- Diphenoxylate + atropine: 5 + 0.05 mg orally3 to 4 times daily initially (decrease dose as soon as symptoms improve)

- Codeine phosphate: 30–60 mg orally up to 4 times daily
- Bismuth subsalicylate: 525 mg every 30–60 min, up to 8 doses a day for up to 48 hours.

Adsorbents, such as kaolin, have been used to treat mild nonspecific acute diarrhea, although little evidence supports efficacy. They should not be used in children under the age of 12 without a physician recommendation; they can interfere with absorption of other drugs.

Antibiotics are rarely indicated in uncomplicated infective diarrhea, except to treat properly diagnosed enteric infections or *C. Difficile* colitis.

Probiotics, nonpathogenic organisms that confer therapeutic or preventive health benefits, are controversial in the treatment of diarrhea. In children, they may shorten the course of mild viral diarrhea. They have also been used in preventing antibiotic-associated diarrhea.

Further reading

DuPont HL (1997). Guidelines on acute infectious diarrhea in adults. The Practice Parameters Committee of the American College of Gastroenterology. *Am J Gastroenterol* **92**:1962–1975.

Fine KD, Schiller LR (1999). AGA technical review on the evaluation and management of chronic diarrhea. *Gastroenterology* **118**:1464–1486.

Manatsathit S, Dupont HL, Farthing M, et al. (2002). Guideline for the management of of acute diarrhea in adults. *J Gastroenterol Hepatol* **17**(Suppl):S54–S71.

Gastroesophageal reflux disease

Gastroesophageal reflux disease (GERD) describes the symptoms or mucosal damage that occurs with abnormal reflux into the esophagus. Gastric acid, pepsin, bile acids, and pancreatic enzymes may promote damage if present in the esophagus.

Reflux may be related to decreased lower esophageal sphincter (LES) pressure or function. Certain foods and medications may worsen GERD symptoms. Medications that have been associated with a lowering of LES pressure include the following:

- Anticholinergics
- Dihydropyridine calcium-channel blockers
- Dopamine
- Estrogen
- Isoproterenol
- Nicotine
- Nitrates
- Phentolamine
- Progesterone
- Opioids (e.g., morphine, meperidine)
- Theophylline

Signs and symptoms

Symptoms include heartburn, regurgitation, or both, most frequently occurring after meals. Symptoms may be exacerbated by bending over, lying down, or exercising. Diagnosis is made on the basis of symptoms.

If the patient has typical symptoms, empiric therapy can be instituted, including lifestyle changes and medical therapy. If the patient does not respond to therapy or has alarm symptoms (e.g., difficult or painful swallowing, bleeding, weight loss, or anemia) or is at risk for Barrett's esophagus, then an endoscopic procedure with or without a biopsy may be considered.

Treatment

Treatment of GERD depends on symptom frequency and severity, as well as the presence of complications. Symptomatic GERD patients without esophagitis should be treated the same as those with erosive esophagitis.

First-line therapy for intermittent symptoms

Lifestyle modification includes decreased dietary fat intake, weight loss and smoking cessation as appropriate, elevation of the head of the bed, and avoidance of recumbency 3 hours after a meal, although there is a paucity of data to support the effectiveness of these actions.

Coffee, tea, colas, alcohol, peppermint, chocolate, and potentially onion and garlic may lower the LES pressure. They should be avoided if ingestion results in symptoms.

For as-needed, self-directed patient treatment, antacids, alginic acid, and OTC histamine-2 receptor antagonists (H2RAs) (see Table 15.64) are the initial treatment options. Antacids quickly neutralize the esophageal pH but have a short duration of action; the potential for drug interactions must also be considered. Alginic acid forms a viscous solution that floats

Table 15.64 OTC preparations for intermittent use in GERD

Product	Dosage form	Dosage	Relief onset/ duration
Antacids			
Magnesium/ aluminum hydroxide (Maalox®)	Suspension (also contains simethicone)	30 mL after meals and bedtime as needed, up to every hour	<5 minutes/ 20–30 minutes
Aluminum hydroxide/ magnesium carbonate/alginic acid (Gaviscon®)	Suspension Chewable tablets	15–30 mL after meals and bedtime as needed 2–4 tablets four times daily	<5 minutes/ 20—30 minutes
Calcium carbonate (Tums®, Alka-mints chewable antacid)	Tablets (as calcium carbonate)	500 mg: 2–4 tablets up to 15 tablets daily 750 mg: 2–4 tablets up to 10 tablets daily 1000 mg: 2–3 tablets up to 7 tablets daily Don't exceed 7.5 g calcium carbonate	<5 minutes/ 20–30 minutes
OTC H2RAs (not to be taken longer than 14 days without prescriber supervision)			
Cimetidine (Tagamet HB®)	Tablets, suspension	200 mg up to twice daily	30–45 minutes/ 4–10 hours
Famotidine (Pepcid AC®)	10 mg: tablets, chewable tablets, gelcaps 20 mg: extra-strength tablets	1 tablet up to twice daily	30–45 minutes/ 4–10 hours
Nizatidine (Axid AR®)	75 mg tablets	1 tablet up to twice daily	30–45 minutes/ 4–10 hours
Ranitidine (Zantac®)	75 mg tablets 150 mg tablets	1 tablet up to twice daily	30–45 minutes/ 4–10 hours
Combination OTC H2RA and antacid products			
Famotidine/ calcium carbonate/ magnesium hydroxide (Pepcid Complete®)	Chewable tablets: 10 mg famotidine/800 mg calcium carbonate/165 mg magnesium hydroxide	Up to 2 tablets daily	<5 minutes/ 8–10 hours
PPI (approved for 14 days of OTC treatment without prescriber supervision)			
Omeprazole (Prilosec OTC®)	Delayed-release tablet	20 mg daily	2–3 hours/12–24 hours

on the surface of the gastric contents, forming a protective barrier when contents are refluxed.

H2RAs inhibit the release of gastric acid and while differences do exist in the pharmacology of the H2RAs, in general, they may be used interchangeably and are especially useful when taken prior to an event that may result in reflux symptoms.

A combination product containing a H2RA and antacid is available combining the quick onset of antacids but the longer relief duration associated with the H2RAs.

Omeprazole is also available OTC and is approved for the short-term use of heartburn symptoms. One to four days may be needed to see the full effect. If symptoms persist despite intermittent use of these agents, continuous treatment may be necessary.

First-line treatment for continuous therapy

Lifestyle modifications should be continued or instituted. Patients should avoid medications that may irritate esophageal mucosa including alendronate, aspirin, iron, NSAIDs, quinidine, and potassium chloride.

Treatment options include proton pump inhibitors (PPIs) and H2RAs. Initial therapy with H2RAs in divided doses may be effective in some patients with mild to moderate GERD. PPIs (see Table 15.65) provide better symptomatic relief and esophageal healing than that with H2RAs.

Most PPIs should be taken before breakfast if used once daily or prior to breakfast and supper if taken twice daily. PPIs are generally used for healing in erosive gastritis. The dose used may be similar or higher than when treating uncomplicated GERD, but patients generally require a longer treatment course.

GERD is a chronic condition. Many patients will require maintenance therapy with continuous acid suppression at the lowest effective dose. On-demand maintenance therapy, when the drug is taken for as many days as needed for symptom control, may be effective in some patients.

Adjunctive therapy

Promotility agents including metoclopramide 10–15 mg 4 times daily before meals, bethanechol 0.3–0.6 mg/kg/day in 3–4 divided doses, or baclofen in a 40 mg single dose have been used as adjunctive therapy. They can be associated with significant side effects and are not ideal for monotherapy.

Second-line therapy

- Antireflux surgery
- Endoscopic procedures

Complications

Complications of GERD include the following:

- Esophageal ulcers
- Hemorrhage
- Esophageal strictures
- Barrett's esophagus
- Esophageal adenocarcinoma

Table 15.65 Prescription medications for GERD

Product	Dosage form	Dosage	
		GERD	Erosive esophagitis
H2RA (not as effective as PPIs for erosive esophagitis)			
Cimetidine (Tagamet®)	Tablets, solution, injection	400 mg twice daily	800 mg twice daily or 400 mg 4 times daily
Famotidine (Pepcid®)	Tablets, oral disintegrating, solution, injection	20 mg twice daily	No FDA indication
Nizatidine (Axid®)	Capsules, solution	150 mg twice daily	No FDA indication
Ranitidine (Zantac®)	Tablets, effervescent tablets, capsules, solution, injection	150 mg twice daily	150 mg 4 times daily
PPIs (may be taken twice daily for healing of erosive esophagitis)			
Esomeprazole (Nexium®)	Capsules, suspension, injection	20 mg daily	20–40 mg daily
Lansoprazole (Prevacid®)	Oral disintegrating tables, capsules, suspension, injection	15–30 mg daily	30 mg daily
Rabeprazole (Aciphex®)	Tablets	20 mg daily	20 mg daily
Pantoprazole (Protonix®)	Tablets, suspension, injection	40 mg daily	40 mg daily
Omeprazole (Prilosec®)	Capsules	20 mg daily	20 mg daily

Further reading

DeVault KR, Castell DO (2005). Updated guidelines for the diagnosis and treatment of gastro-esophageal reflux disease. *Am J Gastroenterol* **100**:190–200.

Falk GW, Fennerty MB, Rothstein RI (2006). AGA Institute technical review on the use of endo-scopic therapy for gastroesophageal reflux disease. *Gastroenterology* **131**:1315–1336.

Tytgat GN, McColl K, Tack J, et al. (2008). New algorithm for the treatment of gastro-oesophageal reflux disease. *Aliment Pharmacol Ther* **27**:249–256.

Vakil N, van Zanten SV, Kahrilas P, Dent J, Jones R, and the Global Consensus Group (2006). The Montreal definitions and classification of gastroesophageal reflux disease: a global evidence-based consensus. *Am J Gastroenterol* **101**:1900–1920.

Helicobacter pylori infections

Helicobacter pylori (*H pylori*) is a gram-negative bacteria that resides in the mucosal lining of the stomach. It produces urease to survive in the acidic environment, and this activity forms the basis for some tests used to detect the presence of the organism.

It causes a low-grade inflammation and gastroduodenal damage resulting in chronic gastritis, peptic ulcer disease (PUD), and gastric malignancies. It is present in most cases of uncomplicated duodenal ulcers. Some suggest that *H. pylori* is associated with iron deficiency anemia and idiopathic thrombocytopenic purpura.

Most patients infected with *H pylori* will be asymptomatic, and it may be present for decades before a patient presents with one of the GI conditions listed above. Patients with active or a documented past history of peptic ulcer disease or gastric mucosa-associated lymphoid tissue (MALT) lymphoma should be tested.

Testing and treatment of positive results in patients under the age of 55 years with uninvestigated dyspepsia with no alarm symptoms are recommended. Testing for *H pylori* should be done only if treatment is offered for positive results.

Invasive and noninvasive tests can be used to identify *H pylori*. The test used depends on whether the patient undergoes upper endoscopy and on an understanding of the individual tests. Urease tests performed either during endoscopy or noninvasively may be falsely negative if a patient has had a recent GI bleed or has received PPIs, H2RAs, antibiotics, or bismuth-containing compounds.

Signs and symptoms

The presenting signs and symptoms will depend on the concurrent condition—e.g., patients with peptic ulcers may present with symptoms ranging from mild epigastric pain to life-threatening upper GI bleeding.

Treatment

Testing for *H pylori* should be performed before treatment with antibiotics. Eradication of *H pylori* is associated with better duodenal ulcer healing rates, a decrease in recurrent bleeding, and a decrease in gastric ulcer recurrence.

For localized MALT lymphoma, treatment is associated with tumor regression in over 50% of patients. Multiple therapeutic regimens are used. The individual regimen chosen depends on cost, resistance rates, potential side effects, and ease of administration.

Once the patient has completed treatment, it is appropriate to check for infection eradication in patients with a documented *H. pylori*–associated ulcer or MALT lymphoma, in patients with persistent dyspeptic symptoms who were *H pylori* positive and received treatment, and after early gastric cancer resection. This is generally done 4–6 weeks after treatment with a noninvasive test unless endoscopy is indicated for another reason.

If the urease breath or fecal antigen test is used the patient should be off PPIs for 1–2 weeks, and off antibiotics and bismuth for 4 weeks.

First-line therapy

The regimen most frequently used is triple therapy with a PPI and two antibiotics. It is helpful to ask patients about their previous use of a macrolide or metronidazole before deciding on the regimen. In patients who have not received a macrolide, amoxicillin and clarithromycin are the preferred antibiotics.

In penicillin-allergic patients, metronidazole may be used in place of amoxicillin, but resistance is associated with this agent and substitution for amoxicillin may decrease treatment effectiveness. Two weeks of therapy may be more effective than shorter courses of therapy. See Table 15.66 for regimens.

Another option is a combination of a PPI or H2RA with bismuth, metronidazole, and tetracycline. Combination with a PPI is preferred over an H2RA, as this provides better efficacy in patients with metronidazole-resistant strains of *H pylori*. This regimen involves a higher pill burden and an increased frequency of administration but may be considered first-line therapy especially in cases of clarithromycin resistance.

Combination products containing bismuth, metronidazole, and tetracycline are available and may decrease pill burden compared to that with prescribing the medications individually. In addition, bismuth, metronidazole, and tetracycline and amoxicilin, lansoprazole, and clarithromycin are available as a package in the United States to simplify prescribing.

Second-line therapy

A PPI and either amoxicillin or clarithromycin for 2 weeks have been approved by the FDA, but eradication rates are significantly less than with PPI-based triple therapy. These regimens may be an alternative in patients who do not tolerate metronidazole or clarithromycin.

Sequential therapy with a PPI and amoxicillin initially followed by a PPI, clarithromycin and tinidazole is also recommended as second-line therapy, although more data are needed in patients in the United States. Substitution of metronidazole for tinidazole in the sequential regimen has not been established.

Adjunct therapy

Probiotics may decrease side effects such as diarrhea from the treatment regimen and may be useful as adjunctive therapy. They should not replace standard therapy.

Complications

Treatment failure can be seen in situations of poor compliance or organism resistance. Smoking, alcohol consumption, and diet may also affect successful treatment. The following are strategies that may be used in cases of treatment failure.

Eradication failure

Retreatment regimens that are the same as the initial therapy should be avoided and regimens containing two new antimicrobial may be more effective than those with only one new antimicrobial. The length of therapy should generally be 2 weeks for retreatment regimens. Bismuth in

Table 15.66 *Helicobacter pylori* treatment regimens

Drug 1	Drug 2	Drug 3	Drug 4	Duration of therapy
PPI-based regimens in patients not allergic to penicillin and who have not previously received a macrolide				
Lansoprazole 30mg twice daily	Amoxicillin 1 g twice daily	Clarithromycin 500 mg twice daily		10–14 days
Omeprazole 20mg twice daily	Amoxicillin 1 g twice daily	Clarithromycin 500 mg twice daily		10–14 days
Pantoprazole 40 mg twice daily	Amoxicillin 1 g twice daily	Clarithromycin 500 mg twice daily		10–14 days
Rabeprazole 20mg twice daily	Amoxicillin 1 g twice daily	Clarithromycin 500 mg twice daily		10–14 days
Esomeprazole 40mg once daily	Amoxicillin 1 g twice daily	Clarithromycin 500 mg twice daily		10–14 days
PPI-based triple therapy in patients who are allergic to penicillin, have not received a macrolide, or are unable to tolerate a quadruple bismuth-based therapy				
PPI, doses as above	Metronidazole 500 mg twice daily	Clarithromycin 500 mg twice daily		10–14 days
Sequential-based therapy				
PPI, doses as above (days 1–10)	Amoxicillin 1 g twice daily (days 1–5)	Clarithromycin 500 mg twice daily (days 6–10)	Tinidazole 500 mg twice daily (days 6–10)	10 days total
Bismuth quadruple-based regimens				
PPI, doses as above	Bismuth 525 mg 4 times daily	Metronidazole 250–500 mg 4 times daily	Tetracycline 500 mg 4 times daily	14 days
Ranitidine 150 mg twice daily	Bismuth 525 mg 4 times daily	Metronidazole 250–500 mg 4 times daily	Tetracycline 500 mg 4 times day	14 days

combination with tetracycline, a PPI, and a higher dose of metronidazole may be considered if a bismuth regimen was not used as initial therapy.

Another rescue regimen is twice-daily pantoprazole 40 mg, amoxicillin 1 g, and levofloxacin 250–500 mg for 10 days; the community resistance patterns to levofloxacin must be considered prior to use. A regimen of pantoprazole 80 mg and amoxicillin 1–1.5 g with rifabutin 150 mg once daily for 12 days has been used in patients who failed a regimen containing a PPI, clarithromycin, and amoxicillin.

Culture and sensitivity testing for resistant organisms is not generally recommended unless the patient has failed two treatment courses.

Resistance

H pylori is intrinsically resistant to vancomycin, trimethoprim, and sulfonamides. Resistance to metronidazole and clarithromycin has been reported, with metronidazole resistance being more common. Resistance to metronidazole may be overcome by using the 500 mg dose or using it in combination with bismuth.

Patients with clarithromycin resistance should be not treated with a two-antibiotic regimen containing clarithromycin. In patients with clarithromycin resistance, the sequential therapy regimen listed in Table 15.66 appears to overcome clarithromycin resistance.

Further reading

Chey WD, Wong BCY, the Practice Parameters Committee of the American College of Gastroenterology (2007). America College of Gastroenterology guideline on the management of *Helicobacter pylori* infection. *Am J Gastroenterol* **102**:1808–1825.

Malfertheiner P, Megraud F, O'Morain C, et al. (2007). Current concepts in the management of *Helicobacter pylori* infection: the Maastricht III consensus report. *Gut* **56**:772–781.

Talley NJ, American Gastroenterological Association (2005). AGA medical position statement: evaluation of dyspepsia. *Gastroenterology* **129**:1753–1755.

Talley NJ, Vakil N. Practice Parameters Committee of the American College of Gastroenterology (2005). Guidelines for the management of dyspepsia. *Am J Gastroenterol* **100**:2324–2337.

Hepatic encephalopathy

Hepatic encephalopathy (HE) is a disturbance of central nervous system (CNS) function resulting from liver dysfunction. HE is a diagnosis of exclusion; other neurological and metabolic causes of altered mental status should be ruled out.

HE is classified into three types: type A occurs in acute liver failure, type B is associated with portal-systemic bypass but no intrinsic hepatocellular disease, and type C is associated with portal hypertension and cirrhosis.

Type C is most commonly seen and associated with acute, chronic, or recurrent symptoms. While the pathophysiology of type C HE is not entirely understood, it is associated with portosystemic shunting and increased levels of ammonia. In many cases of acute HE, a precipitating factor can be identified as the following:

- Gastrointestinal bleeding
- Hypokalemia
- Dehydration (evaluate use of diuretics used to treat ascites)
- Metabolic alkalosis
- Hypoxia
- Hypoglycemia
- Infections, including spontaneous bacterial peritonitis and pneumonia
- Constipation
- Drugs affecting the CNS, e.g., alcohol, sedatives, tranquilizers, and benzodiazepines
- Primary hepatocellular carcinoma
- Vascular occlusion
- Excess dietary protein
- Presence of a transjugular intrahepatic portosystemic shunt (TIPS)
- Zinc deficiency

Signs and symptoms

In addition to the laboratory and physical findings associated with liver failure, patients with HE may have mild to severe changes in level of consciousness, intellectual function, personality, behavior, and neuromuscular abnormalities.

Symptoms include shortened attention span, gross disorientation, hypersomnia, insomnia, lethargy, apathy, depression, slurred speech, bizarre behavior, stupor, and, in severe cases, coma. A flapping tremor or asterixis can be seen and is often used to judge therapy effectiveness.

Treatment

Type A encephalopathy associated with acute liver failure is less common than type C. Recommendations for treating type A–associated HE includes intensive care monitoring, management of cerebral edema, multisystem organ support, and early consideration of liver transplantation.

The management of type C–associated encephalopathy is the focus of this chapter. Potential precipitating factors should be identified and treated. Benzodiazepines should not be used for insomnia in patients at risk for chronic HE symptoms and medications associated with HE should be withheld during acute HE episodes.

Measures to decrease ammonia production and increase elimination, including use of antibiotics and laxatives, are the mainstay of treatment of acute and chronic HE associated with chronic liver disease. After treatment of the acute episode, consideration should be given to preventive therapy, as cirrhotic patients who develop HE are at risk for subsequent episodes.

First-line treatment

Nutrition

Protein may be withheld during the first 1–2 days of acute HE treatment, but withholding protein for prolonged periods should be avoided. Patients can become malnourished if protein is restricted or withheld. Once treatment has been initiated, increasing protein intake to a goal of 1–1.5 g protein/kg/day as tolerated is appropriate.

Vegetable and dairy sources of protein contain nonabsorbable fiber and a higher calorie-to-nitrogen ratio, and may be used in patients if tolerated. Although the use of branched-chain amino acid (BCAA) specialty products is controversial, oral BCAA feedings may be better tolerated than a regular protein diet in some individuals who are severely protein intolerant.

Laxatives

Various laxatives may be used, but the vast majority of experience is with lactulose, even though current evidence-based medicine standards for use are not met with this agent. In acute HE, 30–45 mL may be given orally or by nasogastric tube hourly until an improvement in patient symptoms is seen. Rectal enemas are an alternative; 300 mL lactulose is mixed with 700 mL water and the patient should retain the mixture for 1 hour.

In chronic HE, the starting dose is 15–45 mL twice or three times daily and titrated to 2–3 soft bowel movements a day.

Adjunctive therapy

In patients with a documented zinc deficiency, zinc 200 mg twice daily should be administered.

Supportive care should be considered in acute HE, including fall prevention in hospitalized patients, prevention of aspiration and endotracheal intubation in patients with significant HE, and decubitus ulcer prevention.

Flumazenil may provide short-term benefit in acute HE. Although the routine use of this agent is not recommended, a 1 mg IV bolus dose may be useful in patients who have received benzodiazepines.

Second-line therapy

Alternative therapy for HE includes various antibiotics, which should be reserved for patients who do not respond to or tolerate lactulose. Oral neomycin is no longer frequently used because of the potential for ototoxicity and nephrotoxicity.

Oral metronidazole in doses of 250 mg twice daily may be used short term as an alternative to or in conjunction with lactulose. It should not be used for longer periods because of the risk of peripheral neuropathy.

Rifaxamin in oral doses of 400 mg three times daily shows a trend toward increased efficacy compared to lactulose or neomycin in treating chronic HE, and it may be better tolerated than lactulose. It has been studied alone and in combination with lactulose. However, rifaxamin is expensive and has an orphan indication for this use.

Other options for refractory chronic HE include the following:

- Bromocriptine 30 mg orally twice daily
- Occlusion of large, spontaneous portal-systemic shunts
- Orthotopic liver transplantation

Further reading

Blei AT, Cordoba J, and The Practice Parameters Committee of the American College of Gastroenterology (2001). Hepatic encephalopathy. *Am J Gastroenterol* **96**:1968–1976.

deMelo RT, Charneski L, Hilas O (2008). Rifaximin for the treatment of hepatic encephalopathy. *Am J Health Syst Pharm* **65**:818–828.

Polson J, Lee WM (2005). AASLD position paper: The management of acute liver failure. *Hepatology* **41**:1179–1197.

Stravitz RT, Kramer AH, Davern T, and the Acute Liver Failure Study Group (2007). Intensive care of patients with acute liver failure: recommendations of the US Acute Liver Failure Study Group. *Crit Care Med* **35**:2498–2508.

Hepatitis

Viral hepatitis is a term that describes several unique diseases, each caused by a unique virus. The viruses are not related except in that they all cause hepatitis.

There are three major viruses causing hepatitis in the United States:

- Hepatitis A virus (HAV)
- Hepatitis B virus (HBV)
- Hepatitis C virus (HCV)

Other viruses include the hepatitis D virus, which needs HBV present in order to function; hepatitis E virus; and cytomegalovirus (CMV), which can cause acute hepatitis.

Hepatitis A

Background

- RNA virus
- Estimated 32,000 cases in the United States in 2006
  - Higher prevalence in Mexico, South America, Africa, southern Asia
- Transmission is fecal–oral route
  - Usually through close contact with an infected person such as a household member
  - Can cause outbreaks when a group of people is exposed to fecally contaminated food or water

Course of disease

- Average incubation period is 30 days
- The early (prodromal) phase of infection can initially result in flu-like symptoms, nausea, malaise, anorexia, and other general symptoms. Abdominal pain and vomiting can occur as the infection progresses to the acute phase, and some patients have jaundice accompanied by itching. Jaundice is less common in children than in adults. The incidence corresponds with age.
- Lab tests
  - Elevated liver enzymes, bilirubin
  - +Anti-HAV IgM indicates active infection
- Hepatitis symptoms can last up to 9 months, but are generally much shorter.
- Chronic infection does not occur.
- Mortality is due to fulminant hepatitis, but is uncommon.

Treatment

- Antiviral therapy is not effective.
- Symptomatic management is the only therapy.

Prevention

Vaccination

- Recommended for all children at 1 year of age
- Also recommended for IV drug users, travelers to endemic areas, homosexual males, people with liver disease, and patients with clotting factor disorders

- Two vaccines
  - Havrix®
    —Dose = 720 ELISA units for age <18 years, 1440 ELISA units for those age ≥18. Repeated doses given 6–12 months later
  - Vaqta®
    —Dose = 25 units for age <18 years, 50 units for those ≥18. Repeated doses given 6–18 months later

Prophylaxis

- Immunoglobulin (Ig) or HAV vaccine can be given to patients who either have been or may be exposed to HAV and are not immune.
- Not needed if patient has received HAV vaccine at least 1 month prior to exposure
- HAV vaccine preferred for patients aged 1–40 years
- Ig given to other patients
- Dose = 0.02 mL IM x1 for short-term pre-exposure or post-exposure, 0.06 mL IM x1 for longer-term (3–5 months) pre-exposure

Hepatitis B

Background

- DNA virus
- Estimated 46,000 new cases in the United States in 2006
  - High prevalence in Africa, Brazil, China, and southeastern Asia
- Transmission is by sexual contact and is blood-borne
  - Sexual spread is most common
  - Can be spread through needlesticks

Course of disease

The average incubation period is 3 months. HBV causes acute disease in 30%–50% of patients 5 years of age and older, but infrequently in younger patients. Chronic infection is more common in younger patients. Acute disease presents similarly to HAV.

Most patients clear the virus after acute infection regardless of whether they are symptomatic, but some progress to chronic infection. Some patients who develop chronic infection eventually progress to chronic active hepatitis, then to cirrhosis, then to hepatocellular carcinoma.

Serology is useful in charting patient progress and infectivity:

- HBsAg (surface antigen) appears first, shows that patient is infectious
- HBeAg (core antigen) shows a high degree of infectivity, increased risk of progression
- Anti-HBs (antibody against surface antigen) indicates recovery and cure, or immunity by vaccination
- Anti-HBe (antibody against core antigen) predicts recovery is occurring
- IgM anti-HBc (acute antibody against core antigen) shows active infection
- HBV-DNA (DNA of virus) shows active infection

Treatment

There is no effective treatment of acute HBV infection. Chronic infection can be treated with antiviral drugs and interferon. Treatment is started in the chronic infectious stage with elevated ALT levels.

First-line option: antivirals

- Lamivudine (3TC): 100 mg once daily
- Entecavir: 0.5 mg once daily for 3TC-naïve patients, 1 mg once daily for 3TC-refractory patients
- Adefovir: 10 mg once daily
- Telbivudine: 600 mg once daily
- Antivirals are generally well tolerated

First-line option: interferon

- Pegylated interferon-α_{2a} (IFN-α_{2a}) injected subcutaneously once weekly
- High incidence of adverse effects, including depression, arthralgias, nausea, musculoskeletal pain, anxiety, and others

Second-line options

- Combination therapy with two antivirals or an antiviral and interferon
- Emtricitabine (FTC): 200 mg once daily
- Tenofovir (TDF): 300 mg once daily

Treatment for patients with HBV and cirrhosis

- Compensated cirrhosis: adefovir or entecavir
- Uncompenated cirrhosis: lamivudine + adefovir OR entecavir + adefovir
  - Prognosis is grim without transplant

Prevention

Vaccination

- Two single-antigen vaccines are available, Recombivax HB® and Engerix-B®. Multiple-antigen combination products that contain HBV vaccine also exist.
- Vaccination is given to all infants within a few days of birth and to other susceptible populations.

Prophylaxis

- Post-exposure prophylaxis can be given to unvaccinated people after a needlestick (occupational injury) or babies born to mothers with HBV.
- Occupational exposures do not require therapy if the person was vaccinated with a known response.
- If unvaccinated occupational exposure:
  - Give hepatitis B immunoglobulin (HBIG) 0.06 mL/kg IM x1 and start vaccination if patient is unvaccinated
  - Test patient for anti-HBs if vaccinated, give HBIG if inadequate immunity + HBV vaccine
- For perinatal transmission:
  - Give HBIG 0.5 mL IM x1 and start vaccination

Hepatitis C

Background

- This an RNA virus, so HBV antivirals are inactive against it.
- Estimated 19,000 new cases in the United States in 2006
- Higher prevalence in same areas as HBV
- Transmission is primarily blood-borne. HCV can be spread sexually, but is uncommon. IV drug users are at highest risk.

- Viral genotype predicts treatment efficacy; type 1 is the most difficult to treat and is unfortunately the most common type in the United States.

Course of disease

The incubation period is 1–5 months. Symptoms of acute infection occur in 20%–30% of patients and are similar to those of other viral hepatitis.

Most patients (75%–85%) develop chronic infection. Most of these patients develop chronic liver disease, which can progress to cirrhosis and possibly death. Progression to cirrhosis can take 20–30 years, but is accelerated in patients coinfected with HIV.

Chronic disease is marked by elevated LFTs and positive HCV-RNA assays.

Treatment

Acute disease cannot be treated. Chronic disease can be treated with interferon and ribavirin in combination.

- Pegylated IFN-α_{2a} 180 mcg SC every week

OR

- Pegylated INF-α_{2b} 1.5 mcg/kg SC every week

AND

- Ribavirin 1000 mg PO daily (weight <75 kg) or 1200 mg PO daily (weight ≥75 kg)

The duration of therapy is 24 weeks for genotypes 2 or 3, 48 weeks for genotype 1.

- If no virologic response by week 12 for genotype 1, consider stopping therapy since likelihood of success is low
  - Adverse effects of IFN are significant (see First-Line Option: Interferon, p. 526). Adverse effects of ribavirin include hemolytic anemia, neutropenia, and thrombocytopenia. Hemolytic anemia is to be expected, and dose reduction is warranted if hemoglobin (Hb) is <10 mg/dL. Ribavirin is pregnancy category X.
  - Patients with advanced HCV cirrhosis may be candidates for liver transplantation

Further reading

Department of Health and Human Services, Centers for Disease Control and Prevention, Division of Viral Hepatitis. http://www.cdc.gov/hepatitis

Dienstag JL, McHutchison JG (2006). American Gastroenterological Association medical position statement on the management of hepatitis C. *Gastroenterology* **130**(1):225–230.

Keefe EB, Dieterich DT, Han SB, et al. (2006). A treatment algorithm for the management of chronic hepatitis B virus infection in the United States: an update. *Clin Gastroenterol Hepatol* **4**(8):936–962..

Inflammatory bowel disease

Inflammatory bowel disease (IBD) encompasses both ulcerative colitis (UC) and Crohn's disease (CD); both disorders are associated with inflammation in the GI tract. The distribution and depth of inflammation vary between the diseases.

UC is limited to the mucosal layer of the colon and rectum and generally extends in a continuous pattern. Inflammation in CD is segmental and asymmetric, and may be transmural. It most commonly involves the ileum and colon. The inflammatory process is mediated by proinflammatory cytokines including interleukins and tumor necrosis factor (TNF).

NSAIDs are known to exacerbate both disorders. Smoking exacerbates CD but is protective in UC.

Signs and symptoms

Ulcerative colitis

Symptoms of UC may include diarrhea (constipation may be seen with proctitis), rectal bleeding, abdominal pain and cramping, tenesmus, weight loss, crypt abscesses, arthritis, anal fissures, dehydration, fever, tachycardia, and anemia.

Crohn's disease

Symptoms of CD include diarrhea, rectal bleeding, abdominal pain and cramping, bowel obstruction, weight loss, malnutrition, pallor, fatigue and malaise, anemia, night sweats, nausea and vomiting, fever, tachycardia, arthritis, abdominal mass and tenderness, perianal fistula, and abscesses.

Diagnosis is made on clinical grounds and supported by appropriate laboratory, radiographic, endoscopic, and pathologic findings. It may not be possible to distinguish between UC and CD.

Treatment

The treatment for active disease in both UC and CD depends on the location, extent, and severity of the inflammation. Both diseases are characterized by exacerbations and remission. Surgery is curative in UC, although it is not the treatment of initial choice. Surgery may be necessary for massive hemorrhage, perforation, obstruction, abscesses, unresponsive fulminant disease, or carcinoma.

CD is not surgically or medically curable; surgery may be necessary to treat complications. Maintenance therapy should be considered to maintain remission.

Crohn's disease

Mild–moderate disease

It is seen in ambulatory patients able to tolerate oral feedings who are adequately hydrated. There are no signs of high fevers, abdominal tenderness, painful mass or obstruction, or significant weight loss.

First-line therapy for ileal, ileocolonic, or colonic disease is as follows:

- Aminosalicylate preparations (see Table 15.67), or budesonide controlled ileal release (distal ileal and/or right colonic disease only) 9 mg/day; may taper every 3–4 weeks to 6 mg daily and then 3 mg daily

Alternative therapies for ileal, ileocolonic, or colonic disease include the following:

- Ciprofloxacin 1 g/day in divided doses
- Metronidazole 10–20 mg/kg/day in patients not responding to aminosalicylate preparations
- Prednisone in patients not responding to budesonide

Moderate–severe disease

This is seen in patients who fail to respond to mild–moderate treatment, or who present with fevers, significant weight loss, abdominal pain and tenderness, intermittent nausea and vomiting, or significant anemia.

First-line therapy should be continued until resolution of symptoms and resumption of weight gain.

- Prednisone 40–60 mg/day x7–28 days, taper by 5–10 mg weekly until 20 mg/day, then 2.5–5 mg weekly until completion
  - Some patients will become steroid dependent.
- Budesonide (for distal ileal and/or right colonic disease only), dose as above
- Treatment of abscesses includes broad-spectrum antibiotics and drainage.

Adjunctive therapy includes the following:

- Smoking cessation, if applicable.
- Azathioprine 2–2.5 mg/kg/day or 6-mercaptopurine (6-MP) 1–1.5 mg/kg/day; effect may take 3 or more months
- Methotrexate 25 mg SC or IM weekly has been used to facilitate steroid tapering in steroid-dependent patients. It is contraindicated in pregnancy.
- Natalizumab 300 mg IV every 4 weeks. It should not be used in conjunction with azathioprine, 6-MP, cyclosporine, methotrexate, or agents affecting TNF. It is associated with progressive multifocal leukoencephalopathy and is considered last-line therapy. It is currently available through a special distribution program.
- Anti-TNF-α agents
  - Infliximab IV 5 mg/kg at 0, 2, and 6 weeks then every 8 weeks for maintenance if effective. The development of infliximab antibodies is associated with a reduced duration of response and an increased risk of infusion reactions. Concurrent steroids may decrease antibody development.
  - Adalimumab may be used if there is inadequate response to conventional therapy or in those patients who have lost response or are intolerant of infliximab. Approved dosage is 160 mg on day 1 (or 80 mg on days 1 and 2) followed by 80 mg on day 15 with maintenance therapy of 40 mg every 2 weeks.
  - Certolizumab pegol 400 mg SC at 0, 2, and 4 weeks followed by 400 mg SC every 4 weeks.

Severe–fulminant disease

This is seen in patients symptomatic after oral steroid treatment, or in patients presenting with high fevers, persistent vomiting, intestinal obstruction, rebound tenderness, cachexia, or abscess. Patients should be hospitalized for treatment.

First-line therapy includes the following:

- Methylprednisolone 40–60 mg IV/day (divided doses or continuous infusion); symptoms typically respond in 7–14 days
- Enteral or parenteral nutrition if unable to obtain nutritional goals with oral feedings after 5–7 days or with evidence of bowel obstruction

Adjunctive therapy includes the following:

- Fluid, electrolyte, and red blood cell repletion as appropriate.
- Surgical consult for obstruction or tender abdominal mass, with antibiotics and drainage for an abscess
- Smoking cessation if applicable

Second-line therapy (if patients fail to respond to steroids) is as follows:

- IV infliximab 5 mg/kg/dose at 0, 2, and 6 weeks followed by maintenance therapy if patient responds
- High-dose IV cyclosporine.
- IV tacrolimus.

Therapy for perianal disease includes surgical drainage and antibiotics for abscesses, and metronidazole with or without ciprofloxacin, or azathioprine or 6-MP, or infliximab or adalimumab for fistulas.

CD maintenance therapy

Steroids should not be used as long term therapy to prevent relapse of disease.

First-line therapy includes the following:

- Azathioprine 2.5 mg/kg daily or 6-MP 1.5 mg/kg daily, regardless of disease location.
- Methotrexate 15–25 mg IM weekly in patients who respond to induction therapy with methotrexate. It is contraindicated in pregnancy.
- Aminosalicylate preparations after ileocolonic resections to prevent relapse. Aminosalicylates have not been shown to be effective in medically induced remission.
- Infliximab 5 mg/kg/dose every 8 weeks; dose may be increased to 10mg/kg/dose if response wanes
- Metronidazole 20 mg/kg/day for short-term maintenance
- Budesonide for 3 months in mild to moderate ileoceccal disease is effective for short-term maintenance.
- Smoking cessation if applicable.

Ulcerative colitis

The location of the disease is characterized as distal, e.g., below the splenic flexure and amendable to topical therapy, or extensive, e.g., extends proximal to the splenic flexure and requires systemic therapy.

Severity is classified as mild, e.g., <4 stools/day with or without blood, no systemic signs of toxicity, and normal ESR; moderate, e.g., 4–6 stools/day and minimal signs of toxicity; severe, e.g., >6 stools/day, signs of toxicity such as fever, tachycardia, anemia, or elevated ESR; or fulminant, e.g., >10 stools/day with continuous bleeding, toxicity, abdominal tenderness and distension, and colonic dilation.

Mild–moderate distal colitis

First-line therapy for induction (dependent on patient preference):

- Topical mesalamine.
- Combination of oral and topical mesalamine; this is more effective than topical mesalamine alone
- Oral aminosalicylates alone (see Table 15.67); they are less effective than topical mesalamine
- Topical steroids—hydrocortisone 10% foam or 100 mg.

Table 15.67 Aminosalicylate preparations (dosages are for both UC and CD unless otherwise specified)

Product, dosage form	Mechanism of release	Dosage	Site of action
Sulfasalazine 500 mg regular- and delayed-release tablet	Cleavage of azo bond by colonic bacteria	Induction: 4–6 g daily in divided doses Maintenance: 2–4 g daily in divided doses	Colon
Mesalamine (Asacol®) 400 mg	Delayed release at pH ≥7	Induction: 2.4–4.8 g daily in divided doses Maintenance: 1.6–4.8 g daily in divided doses	Terminal ileum and colon
Mesalamine (Pentasa®) 250 mg and 500 mg capsule	Controlled-release microgranules	Induction: 2–4 g daily in divided doses Maintenance: same	Small bowel and colon
Mesalamine (Canasa® 1 g) suppository	Suppository	Induction: 1 g daily (UC) Maintenance: 0.5–1 g daily (UC)	Rectum
Mesalamine (Rowasa®) 4 g/60mL	Suspension	Induction: 1–4 g daily (UC) Maintenance: 1–4 g up to every 3 days (UC)	Distal left colon and rectum
Mesalamine (Lialda®) 1.2 g tablet	Delayed release at pH ≥7, prolonged release throughout colon	Induction: up to 4.8 g daily Maintenance: same	Terminal ileum and colon
Olsalazine (Dipentum®) 250 mg tablet	Cleavage of azo bond by colonic bacteria	Induction: not recommended Maintenance: 1 g daily in divided doses	Colon
Balsalazide (Colazal®) 750 mg capsule	Cleavage of azo bond by colonic bacteria	Induction: 6.75 g daily in divided doses Maintenance: same	Colon

Second-line therapy consists of
- Prednisone orally 40–60 mg daily

First-line therapy for maintenance of remission includes the following:
- Proctitis: mesalamine suppositories
- Left-sided colitis: mesalamine enemas
- Oral mesalamine is also effective and may be used.
- Combination therapy with oral and topical mesalamine is more effective than either agent alone.

Mild–moderate extensive colitis

First-line therapy for induction of remission:
- Oral aminosalicylate with or without topical therapy; response is seen in 4 weeks

Second-line therapy consists of
- Transdermal nicotine patch 15–25 mg daily

Refractory disease treatment includes the following:
- Prednisone 20–60 mg daily until response, followed by tapering 5–10 mg weekly until 20 mg/day, then 2.5–5 mg weekly until completion. Some patients will become steroid dependent.
- Azathioprine 1.5–3 mg/kg/day or 6-MP 1–1.5 mg /kg/day in steroid-unresponsive patients who do not need IV therapy
- Infliximab 5 mg/kg/dose IV at 0, 2, and 6 weeks followed by maintenance if effective
- Combination therapy with infliximab and an antimetabolite may be appropriate.

Remission maintenance options include the following:
- Oral aminosalicylates (see Table 15.67)
- Azathioprine or 6-MP
- Infliximab 5 mg/kg every 8 weeks

Maximum length of therapy has not been established, although experts recommend indefinite treatment.

Severe colitis

First-line therapy for active disease includes the following:
- IV steroids equivalent to 300 mg hydrocortisone or 60 mg methylprednsiolone for 7–10 days
- Colectomy or IV cyclosporine 2–4 mg/kg/day is indicated if adequate response is not obtained.
- Avoid medications with anticholinergic or narcotic properties.
- Broad-spectrum antibiotics may be used in cases of toxic megacolon.

Remission maintenance options include the following:
- Azathioprine or 6-MP 2–3 mg/kg/day or 6-MP 1–1.5 mg/kg/day
- Oral cyclosporine may be used short term until azathioprine or 6-mercaptopurine takes effect.
- Infliximab 5 mg/kg/dose every 8 weeks; dose may be increased to 10 mg/kg/dose if response wanes.

Drug therapy complications

- Peripheral neuropathy occurs with long-term metronidazole use.
- Dose-dependent secretory diarrhea is associated with olsalazine and it is not the preferred agent for induction of remission.
- Neutropenia is seen with azathioprine and 6-MP. Genetic polymorphisms may be responsible and the FDA recommends TPMT genotype/phenotype be obtained prior to initiation of therapy to avoid toxicity in patients with low enzymatic activity. A CBC with differential should be monitored routinely during therapy.
- Complications of infliximab include development of antibodies, reactivation of latent tuberculosis (TB), and development of fungal infections. Concurrent use with azathioprine or 6-MP has been associated with hepatosplenic lymphoma. It should be avoided in patients with a history of malignancy, with severe CHF, demyelinating disorders, or active infection, or in patients with a known hypersensitivity to the agent.
- Osteoporosis is seen with long-term steroid use. Consider obtaining bone mineral density testing and using concurrent calcium and vitamin D and potentially bisphosphonates.
- *Pneumocystis carinii* infections are seen in patients on cyclosporine. Patients should receive prophylaxis against the infection.

Further reading

Hanauer SB, Sandborn W, and the Practice Parameters Committee of the American College of Gastroenterology (2001). Management of Crohn's disease in adults. Am J Gastroenterol **96**(3):635–643.

Kornbluth A, Sachar DB (2004). Ulcerative colitis practice guidelines in adults (update): American College of Gastroenterology, Practice Parameters Committee. *Am J Gastroenterol* **99**(7):1371–1385.

Lichtenstein GR, Abreu MT, Cohen R, Tremaine W, American Gastroenterological Association (2006). American Gastroenterological Association Institute technical review on corticosteroids, immunomodulators, and infliximab in inflammatory bowel disease. *Gastroenterology* **130**(3):935–987.

Management of nausea and vomiting

Definition

Nausea and vomiting are common and distressing symptoms, which can lead to the following clinical conditions:

- Poor hydration and nutrition
- Weight loss
- Depression
- Increased length of stay
- Poor adherence to oral medicines

Most cases are acute; patients with symptoms for greater than a month are classified as having chronic nausea and vomiting.

Causes of nausea and vomiting

- Infectious causes—e.g., viral or bacterial gastroenteritis, otitis media
- Medications
  - Cancer chemotherapy
  - NSAIDs
  - Dopamine agonists—e.g., l-dopa, bromocriptine
  - Cardiovascular drugs—e.g., digoxin, antiarrhytmics, antihypertensives
  - Antibiotics—e.g., erythromycin, tetracycline, sulfonamides
  - CNS active—e.g., nicotine, narcotics, anticonvulsants, ethanol
  - Hormonal—e.g., oral antidiabetics, oral contraceptives
  - Anesthetics—e.g., nitrous oxide and volatile inhaled anesthetics
- Postoperative
- Metabolic
  - Pregnancy
  - Other: uremia, hyper- or hypoparathyroidism, hypercalcemia
- CNS
  - Emotional and anxiety
  - CNS lesions
  - Vestibular
  - Migraines
  - Seizures
  - Increased intracranial pressure.
- Disorders of the GI tract
  - Constipation
  - Obstruction
  - Gastrointestinal tumors
  - Pancreatitis
- Miscellaneous—e.g., myocardial infarction, heart failure, starvation, diabetic ketoacidosis, adrenal insufficiency

Management of nausea and vomiting requires accurate diagnosis of the cause, and knowledge of control pathways and the ways in which anti-emetics work.

Four steps to managing nausea and vomiting

- Identify the cause. This is not always easy because nausea and vomiting are often multifactorial. It is important, however, because antiemetics are not equally effective against all types of nausea and vomiting. Take an accurate and detailed history, including prescribed and over-the-counter (OTC) drugs.
- Remove or correct cause if possible—e.g., stop NSAIDs and prescribe laxatives if patient is constipated.
- Correct complications—e.g., dehydration, electrolyte abnormalities, acid–base and metabolic disturbances.
- Treat according to cause—start appropriate treatment according to diagnosis (Table 15.68). In some cases, such as appendicitis, antiemetics may not be the treatment of choice. About 10% of cases require more than one drug. Preferably, these should be from different groups (but anticholinergics antagonize the prokinetic effect of metoclopramide). Parenteral administration should be considered for severe intractable episodes whereas oral antiemetics are appropriate for mild nausea and uncomplicated vomiting. See Table 15.68 for recommended drugs.

Specialist advice should be sought for patients with chemotherapy-induced or radiotherapy-induced nausea and vomiting or bowel obstruction. Guidelines are available and provide recommendations based on emetogenicity of the chemotherapy regimen and type of radiation. Agents for anticipatory nausea and vomiting are also discussed.

Review the patient's condition frequently and regularly—if nausea and vomiting persist, change from oral to parenteral administration, increase dose, or try drugs from a different therapeutic class. Allow a 24-hour trial of each intervention before trying another option.

Postoperative nausea and vomiting (PONV)

PONV is a highly undesirable complication of surgery that can occur in up to 70% of high-risk cases. In addition to the consequences described above, severe retching and vomiting postoperatively can put tension on suture lines, cause formation of hematomas, and increase postoperative pain.

Patients at high risk for PONV include females, nonsmokers, obese patients, and those with a history of motion sickness. Additional risk factors for PONV are as follows:

- Use of inhalation anesthetics, e.g., isoflurane, enflurane
- Duration of anesthesia
- Use of opioids
- Use of nitrous oxide
- Abdominal surgery, notably laparoscopic procedures
- Perioperative dehydration

For nonemergency surgery, good preoperative care can reduce risk of PONV:

- Identify risk factors and correct or minimize them wherever possible.
- Employ strategies to reduce baseline risk, including use of regional anesthesia, use of propofol for induction and maintenance of anesthesia, intraoperative oxygen use, hydration, and minimizing the use of neostigmine, volatile anesthetics, or nitrous oxide.

Table 15.68 Treatments according to diagnosis

Cause	First-line drug group	First-line treatment	Second-line treatment	Other treatment
Heartburn/ gastritis	Antacids	Aluminum/ magnesium hydroxide	Ranitidine	Dietary manipulation Omeprazole
Gastro-paresis	Prokinetic	Metoclopramide‡	Erythromycin	Dietary manipulation Procholperazine Cyclizine Ondansetron Tricyclic antidepressants
Pregnancy	Vitamins*/ antihistamine	Pyridoxine/ doxylamine	Promethazine Dimenhydrinate Metoclopramide Trimetho-benzamide	Dietary manipulation Acupressure/ acupuncture Psychotherapy Methylprednisone** Ondansetron
Motion sickness	Antihistamine	Diphenhydramine Meclizine	Scopolamine patch	Accupressure (e.g., Seabands)
CNS	Antihistamine/ anticholinergic†	Cyclizine Meclizine	Procholo-perazine Pormethazine	Dexamethasone
Psycho-logical Emotional	Anxiolytic	Diazepam	Midazolam Lorazepam	Reassurance

* Use of multivitamins at conception decreases the incidence of nausea and vomiting during pregnancy.

† Anticholinergic side effects can increase obstruction.

‡ At high doses, metoclopramide acts as a 5-HT_3 antagonist.

** Avoid before 10 weeks of gestation because of risk for tetratogenic effects.

- Accupressure wristbands may be effective for short surgical procedures if applied prior to induction of anesthesia.

Assess unavoidable risk factors:

- For patients at low risk for PONV, no prophylaxis is necessary unless there is significant medical risk from vomiting, e.g., aspiration in a jaw-wiring procedure.
- For patients at moderate risk of PONV, consider monotherapy in adults or combination therapy in children or adults.
- For patients at high risk of PONV, give two or three antiemetics from different classes.

- If prophylaxis of PONV is undertaken, droperidol, prochlorperazine, promethazine, hydroxyzine, and the 5-HT_3 antagonists, e.g., ondansetron, dolasetron, and granisetron should be given at the end of surgery. Transdermal scopolamine and dexamethasone should be given at least 4 hours before the end of surgery and before induction, respectively.
- Droperidol, while effective for preventing PONV, carries a black box warning regarding the potential for QT prolongation and torsades de pointes development. It should not be used in patients with a prolonged QT interval or in those with the potential for developing a prolonged QT interval as in heart failure or if they are taking other medications known to prolong the QT interval. A 12 lead ECG is recommended prior to use.

If the patient experiences PONV, he or she should be assessed for contributing factors such as abdominal obstruction, surgical complications, and opiate use prior to using rescue medications. If the patient did not receive prophylaxis, a 5-HT_3 antagonist should be used. If the patient experiences PONV despite prophylaxis, an additional antiemetic from a different class should be given.

Drug points

- Avoid metoclopramide in younger (≤30-year-old) patients, especially at higher doses, because of risk of dystonic reactions.
- Long-term metoclopramide, prochlorperazine, and haloperidol use can cause extrapyramidal side effects in older patients.
- Promethazine and prochlorperazine are associated with rare reactions such as neuroleptic malignant syndrome and cholestataic jaundice.
- Anticholinergics antagonize the prokinetic effect of metoclopramide.
- Anticholinergics can cause a "high" in some patients. Avoid their use in patients with a current or past history of drug misuse.
- Tolerance to opioid-induced nausea and vomiting usually develops after 7–10 days. A prophylactic antiemetic can be used initially and the continued need reviewed after 7–10 days.
- Cannabinoids and the neurokinin-1 receptor antagonist aprepitant are also used in certain situations, such as for chemotherapy-induced nausea and vomiting.

Further reading

American College of Obstetrics and Gynecology (2004). ACOG Practice Bulletin: nausea and vomiting of pregnancy. *Obstet Gynecol* **103**:803–815.

American Gastroenterological Association (2001). American Gastroenterological Association Medical position statement: nausea and vomiting. *Gastroenterology* **120**:261–262.

American Gastroenterological Association (2001). AGA technical review on nausea and vomiting. *Gastroenterology* **120**:263–286.

Gan TJ, Meyer T, Apfel CC, et al. (2003). Consensus guidelines for managing postoperative nausea and vomiting. *Anesth Analg* **97**:62–71.

Gan TJ, Meyer T, Apfel CC, et al. (2007). Society for Ambulatory Anesthesia guidelines for the management of postoperative nausea and vomiting. *Anesth Analg* **105**:1615–1628.

Kris MG, Hesketh PJ, Somerfield MR, et al. (2006). American Society of Clinical Oncology guideline for antiemetics in oncology: Update 2006. *J Clin Oncol* **24**:2932–2947.

Basic microbiology

Microorganisms are classified in many ways. The most important classifications are as follows:

- Category—viruses, bacteria, fungi, and protozoa
- Genus— the second most specific grouping that the microorganism belongs to, such as *Staphylococcus*
- Species—the specific name, such as *Staphylococcus aureus*

To correctly name a microorganism, both the genus and the species name must always be used, e.g., *Staphylococcus aureus* and *Haemophilus influenzae*. The genus name may be abbreviated with its first initial, as in *S. aureus* and *H. influenzae*. Some common bacteria are abbreviated informally, such as "*H. flu*".

Identifying microorganisms

To correctly diagnose and treat an infection, the microorganism must be identified. This is usually done by examining samples of blood, sputum, wound sites, feces, and other sites in various ways.

Microscopy

The sample is examined under the microscope. Sometimes the organism can easily be seen and identified, as with some helminths (worms) and their ova (eggs).

Dyes are used to stain cells so that they can be seen more easily. In differential staining, cells with different properties stain differently and can be distinguished.

Bacteria are divided into two groups according to whether they stain with the Gram stain. The difference between gram-positive and gram-negative bacteria lies in the permeability of the cell wall when treated with a purple dye followed by a decolorizing agent. Gram-positive cells retain the stain, whereas gram-negative cells lose the purple stain and appear colorless, until stained with a pink counterstain, which also stains the background pink (see Fig. 15.5).

Since gram-positive organisms stain purple against this pink background, they are somewhat easier to see. However, if the Gram stain is not performed correctly, gram-negative organisms can stain purple (if under-decolorized) and gram-positive ones can show as pink (if over-decolorized).

Some bacteria can stain either way, such as *Acinetobacter* species, which are generally gram-negative but may stain as gram-positive. Other organisms, such as fungi, may also be revealed by a Gram stain.

Mycobacteria have waxy cell walls and do not readily take up the Gram stain. Thus a different staining technique is used and the sample is tested to see if it withstands decolorization with acid and alcohol. Mycobacteria retain the stain and thus are known as acid-fast bacilli (AFB), whereas other bacteria lose the stain.

Examination of stained films allows the shape of the cells to be seen, which can aid in identification.

Bacteria are classified as follows:

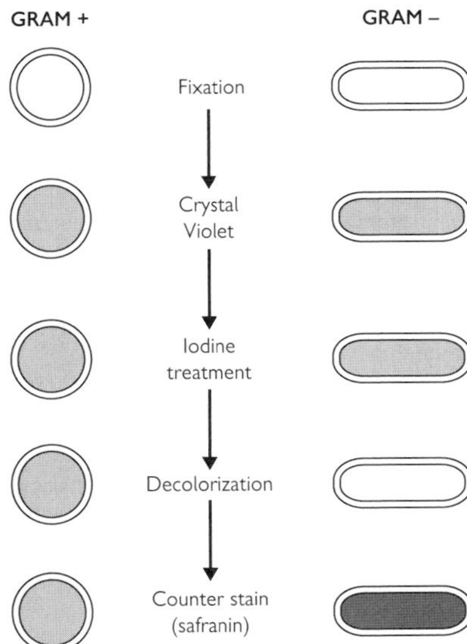

Figure 15.5 The Gram staining procedure.

- Cocci (spherical, rounded)—e.g., streptococci
- Bacilli (straight rod)—e.g., *Pseudomonas* species
- Spirochetes (spiral rod)—e.g., *Treponema* species
- Vibrios (curved, comma-shaped)—e.g., *Vibrio cholerae*

Coccobacilli also exist, such as *Acinobacter* and *Moraxella* species. Since they resemble both cocci and bacilli to a certain extent, they may be reported as cocci, bacilli, or coccobacilli.

For most sites of infection, Gram stains also reveal important data about how the host is reacting to a suspected infection. White blood cells (WBCs) can also be seen on Gram stain—high numbers of WBCs increase the index of suspicion that an infection is present, whereas low or no WBCs can substantially decrease clinical suspicion.

The major exception to this is with blood cultures, where Gram stains are only performed on bacteria that are cultured, not the initial sample, where red blood cells would dominate the stain.

Culture

Bacteria and fungi can be grown on the surface of solid, nutrient media. Colonies of many thousands of the microorganism can be produced from a single cell. Colonies of different species often have characteristic appearances, which aid in identification.

For most species, it takes 12–48 hours for a colony to develop that is visible to the naked eye. Some organisms (e.g., mycobacteria, such as *Mycobacterium tuberculosis*) multiply much more slowly and can take several weeks to develop.

Gram stains and culturing are *both* important for diagnosing an infection. Gram stains give information about what the site of infection is like, whereas cultures report on the type of organisms that are present. Interpreting one without the other can be problematic.

For example, patients on ventilators almost invariably become colonized with bacteria at some point. Once this occurs, they will have positive sputum cultures for those bacteria, even though the bacteria may not be causing infection. A Gram stain showing many WBCs and the bacteria is more indicative of infection (pneumonia, in this case) than a Gram stain with no WBCs, which may demonstrate that colonization has taken place.

Samples can be grown in an environment in which O_2 has been excluded. Bacteria that grow in the absence of O_2 are known as *anaerobes*, and bacteria that need O_2 to grow are *aerobes*. Some bacteria can grow in both environments, though they generally prefer one or the other.

Bacteria are often described as a combination of their Gram staining, shape, and anaerobic or aerobic characteristics. This helps to narrow the range of bacteria under consideration before lengthier tests identify the individual organism (see Table 15.69).

Other tests used to identify the organism include the following:

- Detection of microbial antigen
- Detection of microbial products, e.g., toxin produced by Clostridium difficile
- Gene probes
- Polymerase chain reaction (PCR)

Discussion of these tests is beyond the scope of this section. For further information, the reader is referred to microbiology texts.

Table 15.69 Examples of pathogens from various types of bacteria

Gram-positive cocci	**Gram-negative cooci**
Staphylococci	*Neisseria meningitidis* (meningitis)
Coagulase positive, e.g., *S. aureus*	*Neisseria gonorrheae* (gonorrhea)
Coagulase negative, e.g., *S. epidermidis*	*Moraxella catarrhalis*
Streptococci*	**Gram-negative bacilli (rods)**
β-hemolytic streptococci	Enterobacteriaceae
S. pyogenes (group A)	*Escherichia coli*
S. agalactiae (group B)	*Shigella species*
α-hemolytic streptococci	*Salmonella* species
Viridans group streptococci	*Citrobacter freundii, C. koseri*
S. pneumoniae (pneumococcus)	*Klebsiella pneumoniae, K. oxytoca*
Enterococci (nonhemolytic)†	*Enterobacter aerogenes, E. cloacae*
E. faecium	*Serratia marcesens*
E. faecalis	*Proteus mirabilis/vulgaris*
Anaerobic streptococci	*Morganella morganii*
Gram-positive bacilli (rods)	*Providencia* species
Aerobes	*Yersinia enterocolitica, Y. pestis*
Bacillus anthracis (anthrax)	*Y. paratuberculosis*
Corynebacterium diphtheriae	*Pseudomonas aeruginosa*
Listeria monocytogenes	*Haemophilus influenzae*
Nocardia species	*Brucella species*
Anaerobes	*Bordetella pertussis*
Clostridium species	*Pasterurella multocida*
C. botulinum (botulism)	*Vibrio cholerae*
C. perfringens (gas gangrene)	*Camphylobacter jejuni*
C. tetani (tetanus)	**Anaerobes**
C. difficile (diarrhea)	*Bacteroides* (wound infections)
Actinomyces	*Fusobacterium*
Actinomyces israeli, A. naeslundii	*Helicobacter pylori* (peptic ulcer disease)
A. odontolyticus, A.viscosus	**Mycobacteria**
Obligate intracellular bacteria	*Mycobacterium tuberculosis*
Chlamydia trachomatis	*M. bovis*
C. psittaci	*M. leprae (leprosy)*
C. pneumoniae	**"Atypical" mycobacteria**
Coxiella burnetii	*M. avium intracellulare*
Bartonella	*M. scrofulaceum, M. kansasii*
Ehrlichia	*M. marinum, M. malmoense*
Rickettsia (typhus)	*M. ulcerans, M. xenopi, M. gordonae*
Legionella pneumophilia	*M. fortuitum, M. chelonae, M.flaverscens*
Mycoplasma pneumoniae	*M. smegmatis-phlei*
	Spirochetes
	Treponema (syphilis; yaws; pinta)
	Leptospira (Weil disease; canicola fever)
	Borrelia (relapsing fever; Lyme disease)

*Streptococci are classified according to hemolytic pattern: α-, β-, or nonhemolytic) or by Lancefield antigen (A–G), or by species (e.g., *S. pyogenes*). There is crossover among these groups; the above is a generalization for the chief pathogens.

†Clinically, epidemiologically, and in treatment, enterococci behave unlike other streptococci.

Adapted with permission from Longmore M, Wilkinson IB, Rajagopalan S (2004). *Oxford Handbook of Clinical Medicine*, 6th ed. Oxford: Oxford University Press.

Modes of action of antimicrobials

To avoid unwanted toxic effects on human cells, most antimicobials have a mode of action that affects bacterial but not mammalian cells. The term for this property is *selective toxicity*.

There are many possible sites of action of antimicrobial agents. However, the most common mechanisms are as follows:

- Inhibition of cell-wall synthesis
- Alteration of the cell membrane
- Inhibition of protein synthesis
- Inhibition of nucleic acid synthesis

Inhibition of cell-wall synthesis

- Mammalian cells do not have a cell wall (only a cell membrane), so this mode of action does not affect mammalian cells.
- Penicillins, cephalosporins, and other beta-lactam antimicrobials interfere with the synthesis of a substance called peptidoglycan, which is an essential component of bacterial cell walls. Bacteria grow by continuously breaking down and reassembling the cell wall. Beta-lactams inhibit peptidoglycan synthesis, so the reassembly process is blocked, leading to cell lysis and cell death.
- Some antimicrobials active against *M. tuberculosis* work on the cell wall as well. Isoniazid and pyrazinamide inhibit different enzymes that are essential for synthesis of mycolic acids and the mycobacterial cell wall. Ethambutol works on another component of the mycobacterial cell wall called arabinogalactan to inhibit cell-wall synthesis.

Inhibition of protein synthesis

- The mechanism of protein synthesis is similar in bacterial and mammalian cells, but there are differences in ribosome structure (involved in protein synthesis) and other target sites. This decreases the risk of toxicity to mammalian cells.
- Tetracyclines, glycylcyclines, aminoglycosides, macrolides, streptogramins, lincosamides, oxazolidinones, and chloramphenicol all work by inhibiting synthesis of proteins essential to the growth and reproduction of bacteria.
- Most of these agents work by interfering with the binding of new amino acids onto peptide chains or by preventing the assembly of proteins.
- Aminoglycosides cause the misreading of messenger RNA (mRNA) and cause nonfunctional proteins to be created.

Inhibition of nucleic-acid synthesis

- Sulfonamides are structural analogues of para-amino benzoic acid (PABA). PABA is an essential precursor in bacterial synthesis of folic acid, which is necessary for the synthesis of nucleic acids. Mammalian cells are not affected, as they use exogenous folic acid.
- Trimethoprim is an inhibitor of dihydrofolic acid reductase, an enzyme that reduces dihydrofolic acid to tetrahydrofolic acid. This is one of the stages in bacterial synthesis of purines and, thus, DNA. Trimethoprim

inhibits dihydrofolic acid reductase 50,000 times more efficiently in bacterial cells than in mammalian cells.

- Sulfonamides and trimethoprim produce sequential blocking of folate metabolism and are synergistic when used together. The sulfonamide sulfamethoxazole is frequently used together with trimethoprim in a 5:1 ratio combination product (Bactrim®, Septra®).
- Bacteria use an enzyme called DNA gyrase to make the DNA into a small enough package to fit into the cell. This is called *supercoiling*. The quinolones inhibit DNA gyrase and supercoiling, leading to damage to the DNA and cell death.
- Rifampin inhibits bacterial RNA synthesis by binding to RNA polymerase; mammalian RNA polymerase is not affected.
- Nitroimidazoles (e.g., metronidazole) cause the DNA strand to break (cleavage).

Selection and use of antimicrobials

To treat or not to treat

The presence of microorganisms in a sample does not necessarily mean that there is infection. The human body hosts a wide range of microorganisms (mostly bacteria), but these rarely cause infection in an immunocompetent host. These organisms are known as *commensals* and some have an important role in host defenses.

For example, *C. difficile* is a pathogen that is normally suppressed by normal bowel flora. Eradication of the bowel flora (by broad-spectrum antibiotics) allows overgrowth of *C. difficile*, leading to diarrhea and sometimes pseudomembraneous colitis. Indiscriminate drug therapy can thus increase the risk of other infection.

Some organisms might be commensals in one part of the body and pathogens in another. *Escherichia coli* is part of the normal bowel flora, but if it gets into the bladder it can cause urinary tract infection.

Some pathogenic organisms can reside on the host without causing infection. This is known as *colonization,* and signs and symptoms of infection are absent. A skin or nasal swab positive for methicillin-resistant *S. aureus* (MRSA) does not usually require treatment in the absence of symptoms of infection.

Some infections are self-limiting and resolve without treatment. Many common viral infections resolve without treatment and, in any case, most do not have specific antiviral drugs that are effective.

Choice of therapy

If infection is confirmed or strongly suspected, appropriate therapy must be selected. Ideally, the pathogen is identified before antimicrobial therapy is started. However, identification of an organism by the laboratory through conventional methods usually takes a minimum of 24 hours and antimicrobial sensitivity tests can take a further 24 hours.

For some slow-growing organisms, such as mycobacteria, culture and sensitivity results can take several weeks. Thus, in most cases, therapy will be started using "best-guess" (empiric) antimicrobials and tailored after culture and sensitivity results are known (see Fig. 15.6).

Whenever possible, samples for culture and sensitivity tests should be taken before starting antimicrobial therapy so that growth is not inhibited. However, this delay might not be possible in very sick patients, such as those with suspected bacterial meningitis.

Factors that should be taken into account when selecting an antimicrobial are described below.

Clinical

- Does the patient have an infection that needs to be treated?
- Diagnosis or likely source of infection
- Anatomical site of infection
- Severity or potential severity of infection (and possible consequences, e.g., loss of prosthetic joint)

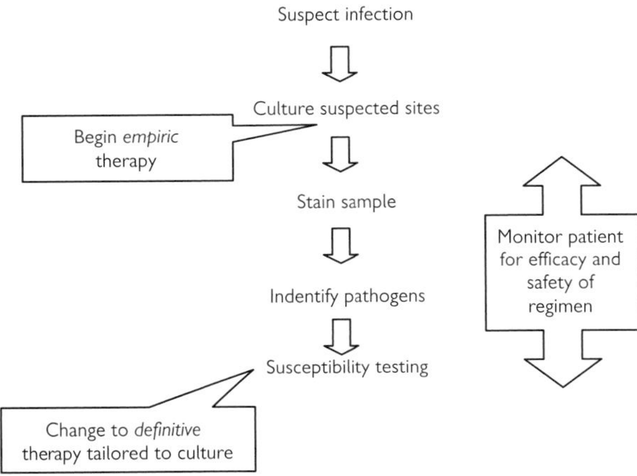

Figure 15.6 General approach to the treatment of infectious diseases.

- Patient's underlying condition (if any) and vulnerability to infection, e.g., neutropenic patients are more susceptible to sepsis
- Patient-specific factors, e.g., allergies, concurrent disease states, and renal function
- Does the infection require empiric therapy or can antimicrobials be delayed until culture and sensitivity results are available?
- Foreign material, necrotic tissue, and abscesses are relatively impervious to antimicrobials. Abscesses should be drained and necrotic tissue debrided. If possible, foreign material should be removed.

Microbiology

- What are the pathogens?
- Empiric therapy is based on presumed pathogens, according to epidemiology and knowledge of probable infecting organisms for the site of infection (see Table 15.70).
- Definitive therapy is based on pathogens identified by microscopy or culture.
- Sensitivity of organisms to antimicrobial agents (see Table 15.71)
- National and local resistance patterns
- Culture and sensitivity data

Pharmaceutical

Evidence of clinical efficacy

- Against the organism
- At the site of infection

Table 15.70 Common infectious diseases and empiric antibiotic therapy

Disease	Common pathogens	Typical empiric treatment
Meningitis	*Streptococci pneumoniae, Neisseria meningitis, Haemophilus influenzae.* Neonates: *Streptococcus agalactiae, Listeria monocytogenes.* Elderly, immunocompromised: *L. monocytogenes.* Neurosurgery: staphylococci, gram-negative rods (GNRs)	Ceftriaxone or cefotaxime + vancomycin. Add ampicillin IV in neonates, elderly, and immunocompromised for *L. monocytogenes.* Neurosurgery: ceftazidime or cefepime + vancomycin
Urinary tract infections (UTIs)	*E. coli*, other enteric GNRs, *Staphylococcus saprophyticus.* Hospital-acquired UTIs may involve *Pseudomonas aeruginosa* and enterococci.	*Cystitis* Trimethoprim/sulfamethoxazole, ciprofloxacin, levofloxacin, nitrofurantoin *Pyelonephritis* Ceftriaxone , cefotaxime, ciprofloxacin, levofloxacin
Otitis media	*S. pneumoniae, H. influenzae, Moraxella catarrhalis,* viruses	Amoxicillin/clavulanate, amoxicillin. Many patients do not require antibacterial therapy
Pharyngitis/ tonsillitis	*Streptococcus pyogenes*	Penicillin V (if positive for *Streptococcus*)
Sinusitis	*S. pneumoniae, H. influenzae, M. catarrhalis, Staphylococcus aureus,* anaerobes	Amoxicillin, trimethoprim/sulfamethoxazole
Pneumonia, community acquired (CAP)	*S. pneumoniae, H. influenzae, M. catarrhalis,* atypical pathogens such as *Mycoplasma pneumoniae, S. aureus.* CAP that develops with concurrent influenza is usually caused by *S. aureus*	*Inpatient* Ceftriaxone + azithromycin or a fluoroquinolone (not ciprofloxacin) *Outpatient* Azithromycin, clarithromycin, or a fluoroquinolone (not ciprofloxacin)

Pneumonia, hospital acquired (HAP)	Early onset (3–5 days in hospital): *S. pneumoniae, H. influenzae, M. catarrhalis*, methicillin-susceptible *S. aureus* (MSSA)	Ceftriaxone, cefotaxime, ampicillin/sulbactam, levofloxacin, moxifloxacin, or ertapenem
	Late onset (≥5 days): *Pseudomonas aeruginosa*, methicillin-resistant *S. aureus* (MRSA), *Acinetobacter baumanni*	Piperacillin/tazobactam, ceftazidime, cefepime, meropenem, or imipenem PLUS Tobramycin, amikacin, gentamicin, ciprofloxacin, or levofloxacin PLUS (if MRSA suspected) Vancomycin or linezolid
Endocarditis	*S. aureus* (MSSA or MRSA), *S. epidermidis*, viridans group streptococci, enterococci	Vancomycin
Cellulitis	*S. pyogenes, S. aureus* (particularly if an abscess is involved) MSSA has predominated, but MRSA is becoming prevalent in many community settings.	Inpatient: vancomycin or cefazolin Outpatient: cephalexin if streptococci or MSSA suspected; clindamycin, trimethoprim/sulfamethoxazole, doxycycline, minocycline, linezolid if MRSA is suspected If cause is not clear, clindamycin is a reasonable choice or combination therapy. Abscesses must be drained.
Septic arthritis	Monoarticular: *S. aureus*, streptococci Polyarticular: *Neisseria gorrorhoeae*	Monoarticular: vancomycin ± ceftriaxone Polyarticular: ceftriaxone
Osteomyelitis	*S. aureus*, streptococci, GNRs	Vancomycin, antistaphylococcal penicillin, cefazolin, or clindamycin. Organism identification is key to correct pharmacotherapy and osteomyelitis is generally not an emergency, so collecting culture results before therapy is important.

Table 15.70 *(Contd.)*

Disease	Common pathogens	Typical empiric treatment
Febrile neutropenia	*S. epidermidis, S. aureus, P. aeruginosa, E. coli, Klebsiella pneumoniae*, other GNRs, fungi	Cefepime, ceftazidime, imipenem, meropenem, or piperacillin/tazobactam. Add vancomycin if gram-positive pathogens (e.g., MRSA) are suspected.
Appendicitis	*E. coli, K. pneumoniae, Enterobacter spp.*, other GNRs, anaerobes	Cefoxitin, cefotetan, ampicillin/sulbactam. If appendix ruptured or is gangrenous: piperacillin/tazobactam, ertapenem, imipenem, meropenem
Peritonitis	*E. coli, K. pneumoniae, Enterobacter spp.*, other GNRs, anaerobes	Ceftriaxone, ciprofloxacin, levofloxacin
Invasive candidemia (fungal infection)	Candida albicans, Candida glabrata	Caspofungin, micafungin, anidulafungin, or fluconazole

Table 15.71 Invitro activity of antibacterials

✓ = usually sensitive ? = variable sensitivity X = usually resistant or inappropriate therapy

Note: These are generalizations. There are major differences between countries, areas and hospitals. Check local Public Health or Microbiology laboratories for local sensitivity patterns. Antibacterials may not be licensed to treat the bacteria for which they are active.

	Gram positives								Anaerobes			Gram negatives									Atypicals		
	Staphylococcus aureus MSSA	*Staphylococcus aureus* MRSA	*Staphylococcus epidermidis*	*Hemolytic streptococci (Strep A, C, G and Strep B)*	*Enterococcus faecalis*	*Enterococcus faecium*	*Streptococcus pneumoniae*	*Listeria monocytogenes*	*Clostridium perfringens*	*Clostridium difficile*	*Bacteroides fragilis*	*Neisseria meningitidis*	*Neisseria gonorrhoeae*	*Haemophilus influenzae*	*Escherichia coli*	*Klebsiella spp*	*Proteus mirabilis*	*Proteus vulgaris*	*Pseudomonas aeruginosa*	*Moraxella catarrhalis*	*Legionella spp*	*Mycoplasma pneumoniae*	*Chlamydia spp*
Penicillins																							
Penicillin V (oral)	X	X	X	✓	✓	?	✓	X	✓	X	X	X	?	X	X	X	X	X	X	X	X	X	X
Penicillin G (parenteral)	X	X	X	✓	✓	?	✓	✓	✓	X	X	✓	?	X	X	X	X	X	X	X	X	X	X
Ampicillin/ Amoxicillin	X	X	X	✓	✓	?	✓	✓	✓	X	X	✓	?	?	?	X	✓	✓	X	X	X	X	X
Amoxicillin/clavulanate	✓	X	✓	✓	✓	?	✓	X	✓	X	✓	X	?	✓	✓	?	✓	✓	X	✓	X	X	X
Oxacillin	✓	X	?	✓	X	X	✓	X	X	X	X	X	X	X	X	X	X	X	X	X	X	X	X
Piperacillin/ tazobactam	✓	X	?	✓	✓	?	✓	X	✓	X	✓	✓	✓	✓	✓	✓	✓	✓	✓	X	X	X	X
Cephalosporins																							
Cefazolin/Cephalexin	✓	X	?	✓	X	X	✓	X	X	X	X	X	X	X	✓	?	✓	X	X	X	X	X	X
Cefotaxime	✓	X	?	✓	X	X	✓	X	X	X	X	✓	?	✓	✓	✓	✓	✓	X	✓	X	X	X
Cefuroxime	✓	X	?	✓	X	X	✓	X	X	X	X	X	?	✓	✓	✓	✓	✓	X	✓	X	X	X
Ceftriaxone	✓	X	?	✓	X	X	✓	X	X	X	X	✓	✓	✓	✓	✓	✓	✓	X	✓	X	X	X
Ceftazidime	?	X	?	✓	X	X	?	X	X	X	X	?	?	✓	✓	✓	✓	✓	✓	✓	X	X	X

Table 15.71 *(Contd.)*

	Gram positives								Anaerobes			Gram negatives									Atypicals		
	Staphylococcus aureus MSSA	*Staphylococcus aureus* MRSA	Staphylococcus epidermidis	*Haemolytic streptococci (Strep A, C, G and Strep B)*	*Enterococcus faecalis*	*Enterococcus faecium*	*Streptococcus pneumoniae*	*Listeria monocytogenes*	*Clostridium perfringens*	*Clostridium difficile*	*Bacteroides fragilis*	*Neisseria meningitidis*	*Neisseria gonorrhoeae*	*Haemophilus influenzae*	*Escherichia coli*	*Klebsiella spp*	*Proteus mirabilis*	*Proteus vulgaris*	*Pseudomonas aeruginosa*	*Moraxella catarrhalis*	*Legionella spp*	*Mycoplasma pneumoniae*	*Chlamydia spp*
Carbapenems																							
Ertapenem	✓	X	✓	✓	?	X	✓	?	✓	X	✓	✓	✓	✓	✓	✓	✓	✓	X	✓	X	X	X
Meropenem/ Imipenem	✓	X	✓	✓	?	?	✓	X	✓	X	✓	✓	✓	✓	✓	✓	✓	✓	✓	✓	X	X	X
Macrolides/ Lincosamides																							
Azithromycin	✓	X	X	✓	X	X	✓	X	✓	X	X	✓	?	✓	X	X	X	X	X	✓	✓	✓	✓
Erythromycin	✓	X	?	✓	X	X	✓	X	X	X	X	✓	?	?	X	X	X	X	X	✓	✓	✓	✓
Clarithromycin	✓	X	X	✓	X	X	✓	X	✓	X	X	X	?	✓	X	X	X	X	X	✓	✓	✓	✓
Clindamycin	✓	X	X	✓	X	X	✓	X	✓	X	✓	X	X	X	X	X	X	X	X	X	X	X	X
Aminoglycosides																							
Amikacin	✓	✓	?	X	✓[1]	X	X	✓[1]	X	X	X	X	X	✓	✓	✓	✓	✓	✓	✓	✓	X	X
Gentamicin	✓	✓	?	X	✓[1]	✓[1]	X	✓[1]	X	X	X	X	X	✓	✓	✓	✓	✓	✓	✓	✓	X	X
Diaminopryimidines and sulphonamides																							
Trimethoprim/ sulfamethoxazole	✓	?	?	?	X	X	✓	X	X	X	X	✓	?	?	✓	✓	✓	X	X	✓	✓	X	✓
Trimethoprim	?	?	?	?	✓	X	?	X	X	X	X	?	X	?	✓	✓	X	X	X	X	✓	X	X
Quinolones																							
Ciprofloxacin	✓	X	✓	X	X	X	X	X	X	X	X	✓	✓	✓	✓	✓	✓	✓	✓	✓	✓	✓	✓
Levofloxacin	✓	X	✓	?	✓	X	✓	X	✓	X	X	✓	✓	✓	✓	✓	✓	✓	✓	✓	✓	✓	✓
Moxifloxacin	✓	X	✓	✓	✓	?	✓	X	✓	X	?	✓	✓	✓	✓	✓	✓	✓	X	✓	✓	✓	✓
Glycopeptides																							
Vancomycin (IV)	✓	✓	✓	✓	✓	?	✓	✓	✓	X[3]	X	X	X	X	X	X	X	X	X	X	X	X	X
Nitromidazoles																							
Metronidazole	X	X	X	X	X	X	X	X	✓	✓	✓	X	X	X	X	X	X	X	X	X	X	X	X
Oxazolidinones																							
Linezolid	✓	✓	✓	✓	✓	✓	✓	✓	✓	?	?	X	X	?	X	X	X	X	X	X	X	X	✓
Tetracyclines																							
Doxycycline	✓	?	X	?	X	X	✓	✓	✓	X	?	✓	?	✓	✓	?	X	X	X	✓	✓	✓	✓

	Gram positives								Anaerobes			Gram negatives									Atypicals		
	Staphylococcus aureus MSSA	*Staphylococcus aureus* MRSA	*Staphylococcus epidermidis*	*Haemolytic streptococci* (*Strep A, C, G and Strep B*)	*Enterococcus faecalis*	*Enterococcus faecium*	*Streptococcus pneumoniae*	*Listeria monocytogenes*	*Clostridium perfringens*	*Clostridium difficile*	*Bacteroides fragilis*	*Neisseria meningitidis*	*Neisseria gonorrhoeae*	*Haemophilus influenzae*	*Escherichia coli*	*Klebsiella spp*	*Proteus mirabilis*	*Proteus vulgaris*	*Pseudomonas aeruginosa*	*Moraxella catarrhalis*	*Legionella spp*	*Mycoplasma pneumoniae*	*Chlamydia spp*
Miscellaneous																							
Chloramphenicol	?	×	×	✓	?	?	✓	×	?	×	✓	✓	✓	✓	✓	?	?	?	×	✓	✓	✓	✓
Daptomycin	✓	✓	✓	✓	✓	✓	✓	×	×	×	×	×	×	×	×	×	×	×	×	×	×	×	×
Quinupristin/dalfopristin (Synercid®)	✓	✓	✓	✓	×	✓	✓	✓	✓	?		×	✓	?	×	×	×	×	×	✓	✓	✓	✓

[1] Sensitive if used synergistically with penicillins/glycopeptides

[2] IV vancomycin ineffective for *Clostridium difficile*

Bactericidal vs. bacteriostatic agents

- Bactericidal drugs are preferred in settings of inadequate host response, such as meningitis and neutropenia.
- Bacteriostatic drugs rely on phagocytes to eliminate the organisms and are adequate in most clinical infections.

Spectrum of activity

- Broad-spectrum antimicrobials might be required in empiric therapy or mixed infection.
- Narrow-spectrum antimicrobials are preferred if the organism has been identified.
- Indiscriminate use of broad-spectrum antimicrobials increases the risk of development of drug resistance and superinfection, such as *C. difficile* infection.
- Several antibiotics may be needed as empiric therapy if many types of organisms can cause the same infection, as in hospital-acquired pneumonia.

Appropriate route of administration

- Topical antimicrobials should be avoided except for superficial infections.
- Oral therapy is preferred in most settings and many antimicrobials have good bioavailability.
- IV therapy might be necessary in the following circumstances:
  - The necessary drug has poor oral bioavailability.
  - The patient is unconscious or unable to take oral drugs, as in states of poor absorption.
  - The infection is severe and the patient is acutely ill.
- Conversions from IV to oral antibiotic therapy are common. They can generally be categorized three ways:
  - *Equivalent*—the IV drug is exchanged for an equivalent oral dose of the same drug
  - *Parallel*—the IV drug is exchanged for a well-absorbed, equally effective antibiotic that is not the same as the IV drug.
  - *Step-down*—the IV drug is exchanged for a less-well absorbed, possibly narrower spectrum of activity oral drug. When step-down therapy is used, it is important that the patient is stable and has shown improvement from the infection.

Patient factors

- Adherence—will the patient take the medication?
- Concomitant disease states—does the patient have diseases that impair antibiotic efficacy, such as cancer and diabetes?

Pharmacokinetics

- Tissue penetration—will the antimicrobial get to the site of infection?
- Clearance in liver or kidney impairment
- Drug interactions

Adverse effects

- Avoid likely adverse effects that will result in patient harm, if possible. For example, nephrotoxic drugs such as aminoglycosides should be

avoided in patients with renal dysfunction. However, in the setting of severe infection, sometimes it is necessary to administer these drugs anyway.
- Ask patients about their allergy history. Be sure to inquire about the type of allergy that patients report. Many mild adverse effects (such as diarrhea or nausea) are labeled as allergies, leading to patients receiving less-preferred agents.

Duration of therapy
- Durations of therapy need to be long enough to ensure efficacy but short enough to decrease likelihood of resistance and adverse effects.
- Some infections have well-defined short durations of therapy, such as uncomplicated cystitis (urinary tract infection), which is often treated for 3 days.
- Infections involving poorly perfused tissue, such as bone, synthetic material, and heart valves, may require weeks to months of therapy.

Combination antimicrobial therapy

Combination antimicrobial therapy is prescribed for certain indications:
- To give a broad spectrum of activity in empiric therapy—especially in high-risk situations, such as neutropenic fever or nosocomial sepsis
- To treat a mixed infection, if one drug does not cover all possible pathogens
- To achieve a synergistic effect and increase efficacy, e.g., ampicillin and gentamicin in treatment of enterococcal endocarditis. Relatively low doses of gentamicin are used, decreasing the risk of nephrotoxicity.
- To decrease the probability of the emergence of drug resistance. The treatment of TB requires a minimum of two drugs, and antiretroviral pharmacotherapy for HIV requires a minimum of three drugs.
- To restore or extend the spectrum of activity by including an enzyme inhibitor, e.g., piperacillin (a beta-lactam) and tazobactam (a beta-lactamase inhibitor). Tazobactam coadministration allows piperacillin to work against bacteria that could otherwise destroy it.

Penicillin and hypersensitivity with other beta-lactams

Up to 10% of people are allergic to penicillins. A large majority of patients who report a penicillin allergy are negative by skin testing, however, which evaluates IgE-mediated sensitivity. It has been widely reported that 10% of people who are allergic to penicillin are also allergic to cephalosporins, though this is an overestimate.

Cross-reactivity between cephalosporins and penicillins is not common but needs to be taken seriously because it does occur. Early estimates of cross-reactivity between penicillin and carbapenem allergies have also been shown to be an overestimate.

If a patient had a serious, IgE-mediated reaction to a penicillin, such as hives, difficulty breathing, or anaphylaxis, then beta-lactams should be avoided if possible (with the possible exception of aztreonam). If the penicillin allergy is relatively mild, such as rash without hives, then other beta-lactams can be prescribed cautiously.

Some patients state that they have had an allergic reaction when they have really only had nausea or a headache. This is not drug allergy, and it is safe to use penicillins and other beta-lactams in these patients.

Ampicillin and amoxicillin can cause rashes in patients who have had glandular fever or leukemia or are HIV positive. This is not a true allergic reaction; penicillins can be used in these patients.

Monitoring therapy

It is essential to monitor and review antimicrobial therapy regularly, to ensure that treatment is working, de-escalate to more narrow-spectrum antibiotics as culture results return, and avoid inappropriate continuation of therapy.

The pharmacist should monitor the following parameters:

- Temperature should revert to normal (~98.6°F for most patients). Note: drug hypersensitivity is a common cause of persistent pyrexia.
- Pulse, BP, and respiratory rate revert to normal
- Normalization of white cell count
- Resolution of symptoms such as local inflammation, pain, malaise, GI upset, headache, and confusion, as appropriate for the infection

Reasons for treatment failure

- Wrong antimicrobial
- Wrong diagnosis
- Drug resistance
- The isolated organism is not the cause of the disease.
- Treatment started too late
- The wrong dose, duration, or route of administration
- Lack of patient adherence
- Inadequate source control (e.g., infected catheter not removed)
- Inadequate host defenses

Antimicrobial prophylaxis

Indiscriminate and prolonged courses of antimicrobials should be avoided. However, in some situations short- or long-term antimicrobial prophylaxis is appropriate to prevent infection (and thus further courses of antimicrobials).

Surgical prophylaxis

Antibacterial drugs are given to decrease the risk of the following:

- Wound infection after potentially contaminated surgery, such as GI or genitourinary surgery and penetrating abdominal trauma
- Infection of implanted material, such as prosthetic joints
- Endocarditis in patients with damaged or prosthetic heart valves who are undergoing high-risk procedures, such as dental surgery. This has not been proven to be effective, and new guidelines de-emphasize this common practice.

It is important that there are adequate concentrations of antibacterials in the blood *at the time of incision* ("knife-to-skin time") and *throughout* surgery. Thus, it is important to administer antibacterials at an appropriate time (usually 30–60 minutes) before surgery starts and repeat doses of short-acting antibacterials if surgery is delayed or prolonged.

It is rarely necessary to continue antibacterials after wound closure. More prolonged therapy is effectively treatment rather than prophylaxis.

Cephalosporins (with metronidazole if anaerobic coverage is necessary) are the antibacterials most commonly used for surgical prophylaxis. Vancomycin is used for patients with proven or suspected MRSA colonization. Drugs are usually administered by IV infusion to ensure adequate levels at the critical time.

Medical prophylaxis

Medical prophylaxis is appropriate for specific infections and for high-risk patients, as follows:

- Contacts of sick patients, e.g., meningitis and TB
- Immunosuppressed patients, e.g. organ-transplant recipients, HIV-positive patients, and splenectomy patients
- Malaria
- Postexposure prophylaxis, following exposure to HIV or hepatitis B

Further reading

Bratzler DW, Houck PM, et al. (2004). Antimicrobial prophylaxis for surgery: an advisory statement from the National Surgical Infection Prevention Project. *Clin Infect Dis* **38**:1706–1715.

Optimizing antimicrobial use

As the pace of new antimicrobial development has slowed, the need to optimize use of current antimicrobials has increased. Guidelines published by the Infectious Diseases Society of America emphasize the role that pharmacists have in antimicrobial stewardship, particularly on multidisciplinary teams in hospitals.

Pharmacists outside of these teams can play also a major role in improving antimicrobial use by evaluating prescriptions for appropriateness, informing patients about the role of antimicrobial therapy (or lack of it), and answering common questions about infectious diseases. For example, as first-line health-care practitioners, community pharmacists can be instrumental in educating patients about recommended vaccinations or that not every sniffle requires an antibiotic.

Strategies for antimicrobial stewardship

- Emphasize the establishment of a correct diagnosis, to avoid treating patients who are not truly infected
- De-escalation of empiric broad-spectrum to narrow-spectrum therapy as culture results become available
- Control sources of infections as appropriate, such as draining abscesses and removing infected invasive devices such as catheters
- Use improved systems for resistance testing and better communication of resistance data in hospital and community settings, to enable better directed therapy
  - Avoid continued use of ineffective drugs
  - Re-culture patients without clinical improvement
- Speed the diagnosis of infection, to decrease the amount of unnecessary empiric therapy
- Ensure that empiric therapy considers the following adjustments, as necessary:
  - Therapy is stopped if infection is ruled out.
  - Therapy is changed, as necessary, when culture results are available.
- Produce antimicrobial prescribing policies and promote adherence to guidelines
- Avoid unnecessary or prolonged use of broad-spectrum antimicrobials
- Appropriate use of antimicrobials for surgical prophylaxis, including avoiding prolonged courses
- Improve patient education, emphasizing the correct use of antimicrobials and that some infections do not require antimicrobial therapy

Points to consider when reviewing a prescription for an antimicrobial

- Is it the right choice for the infection (or appropriate empiric therapy)?
- Does it comply with local policies and restrictive practices?
- Could a narrower-spectrum antimicrobial be used?
- Will the antimicrobial be distributed to the target (infected) organ?
- Is the dose correct, taking into account the following:
  - Renal impairment

    - Type of infection
    - Patient weight
- Are therapeutic drug monitoring (TDM) and subsequent dose adjustments required?
- Is the route of administration appropriate?
- Is the duration of therapy appropriate?
- Does the patient understand the dosing instructions and importance of completing the course?

Further reading

Dellit TH, Owens RC, McGowan JE, et al. (2007). Infectious Diseases Society of American and Society for Healthcare Epidemiology of America guidelines for developing an institutional program to enhance antimicrobial stewardship. *Clin Infect Dis* **44**:159–177.

MacDougall C, Polk RE (2005). Antimicrobial stewardship programs in health care systems. *Clin Microbiol Rev* **18**(4):638–656.

Antimicrobial resistance

Resistance is an almost inevitable consequence of antimicrobial use. While bacteria, viruses, or other microorganisms reproduce, mutations can spontaneously occur. These mutations might provide some protection against the action of certain antimicrobials. "Survival of the fittest" means that when these microorganisms are exposed to antimicrobials, the fully sensitive ones are suppressed but resistant ones survive, reproduce, and become the dominant strain.

Mutations that lead to resistance may or may not also lead to decreased microbial fitness, in which the organism is more resistant to antimicrobials but at an expense to its normal physiology, such as slowed growth. Partially for this reason, health-care settings with higher degrees of antibiotic use, such as hospitals, have higher degrees of resistance than those with less antibiotic use, such as in most community settings.

Many clinicians find antimicrobial resistance confusing, but there are only a few basic mechanisms by which the vast majority of resistance is conferred.

Mechanisms of resistance

1. Decreased intracellular concentrations

Through this mechanism, less antibiotic is available to affect the microorganism. There are two ways through which this can happen:

1) Change in cell-wall permeability decreases the ability of the antibiotic to enter the cell.
   - The relatively simple cell wall of gram-positive bacteria makes them inherently more permeable; therefore this resistance mechanism is more common in gram-negative bacteria.

2) Efflux pumps
   - These pumps are thought to contribute to normal functions of cells, but they can also pump antimicrobials from the cell.

2. Enzymatic inactivation

Beta-lactamases, which destroy various beta-lactams, are the most notable example of this.

3. Target site alterations

- Alteration of penicillin-binding proteins leads to resistance to penicillins.
- Changes in the structure of the enzyme reverse transcriptase in HIV leads to resistance to reverse transcriptase inhibitors.

Microorganisms can develop multiple resistance mechanisms and express them simultaneously. Sometimes just one type of resistance does not lead to antibiotic failure, and multiple mechanisms are required for clinically relevant resistance.

Implications of antimicrobial resistance

Antimicrobial resistance leads to the following:

- Increased morbidity
  - Patients might be sicker for longer.
  - Increased length of hospital stay

  - Alternative antimicrobials may have more adverse effects
  - Residential placements might be difficult given the risk of transmission
  - Isolation and institutionalization
- Mortality
  - Higher rates of incorrect empiric therapy are seen with resistant organisms.
  - Choosing an ineffective empiric therapy can lead to higher mortality in many infections.
- Cost
  - Newer, potentially more expensive antimicrobials might have to be used.
  - Extended hospital stay
  - More nursing time
  - In some cases, equipment might have to be discarded.

New strains of resistant bacteria are appearing at an alarming rate. Within the hospital environment, MRSA has been a problem for many years but the emergence of vancomycin-resistant *Staphylococcus aureus* (VRSA) and community-associated MRSA (CA-MRSA) is of significant concern. Other increasingly problematic resistant organisms include the following:

- Vancomycin-resistant enterococci (VRE)
- Gram-negative bacilli that produce extended-spectrum beta-lactamases (ESBLs), such as *Klebsiella pneumoniae*
- *Acinetobacter baumanii*

At present, there are agents available to treat most of these resistant organisms, but they tend to be expensive and some have a higher risk of side effects. The production of new drugs is not keeping up with development of new resistant bacteria and the possibility of resistant species emerging for which there is no antibacterial therapy available is very real.

Measuring resistance

In vitro resistance tests generally require the organism to be cultured in the presence of antimicrobials.

Disk diffusion

Disk diffusion involves culturing bacteria on an agar plate that has had samples (impregnated disks) of antibiotic placed on it. If there is no growth around the antibiotic disk within a predetermined range, the bacteria are considered susceptible to the antibiotic, but if the bacteria grow around the sample within the range, this means they are resistant to an extent. The degree of susceptibility is determined by the *zone of inhibition* —larger zones show greater susceptibility.

Broth dilution

The gold standard of susceptibility testing is broth dilution. This involves inoculating a culture medium that contains serial dilutions of antibiotic solution with the bacteria of interest. Each concentration is twice as high as the next, and the lowest concentration with no visible growth is the minimum inhibitory concentration (MIC). The MIC is then compared to a table of standards to determine whether it falls within the range of susceptible.

Broth dilution can be performed by automatic systems, and many hospitals use these systems for simplicity.

E-test

The E-test works on principles similar to those of disk diffusion, but here an impregnated strip containing a single antibacterial at increasing concentrations along it is placed on an agar plate that has been inoculated with bacteria. The antibiotic within the strip inhibits bacterial growth to various extents depending on the concentration.

The number at which growth intersects with the E-test is the MIC. E-tests are easily performed and may be used to supplement data learned by other resistance testing.

Fungal susceptibility testing

The above techniques are also used to determine antifungal susceptibility, although fewer institutions perform this testing regularly for fungi. The fungi most often tested are species of yeasts in the *Candida* genus.

HIV resistance testing

Antiviral susceptibility testing is problematic and most frequently performed with HIV. Two types of HIV susceptibility testing are available: phenotypic and genotypic.

Phenotypic testing involves culturing the HIV virus and testing its susceptibility to various antiretrovirals. In genotypic testing, samples of the virus obtained from the patient are tested for the presence of certain mutations that predict antiretroviral resistance. This allows the clinician to determine which drugs are most likely to work for the patient.

Risk factors for antimicrobial resistance

Excessive and inappropriate antimicrobial use results in selective pressures that facilitate the emergence of resistant microorganisms. It has been estimated that up to 50% of antimicrobial use is inappropriate. Unnecessary antimicrobial use contributes to resistance without any clinical gain. This includes the following:

- Use of antimicrobials for infection that is trivial or self-limiting
- Use of antibacterials to treat infection of viral origin, such as the common cold
- Overly long antimicrobial prophylaxis or treatment courses

Even appropriate antimicrobial therapy is increasing worldwide, for the following reasons:

- Higher numbers of severely ill hospital patients
- More frequent use of invasive devices and procedures
- Presence of more severely immunocompromised patients in hospitals and the community, due to an organ transplantation, successful cancer therapy, and other reasons

Strategies to decrease or contain antimicrobial resistance include the following:

- Prevention of infection through the following mechanisms:
  - Vaccination
  - Prophylaxis in appropriate populations
  - Careful use of invasive devices.
  - Good hygiene
- Limiting dissemination of antimicrobial-resistant organisms
- Limiting antimicrobial use to when necessary
- De-escalation of empiric broad-spectrum therapy

Further reading

Department of Health and Human Services, Centers for Disease Control and Prevention, Antibiotic Resistance. Available at : http://www.cdc.gov/drugresistance/index.htm

Madaras-Kelly K (2003). Optimizing antibiotic use in hospitals: the role of population-based antibiotic surveillance in limiting antibiotic resistance. *Pharmacotherapy* **23**(12):1627–1633.

Nicasio AM, Kuti JL, Nicolau DP. (2008). The current state of multidrug-resistant gram-negative bacilli in North America. *Pharmacotherapy* **28**(2):235–249.

Shlaes DM, Gerding DN, John JF Jr, et al. (1997). Society for Healthcare Epidemiology of America and Infectious Diseases Society of America Joint Committee on the Prevention of Antimicrobial Resistance: guidelines for the prevention of antimicrobial resistance in hospitals. *Clin Infect Dis* **25**:584–599.

Infection control

Infection control is important in hospital and community residential facilities for the following reasons:

- To prevent cross-transmission of infection
- To prevent the spread of resistant microorganisms

Special attention should be paid to infection control in areas where patients are most vulnerable and antimicrobial resistance is most likely:

- Intensive care units
- Neonatal units
- Burns wards
- Vascular wards
- Units treating immunocompromised patients

Special attention should also be paid to infection control where procedures or devices make patients more vulnerable:

- Urinary catheters
- Intravascular devices
- Surgical procedures
- Respiratory care equipment
- Enteral or parenteral feeding

Infection control should be an integral part of the culture of any institution. This requires the following considerations:

- An infection control lead clinician or nurse oversees infection control practice.
- There are written procedures for infection control.
- Staff education and training on infection control procedures are provided.
- There are adequate supplies and facilities, such as the availability of aprons and gloves, particularly in areas of isolation.
- Additional infection control requirements, as necessary, for individual patients are documented.
- Health-care staff are immunized (or offered immunization) for hepatitis B, varicella, and influenza.
- There are written procedures for managing occupational exposure to blood-borne viruses and staff are made aware of these procedures.

Universal precautions

Strict attention to hygiene is essential. All body fluids and contaminated equipment, including linen, from all patients should be handled as if infected. This is known as *universal precautions* and includes taking appropriate measures to ensure the following:

- Prevent contamination, e.g., wearing apron and gloves and bagging dirty linen
- Dispose of waste safely, e.g., use of clinical waste bins and sharps boxes
- Protect staff against occupational exposure to blood-borne viruses (e.g., hepatitis B and C, and HIV)

Isolation of patients

It might be necessary to treat patients in isolation in the following circumstances:

- They are a potential source of resistant or dangerous infection, such as with MRSA, *C. difficile* diarrhea, tuberculosis, and multidrug-resistant gram-negative organisms.
- They are particularly vulnerable to infection, e.g., severely neutropenic patients and those with transplanted organs. These patients may be placed in units with more strict infection-control procedures to protect them from otherwise routine exposures that could be dangerous.

Isolation procedures include the following:

- Treating patients with diseases that can be spread via respiratory droplets (e.g., tuberculosis, influenza) in negative-pressure rooms, where air from the inside of the room does not enter the hallway
- Labeling rooms of patients with resistant organisms to warn health-care practitioners and visitors that extra precautions must be taken
- Wearing protective clothing when in contact with the patient. This includes staff who might be in contact with the patient elsewhere in the hospital.
- Ensuring that gowns, gloves, and other disposables are disposed of safely (usually bagged within the room) and are only used once
- Ensuring that visitors take appropriate measures to prevent cross-contamination—e.g., hand washing and wearing protective clothing for particularly vulnerable patients

Ultimately, no single precaution is as important as hand hygiene. Hand-washing can prevent the transmission of most resistant organisms from patient to patient. Alcohol-based solutions that are less time intensive than hand-washing are available in many health-care settings, but they do not work better than soap and water for most infections.

C. difficile spores are particularly resistant to these solutions, thus soap and water hand-washing should be performed by hospital personnel in contact with these patients.

Further reading

U.S. Department of Health and Human Services, Centers for Disease Control and Prevention. Infection Control Guidelines. Available at: http://www.cdc.gov/ncidod/dhqp/guidelines.html

Human immunodeficiency virus (HIV) and acquired immune deficiency syndrome (AIDS)

The acquired immune deficiency syndrome (AIDS) is caused by the retrovirus, human immunodeficiency virus (HIV). HIV attacks and destroys the CD4 lymphocyte, leading to a state of severe immunosuppression. AIDS is defined by the Centers for Disease Control and Prevention (CDC) as a CD4 cell count of <200 cells/mm^3 or a total percentage of CD4 lymphocytes <14%.

Epidemiology

In 2007, 33.2 million persons were living with HIV worldwide. Of these, 22.5 million persons were in Sub-Saharan Africa, with only 1.3 million persons in the United States. Newly infected HIV cases accounted for 2.5 million cases.

Pathogenesis

HIV attacks the CD4 cell by binding to the CD4 and the chemokine receptors. The chemokine receptor may be a CCR5, CXCR4, dual tropic (both receptors present), or mixed tropic. Once receptor binding has completed, HIV fusion occurs and the virus enters the CD4 cell. HIV then completes the replication cycle by using three enzymes: reverse transcriptase, integrase, and protease.

Reverse transcriptase allows the retrovirus to convert to the DNA provirus. Integrase incorporates the DNA provirus into the host genome. HIV protease is the final step in the life cycle, cleaving the gag-pol polypeptide into an infectious virion.

Highly active antiretroviral therapy (HAART)

The U.S. Department of Health and Human Services has developed an evidence-based guideline for clinicians on the treatment of adult and adolescent patients with HIV. The basis for treating HIV/AIDS is with antiretroviral therapy (see Table 15.72).

HAART is a combination of at least three different agents from two antiretroviral classes (see Table 15.73).

HAART should be initiated in the following patients:

- History of AIDS-defining illness
- CD4 count <350 cells/mm^3
- Pregnant women
- Persons with HIV-associated nephropathy
- Persons co-infected with hepatitis B virus (HBV), when HBV treatment is indicated (Treatment with fully suppressive antiviral drugs active against both HIV and HBV is recommended.).

For patients with CD4 counts >350 cells/mm^3, HAART initiation should be based on patient-specific issues as well as balancing the risks and benefits of early HAART use.

Table 15.72 FDA-approved antiretrovirals

Mechanism of action	Medication brand (generic)	Common dosage*	Elimination	Common adverse reactions
CCR5 inhibition	Maraviroc (Selzentry)	300 mg twice daily	Hepatic	Bronchitis, fever, hepatitis, rash
Fusion inhibition	Enfuvirtide (Fuzeon)	90 mg injection twice daily	Catabolic degradation	Injection site reactions
NRTIs	Abacavir (Ziagen)	600 mg once daily	Alcohol dehydrogenase	Hypersensitivity reaction
	Didanosine (Videx EC)	400 mg once daily (dose adjust for weight <60 kg)	Renal	Hepatitis, pancreatitis, peripheral neuropathy
	Emtricitabine (Emtriva)	200 mg once daily	Renal	Hyperpigmentation
	Lamivudine (Epivir)	300 mg once daily	Renal	Well tolerated
	Stavudine (Zerit)	40 mg twice daily (dose adjust for weight <60 kg)	Renal	Peripheral neuropathy
	Tenofovir (Viread)	300 mg once daily	Renal	GI intolerance, renal insufficiency
	Zidovudine (Retrovir)	300 mg twice daily	Renal; hepatic glucuronidation	Bone marrow suppression, GI intolerance, fatigue
NNRTIs	Delavirdine (Rescriptor)	400 mg three times daily	Hepatic	Rash, hepatitis
	Efavirenz (Sustiva)	600 mg once daily	Hepatic	Rash, hepatitis, CNS dysphoria
	Etravirine (Intelence)	200 mg twice daily	Hepatic	Rash
	Nevirapine (Viramune)	200 mg once daily for 14 days then 200 mg twice daily	Hepatic	Rash, hepatitis

Table 15.72 (*Contd.*)

IIs	Raltegravir (Isentress)	400 mg twice daily	Hepatic glucuronidation	GI intolerance
PIs	Atazanavir (Reyataz)	300 mg once daily with 100 mg ritonavir once daily	Hepatic	GI intolerance, hepatitis, indirect hyperbilirubinemia
	Darunavir (Prezista)	600 mg twice daily with 100 mg ritonavir twice daily	Hepatic	GI intolerance, hepatitis, hyperlipidemia, rash
	Fosamprenavir (Lexiva)	700 mg twice daily with 100 mg ritonavir twice daily	Hepatic	GI intolerance, hepatitis, hyperlipidemia, rash
	Indinavir (Crixivan)	800 mg every 8 hours	Hepatic	GI intolerance, hepatitis, hyperlipidemia, nephrolithiasis
	Lopinavir/ritonavir (Kaletra)	400 mg/100 mg twice daily	Hepatic	GI intolerance, hepatitis, hyperlipidemia
	Nelfinavir (Viracept)	1250 mg twice daily	Hepatic	GI intolerance, hepatitis, hyperlipidemia
	Ritonavir (Norvir)	100–200 mg once or twice daily	Hepatic	GI intolerance, hepatitis, hyperlipidemia
	Saquinavir (Invirase)	1000 mg twice daily with 100 mg ritonavir twice daily	Hepatic	GI intolerance, hepatitis, hyperlipidemia
	Tipranavir (Aptivus)	500 mg twice daily with 200 mg ritonavir twice daily	Hepatic	GI intolerance, hepatitis, hyperlipidemia, intracranial hemorrhage (rare), rash

Data from Panel on Antiretroviral Guidelines for Adult and Adolescents. Guidelines for the use of antiretroviral agents in HIV-1-infected adults and adolescents. Department of Health and Human Services. January 29, 2008; 1–128. Accessed June 22, 2008, from: http://www.aidsinfo.nih.gov/ContentFiles/AdultandAdolescentGL.pdf

* Note: All antiretrovirals may have altered dosing requirements when used as a part of HAART regimen. Drug interactions must be taken into consideration. The reader is referred to www.aidsinfo.nih.gov for a more detailed description of drug–drug interactions dosing requirements. Combination products are also available and are commonly used to improve medication adherence.

Table 15.73 HAART classifications

- CCR5 inhibitors
- Fusion inhibitors
- Reverse transcriptase inhibitors
- Nucleoside/tide reverse transcriptase inhibitors (NRTIs)
- Non-nucleoside reverse transcriptase inhibitors (NNRTIs)
- Integrase inhibitors (IIs)
- Protease inhibitors (PIs)

Data from: Panel on Antiretroviral Guidelines for Adult and Adolescents. Guidelines for the use of antiretroviral agents in HIV-1-infected adults and adolescents. Department of Health and Human Services. January 29, 2008; 1–128. Accessed June 22, 2008, from: http://www.aidsinfo.nih.gov/ContentFiles/AdultandAdolescentGL.pdf

HAART should be initiated with either one NNRTI and two NRTIs or a boosted PI with two NRTIs.

Preferred regimens (based on ease of use, efficacy and tolerability)

- Efavirenz OR
- Atazanavir/ritonavir OR
- Fosamprenavir/ritonavir twice daily OR
- Lopinavir/ritonavir twice daily WITH
  - Emtricitabine or lamivudine WITH
  - Abacavir OR
  - Tenofovir

Alternative regimens

- Nevirapine OR
- Atazanavir OR
- Fosamprenavir OR
- Fosamprenavir/ritonavir once daily OR
- Lopinavir/ritonavir once daily OR
- Saquinavir/ritonavir WITH
  - Emtricitabine OR lamivudine WITH
  - Didanosine OR
  - Zidovudine

Further reading

CDC. 1993 Revised classification system for HIV infection and expanded surveillance case definition for AIDS among adolescents and adults. MMWR 1992, 41 (No. RR-17).

Panel on Antiretroviral Guidelines for Adult and Adolescents. Guidelines for the use of antiretroviral agents in HIV-1-infected adults and adolescents. Department of Health and Human Services. January 29, 2008; 1–128. Available at http://www.aidsinfo.nih.gov/ContentFiles/AdultandAdolescentGL.pdf.

World Health Organization (2007). 2007 AIDS epidemic update. Joint United Nations Programme on HIV/AIDS (UNAIDS) and World Health Organization (WHO).

Opportunistic infections —HIV/AIDS

HIV infection results in a destruction of the CD4 lymphocytes and a chronic immunosuppressive state with the development of AIDS. The CDC defines AIDS as a CD4 count <200 cells/mm^3 or total CD4 percentage <14%.

Opportunistic infections (OIs) are the result of this generalized immunosuppression and occur with a higher severity and frequency. In the pre-highly active antiretroviral therapy (HAART) era, AIDS-associated morbidity and mortality resulted primarily from the development and progression of OIs. The incidence of OIs has declined dramatically since the introduction of HAART in 1996.

A consensus guideline supported by the National Institutes of Health (NIH), the CDC, and the HIV Medicine Association of the Infectious Diseases Society of America provides an evidence-based medicine approach for when pharmacotherapy interventions should be implemented for OI prevention and treatment.

Definitions

- *Primary prophylaxis:* The use of pharmacotherapy to prevent the first episode of an OI
- *Treatment of an OI:* The acute pharmacological management of an OI
- *Secondary prophylaxis* or *chronic maintenance therapy:* The prevention of a second occurrence or the use of pharmacotherapy to prevent the recurrence of an OI

Pneumonia

Bacterial pneumonia

- Higher incidence in the HIV-infected population
- Similar microbiologic etiology to that of non-HIV-infected patients, with some additional considerations:
- *Mycobacterium* tuberculosis
- *Pseudomonas aeruginosa*
- *Staphylococcus aureus*

Prevention recommendations

- Single dose of the 23-valent polysaccharide pneumococcal vaccine
  - If CD4 >200 cells/mm^3
  - <5 years since last dose unless CD4 <200 cells/mm^3 at time of administration

Influenza

Prevention recommendations

- Inactivated influenza vaccine annually
- Vaccinate all HIV-infected patients regardless of CD4 count

Pneumocystis jiroveci pneumonia (PCP)

- A fungus with protozoal characteristics
- Highest incidence with the following:
  - CD4 <200 cells/mm^3
  - CD4 percentage <14%
  - History of oropharyngeal candidiasis, or any AIDS-defining illness

Primary prevention

- Trimethoprim/sulfamethoxazole (TMP/SMX) single strength or double strength orally once daily (first-line)
- Dapsone 100 mg orally once daily (alternative, must be glucose-6-phosphate dehydrogenase [G6PD] deficiency negative)
- Atovaquone 1500 mg orally once daily (alternative)
- Aerosolized pentamidine 300 mg once monthly (alternative).

Treatment (duration 21 days)

- TMP/SMX, IV or oral, 15–20 mg/kg/day of trimethoprim component (divided in 3 to 4 daily doses) (first-line)
- Pentamidine 4 mg/kg IV once daily (alternative)
- Clindamycin 450–600 mg IV or oral, 3 to 4 times daily with primaquine 1–2 tablets orally once daily (alternative)
- TMP 15 mg/kg/day orally (divided in 3 to 4 daily doses) with dapsone 100 mg orally once daily (alternative)
- Atovaquone 750 mg orally twice daily (alternative for mild to moderate cases only)
- Addition of corticosteroids if high severity
  - paO_2 <70 mmHg OR
  - Arterial–alveolar gradient >35 mmHg
    —Prednisone 40 mg twice daily, days 1–5
    —Prednisone 40 mg once daily, days 6–10
    —Prednisone 20 mg once daily, days 11–21

Secondary prophylaxis (same as primary prevention)

Toxoplasma gondii encephalitis

- This is a protozoal infection primarily from reactivation of latent infection. The highest incidence of infection is among those with
- CD4 <100 cells/mm^3, and
- Toxoplasma IgG+

Primary prevention

- TMP/SMX DS orally once daily
- Dapsone 50 mg orally once daily with pyrimethamine 50 mg and leucovorin 25 mg orally once weekly (alternative).

Treatment (6 weeks)

- Sulfadiazine 1000 mg (<60 kg) or 1500 mg (≥60 kg) orally every 6 hours (preferred), with
- Pyrimethamine 200 mg loading dose orally, then 50 mg (<60 kg) or 75 mg (≥60 kg), with
- Leucovorin 10–25 mg orally once daily

Clindamycin 600 mg orally every 6 hours with the above treatment doses of pyrimethamine and leucovorin may be used as an alternative to sulfadiazine for sulfa-allergic patients.

Chronic maintenance therapy

- Sulfadiazine 2000–4000 mg orally daily divided into 2–4 daily doses, with
- Pyrimethamine 25–50 mg orally once daily, with
- Leucovorin 10–25 mg orally once daily

Clindamycin 300 mg orally every 6 hours with the above chronic maintenance doses of pyrimethamine and leucovorin may be used as an alternative to sulfadizine for sulfa-allergic patients

Disseminated *Mycobacterium avium* complex

- Multi-organ infection
- Diagnosis is a combination of signs and symptoms of active infection and positive cultures from sterile body fluids:
  - Blood
  - Bone marrow
  - Liver
  - Lymph nodes
- Highest incidence of infection with a CD4 <50 cells/mm^3

Primary prevention

- Azithromycin 1200 mg orally once weekly
- Clarithromycin 500 mg orally twice daily (Note: Use of either of these macrolide regimens will also be prophylactic against Bartonellosis.)

Treatment (12 months to indefinite treatment; depends on post-HAART immune reconstitution)

- Clarithromycin (drug of choice) 500 mg orally twice daily, or
- Azithromycin 500–600 mg orally once daily, with
- Ethambutol 15 mg/kg orally once daily, and ±
- Rifabutin 150–600 mg orally 3 times weekly or daily (dosing based on concomitant HAART regimen)

Chronic maintenance therapy

This is the same as treatment recommendations.

Mucocutaneous candidiasis

- Highest incidence with CD4 <200 cells/mm^3
- Primary sites of infection
  - Oropharyngeal or
  - Esophageal

Primary prevention

This is generally not recommended for the following reasons:

- Development of azole-resistant *Candida* species
- Drug–drug interactions
- Expense

Treatment

Oropharyngeal candidiasis (duration 7–14 days)

- Topical therapy including:
  - Clotrimazole troches 10 mg orally 5 times daily
  - Nystatin suspension 5 mL orally four to five times daily
  - Fluconazole 100 mg orally daily

Esophageal candidiasis (duration 14–21 days)

- Fluconazole 100–400 mg IV or orally daily

- Alternative therapies may be used (especially when fluconazole-resistant *Candida species* are suspected):
  - Amphotericin
  - Echinocandins
  - Itraconazole
  - Posaconazole
  - Voriconazole

Secondary prophylaxis

This is only recommended for patients with frequent or severe cases and is the same as treatment recommendations.

Cryptococcus

- Highest incidence with CD4 <50 cells/mm^3
- Primary sites of infection:
  - Meningitis (most common presentation)
  - Pneumonia

Primary prevention

- This is generally not recommended for the following reasons:
- No mortality benefit
- Development of treatment-resistant species
- Drug–drug interactions
- Expense

Treatment (minimum of 10 weeks)

- Amphotericin B deoxycholate 0.7 mg/kg IV daily for 2 weeks, or
- Amphotericin (lipid formulation) 4–6 mg/kg IV daily for 2 weeks, with
- Flucytosine 100 mg/kg/day orally (divided in four daily doses) for 2 weeks

After completion of the initial 2 weeks of therapy with sterilization of the cerebrospinal fluid, begin treatment with the following:

- Fluconazole 400 mg orally for 8 weeks

Chronic maintenance therapy

- Fluconazole 200 mg orally daily

Cytomegalovirus (CMV)

Disease usually occurs as reactivation of latent infection. It takes the following forms:

- Disseminated or
- Localized end-organ
  - Retinitis
  - Colitis
  - Esophagitis
  - Pneumonitis
  - Neurological manifestations
    —Dementia
    —Ventriculoencephalitis
    - Ascending polyradiculomyelopathy

- Highest incidence of infection
- CD4 <50 cells/mm,[3] and
- CMV IgG+

Primary prevention

This is generally not recommended for the following reasons:

- Development of CMV-resistant species
- No mortality benefit
- Expense

Treatment

- Retinitis (duration 14–21 days): for immediate site-threatening disease, a combination of the following:
  - IV ganciclovir 5 mg/kg twice daily, or oral valganciclovir 900 mg twice daily, with
  - Intraocular ganciclovir implant

Alternative options include IV foscarnet, IV cidofovir, or combination regimens, which depend on individual patient factors:

- Colitis/esophagitis (duration 21–28 days)
  - IV ganciclovir 5 mg/kg twice daily, or
  - IV foscarnet 90 mg/kg twice daily
  - Oral valganciclovir 900 mg twice daily if patient is able to ingest or absorb medication
- Pneumonitis
  - Similar to above regimens if patient is not responding to other co-infecting pathogens
- Neurological manifestations
  - IV ganciclovir 5 mg/kg twice daily with IV foscarnet 90 mg/kg twice daily

Secondary prevention

- Retinitis
  - IV ganciclovir 5 mg/kg once daily or
  - Oral valganciclovir 900 mg once daily
- Colitis/esophagitis
  - Not generally recommended
- Pneumonitis
  - Guidelines not established
- Neurological manifestations
  - IV ganciclovir 5 mg/kg once daily, or
  - Valganciclovir 900 mg once daily, and
  - IV foscarnet 90 mg/kg once daily

Hepatitis B virus

Primary prevention

All patients should be offered vaccine, regardless of current CD4 count.

- Three-dose IM vaccine series at 0, 1, and 6 months with either of the following:
  - Engerix-B (20 mcg/mL), or
  - Recombivax (10 mcg/mL)

Test for immunologic response at 1 month after completing series and repeat if inadequate response.

Immune reconstitution

Primary or secondary prophylaxis may be discontinued if the HIV-positive patient has immune reconstitution while receiving HAART. The reader is referred to the OI guidelines for specific recommendations.

Further reading

Guidelines for prevention and treatment of opportunistic infections in HIV-infected adults and adolescents. Recommendations of the National Institutes of Health (NIH), the Centers for Disease Control and Prevention (CDC), and the HIV Medicine Association of the Infectious Diseases Society of America. June 18, 2008, 1–286. Available at: www.aidsinfo.nih.gov/contentfiles/Adult_OI.pdf.

HIV post-exposure prophylaxis (PEP)

HIV transmission may occur via occupational (health-care personnel [HCP]) or nonoccupational exposures.

Occupational

There are only six documented cases of HIV transmission related to HCP occupational exposures. HCP exposures are classified as percutaneous (direct venipuncture or sharp instrument) or mucous membrane with or without nonintact skin.

The highest risk occurs with exposure to blood, tissue, or other infectious fluids including semen, vaginal or cervical secretions. Body fluids also considered infectious include cerebrospinal, synovial, pleural, peritoneal, pericardial, and amniotic fluids.

The risk of HIV transmission when exposed to blood via either percutaneously or mucous membrane is 0.3% and 0.09%, respectively. No definitive data are available for exposures to other body fluids, but the risk is thought to be significantly reduced compared to that of blood exposure.

The highest risk of HIV transmission occurs with a larger quantity of exposed blood (visible blood on needle), direct entry into an artery or vein, or a deep injury. PEP regimens are offered if an exposed health-care provider presents within the first 24 hours after exposure.

PEP pharmacotherapy regimens (28 days duration)

- Two-drug regimens; include two nucleoside/tide analogs (preferred)
  - Emtricitabine or lamivudine with either
  - Tenofovir or
  - Zidovudine
- Three-drug regimens; include two-drug regimen PLUS (preferred)
  - Lopinavir/ritonavir

Alternative regimens are available depending on the source patient's antiretroviral history and genotypic resistance pattern, but consultation with an expert in infectious diseases is recommended. For standard dosing recommendations, the reader is referred to the unit in this chapter on HIV management (HIV and AIDS, p. 566).

Whether a two- or three-drug regimen is recommended depends on the type of occupational exposure.

Percutaneous exposure

Less severe injury (solid needle or superficial injury)

- Two-drug regimen recommended if source patient has the following:
  - Asymptomatic HIV
  - Low HIV viral load (defined as <1500 copies/mL)
- Three-drug regimen recommended if source has the following:
  - Symptomatic HIV
  - High HIV viral load
  - AIDS
- If the source patient has an unknown HIV status (patient expired) or the source is unknown (needlestick from a sharps container) with no available body fluids for analysis:

    - No PEP is recommended
    - Consider two-drug regimen with discussion of benefits and risks to exposed HCP.
- If the source patient is HIV negative:
    - No PEP is recommended.

More severe injury

This type of injury involves a large-bore hollow needle, deep puncture, visible blood on the device, or a needle placed in the source patient's artery or vein.

- Three-drug regimen recommended for both
    - Asymptomatic HIV and
    - Symptomatic HIV
- If the source patient's HIV status is unknown, or body fluids are not available for testing:
    - No PEP is recommended.
    - Consider two-drug regimen with discussion about benefits and risk.
- If the source patient is HIV negative:
    - No PEP is recommended.

Mucous membrane and nonintact skin exposure

Small volume (a few drops)

- Two-drug regimen optional for either asymptomatic or symptomatic HIV
- Consider treatment based on discussion regarding benefits and risk.
- If the source patient's HIV status is any of the following:
    - Unknown (patient expired)
    - No available body fluids for analysis (blood splash from improperly disposed waste)
    - HIV negative
    - No PEP warranted

Counseling throughout the PEP treatment course and repeat HIV testing should be made available to all patients at the following intervals:

- Baseline
- 6 weeks
- 12 weeks
- 6 months

Resources available to case patients

- PEPline at http://www.ucsf.edu/hivcntr/Hotlines/PEPline
- Telephone: 888-448-4911

Nonoccupational

HIV exposure from high-risk behaviors including injection drug use, nonprotected sexual encounters, or exposure to other infectious body fluids may lead to HIV transmission. Abstinence, consistent safe sexual practices, and/or avoidance of using nonsterile injection devices are the most effective HIV prevention methods.

Nonoccupational HIV exposures are classified as mucosal, percutaneous, or parenteral contact with infectious body fluids including: blood, semen, vaginal/rectal secretions, breast milk, or other bloody fluid. Nonoccupational PEP (nPEP) regimens are offered if a patient presents within 72 hours after exposure.

nPEP pharmacotherapy regimens (28 days duration)

- Three-drug regimens (preferred)
  - Include one non-nucleoside reverse transcriptase inhibitor
  - Efavirenz with two nucleoside/tide analogs
  - Emtricitabine or lamivudine with
  - Tenofovir or zidovudine
- Include one protease inhibitor
  - Lopinavir/ritonavir with two nucleoside/tide analogs
  - Emtricitabine or lamivudine with
  - Zidovudine

Substantial HIV exposure

- This involves infectious body fluids with exposure to the following:
  - Eye
  - Mouth
  - Mucous membrane
  - Nonintact skin
  - Percutaneous
  - Rectum
  - Vagina
- Three-drug regimen recommended, if the source patient is HIV positive
- If HIV status unknown, individual discussion of the HIV exposure and antiretroviral risk/benefits should be considered.

Negligible HIV exposure

- This involves body fluids without blood contamination (nasal secretions, urine, saliva, sweat, and tears) with exposure to the following:
  - Eye
  - Mouth
  - Mucous membrane
  - Nonintact skin
  - Percutaneous
  - Rectum
  - Vagina
- No nPEP recommended

Alternative regimens are available depending on the source patient's antiretroviral history and genotypic resistance pattern, but consultation with an expert in infectious diseases is recommended. For standard dosing recommendations, the reader is referred to the unit in this chapter on HIV management (HIV and AIDS, p. 566).

Counseling throughout the nPEP treatment course and repeat HIV testing should be made available to all patients at the following intervals:

- Baseline
- 4–6 weeks
- 12 weeks
- 6 months

All patients should be counseled on risk-reduction behaviors during the follow-up period.

Further reading

Panlilio AL, Cardo DM, Grohskopf LA, Heneine W, Ross CR (2005). Updated U.S. Public Health Service Guidelines for the management of occupational exposures to HIV and recommendations for postexposure prophylaxis (2005). *MMWR Morb Mortal Wkly Rep* **54**(RR09):1–17.

Smith DK, Grohskopf LA, Black RJ, et al. (2005). Antiretroviral postexposure prophylaxis after sexual, injection-drug use, or other nonoccupational exposure to HIV in the United States. *MMWR Morb Mortal Wkly Rep* **54**(RR07):1–20.

Vaccine overview

Vaccines save more lives and prevent more deaths than any other medical advance in the last century. Vaccines are administered to prevent infections from occurring months, years, or decades in the future. Vaccine policies vary according to many factors, such as epidemiology of involved diseases, immunological characteristics of vaccines, sociological characteristics of patients and clinicians, likelihood of adverse effects, and costs associated with each factor.

Vaccination schedules are recommended by the Advisory Committee on Immunization Practices (ACIP) of the CDC. Current ACIP immunization schedules for children 0–6 years of age, 7–18 years of age, and adults are available from the CDC (http://www.cdc.gov/mmwr/). Pharmacists should always check the CDC Web site to determine the most up-to-date vaccination recommendations.

Principles of immunity

Immune-response mechanisms are categorized as humoral or cell-mediated. Humoral immunity involves antibodies, and cell-mediated immunity involves macrophages, other immune-presenting cells, and T lymphocytes.

Active immunity develops in response to infection or after administration of a vaccine or toxoid. Sufficient active immunity may take several weeks or months to induce, after which immunity is generally long-lasting.

Passive immunity is temporary immunity provided by antitoxins or antibodies from other living hosts. Passive immunity provides protection almost immediately but persists with the biological half-life of IgG.

Vaccinations available in the United States are live or inactivated compounds.

- *Live, attenuated vaccines* contain altered, weakened, or avirulent microorganisms that induce active immunity. Live vaccines are contraindicated in immunocompromised patients because of either drug therapy or diseases, and in patients with serious active infection. Caution should also be used when vaccinating individuals who live with immunosuppressed individuals, because of the risk of transmission between the vaccine recipient and the family member.
- *Inactivated vaccines* consist of killed, whole microbes, or isolated microbial components that induce active immunity. Inactivated vaccines are contraindicated in patients with serious active infections, such as tuberculosis. Immunosuppressed patients may not mount an adequate antibody response.

Vaccines for pediatrics

Childhood vaccination prevents 33,000 deaths and 14 million cases of disease, saves $10 billion in direct costs, and saves society $33 million in costs due to disability and lost productivity.

Diphtheria, tetanus, pertussis vaccine

DTaP vaccine is given in children <7 years of age, Tdap in those 11 years and older.

- Inactivated
- *Diphtheria* is caused by *Corynebacterium diphtheriae*, a bacterium of the nose and throat that is spread by coughing and sneezing. Severe illness characterized myocardial and nervous system damage as well as membranous inflammation of the upper respiratory tract and death may occur in those infected.
- *Tetanus* is caused by *Clostridium tetani*, a bacterium found in soil, dust, and manure that results in infection when in it comes into contact with an open wound. Tetanus manifests as neuromuscular dysfunction, rigidity, and painful skeletal muscle spasms. Although cases are infrequent and tetanus is not contagious, approximately 10% of cases are fatal.
- *Pertussis*, or whooping cough, is a highly contagious respiratory tract illness caused by *Bordetella pertussis*. Pertussis can cause serious and often fatal disease in infants under 6 months of age.

Immunization schedule

- DTaP: 0.5 mL intramuscularly (IM) at 2, 4, 6, and 15–18 months of age and then another booster dose between 4 and 6 years of age (before entry in school)
- Tdap: 0.5 mL IM at 11 years of age (before entry into 6th grade)

Poliovirus vaccine (IPV)

- Inactivated
- Enterovirus that results in poliovirus infections, which are generally asymptomatic or mildly symptomatic. Central nervous system involvement and paralysis may occur in 2% of those infected. Poliovirus has been eradicated in the United States but not in Third World countries.
- Immunization schedule: 0.5 mL subcutaneously (SC) or IM at 2, 4, 6–18 months of age and 4–6 years of age

Haemophilus influenzae type B (Hib) vaccine

- Inactivated
- Hib was the most frequent cause of bacterial meningitis in young children prior to universal vaccination policy. Fatality of Hib meningitis was 5%, with 35% of those infected having serious neurological sequelae such as seizures, deafness, and mental retardation.
- Immunization schedule: 0.5 mL IM at 2, 4, 6, and 12–15 months of age

Rotavirus vaccine

- Live
- Leading cause of severe acute gastroenteritis in infants and young children, accounting for 70,000 hospitalizations and 250,000 emergency room visits annually
- Two different vaccines are commercially available:
  - RotaTeq provides provides protection against serotypes G1, G2, G3, G4, and P1.
  - Rotarix provides protection against G1, G3, G4, and G9.

Immunization schedule

- RotaTeq: 2 mL orally at 2, 4, and 6 months of age
- Rotarix: 1 mL orally at 2 and 4 months of age

Measles, mumps, and rubella (MMR) vaccine

- Live, attenuated
- *Measles* is a highly contagious viral infection characterized by full body rash. Measles can cause pneumonia and encephalitis.
- *Mumps* is characterized by swelling of the cheeks and jaw, resulting in salivary gland inflammation. It may lead to aseptic meningitis, deafness, and orchitis.
- *Rubella* is generally mild if contracted but is extremely dangerous to a developing fetus, resulting in blindness, deafness, cardiac or neurological defects, or mental retardation.
- Measles, mumps, and rubella are transmitted through coughing, sneezing, or breathing.
- Contraindication: pregnancy, hypersensitivity to gelatin or neomycin
- Immunization schedule: 0.5 mL SC at 12–15 months and 4–6 years of age

Pneumococcal conjugate vaccine, 7-valent (PCV7)

- Inactivated
- *S. pneumoniae* is the leading cause of invasive disease in infants 1 month to 2 years of age. *S. pneumoniae* is responsible for pneumococcal meningitis and many cases of acute otitis media.
- Vaccine provides protection against *S. pneumoniae* serotypes 4, 6B, 9V, 14, 18C, 19F, and 23.
- Immunization schedule: 0.5 mL IM at 2, 4, 6, and 12–15 months of age

Varicella virus vaccine

- Live, attenuated
- Varicella-zoster virus causes chickenpox, a highly contagious disease of childhood. The primary manifestations are fever and 300–500 maculopapular or vesicular lesions. Although generally mild and self-limiting, varicella may result in complications such as bacterial superinfection, pneumonia, encephalitis, Reye's syndrome, and death.
- Contraindications: hypersensitivity to gelatin, anaphylaxis to neomycin, immunosuppression, pregnancy
- Immunization schedule: 0.5 mL SC at 12–15 months and 4–6 years of age (before entry into school)

Hepatitis A vaccine (HepA) (see Hepatitis unit, p. 524)

- Inactivated
- Immunization schedule: two doses of 0.5 mL between 12 and 24 months of age, given at least 6 months apart.

Hepatitis B vaccine (HepB) (see Hepatitis unit, p. 524)

- Inactivated
- Immunization schedule: 0.5 mL IM at birth, 1–2 and 6–18 months of age

Meningococcal conjugate vaccine (MCV4)

- Inactivated
- *Neisseria meningitidis* causes approximately 2000 cases of meningococcal disease in the United States each year, with a case fatality of 10% for meningitis and 40% for meningococcemia. Of survivors, 20% have permanent disabilities, including hearing loss, neurological damage, and limb amputations. Rates of meningococcal disease are highest in infancy, with a second peak occurring in adolescence and young adulthood.
- Vaccine provides protection against *N. meningitidis* serogroups A, C, Y, and W-135
- Immunization schedule: 0.5 mL IM at 11–12 years of age

Influenza virus vaccine, injection

- Inactivated
- Influenza is a respiratory illness that accounts for approximately 200,000 hospitalizations and 36,000 deaths annually. Young children are considered a high-risk population for developing serious influenza complications (e.g., pneumonia).
- Vaccination formulation is modified annually and provides protection against influenza types A and B.
- Contraindications: anaphylactoid or immediate reactions to eggs

Immunization schedule

- 6–35 months: 0.25 mL IM annually
- ≥36 months: 0.5 mL IM annually
  - Any previously unvaccinated child age 8 years and younger should receive 2 doses (in the amounts above) at least 1 month apart.

Influenza virus vaccine, nasal

- Live, attenuated
- Vaccination formulation is modified annually and provides protection against influenza types A and B.
- Contraindications: anaphylactoid or immediate reactions to eggs, asthmatics, and children 2–17 years of age receiving aspirin

Immunization schedule

- 0.1 mL into each nostril annually
- Children 2–8 years of age who are previously unvaccinated with any influenza virus vaccine should receive 2 doses at least 1 month apart.

Human papillomavirus (HPV) vaccine

- Inactivated
- HPV is responsible for the majority of cervical cancers (types 16 and 18) and genital warts (types 6 nd 11).
- Vaccine provides protection against HPV 6, 11, 16, and 18.
- Indicated for females only

Immunization schedule

- Three 0.5 mL IM injections for females between 9 and 26 years of age
- The second and third doses are given 2 and 6 months after the first injection.

Combination vaccines

A number of manufacturers have combined some of the standard pediatric vaccines into one product to reduce the number of vaccinations required in infants and young children. Consult individual package inserts for components and dosage schedules.

Missed vaccinations

- Recommendations for managing missed vaccinations (catch-up dosing) are provided by the CDC.

Further reading

CDC (2008). Recommended immunization schedules for persons aged 0–18 Years—United States, 2008. MMWR *Morb Mortal Wkly Rep* **57**(01);Q1–Q4.

Grabenstein JD (2008). *ImmunoFacts: Vaccines and Immunologic Drugs*. St. Louis, MO: Wolters Kluwer Health.

Vaccines for adults

Vaccination recommendations for adults are by the Advisory Committee on Immunization Practices (ACIP), the American Academy of Family Physicians, the American College of Obstetricians and Gynecologists, and the American College of Physicians.

Vaccine recommendations for adults are divided into two groups: those that are routinely recommended, and those that are recommended for individuals with select medical conditions.

Tetanus, diphtheria (Td) and tetanus, diphtheria, and acellular pertussis (Tdap) vaccine

- Tetanus and diphtheria (Td) is recommended every 10 years for all adults.
- One dose of Tdap should be substituted for Td to provide protection against pertussis.
- Tdap can be given as close as 2 years to Td in postpartum women, close contacts of infants <12 months of age, and all health-care workers with direct patient contact.

HPV (see HPV in Vaccines for Pediatrics, p. 585)

- Indicated for all women ≤26 years of age who have not previously completed the series.

MMR vaccine

Measles

- All adults born before 1957 are considered immune to measles.
- Adults born during or after 1957 should receive ≥1 dose of MMR unless they have a documented history of measles from a health-care provider diagnosis or laboratory evidence of immunity.
- A second MMR is recommended for the following adults:
  - Those recently exposed to measles or in an outbreak setting
  - Those previously vaccinated with killed measles vaccine
  - Those vaccinated with an unknown type of measles vaccine during 1963–1967
  - College students
  - Workers in a health-care facility
  - Those planning to travel internationally

Mumps

- All adults born before 1957 are considered immune to mumps.
- Adults born during or after 1957 should receive ≥1 dose of MMR unless they have a history of mumps from a health-care provider diagnosis or laboratory evidence of immunity.
- A second MMR is recommended for the following adults:
  - An affected age group during an outbreak
  - College students

- Workers in a health-care facility
- Those planning to travel internationally

Rubella

One dose of MMR vaccine should be administered to women whose rubella vaccination history is unreliable or who lack laboratory evidence of immunity.

Rubella immunity should be determined in all women of childbearing age, regardless of birth year. Women without evidence of immunity should receive MMR vaccine on completion or termination of pregnancy and before discharge from the health-care facility.

Varicella vaccine

Adults without evidence of immunity to varicella should receive 2 doses of vaccine. The second dose is administered 4–8 weeks after the first.

Special consideration for vaccination should be given to those

- With close contact to persons at high risk for severe disease
- At high risk for exposure or transmission (e.g., teachers, child-care employees, staff and residents of institutional settings, adolescents and adults living in households with children, nonpregnant women of child-bearing potential, international travelers)

Influenza vaccine

This vaccine is administered annually to any individual requesting vaccination. Particular emphasis on vaccination should be given to the following individuals:

- Those with chronic cardiovascular or pulmonary disorders
- Those with chronic metabolic diseases including diabetes, renal or hepatic dysfunction, hemoglobinopathies, or immunosuppression
- Those with any condition that compromises respiratory function or handling of respiratory secretions or that can increase aspiration risk
- Women who are pregnant during influenza season
- Health-care personnel and employees of long-term care and assisted-living facilities
- Residents of nursing homes, long-term care, or assisted-living facilities
- Those likely to transmit influenza to persons at high risk (e.g., in home contacts and caregivers of children <59 months of age, or persons with high-risk conditions)

Live, intranasal influenza vaccine can be given to nonpregnant adults ≤49 years of age without high-risk medical conditions who are not contacts of severely immunocompromised persons. Recipients should avoid close contact with immunocompromised people for at least 7 days.

Pneumococcal polysaccharide vaccine, 23-valent

- Inactivated
- For prevention of invasive pneumococcal disease, pneumococcal bacteremia, and other pneumococcal infections
- Provides protection against *S. pneumoniae* types 1, 2, 3, 4, 5, 8, 9, 12, 14, 17, 19, 20, 22, 23, 26, 34, 43, 51, 54, 56, 57, 68, and 70
- For all adults ≥65 years of age

It should also be given to the following adults:
- Those with chronic pulmonary disease (excluding asthma), chronic cardiovascular disease, diabetes, chronic liver disease, chronic alcoholism, chronic renal failure, or nephrotic syndrome
- Those with functional or anatomic asplenia (e.g., sickle cell disease or splenectomy). For elective splenectomy, vaccinate at least 2 weeks before surgery.
- Those with immunosuppressive conditions
- Those with cochlear implants and cerebrospinal fluid leaks
- Alaska Natives, certain American Indian populations
- Residents of nursing homes or other long-term care facilities

Immunization schedule
- 0.5 mL SC or IM single dose
- A second dose is given after 5 years to those with chronic renal failure or nephrotic syndrome, functional or anatomic asplenia, or immunosuppressive conditions, and those >65 years of age who were <65 years of age when they received the first dose and if the dose was 5 years before or longer.

Hepatitis A vaccine (see Hepatitis, p. 524)

This vaccine is for anyone requesting protection against hepatitis A. It should be administered to the following individuals:
- Those with chronic liver disease
- Those who receive clotting factor concentrates
- Men who have sex with men
- Persons who use illegal drugs
- Persons working with hepatitis A virus–infected primates or in laboratory settings with hepatitis A virus
- Persons traveling to or working in countries with highly or intermediately endemic hepatitis A

Immunization schedule
- 1 mL IM three times within 6 months
- The second and third doses are given 1 month and 6 months after the first dose, respectively.

Hepatitis B vaccine (see Hepatitis, p. 524)

This vaccine is for anyone requesting protection against hepatitis B. It should be administered to the following individuals:
- Those with end-stage renal disease including hemodialysis
- Those seeking evaluation or treatment of a sexually transmitted disease (STD)
- Those with HIV
- Those with chronic liver disease
- Health-care personnel and public safety workers exposed to blood or other bodily fluids
- Sexually active persons who are not in long-term, mutually monogamous relationships
- Current or recent injectable drug-users
- Men who have sex with men

- Household contacts and sexual contacts of persons with hepatitis B virus infection
- Clients and staff members of institutions and nonresidential day care facilities for persons with developmental disabilities
- International travelers to countries with high or intermediate prevalence of chronic hepatitis B virus infection
- All adults at STD treatment facilities, HIV testing and treatment facilities, drug abuse treatment and prevention facilities, health-care settings targeting injection-drug users or men who have sex with men, correctional facilities, and end-stage renal disease programs and dialysis facilities

Immunization schedule

- Adults: 1 mL (10 mcg of Recombivax or 20 mcg of Engerix-B) IM 3 times within 6 months
- The second and third doses are 1 and 6 months after the first dose, respectively.
- Hemodialysis or immunocompromised patients: 40 mcg at each dose

Meningococcal vaccine

- Inactivated
- Commercially available as polysaccharide (MPSV4, Menomune) or conjugate vaccine (MCV4, Menactra)
- For prevention of invasive meningococcal disease, caused by *N. meningitidis* types A, C, Y, and W-135

This vaccine is recommended for the following individuals:

- Adults with anatomic or functional asplenia or terminal complement component deficiencies
- First-year college students living in dormitories
- Laboratory personnel routinely exposed to isolates of *N. meningitides*
- Military recruits
- Persons who travel to or live in countries in which meningococcal disease is hyperendemic or endemic (Sub-Saharan Africa between December and June)
- MCV4 is the recommended product for those ≤55 years of age with the above indications.
- Immunization schedule: 0.5 mL IM single dose
- Revaccination after 3–5 years may be appropriate for those previously vaccinated with MPSV4 and who remain at increased infection risk.

Zoster vaccine

- Live, attenuated
- Herpes zoster or shingles is associated with reactivation of dormant varicella zoster virus and manifests as painful, vesicular cutaneous lesions.
- For all adults 60 years of age and older, regardless of herpes zoster history

- Contraindications: anaphylactic or anaphylactoid reaction to gelatin or neomycin, immunodeficiency, and pregnancy
- Immunization schedule: 0.65 mL SC single dose

Vaccines for travelers

- The CDC provides vaccine recommendations for international travelers based upon the area to which travel will occur. These guidelines are located at: http://wwwn.cdc.gov/travel/default.aspx

Further reading

CDC (2008). Recommended adult immunization schedule—United States, October 2007–September 2008. *MMWR Morb Mortal Wkly Rep* **56**(41);Q1–Q4.

Grabenstein JD (2008). *ImmunoFacts: Vaccines and Immunologic Drugs*. St. Louis, MO: Wolters Kluwer Health.

Alzheimer's disease

Alzheimer's disease (AD) is the most common form of dementia, accounting for up to 70% of cases. It is a progressive and fatal disease characterized by the destruction of neurons in the brain, leading to problems with memory, thinking, and behavior. Approximately 5 million Americans currently suffer from the disease and it is now the sixth leading cause of death in the United States.

AD is diagnosed according to clinical criteria from the DSM-IV (*Diagnostic and Statistical Manual of Mental Disorders*, fourth edition). Diagnosis should also include a complete medical history, physical and neurological exam, laboratory tests, and possibly imaging, such as computerized tomography (CT) or magnetic resonance imaging (MRI). The definitive diagnosis of AD can only be made on autopsy with the presence of lesions known as plaques and tangles.

Warning signs of AD

- Memory loss
- Difficulty performing routine tasks
- Language difficulties
- Disorientation to place and time
- Impaired judgment
- Difficulty with abstract thinking
- Misplacing things in unusual places
- Changes in mood or behavior
- Personality changes
- Loss of initiative

Disease progression

AD is a progressive disease, with death occurring an average of 4 to 6 years after diagnosis. The cause is unknown, although increasing age is the biggest risk factor. Although specific symptoms may vary among individuals, the general stages of the disease are consistent.

The stages of AD begin with no or very mild cognitive decline and progress to very severe cognitive decline. Patients in the final stage of AD are unable to perform activities of daily living (ADLs) independently, they lose their ability to walk, their muscles become rigid, they have difficulty holding their head up, and their swallowing becomes impaired.

Treatment

There is no cure for AD, but medications can slow the worsening of symptoms. Other medications can be used to treat the behavioral and psychiatric symptoms of AD.

Cholinesterase inhibitors

Cholinesterase inhibitors prevent the metabolism of acetylcholine, a neurotransmitter involved in memory and other thought processes. There are currently three cholinesterase inhibitors available for the treatment of AD.

- Donepezil, approved to treat all stages of AD. The usual dose is 5–10 mg/day.
- Galantamine, approved to treat mild to moderate stages of AD. The usual dose is 16–24 mg/day.
- Rivastigmine is also approved to treat mild to moderate stages of AD. The usual oral dose is 6–12 mg/day in two divided doses. It is also available in a transdermal patch dosed 4.6 or 9.5 mg/24 hours.

N-methyl-D-aspartate (NMDA) receptor antagonist

Glutamate is an excitatory neurotransmitter involved in many cognitive functions of the brain, including processing of information and memory storage. It works on the NMDA receptors.

Overstimulation of NMDA receptors by excess glutamate occurs in AD and leads to destruction of neurons. NMDA receptor antagonist partially blocks these receptors and protects the cells from excess glutamate.

- Memantine is the only NMDA receptor antagonist available. It is approved for treatment of moderate to severe AD. The usual dose is 20 mg/day in two divided doses.

Adjunctive therapies

- Vitamin E has been suggested as a neuroprotective agent in patients with AD, but supporting evidence is very limited and recent data suggest an increase in mortality in patients receiving vitamin E for other diseases.
- Antidepressants, typically SSRIs, can be used for depressive symptoms (see Depression unit in this chapter, p. 674)
- Anxiolytics, typically benzodiazepines, can be used for agitation and restlessness (see Anxiety unit in this chapter, pp. 670–1)
- Antipsychotics, typically newer generation agents, can be used for hallucinations, delusions, and psychosis.
- Herbal agents have been promoted for the treatment of AD, but scientific evidence supporting these claims is lacking

Further reading

American Psychiatric Association. Practice guideline for the treatment of patients with Alzheimer's disease and other dementias. Available at: www.psychiatryonline.com

Headaches

Headaches are one of the most common pain complaints seen in family practice medicine and the most common reason for patient visits to a neurologist.

There are two types of headache, primary and secondary. Primary headaches include migraines, tension-type, and cluster headaches. Secondary headaches are caused by other conditions, such as dental pain.

Most headaches are the primary type and affect 3 times as many women as men (18% vs. 6%, respectively) in the United States. They can be difficult to treat, and many primary headache sufferers report dissatisfaction with therapy and a decrease in quality of life.

Treatment of primary headache includes treatment for acute attacks and, when appropriate, preventative treatment. Treatment and prophylactic regimens vary considerably and management must be individualized to each patient. Therapeutic regimens should be based on the frequency and severity of attacks, the degree of temporary disability, and the associated symptoms, such as nausea and vomiting.

Goals of treatment

Acute treatment

- Treat attacks rapidly and consistently without recurrence
- Restore the patient's ability to function
- Minimize the use of back-up and rescue medications
- Optimize self-care and reduce subsequent use of resources
- Be cost-effective for overall management
- Have minimal or no adverse events

Long-term management

- Reduce attack frequency and severity
- Reduce disability
- Improve quality of life
- Prevent headache
- Avoid escalation of headache medication
- Educate and enable patients to manage their disease

Nonpharmacological treatments

Cognitive and behavior techniques (e.g., biofeedback, relaxation training) may be useful in the prevention of headaches.

Pharmacological treatment of acute attacks

Key points

There is no definitive algorithm for the treatment of primary headache. For mild to moderate headache, NSAIDS or combination products containing aspirin, acetaminophen, and caffeine may be effective. More severe headaches may require the use of serotonin ($5HT_1$) agonists (triptans), dihydroergotamine (DHE), or ergotamine. Opioid analgesics may be effective, but excess sedation, overuse headaches, and abuse potential must be considered with these agents.

Butalbital-containing products should be limited because of medication-overuse headaches and withdrawal.

Oral or injectable antiemetics may be used for the treatment of nausea associated with primary headache. Non-oral analgesic medication may also be necessary.

Preventative treatment

There are a number of medications that have been used for prophylaxis against primary headaches. However, definitive supportive data are minimal and recommendations are based on expert consensus rather than clinical evidence. Medications with the highest level of proven efficacy include the following:

- Divalproex sodium 500–1500 mg/day
- Amitriptyline 30–150 mg/day
- Propranolol 80–240 mg/day
- Timolol 20–30 mg/day

Other, less-proven therapies include, but are not limited to, select calcium channel blockers (verapamil, nimodipine, and diltiazem), some beta-blockers, NSAIDs, and certain anticonvulsants (gabapentin, topiramate, and tiagabine).

Key points

- Use the lowest effective doses of medications.
- Allow for an adequate trial of medication to determine effectiveness—a minimum of 2–3 months.
- Use long-acting formulations to improve compliance whenever possible.
- Avoid overuse of certain medications (e.g., ergotamine; maximum dose is 6 mg/24 hours or 10 mg/week) that could interfere with effectiveness.

Further reading

Matchar DB, Young WB, Rosenberg JH, et al. Evidence-based guidelines for migraine headache in the primary care setting: pharmacological management of acute attacks. Practice guidelines. Available at: www.aan.com

Ramadan NM, Silberstein SD, Freitag FG, et al. Evidence-based guidelines for migraine headache in the primary care setting: pharmacologic management for prevention of migraine. Practice guidelines. Available at: www.aan.com

Snow V, Weiss K, Wall EM, et al. (2002). Pharmacologic management of acute attacks of migraine and prevention of migraine headache. *Ann Intern Med* **137**:840–849.

Multiple sclerosis

Multiple sclerosis (MS) is a chronic, recurrent inflammatory autoimmune disorder of the central nervous system (CNS). It is characterized by demyelination and axonal damage in multiple areas of the brain, resulting in the hallmark lesions in the brain. Symptoms vary based on the location of plaques in the brain.

MS affects approximately 400,000 Americans and is most often diagnosed in young women of childbearing age. The exact cause is unknown, although it is thought to be a combination of genetic, environmental, and immunological causes.

Common symptoms of MS include fatigue, numbness, gait and balance difficulties, bowel and bladder dysfunction, vision loss, dizziness and vertigo, sexual dysfunction, pain, depression, and spasticity.

Four types of MS

- Relapsing-remitting MS (RRMS) is the most common type, occurring in 85% of patients. It is characterized by exacerbations of the disease, known as relapses, followed by periods of partial or complete remission.
- Secondary-progressive MS (SPMS) can develop following RRMS, in which patients no longer experience exacerbations but rather a steady decline in function.
- Primary-progressive MS (PPMS) is characterized by a steady decline in function from the onset of disease without relapses or remissions.
- Progressive-relapsing MS (PRMS) begins with a steady decline in function but can also have periodic exacerbations.

Treatment of acute exacerbations

Corticosteroids are the mainstay of treatment. Intravenous methylprednisolone 500–1000 mg/day for 3–10 days is recommended for acute attacks.

Treatment of the disease (see Table 15.74)

There is no cure for MS. Treatment is aimed at altering the course of the disease to minimize frequency and severity of relapses and slow progress of the disease. Disease-modifying drugs (DMD) should be initiated as early in the disease as possible. There are two categories of DMD, immunomodulators and immunosuppressants.

Immunomodulators

- Interferon-β-1a (Avonex, Rebif)
- Interferon-β-1b (Betaseron)
- Glatiramer acetate (Copaxone)
- Natalizumab (Tysabri)

The interferon-β products and glatiramer acetate are first-line treatment for RRMS.

Natalizumab is indicated only as monotherapy for patients who cannot tolerate first-line agents. A serious and potentially fatal side effect, progressive multifocal leukoencephalopathy (PML), limits its use and both

Table 15.74 Medications used for treatment of MS

Immunomodulating drugs	Usual dose/route of delivery	Adverse effects
Avonex®	30 mcg IM; once weekly	Flu-like symptoms, nausea, infection, elevated hepatic enzymes, leukopenia, chest pain, rash Less common: anaphylaxis, autoimmune disorders, psychiatric symptoms, cardiomyopathy
Betaseron®	250 mcg SC; every other day	Edema, flu-like symptoms, nausea/diarrhea, rash, neutropenia, leukopenia, elevated hepatic enzymes, chest pain Less common: anaphylaxis, hepatic failure, cardiomyopathy, psychosis, seizure
Copaxone®	20 mg SC; once daily	Vasodilation, chest pain, nausea/diarrhea, infection, flu-like symptoms, rash Less common: anaphylactoid reaction
Ribif®	44 mcg SC; 3 times weekly	Same as Avonex
Tysabri®	300 mg IV infusion; every 4 weeks	Flu-like symptoms, infection, diarrhea, rash Less common: anaphylaxis, PML
Immunosuppressant drug		
Mitoxantrone	12 mg/m^2 IV infusion; 4 times a year, lifetime maximum 8–12 doses over 2–3 years	Edema, arrhythmia, fatigue, menstrual disorder, nausea, diarrhea, myelosuppression, elevated hepatic enzymes Less common: cardiotoxicity, anaphylaxis, extravasation and phlebitis at infusion site

prescribers and patients must be enrolled in TOUCH, a restricted distribution program.

Immunosuppressants

Mitoxantrone is effective for worsening RRMS and progressive MS. It is used in conjunction with interferons or glatiramer. Risk of cardiotoxicity warrants regular cardiac function testing with this medication.

Alternative therapies

Additional therapies that are sometimes used but lack definitive supportive evidence of efficacy include: cyclophosphamide, methotrexate, azathioprine, cyclosporine, and mycophenolate.

Symptom management

Symptoms of MS vary among patients and treatment should be directed at individualized problems. Common symptoms for which treatment exists include spasticity, for which baclofen, tizanidine, and benzodiazepines are often used. Bladder dysfunction is commonly treated with antichoinergic agents and/or alpha-blockers.

Modafinil or amantidine are first-line agents for treatment of MS-related fatigue. Neurogenic pain is usually treated with gabapentin or pregabalin.

Depression is common among MS patients and is typically treated with an SSRI or tricyclic antidepressant (See Depression unit in this chapter, p. 674).

Further reading

Report of the Therapeutics and Technology Assessment Subcommittee of the American Academy of Neurology and the MS Council for Clinical Practice Guidelines. Disease modifying therapies in multiple sclerosis. Accessed August 29, 2008, from: www.aan.com.

www.nationalmssociety.org

Myasthenia gravis

Myasthenia gravis (MG) is an autoimmune disorder caused by antibodies to muscle acetylcholine receptors (AChR) at the neuromuscular junction. Loss of these receptors prevents normal neuromuscular transmission of nerve impulse and results in muscle fatigue and weakness. The amount of weakness fluctuates, often worsening after activity and improving with rest.

The prevalence of the disease in the United States is approximately 20 per 100,000 people and may be underdiagnosed. Patients of all ages, races, and gender can be affected. The exact cause of the disease is unknown, but it is believed to have a genetic component.

Symptoms

Patients often present with weakness of the bulbar and facial muscles. They can have difficultly chewing and swallowing, and weight loss is common upon presentation. Weakness can also be present in upper and/or lower extremities. It can remain localized, or spread to other muscle groups. In acute exacerbations, respiratory muscles can be affected and patients may need to be mechanically ventilated.

Onset of symptoms can be acute or subacute, and patients can have exacerbations of the disease. Myasthenic crises can be life threatening and are characterized by bulbar or respiratory weakness. On the other hand, cholinergic crises can mimic exacerbations of the disease but are caused by excessive acetylcholinesterase inhibition leading to depolarization of the neuromuscular junction, blocking neurotransmitters and thereby increasing weakness.

Diagnosis

- Presence of serum AChR antibodies is diagnostic and is positive in about 85% of MG patients.
- Anti-MuSK antibodies are present in 40%–70% of those patients who are seronegative for AChR antbodies.
- Electromyography (EMG) studies can be useful.
- Edrophonium chloride (Tensilon®) has been inconsistently available for testing because of marketing issues.

Once the diagnosis is made, CT or MRI of the chest should be done to evaluate the thymus gland. Thymomas occur in about 10% of patients with MG and may contribute to symptoms of the disease.

Treatment

Acute exacerbations

- Immune globulin intravenously (IgIV), 2 g/kg usually given in 2–5 divided doses.
    - Adverse effects include acute renal failure, infusion-related reactions, anaphylaxis, thrombotic events, arthralgia, myalgia, pulmonary edema, rash, nausea and diarrhea.
- Plasmapheresis, 4–5 exchanges over 8–10 days

Disease management

Pyridostigmine is an acetylcholinestease inhibitor that prevents the breakdown of acetylcholine in the neuromuscular junction, prolonging its availability to activate the AChR. Dosing must be individualized and can range from 60 to 1500 mg/day in divided doses; the average dose is 600 mg/day in 5–6 doses.

Adverse effects reflect increased response of parasympathetic system and include nausea and diarrhea, abdominal pain, urinary urgency, excess salivation and sweating, increased bronchial secretions, and cholinergic crisis.

Immunosuppressants, such as prednisone or azathiaprine, may be used to suppress the immune system. Prednisone is typically dosed 60 mg daily for several months with a slow taper to follow.

Steroids may cause a transient increase in symptoms when initiated and should be given under carefully monitored conditions (e.g., hospitalized patient). Other side effects include nervousness, increased appetite, headache, hyperglycemia, osteoporosis, psychosis, and hypothalamic–pituitary–adrenal (HPA) axis suppression.

Azathiaprine 50 mg daily is the usual starting dose with titration up to 2–3 mg/kg/day. Adverse effects include myelosuppression, nausea, vomiting, diarrhea, hepatotoxicity, rash, and hypersensitivity reactions.

Thymectomy is performed in patients with a thymoma.

Medications to be avoided in MG

Exposure to a wide variety of medications can exacerbate symptoms of MG, thus caution must be exercised when prescribing medications to patients with MG. The list of medications to be avoided in this patient population is long, and much of it is based on anecdotal case reports or theorized mechanisms of action of medications.

A thorough and up-to-date list can be found on the MG Foundation of America Web site at www.myasthenia.org, reference document "Medications and Myasthenia Gravis (A Reference for Health Care Professionals)."

Further reading

Myasthenia Gravis Foundation of America, Inc. Educational material for healthcare professionals. www.myasthenia.org.

Parkinson's disease

Parkinson's disease (PD) is a progressive neurodegenerative disorder characterized by two or more of the following: tremor, rigidity, bradykinesia, or postural instability. Onset of the disease is variable and can occur somewhere between 50 and 80 years of age. It affects more men than women.

The exact cause of PD is unknown but the mechanism of the disease is due to a loss of dopamine neurons in the substantia nigra of the basal ganglia. The normal dopamine–acetylcholine balance in the brain is disturbed and a resultant increase in acetylcholine occurs. This leads to muscles that are overly tense, causing tremor, rigidity, and slowness of movement. Additionally, Lewy bodies can be found in cells in the substantia nigra upon autopsy.

Drug-induced parkinsonism syndrome can occur and must be ruled out when diagnosing the disease. Medications that block dopamine receptors, such as older neuroleptic agents (e.g., haloperidol), have been implicated.

Other movement disorders can also mimic PD. A levodopa challenge is the definitive diagnostic tool when PD is suspected based on history and clinical symptoms.

Staging

Hoehn and Yahr classification scale

- Stage 1: unilateral involvement, minimal or no functional impairment
- Stage 2: bilateral involvement, no impairment of balance
- Stage 3: postural imbalance, some restriction in activities
- Stage 4: severely disabled, require assistance for standing and walking
- Stage 5: severely disable, confined to bed or wheelchair

Treatment

There is no definitive treatment for PD. Strategies to manage symptoms and slow the progression of disease are employed. Most drug treatments are aimed at increasing levels of dopamine or opposing excess acetylcholine in the brain.

Medications increasing levels of dopamine

Oral dopamine agonists (DA)

DAs such as pramipexole and ropinirole directly stimulate striatal dopamine receptors. Usual doses of pramipexole are 1.5–4.5 mg/day in 3 divided doses. Ropinirole is dosed anywhere from 0.75 to 24 mg/day in divided doses for immediate-release tablets and once daily for extended-release tablets.

Apomorphine is another DA that is given in late stages of the disease. Apomorphine 2–6 mg is given subcutaneously for "off" episodes.

Bromocriptine is an older, ergot-derived DA that is rarely used anymore in PD because of side effects. When used, doses of bromocriptine average 2.5–40 mg/day in 2 divided doses.

Common adverse effects of dopamine agonists include nausea, orthostatic hypotension, dizziness, somnolence, and hallucinations.

Levodopa

Levodopa is a precursor to dopamine and can be given exogenously to supplement dopamine levels. It is given in combination with carbidopa, a peripheral decarboxylase inhibitor, which prevents its breakdown in the periphery before crossing the blood–brain barrier.

Doses and dosing intervals for levodopa/carbidopa vary widely and must be individualized to the patient. Average doses of levodopa are 400–1600 mg daily in 3 to 6 divided doses. Adverse effects include dizziness, nausea and vomiting, orthostatic hypotension, on–off phenomenon, agitation, and dyskinesias. Levodopa or DAs are usually first-line treatment for symptoms of PD.

Catechol-O-methyltransferase (COMT) inhibitors

COMT inhibitors prevent the breakdown of levodopa in the periphery and are used in combination with levodopa/carbidopa to extend the half-life of levodopa.

Entacapone is the COMT inhibitor of choice. It is given concomitantly with doses of levodopa/carbidopa (200 mg/dose, maximum of 1600 mg/day). Common side effects include diarrhea, nausea, somnolence, and hallucinations.

Tolcapone, another COMT inhibitor, is reserved for patients who cannot tolerate entacapone. It carries a risk of fatal hepatotoxicity and careful monitoring of the patient must be performed.

Monoamine oxidase type B (MAO-B) inhibitors

MAO-B inhibitors prevent the breakdown of dopamine in the striatum. Selegiline has been available for decades and has some beneficial effect early in the disease, but its effects are not sustained.

Rasagiline is a new, second-generation, MAO-B inhibitor. It is more selective in its MAO-B inhibition, making it useful in both early and late parts of the disease process. It is also thought to have some neuroprotective benefit, but that has yet to be proven.

Selegiline 10 mg/day in 2 divided doses (breakfast and lunch) or 1.25–2.5 mg once daily of the orally disintegrating tablet is the recommended dosing. Rasagiline 0.5–1 mg daily is recommended.

Common adverse effects include nausea, vomiting, orthostatic hypotension, hallucinations, confusion, and dizziness.

Amantadine

Amantadine is an antiviral agent that also has the ability to augment dopamine release and inhibit reuptake. Its benefits are mild and not sustained. It is only used early in the disease process. Doses of 200–400 mg/day in 2 divided doses are typical.

Adverse effects include dizziness, orthostatic hypotension, agitation, and insomnia.

Medications decreasing levels of acetylcholine

Anticholinergic agents such as benztropine and trihexyphenidyl are used in early PD for resting tremor. Because of side effects, they are not frequently used anymore and should be avoided in elderly patients.

Nonpharmacological treatment

Deep brain stimulation with surgically implanted electrodes and a pulse generator has benefit in select patients with advanced disease.

Complications of treatment

Motor fluctuations occur as the disease progresses and are characterized by wearing off of the medication, sudden on–off fluctuations, and motor freezing. Rasagiline and entacapone have demonstrated effectiveness in reducing off time. Pramipexole, ropinirole, apomorphine, and selegiline may also be effective.

Levodopa-induced dyskinesias are also common after long-term use of the medication and can be difficult to differentiate from symptoms of PD. Therapeutic regimens must be individualized to maximize symptom control and reduce off time.

Nonmotor complications of PD

Nonmotor symptoms of PD can also cause significant disability but are often underrecognized. Common symptoms include depression, dementia, psychosis, and autonomic dysfunction. Eighty-eight percent of patients with PD have at least one nonmotor symptom, and often more than one is present.

Further reading

Miyasaki JM, Shannon K, Voon V, et al. (2006). Practice parameter: Evaluation and treatment of depression, psychosis, and dementia in Parkinson disease (an evidence-based review). *Neurology* **66**:996–1002.

Pahwa R, Factor SA, Lyons KE, et al. (2006). Practice parameter: Treatment of Parkinson disease with motor fluctuations and dyskinesia (an evidence-based review). *Neurology* **66**:983–995.

Suchowersky O, Gronseth G, Perlmutter J, et al (2006). Practice parameter: Neuroprotective strategies and alternative therapies for Parkinson disease (an evidence-based review). *Neurology* **66**:976–982.

Suchowersky O, Reich S, Perlmutter J, et al. (2006). Practice parameter: Diagnosis and prognosis of new onset Parkinson disease (an evidence-based review). *Neurology* **66**:968–975.

Seizure disorder

Seizures disorders are one of the most common disease states encountered by neurologists. Approximately 150,000 Americans suffer a first seizure annually and approximately 50% of them will recur. Recurrence of unprovoked seizures defines epilepsy.

Evaluation of first seizure

- Complete physical and neurological exam and history
- Electroencephalogram (EEG)
- Neuroimaging (CT or MRI)

Additional studies that may be helpful

- Laboratory tests (electrolytes, blood counts, blood glucose)
- Lumbar puncture may (e.g., febrile patient)
- Toxicology screening

Seizure classification

Generalized seizures

- Tonic–clonic (grand mal), loss of consciousness without warning
- Absence (petit mal), brief loss of consciousness without loss of postural tone
- Other (tonic, clonic, myoclonic)

Partial seizures

- Simple partial, single or limited muscle group involved, usually no loss of consciousness
- Complex partial, impaired level of consciousness
- Partial seizures with secondary generalization

Treatment

Treatment should be initiated with one antiepileptic medication with dosing increased until seizures are controlled or adverse effects prevent further increase. If seizures persist, trials of other medications as monotherapy are generally done before the addition of a second agent.

In general, when used for appropriate seizure types, most antiepileptic medications are equally effective. In addition, most agents that are initially approved for adjunctive therapy of partial seizures prove to be effective for other types of seizures and as monotherapy.

Drug interactions

Most antiepileptic medications have multiple drug–drug interactions because of their metabolism through the cytochrome P450 enzyme pathway, affinity for protein binding, and/or altered absorption when given with other medications. It is prudent to review all concurrent medications for potential interactions when initiating or discontinuing antiepileptic medications.

Monitoring

Many of the older antiepileptics (e.g., phenytoin, valproic acid, carbamazepine) have established therapeutic serum concentrations that can be helpful to guide dosing. However, it is important to remember to treat the seizures and not the serum drug level.

The dosing, indications, and adverse effects of the antiepileptic medications are in Table 15.75

Table 15.75 Antiepileptic medications

Medication	Indications[1]	Usual dosing	Adverse effects
Phenytoin	P, GTC, S	Loading dose 15–20 mg/kg IV or oral (in divided doses) Maintenance dose 5–7 mg/kg/day	Nystagmus, diplopia, somnolence, gingival hyperplasia, rash, Stevens-Johnson syndrome (SJS)
Carbamazepine	P, S	400–1600 mg/day in divided doses	Somnolence, diplopia, blood dyscrasias, rash, SJS, hyponatremia
Oxcarbazepine	P, S	600–2400 mg/day in divided doses	Somnolence, diplopia, n/v, hyponatremia, SJS
Phenobarbital	P, GTC, S	90–180 mg/day	Somnolence, ataxia, diplopia, rash, SJS
Valproic acid	GTC, M, A, P, S	Loading dose 20–30 mg/kg IV Maintenance dose 15–60 mg/kg/day	Somnolence, weight gain, thrombocytopenia, hepatic dysfunction, hair loss
Ethosuximide	A	15–40 mg/kg/day	Somnolence, n/v, headache, behavioral changes
Clonazepam	A, P, M	1.5–8 mg/day in 2–3 divided doses	Somnolence, withdrawal symptoms upon abrupt discontinuation
Gabapentin	P, S	900–4800 mg/day in 3 divided doses	Somnolence, ataxia, nystagmus, weight gain
Lamotrigine	GTC, P, S	100–700 mg/day	Somnolence, diplopia, n/v, rash, SJS
Levetiracetam	GTC, P, M	1000–3000 mg/day in divided doses	Somnolence, GI upset, behavioral changes

Table 15.75 (*Contd.*)

Medication	Indications[1]	Usual dosing	Adverse effects
Topiramate	GTC, P, S	200–400 mg/day in divided doses	Somnolence, nervousness, confusion, weight loss
Tiagabine	P	12–56 mg/day in 3 divided doses	Somnolence, n/v, rash
Zonisamide	P	300–600 mg/day in 1–2 doses	Somnolence, confusion, n/v, weight loss, irritability, rash, SJS, agranulocytosis

1 A, absence; GTC, generalized tonic-clonic; P, partial; S, secondarily GTC; M, myoclonic

Further reading

Report of the Quality Standards Subcommittee of the American Academy of Neurology and the American Epilepsy Society. Practice parameter: evaluating an apparent unprovoked first seizure in adults (an evidence-based review). Available at: www.aan.com

Stroke

Stroke is a cardiovascular disease that affects approximately 780,000 Americans each year. Approximately 600,000 of these are first strokes, whereas 180,000 are recurrent attacks.

Types of strokes

- Ischemic stroke: 80% of all strokes
- Hemorrhagic stroke: 20% of strokes

Ischemic stroke

Nonmodifiable risk factors

- Increased age
- Gender: male > female
- Race/ethnicity: African Americans, some Hispanic Americans > whites
- Family history of stroke

Modifiable risk factors

- Hypertension
- Smoking
- Diabetes
- Carotid stenosis
- Atrial filbrillation (AF)
- Sickle cell disease
- Hyperlipidemia

Primary prevention strategies

- Screening and management of hypertension, especially in diabetic patients
- Smoking cessation
- Glycemic control in diabetic patients
- Endarterectomy for high-grade carotid stenosis (consider)
- Antithrombotic therapy (warfarin or aspirin) for patients with AF (consider)
- Management of elevated cholesterol
- Healthy diet, regular exercise, and weight loss for obese patients

Diagnosis

- Patient history and time of symptom onset
- Physical and neurological exam and stroke scale score (National Institutes of Health Stroke Scale [NIHSS])
- Rule out hypoglycemia or other conditions that mimic stroke (e.g., seizure)
- Non-contrast CT of brain to rule out hemorrhage
- CBC, PT/INR
- Basic metabolic profile (BMP)
- ECG

Treatment of acute ischemic stroke

Within 3 hours of symptom onset, consider intravenous thrombolytic therapy with recombinant tissue plasminogen activator (tPA) 0.9 mg/kg, maximum dose 90 mg, 10% given as loading dose over 1–2 minutes. The remaining 90% is given as intravenous infusion over 60 minutes.

Patient eligibility for tPA must be considered on the basis of time of symptom onset, size of stroke, risk of bleeding, and control of arterial hypertension. It is contraindicated when significant risk is present.

Intra-arterial thrombolysis is an option for select patients who are otherwise not eligible for intravenous therapy.

Secondary prevention of ischemic stroke

In addition to the strategies for primary prevention, antithrombotic therapy is recommended for prevention of recurrent stroke. Antiplatelet agents are recommended for noncardioembolic strokes (e.g., large-artery atherosclerosis, small-vessel disease). Aspirin, clopidogrel, or the combination of aspirin and extended-release dipyridimole are all first-line options.

Oral anticoagulation with warfarin is recommended for many types of cardioembolic strokes, including atrial fibrillation, valvular disease, and left ventricular thrombus associated with acute myocardial infarction. The goal INR is generally 2–3, with the exception of those with mechanical prosthetic heart valves, in which case the goal INR is 2.5–3.5.

Hemorrhagic stroke

Intracerebral hemorrhage (spontaneous)

Causes

- Hypertension
- Cerebral amyloid angiopathy
- Vascular abnormalities
- Anticoagulation

Diagnosis

- Non-contrast CT or MRI of brain

Treatment

- Supportive therapy
- Reversal of coagulopathy if present (fresh frozen plasma [FFP], vitamin K)
- Management of elevated intracranial pressure and blood pressure
- Hematoma evacuation in certain cases
- Treatment of seizures, prophylactic therapy considered in certain circumstances
- Management of hyperglycemia

Subarachnoid hemorrhage (aneurysmal)

Risk factors

- Smoking, hypertension

Diagnosis

- Non-contrast CT of brain
- Lumbar puncture if CT is negative
- Cerebral angiography to identify aneurysm

Treatment

- Secure the aneurysm via surgical or endovascular technique.
- Prevent secondary ischemic deficits due to vasospasm.

- Treatment of vasospasm includes induced hypertension, hypervolemia, and hemodilution to improve cerebral perfusion, calcium-channel antagonists (nimodipine PO 60 mg every 4 hours, intra-arterial verapamil or nicardipine injections) to improve dilation of constricted cerebral vessels, and transluminal angioplasty. Consider statin therapy (HMG-CoA reductase inhibitor), although data are limited to small trials with simvastatin 80 mg daily and pravastatin 40 mg daily.

- Ventriculostomy if hydrocephalus present
- Avoid volume contraction in hyponatremia, give isotonic or hypertonic fluids

Further reading

Adams HP, del Zoppo G, Alberts MJ, et al. (2007). Guidelines for the early management of adults with ischemic stroke. *Circulation* **115**:e478–e534.

Broderick J, Connolly S, Feldmann E, et al. (2007). Guidelines for the management of spontaneous intracerebral hemorrhage in adults. *Stroke* **38**:2001–2023.

Sacco RL, Adams R, Albers G, et al. (2006). Guidelines for prevention of stroke in patients with ischemic stroke or transient ischemic attack. *Stroke* **37**:577–617.

Policy for administration and handling of cytotoxic drugs

Cytotoxic drugs are used in the treatment of cancers and certain other disorders. They act by killing dividing cells, by preventing their division. In addition to malignant cells, they also act on normal cells, thus their use poses risks to those who handle them. It is important to ensure the safety of staff and patients who come in contact with these drugs.

- Cytotoxic drugs may only be reconstituted in facilities specifically approved for the purpose.
- Staff who prescribe, clinically screen, reconstitute, label, administer, and dispose of cytotoxic drugs must be appropriately trained and assessed as competent and must follow the local, approved procedures.
- In areas where cytotoxic drug use is infrequent, a risk assessment must be carried out before a cytotoxic drug is requested. This should assess the availability of appropriate equipment and evidence of training, and demonstrate competence in safe administration of the drugs.

Cytotoxic drug procedures

Any area (including inpatient, outpatient, or pharmacy) where cytotoxic drugs are used should have available current information on the type of agents used. This information should include relevant health and safety information (control of substances hazardous to health).

Cytotoxic drugs are occasionally used to treat clinical disorders other than cancer. In such instances, the patient should be referred to a clinical area where cytotoxic drugs are used routinely.

Alternatively, a competent practitioner from such an area can administer the drug in the patient's own area. A trained member of staff must undertake a risk assessment to determine who can administer the drug and under what circumstances.

Prescription, preparation, and reconstitution

All prescriptions must be written legibly and signed in indelible ink. Computer-generated prescriptions must have electronic-signature capability, on either an approved chemotherapy chart or a standard prescription chart.

Chemotherapy should be prescribed by physicians experienced in the treatment of neoplastic disorders. Be aware of local policies stipulating who can prescribe chemotherapy.

The pharmacist-in-charge is responsible for ensuring cytotoxic-drug reconstitution services are provided in appropriate facilities. In exceptional circumstances, they can designate other areas for reconstitution.

Labeling and transportation

Syringes, infusion devices, and infusion fluids containing cytotoxic drugs must be clearly labeled, to identify the potential cytotoxic hazard, and placed inside a sealed plastic bag.

Cytotoxic drugs must be packaged and transported in sealed containers identified as containing cytotoxic drugs. The designated cytotoxic-drug reconstitution service must be notified at once if the integrity of a container received is suspect.

Oral cytotoxic drugs should be transported in the same way as non-cytotoxic medication. Inpatient supplies should be labeled "cytotoxic" on the normal prescription label.

Administration

Relevant clinical laboratory results, as defined by chemotherapy protocols, must be reviewed before administration and appropriate action is taken.

The following checks should be made by two qualified staff members, one of whom must be registered as competent in cytotoxic-drug administration, depending on local policy:

- Visual check of the product (to include signs of leakage, contamination, or breakdown products)
- The drug has been appropriately stored and is within its expiration date.
- Patients must be positively identified using patient identifiers, as determined in the local, approved procedure.

The following prescription details must be checked:

- Protocol
- Dose
- Diluent (if relevant)
- Route of administration
- Frequency

Staff should use personal-protective equipment and clothing if handling and administering cytotoxic drugs. This includes gloves, gown, and protection for the face, either goggles or a mask.

Accidental spillage

All areas in which cytotoxic agents are stored, prepared, and administered should have a spill kit available for use at all times. These kits are usually obtained from the pharmacy department. The kit includes instructions on how to proceed safely. Staff should be familiar with the instructions before handling a spill.

A trained health-care professional should manage the spill immediately. After use, the spillage kit should be replaced. Be familiar with your local policy and location of spillage kits in areas with cytotoxic drugs.

Disposal of product waste

Cytotoxic waste should be disposed of separately from normal clinical waste and marked as being cytotoxic, according to local policy. The incorrect disposal of cytotoxic waste can result in prosecution.

Cytotoxic waste includes vials that have contained cytotoxic drugs, syringes, needles, IV bags, and infusion sets used to administer cytotoxic drugs; and gowns, gloves, and urinary catheters and drainage bags from patients undergoing cytotoxic therapy.

Hospitals have specific policies on the storage and collection of cytotoxic waste to ensure that cytotoxic waste does not enter the normal clinical waste stream.

Disposal of blood and body fluids

Precautions should be taken to prevent occupational skin contact. Because cytotoxic drugs have varying half-lives, specific information about them will be found on Material Safety Data (MSD) sheets. If the information is not specified, it is deemed general practice to apply universal precautions for 48 hours after administration.

Patients and relatives (particularly pregnant mothers) who handle body fluids at home should be given appropriate advice.

Gloves must be worn when handling all body fluids (e.g., blood, urine, feces, colostomy and urostomy bags) during and after the administration of cytotoxic drugs.

Linen contaminated with body fluids and cytotoxic drugs must be handled according to local policy for handling cytotoxic-contaminated waste.

If contamination of the skin, eyes, or mucous membranes is suspected, the area should be rinsed thoroughly with large amounts of water and then washed with soap and water.

Incidents arising from handling and administration of cytotoxic drugs

Any incident involving prescribing, administration, and disposal of cytotoxic drugs must be reported according to the local incident-reporting system. The most probable incident for staff is accidental exposure to the drug during set-up and administration of the drug. This might result from a bag leaking or bursting, or problems with the line in situ.

If there is eye and skin contamination, rinse the affected area with copious amounts of tap water and seek further treatment, if needed. For all cases of staff exposure, the occupational health department should be notified to organize risk assessment and follow-up care plans.

The mostly likely incident for patients is extravasation during treatment. See Principles of Extravasation (Chapter 10, p. 244) for extravasation management.

Handling cytotoxics during pregnancy

Pregnant staff should refer to their local policy with regard to handling cytotoxic drugs, because these groups of drugs are potentially mutagenic, teratogenic, and carcinogenic. A risk assessment must be undertaken for each local area.

See Drugs in Pregnancy (Chapter 10, p. 194) for recommendations on handling potentially teratogenic drugs during pregnancy.

Intrathecal chemotherapy

Refer to Intrathecal Administration of Chemotherapy section in this chapter (p. 626).

Further reading

American Society of Hospital Pharmacists (2006). ASHP guidelines on handling hazardous drugs. *Am J Health Syst Pharm* **63**:1172–1193.

Clinical screening of chemotherapy prescriptions

To the extent possible, the prescribing, preparation, dispensing, and administration of medication should be standardized. Well-designed standardized medication-order forms decrease the number of potential errors by organizing treatment information in a clear, consistent, and uniform format. Except for discontinuing treatment, medication-use systems should not permit health-care providers to transmit or accept orders to start or modify medication that are communicated orally.

Validating chemotherapy orders and prescriptions

- Check that doses have been correctly calculated and prescribed.
- Generic drug names should be used; use generic drug names approved by the U.S. Adopted Names program.
- Check maximum doses according to the protocol.
- Body surface areas are often rounded, do not query a discrepancy unless it is >0.1 m^2 for adults.
- The dosage form should be specified.
- Drug dosages should be expressed in metric notation whenever possible. The word *units* should never be abbreviated.
- For rounding doses, be aware that the exact dose might have to be rounded to account for tablet or vial size.
- Check local policy for variation in the dispensed dose compared with the prescribed dose that has been agreed (often 5% variation is agreed).
- Administration route and rate should be specified.
- Administration schedule and duration of treatment should be included.
- Ensure that the doctor has signed and dated the prescription.
- Ensure that the infusion fluid and volume are stated and appropriate.
- For routes other than IV, ensure that the route is prescribed in full (e.g., *intrathecal*, not *IT*).

Order verification for cycle 1

- Check patient's name, date of birth, and unique identifying code or number.
- Check the date the order was generated, and time and date treatments are to be administered.
- Check patient-specific laboratory values (e.g., height, body weight, BSA) from which dosages are calculated.
- Check that surface area has been calculated correctly (see BSA calculations, p. 208)
- Surface area is often capped at 2 m^2 or 2.2 m^2. Check your local policy.
- Check patient's ideal body weight. If the patient is significantly more or less than their ideal body weight, discuss this with their doctor.

IBW (male) = 50 kg + (2.3 x height in inches over 5 feet)

IBW (female) = 45.5 kg + (2.3 x height in inches over 5 feet)

- Check medication dosages and administration rates as a function of patient-specific factors and the calculated doses and rates to be administered.
- Check patient's treatment against the established protocol.
  - Ensure that it is the intended protocol to be prescribed by checking in the patient's medical record.
  - Check for verification of dose modification or variance from the protocol and identification of the factors on which treatment modifications are based.
  - Confirm the dose per day vs. the dose per cycle with the protocol.
- Interpret critical laboratory values to see if a dose modification is required (e.g., impaired renal function, clotting disorders, and liver function tests).
- Check that the correct drugs have been prescribed and that all calculations have been performed correctly.
- Check the frequency of intended cycles and appropriate interval since any previous chemotherapy.
- Check if there are any drug interactions between the chemotherapy and the patient's regular medication.
- Check patient's allergies and medication sensitivities.
- Check for authorized prescriber's name and signature.

Second and subsequent cycles

- Check that the chemotherapy cycle is correct for the protocol.
- Check that the correct cycle was ordered.
- Check that the drugs were prescribed on the correct days and start dates.
- Check that there has been no significant change in the patient's weight that might significantly change the calculated surface area.
- Check response to previous treatment.
  - Blood indices–hematology and biochemical
  - Tolerability and adverse reactions
- Check to see if any appropriate modifications have been made in relation to a previous response or critical laboratory values (normally in the protocol).

Clinical check

- What type of malignancy does the patient have? Is the chemotherapy appropriate for the malignancy?
- What is the patient's renal and hepatic function? Do any of the doses need adjusting to take this into account?
- Has the patient had any chemotherapy before? Do any of the drugs have a maximum cumulative lifetime dose (e.g., anthracyclines)?
- Other checks include reactions to previous chemotherapy and the extent of disease (need for prehydration or allopurinol).
- Check critical laboratory values—if white cell count, neutrophils, or hemoglobin are above a predefined limit, refer to individual protocols.
- Check to see if any appropriate modifications have been made in relation to previous response or critical tests (normally in protocol).
- Check if any supportive care has been prescribed (e.g., antiemetics).

Medication-order verification system

- Established checkpoints for ensuring that an antineoplastic drug is accurately prescribed, prepared, dispensed, and administered to the patient for whom it was intended have been developed and are incorporated into local multidisciplinary verification processes. These nine established checkpoints are as follows.
- Prescribing
    - Order generated—checkpoint 1
- Preparing
    - Order evaluated—checkpoint 2
    - Product evaluated—checkpoint 3
    - Worksheet setup—checkpoint 4
- Dispensing
    - Patient: product evaluated with patient—checkpoint 5
    - Health-care provider: order evaluated—checkpoint 6
    - Product evaluated—checkpoint 7
- Administration
    - Patient examines labeled instructions—checkpoint 8
    - Health care provider checked with patient—checkpoint 9

Further reading

American Society of Health-System Pharmacists (2002). ASHP guidelines on preventing medication errors with antineoplastic agents. *Am J Health Syst Pharm* **59**:1648–1668.

Cohen MR, Anderson RW, Attilio RM, et al. (1996). Preventing medication errors in cancer chemotherapy. *Am J Health Syst Pharm* **53**:737–746.

Chemotherapy dosing

Cancer chemotherapy drugs often have a narrow therapeutic window between the dose that is effective and the dose that can be toxic. Inappropriate dose reduction reduces chemotherapy efficacy. However, if doses are not reduced in patients with organ dysfunction, this can lead to serious or life-threatening toxicity. It is essential that cytotoxic drugs are dosed correctly and adapted to individual patients to enable the maximum probability of a desired therapeutic outcome, with minimum toxicity.

Before administration of chemotherapy, each patient should be assessed for performance status, renal function, liver biochemistry tests, serum albumin level, and prognosis. Myelosuppression is the most common and dangerous toxicity of cytotoxics, so all patients must have a blood count taken before each cycle of chemotherapy.

Patients should only be administered chemotherapy if their white blood cell count is $>3.0 \times 10^9$/L (or neutrophil count is $>1.5 \times 10^9$/L) and platelet count is $>150 \times 10^9$/L. There can be exceptions to this in some local policies or for patients with hematological malignancies and those undergoing intensive treatment with specialized support.

Doses of cytotoxics are usually calculated on the basis of body surface area (BSA), which is measured in square meters (m^2). The dose is quoted as units (e.g., milligrams, grams, or international units) per square meter. The patient's surface area is calculated using a nomogram from patient height and weight measurements or using one of the following formulas:

$$\text{DuBois formula BSA } (m^2) = \frac{kg^{0.425} \times cm^{0.725} \times 71.84}{10{,}000}$$

$$\text{Simplified formula} = \sqrt{\frac{\text{height (cm)} \times \text{weight (kg)}}{3600}}$$

This practice is derived from the relationship between body size and physiological parameters, e.g., renal function. The performance status of the patient and their renal and liver functions are also taken into account. Prior to each cycle of treatment, toxicities must be recorded using common toxicity criteria.

Doses are modified if the patient experiences toxicity to treatment or changes in body weight occur. The size of the reduction depends on the nature and severity of the toxicity, taking into account whether the chemotherapy is palliative or curative in intent.

Obese patients have physiological changes that affect drug disposition, including blood volume, organ size, and adipose tissue mass. The use of ideal body weight can be considered in these settings. However, the possibility of underdosing needs to be considered in curative patients.

Although it is conventional to prescribe chemotherapy according to body surface area, it is acceptable to use pre-prepared standard doses for commonly used drugs to facilitate bulk preparation and rapid dispensing. This is known as *dose banding*. The rounded dose must be within agreed limits, e.g., within 5% of the calculated dose.

There are, however, some exceptions to doses being calculated on the basis of body surface area. Drugs whose doses can be calculated using other parameters include the following:

- Asparaginase—the dosage is international units/kg body weight or international units/body surface area
- Bleomycin—international units, either per patient surface area or as a fixed dose
- Carboplatin—The Calvert equation can be used to calculate the dose of carboplatin in patients with or without renal impairment (1):

Dose (mg) = target area under the plasma concentration curve (AUC) × (GFR + 25) (AUC usually 4–7)

For example, for a patient with a GFR of 75mL/min, using an AUC of 5, the dose of carboplatin would be as follows:

Dose (mg) = 5(75 + 25) = 500 mg carboplatin

- Cytarabine—dosage in mg/kg for certain indications
- Floxuridine—dosage in mg/kg
- Mitomycin—dosage in mg/kg for certain indications

Frequency of chemotherapy administration

Chemotherapy is administered at various treatment cycles ranging from 1 to 4 weeks. Cycle frequency is based on cancer type and treatment choice. Frequency and duration of treatment cycles continue to evolve and are not absolute. It is important to always verify treatment selection, frequency, and duration with established protocols.

Critical tests for chemotherapy to proceed on time

Chemotherapy should only be administered at the full protocol dose if the hematological and biochemical parameters are within the normal range. Biochemical parameters depend on the excreted route of the drug.

Creatinine clearance should be monitored for renally cleared drugs and liver function tests (LFTs) should be monitored for those drugs metabolized hepatically. Hematological parameters include the white cell count, absolute neutrophil count (>1.5), and platelet count (>150).

If the biochemical or hematological parameters are not within the normal range, dose reduction or delaying of subsequent doses must be considered. Doses are usually reduced by 20%–25% initially. Chemotherapy is usually delayed by a week at a time.

Common toxicity criteria (CTC)

The CTC are a standardized classification developed by the National Cancer Institute (NCI) used for the side effects of chemotherapy drugs. The adverse events are graded from 0 (none) to 5 (death) for all possible side effects.

The CTC are used in cancer clinical trials, adverse drug reporting, and publications to ensure uniform capture of toxicity data. The full table of CTC is available from: http://ctep.cancer.gov/forms/CTCAEv3.pdf.

Treatment guidelines

Oncology is an evolving field of practice. Treatments are becoming more individualized and targeted on the basis of genetics, tumor markers, and staging of disease. The following references provide comprehensive and timely information on cancer statistics and treatments:

- National Comprehensive Cancer Network (NCCN): www.nccn.org/
- American Society of Clinical Oncology: www.asco.org
- Proceedings from the American Society of Hematology and American Society of Oncology Annual meetings: www.hematology.org and www.asco.org
- American Cancer Society: www.cancer.org
- National Cancer Institute: www.cancer.gov

For more detailed information on the management of oncological disorders, refer to the Oxford American Handbook of Oncology.

Intrathecal administration of chemotherapy

Background

Intrathecal chemotherapy is mainly used to treat CNS complications of hematological malignancy. The only chemotherapy drugs that can be given intrathecally are cytarabine, methotrexate, and thiotepa.

However, other noncytotoxic drugs can be administered by this route and include bupivacaine, opioids, baclofen, clonidine, gentamicin, hydrocortisone, and vancomycin.

Fatal neurotoxicity of intrathecal vinca alkaloids

Vincristine and the other vinca alkaloids don't pass through the blood–brain barrier. Vinca alkaloids are NEVER given intrathecally; they are always used intravenously. Peripheral neurotoxicity is one of the main side effects, which increases in a cumulative fashion with the total dose of treatment. Hence, when vinca alkaloids are inadvertently injected into the cerebrospinal fluid the outcome is normally fatal.

The Institute of Safe Medication Practices has received voluntary information from doctors about 8 U.S. cases that resulted in 5 deaths in 30 years.

Safe practice

- To prevent inadvertent mix-up with other drugs, intrathecal chemotherapy should be segregated from IV chemotherapy. The separate delivery and locations for these drugs help assure that IV drugs are never present in the same location as intrathecal medications.
- To facilitate this, intrathecal medications should only be administered in a designated location, such as an anesthetic room, at a standard time by competent, registered staff. In this way, the pharmacy can release intrathecal medications to the doctor immediately before they are needed.
- Also, at least two health professionals should independently verify the accuracy of all intrathecal doses before administration.
- A list of drugs that can be administered intrathecally should be established.
- Intrathecal drugs should be wrapped in a sterile bag, which is then wrapped again in another bag labeled for intrathecal use. The package should not be unwrapped until immediately before injection.
- In many hospitals, the practice is to dilute vincristine to avoid confusion with intrathecal syringes.

Frequently asked questions

Which drugs are contraindicated for use through the intrathecal route?

Vinca alkaloids, e.g., vincristine, vinblastine, and vinorelbine, must never be given by this route.

Explain the intrathecal route of administration?

Chemotherapy is injected into the area of the lower spine into cerebrospinal fluid (CSF). This injection is also termed *spinal* or *subarachnoid*. It is mainly indicated when patients show clinical signs that their disease has spread into the CNS. Drugs can also be administered through an Ommaya reservoir, which is discussed below.

Why have people been given the wrong drug intrathecally?

The main problem occurs when inexperienced health professionals become involved in the process, with the result that the drug vincristine (intended solely for the IV route) is administered in error using the intrathecal route. This leads to immediate neural damage that normally results in death.

How are intrathecal products to be labeled?

The label on the product states that the drug is *intended for intrathecal use only*. The product is packaged and transported in a separate container from other IV chemotherapy products and collected by the person who is going to give the drug.

How should vincristine to be labeled?

USP requires specific caution labeling with the vinca alkaloids. The label will state "FATAL if given intrathecally. FOR IV USE ONLY." In addition, the syringe must be placed into an overwrap (accompanies manufacturer's container), which also has this warning label.

What range of volumes is administered intrathecally?

Generally, the volume administered varies with the dose, but the typical volume tends to be 5 mL.

Who is allowed to administer intrathecal products?

Only physicians or licensed personnel with privileges are allowed to administer chemotherapy products intrathecally. Anesthetists also administer intrathecal products, but are generally not allowed to administer cytotoxic chemotherapy unless there are deemed competent.

What is an Ommaya reservoir?

It is a small plastic dome-like device with a small tube. The reservoir is placed under the scalp and the tube is placed into the ventricles so that it connects with cerebrospinal fluid. The Ommaya reservoir is permanent, unless there are complications.

This device allows certain drugs to be administered into the CSF and allows CSF sampling without repeated need of lumbar puncture. Drug doses may be different when given via lumbar puncture vs. Ommaya reservoir. Be sure to verify the dose with the treatment protocol.

How are intrathecal products administered?

A spinal needle is inserted past the epidural space until the dura is pierced and enters the cerebrospinal fluid, which should flow from the needle. When cerebrospinal fluid appears, care is needed not to alter the position of the spinal needle while the syringe of chemotherapy is being attached. The syringe is attached firmly to the hub of the needle and then injected slowly. When the injection is complete, the needle is removed.

Pertinent points for tasks involving medical staff

Prescribing

Prescription, collection, and administration of intrathecal chemotherapy can only be performed by physicians who are registered after competency assessment. Prescribing should be performed on an approved intrathecal prescription form.

Collecting

The doctor who is to administer the intrathecal chemotherapy should collect the drug in person by presenting the intrathecal prescription and any other chemotherapy prescriptions for that patient. The doctor must check the drug against the prescription before accepting drug. It must be released only by a pharmacist authorized to do so. The drug should be carried to the patient from the pharmacy in a dedicated container.

Administering

Frequently asked questions about administering include the following:

Where can intrathecal chemotherapy be administered?

This should be done only in designated areas.

When can intrathecal chemotherapy be administered?

This should only be done at designated times that have been approved locally, and must be undertaken within normal working hours.

Who checks the intrathecal chemotherapy at the bedside?

This should be done by medical staff authorized to perform this task. A final check must always be done by the administering doctor just before injection.

How should intrathecal chemotherapy be administered?

Access to CSF should be obtained by a standard lumbar puncture procedure to obtain free flow of CSF. Injection of the chemotherapy must only be performed when the physician is confident that the spinal needle is in the intrathecal space. If assistance from an anesthetist is required to perform the lumbar puncture, the chemotherapy must only be injected intrathecally by an authorized doctor, as above.

Pertinent points for pharmacists

Clinically screening prescriptions

Pharmacists must have been assessed as competent and registered to screen chemotherapy. Follow local chemotherapy screening protocol.

Releasing the product to medical staff

Only pharmacists who have been authorized and registered are involved in this process. The doctor who is due to administer the intrathecal product should present the correct prescription to an authorized pharmacist. The product is released providing there is documented evidence that any IV chemotherapy intended on the same day has already been administered.

Supportive care: anemia

Anemia is defined as a decrease in either hemoglobin (Hb) or red blood cells (RBCs), which results in decreased oxygen carrying capacity. Anemia can be divided into three classes: inappropriate RBC destruction, blood loss, or inadequate RBC production. It often occurs from either anticancer treatment or disease-related processes.

Approximately 30% of cancer patients will develop anemia. Therefore, it is considered one of the most common hematological complications associated with malignancy. In addition, 80%–90% of patients experience cancer-related fatigue, and anemia is one of the proposed mechanisms responsible.

Risk factors

- History of transfusion in past 6 months
- History of radiotherapy
- Myelosuppression of current treatment
- Previous myelosuppressive therapy
- Low initial Hb level
- Cardiac history
- Pulmonary disease
- Cerebral vascular disease

Signs and symptoms

- Fatigue
- Weakness
- Tiredness
- Shortness of breath
- Rapid pulse
- Dizziness
- Hypotension
- Brittle nails
- Concave nails

Pharmacologic treatment options

Treatment strategies for managing chemotherapy-associated anemia are often based on symptoms and Hb levels (see Table 15.76). There are currently three erythropoiesis-stimulating agents (ESAs) available on the U.S. market that are approved for treatment of anemia (i.e., epoetin alfa [Epogen, Procrit], darbepoetin [Aranesp]). These agents along with iron supplementation are considered the treatment of choice for managing chemotherapy-induced anemia.

ESA therapy should only be used in those patients with anemia due to concomitant myelosuppressive chemotherapy. Additonally, the product labeling of these agents indicates that they are not to be used in patients receiving myelosuppressive therapy when the anticipated outcome is cure. Specific dosing recommendations including dose increases and reductions for each agent are found in Table 15.77.

Before initiating ESA therapy, it is important to assess iron stores. If deficient, iron stores should be replaced.

Table 15.76 Treatment options for chemotherapy-associated anemia

Description	Hb (≤10 g/dL)	Hb (10–11 g/dL)
Asymptomatic	Iron panel (serum iron, total iron binding capacity, serum ferritin) Consider ESA therapy if not absolute iron deficient	Observation
Symptomatic	Iron panel Consider ESA therapy	Iron panel Consider ESA therapy

Red blood cell transfusions should be used as indicated based on symptoms, institutional policy, and practice guidelines.

Table 15.77 Dosing regimen for ESA therapy

Drug/dose	Response	Action
Epoetin alfa 150 U/kg SC 3 times weekly	No rise in Hb by ≥1 g/dL after 4 weeks	Increase to 300 U/kg SC 3 times weekly
	Hb ~12 g/dL or Hb increases >1 g/dL in 2 weeks	Decrease dose by 25%
	Hb >12 g/dL	Withhold dose until Hb <11 g/dL; restart at a 25% dose reduction
Epoetin alfa 40,000 units SC weekly	No rise in Hb by ≥1 g/dL after 4 weeks	Increase to 60,000 U/kg SC weekly
	Hb ~12 g/dL or Hb increases >1 g/dL in 2 weeks	Decrease dose by 25%
	Hb >12 g/dL	Withhold dose until Hb <11 g/dL; restart at a 25% dose reduction
Darbepoetin alfa 2.25 mcg/kg SC weekly	No rise in Hb by ≥1 g/dL after 6 weeks	Increase dose to 4.5 mcg/kg
	Hb >11 g/dL or Hb increases >1 g/dL in 2 weeks	Decrease dose by 40%
	Hb >12 g/dL	Withhold dose until Hb <11 g/dL; restart at a 40% dose reduction

Abbreviations: mcg/kg, micrograms per kilogram; SC, subcutaneous; U/kg, units per kilogram.

Iron replacement

- If ferritin <30 ng/mL and transferrin saturation <15%:
    - Treat with IV or oral iron supplementation
    - After iron stores increase, reassess Hb and need for ESA therapy
- If ferritin <300 ng/mL and transferrin saturation <20%:
    - Consider ESA therapy
    - Consider oral iron supplementation

Reassessment of ESA therapy

- If no response within 8–9 weeks; discontinue therapy
- Stable Hb (1–2 g/dL from baseline); continue therapy
- Titrate dosage to avoid RBC transfusion; keeping Hb 10 to <12 g/dL
- Discontinue therapy when chemotherapy is complete and anemia has resolved

Treatment considerations

Erythropoietic therapy

Risks

- Thrombotic events
- Potential for decreased survival
- Time to tumor progression likely shortened

Benefits

- Decrease in transfusions
- Gradual improvement in fatigue

Transfusion

Risks

- Viral transmission
- Bacterial contamination
- Transfusion reactions
- Iron overload

Benefits

- Rapid increase in Hb
- Rapid improvement in fatigue

Further reading

National Comprehensive Cancer Network (2009). Practice guidelines for cancer and chemotherapy related anemia: NCCN v.1.2009. Available at: www.nccn.org/professionals/physician_gls/PDF/anemia.pdf.

Rizzo JD, Somerfield MR, Hagerty, KL, et al. (2007). Use of epoetin and darbepoetin in patients with cancer: American Society of Clinical Oncology/American Society of Hematology clinical practice guideline update. *J Clin Oncol* **14**:3396.

Antiemetics for prophylaxis of chemotherapy-induced nausea and vomiting

Nausea and vomiting remain two of the most feared side effects of chemotherapy in cancer patients, with nausea being experienced more often than vomiting. Three types of nausea and vomiting exist: anticipatory, acute (0–24 hours after chemotherapy administration), and delayed (>24 hours after chemotherapy administration).

Antiemetics used to treat nausea and vomiting have different mechanism of action.

Risk factors

- Female
- <30 years of age
- History of motion sickness
- Poor control nausea and vomiting with prior chemotherapy
- Anxiety

Emetogenicity of antineoplastic agents is classified according to degree of incidence, from very low (level 1) to very high incidence (level 5). Emetogenicity is dependent on the type of chemotherapy and the dose.

High emetic risk (emesis frequency >90%; level 5)

- Carmustine >250 mg/m^2
- Cisplatin >50 mg/m^2
- Cyclophosphamide >1500 mg/m^2
- Dacarbazine
- Doxorubicin/epirubicin + cyclophosphamide
- Mechloretamine
- Streptozocin

Moderate emetic risk (emesis frequency 30%–90%; level 3 or 4)

- Actinomycin-D
- Aldesleukin >12–15 million units/m^2
- Azacitadine
- Carboplatin
- Carmustine <250 mg/m^2
- Cisplatin <50 mg/m^2
- Cyclophosphamide <1500 mg/m^2
- Cytarabine >1000 mg/m^2
- Daunorubicin
- Doxorubicin
- Epirubicin
- Ifosfamide
- Idarubicin
- Imatinib
- Irinotecan
- Lomustine
- Methotrexate 250 to >1000 mg/m^2

- Oxaliplatin >75 mg/m^2
- Streptozocin
- Temozolomide

Low emetic risk (emesis frequency 10%–30%; level 2)

- Capecitabine
- Cyclophosphamide (oral)
- Cytarabine 100–200 mg/m^2
- Docetaxel
- Doxorubicin 20–59 mg/m^2
- Doxorubicin (liposomal)
- Etoposide
- 5-flurouracil
- Fludarabine
- Gemcitabine
- Methotrexate >50 mg/m^2 and <250 mg/m^2
- Mitomycin
- Mitoxantrone
- Paclitaxel
- Pemetrexed
- Procarbazine (oral)
- Teniposide
- Topotecan

Minimal emetic risk (emesis frequency <10%; level 1)

- Alemtuzumab
- Asparaginase
- Bevacizumab
- Bleomycin
- Bortezomib
- Busulfan (low dose)
- Cetuximab
- Chlorambucil (oral)
- Dasatinib
- Erlotinib
- Gemtuzumab
- Hydroxyurea
- Lapatinib
- Mercaptopurine
- Methotrexate ≤50 mg/m^2
- Panitumumab
- Rituximab
- Sorafenib
- Sunitinib
- Temsirolimus
- Thioguanine
- Trastuzumab
- Vinblastine
- Vincristine
- Vinorelbine

Considerations when choosing an antiemetic regimen

- Chemotherapy emetic risk, dose, and schedule
- Chemotherapy drug combinations (additive emetic effect)
  - Addition of level 3 or 4 agents increases emetogenicity by 1 level per agent.
  - Addition of one or more level 2 agents increases emetogenicity by 1 level greater than the most emetogenic agent.
  - Level 1 agents do not contribute to total emetogenicity.
- Type of nausea and vomiting being treated
- Risk factors for nausea and vomiting
- Mechanism of action and dosage forms available for each antiemetic
- Adverse effects

Prevention is the best treatment for managing chemotherapy-induced nausea and vomiting. This often requires a combination of antiemetics.

Specific antiemetic recommendations and dosing are provided in Table 15.78.

Breakthrough antiemetics play a very important role in emetic control. These medications allow the patient to prevent and control nausea and vomiting post-chemotherapy (see Table 15.79).

Optimal treatment for anticipatory nausea and vomiting is to prevent emesis before each chemotherapy cycle. Unfortunately, this is not always possible; therefore, benzodiazepines may be necessary to treat this type of nausea and vomiting (see Table 15.80).

Table 15.78 Combination of antiemetics to prevent or reduce chemotherapy-induced nausea and vomiting

Emetogenic potential	Treatment
High emetic risk (>90%) Level 5	$5HT_3$, IV/PO 1 hour before chemotherapy day 1 (e.g., ondansetron 24 mg PO or 8 mg IV, granisetron 2 mg PO or 0.01 mg/kg IV) ***and*** Dexamethasone 8–20 mg IV/PO daily, starting on the morning of chemotherapy and continued days 1–4 (dose reduce to 12 mg when administered with aprepitant or fosaprepitant) ***and*** Neurokinin receptor antagonist (NKA) (aprepitant 125 mg PO 1 hour before chemotherapy or fosaprepitant 115 mg IV on day 1, then aprepitant 80 mg PO on days 2–3) ***and*** As-needed medication for breakthrough nausea and vomiting Agents with high emetic risk also carry a high risk for delayed nausea and vomiting.

Table 15.78 (*Contd.*)

Moderate emetic risk (30%–90%) Level 3 or 4	Day 1 $5HT_3$, IV/PO 1 hour before chemotherapy (e.g., ondansetron 24 mg PO or 8 mg IV, granisetron 2 mg PO or 0.01 mg/kg IV) ***and*** Dexamethasone 8–20 mg IV/PO daily starting on the morning of chemotherapy and continued days 1–4 (dose reduce to 12 mg when administered with aprepitant or fosaprepitant) ± NKA (aprepitant 125 mg PO 1 hour before chemotherapy or fosaprepitant 115 mg IV on day 1) Days 2–3 If aprepitant or fosaprepitant is used on day 1, then continue aprepitant 80 mg PO on days 2–3 ***or*** Dexamethasone 8 PO daily or 4 mg PO bid ***or*** $5HT_3$ daily (e.g., ondansetron 16 mg PO daily or 8 mg PO bid, granisetron 1 mg PO bid) As-needed medication for breakthrough nausea and vomiting
Low emetic risk (10%–30%) Level 2	Dexamethasone 8 mg IV/PO daily ***or*** Prochlorperazine 10 mg PO/IV every 4–6 hours ***or*** Metoclopramide 10 mg–40 mg PO/IV every 4–6 hours All should start morning of chemotherapy As-needed medication for breakthrough nausea and vomiting
Minimal emetic risk (<10%) Level 1	No routine prophylaxis As-needed medication for breakthrough nausea and vomiting

Table 15.79 Breakthrough and adjuvant treatment for chemotherapy-induced nausea and vomiting

- The best strategy is to use an additional agent from a different class of antiemetics.
- It is preferred to schedule the medication first, then as the nausea and vomiting decrease, change to an as-needed basis.
- Dosage-form decisions are very important because of the patient's physical or psychological inability to take medications by mouth.
- At the next chemotherapy treatment, the antiemetic regimen should be changed to a higher level of primary prevention.

Treatment options

- Prochlorperazine 25 mg suppository every 12 hours or 10 mg IV/PO every 4–6 hours
- Metoclopramide 10–40 mg IV/PO every 4–6 hours
- Diphenhydramine 25–50 mg PO/IV every 4–6 hours
- Lorazepam 0.5–2 mg PO every 4–6 hours
- Promethazine 12.5–25 mg PO every 4 hours
- $5HT_3$ antagonist
- Dexamethasone 8 mg PO daily
- Haloperidol 1–2 mg PO every 4–6 hours
- Dronabinol 5–10 mg PO every 3–6 hours

Table 15.80 Treatment of anticipatory nausea and vomiting

- Use optimal antiemetic treatment before each cycle
- Alprazolam 0.5–2 mg PO tid beginning on the night before treatment
- Lorazepam 0.5–2 mg PO on the night before and morning of treatment

Further reading

Chris MG, Hesketh PJ, Somerfield MR, et al. (2006). American Society of Clinical Oncology guideline for antiemetics in oncology: update 2006. *J Clin Oncol* **24**:2932–2947.

National Comprehensive Cancer Network (2009). Practice guidelines for antiemesis: NCCN v.3.2009. Available at: www.nccn.org/professionals/physician_gls/PDF/antiemesis.pdf

Febrile neutropenia

Infections are an important cause of morbidity and mortality in immunocomprised patients. It is estimated that 50%–60% of patients who become febrile have an occult infection. The primary sites of infection are the mouth, esophagus, pharynx, small and large bowel, rectum, sinuses, lung, intravascular access sites, and skin.

Febrile neutropenia is defined as a single temperature of >38.3°C or a temperature >38°C lasting for 1 hour with an absolute neutrophil count (ANC) of < 500 neutrophils/mm^3.

$$ANC = (WBC \times 10^3/mm^3) \times (\%\ bands + \%\ segs)$$

Risk factors

- Myelosuppressive chemotherapy regimen
- Hematopoietic stem cell transplant (HSCT)
- Severe, prolonged neutropenia
- Hematological malignancies
- Myelodysplastic syndrome
- Advanced or refractory malignancy
- Radiation therapy
- High-dose corticosteroids
- Lymphocytic depleting agents (e.g., fludarabine)

Considerations when implementing therapy

Initial evaluation

- Potential sites of infection
- Causative agents

Site-specific history and physical

- Recent antimicrobial therapy (including prophylaxis)
- Previous positive cultures
- Cell lines affected by the chemotherapy regimen
- Last administration of chemotherapy agent
- Family illness
- Recent travel
- Comorbid illnesses
- Drug interactions
- Bactericidal antimicrobial regimen
- Drug allergy
- Clinical instability
- Institutional bacterial-resistant patterns

Pharmacological treatment options (see Table 15.81)

Colony-stimulating factors should be considered in patients with serious infection complications such as invasive fungal infections, pneumonia, and progressive infection (any). Recommendations and dosing are listed in Table 15.82.

Table 15.81 Agents used for treatment of febrile neutropenia

Time since onset	Common pathogens	Treatment
0 to <72 hours	Gram positive Coagulase-negative staphylococci *Streptococcus viridans* *Staphylococcus aureus* *Enterococcus* species Gram negative *Escherichia coli* *Klebsiella* species *Enterobacter* species *Pseudomonas aeruginosa*	Antimicrobial monotherapy (broad spectrum) Piperacillin/tazobactam Imipenem/cilastatin Meropenem Cefepime Antimicrobial combination therapy (broad spectrum) Aminoglycoside + antipseudomonal penicillin ± beta-lactamase inhibitor Aminoglycoside + extended-spectrum cephalosporin Ciprofloxacin + antipseudomonal penicillin
≥72–96 hours without response to previous agent	Resistant gram positive, resistant gram negative, anaerobes	Broad-spectrum antimicrobial ***plus*** Vancomycin (not recommended for empiric therapy, but if at risk for resistant gram-positive infection; reassess in 2–3 days; discontinue if negative cultures) Metronidazole (if not currently on appropriate anaerobic coverage and suspect infection) If initial broad-spectrum antibiotic used could be broadened, such as ceftazidime, pipercillin/tazobactam, or cefepime, switch coverage to a carbapenem. If indicated per culture results Linezolid Daptomycin

Table 15.81 (*Contd.*)

Time since onset	Common pathogens	Treatment
>96 hours without response to previous agents	Fungus (*Candida*, moulds),viral (herpes simplex, varicella zoster, cytomegalovirus)	Broad-spectrum antimicrobial ***plus*** Fluconazole Voriconazole Posaconazole Micafungin Caspofungin Anidulafungin Amphotericin B (including conventional, liposomal, lipid complex) Acyclovir Valacyclovir Valganciclovir Ganciclovir Consider granulocyte colony– stimulating factor or granulocyte-macrophage colony-stimulating factor when patient has a serious infection such as pneumonia or invasive fungal infection. Agent and dosing are patient specific, depending on patient's chemotherapy regimen, type of cancer, HSCT, duration of neutropenia, prophylactic antifungal and/or viral therapy, and site-specific infection.

Renal and/or liver function should be considered when dosing most of these agents.

Initial empiric therapy in a neutropenic patient with sepsis may differ from above.

Update antimicrobial therapy after cultures are reviewed.

Keep broad-spectrum antimicrobial until ANC >500 cells/mcL.

Table 15.82 Dosing and frequency of colony-stimulating factors

Colony-stimulating factor	Dosing
Filgrastim (Neupogen)	5 mcg/kg subcutaneously daily x 14 days or until ANC reaches 10,000 cells/m^3
Pegfilgrastim (Neulasta)	6 mg subcutaneously every 14 days: begin 24 hours after chemotherapy cycle and continue until ANC reaches 10,000 cells/m^3
Sargramostim (Leukine)	250 mcg/m^2/day IV: start 4 days after chemotherapy cycle and continue until ANC ≥1500 cells/m^3

Duration of treatment

- Antimicrobials should be continued until ANC ≥500 cells/m^3 in cases of unknown fever etiology
- Documented infections are treated according to the site, pathogen, and until the ANC ≥500 cells/m^3
- The initial empiric antimicrobial therapy should be continued until ANC >500 cells/mm^3

Evaluation and follow-up

- Continued culture assessment
- Continued site specific assessment
- Continued evaluation of patient's clinical response to therapy

Further reading

National Comprehensive Cancer Network (2008). Practice guidelines for the treatment and prevention of cancer-related infections: NCCN v.1.2008. Available at: www.nccn.org

Hypercalcemia

Hypercalcemia of malignancy occurs in 10%–40% of patients. The detection of hypercalcemia is associated with very poor prognosis (~50% mortality).

There are four types of hypercalcemia associated with cancer: local osteolytic, humoral, 1,25-dihydroxyvitamin D-secreting lymphomas, and ectopic hyperparathyroidism. Humoral is the most common type, and is associated with secretion of parathyroid hormone (PTH)-related protein.

Cancers associated with the release of PTH-related protein are squamous cell, renal cell, endometrial, and breast. Local osteolytic hypercalcemia is most common in bone metastases associated with multiple myeloma, breast cancer, and lymphoma.

Signs and symptoms

- Fatigue
- Muscle weakness
- Depression
- Abdominal pain
- Constipation
- Anorexia
- Nausea/vomiting
- Dizziness
- Polyuria
- Polydipsia
- Pain
- Hallucinations
- Psychosis
- Arrhythmias
- Somnolence
- Coma

Keep in mind that the signs and symptoms associated with hypercalcemia do not correlate well with calcium levels. Normal calcium levels range from 8.5 to 10.5 mg/dL (if low albumin, corrected calcium needs to be calculated):

$$\text{Calcium}_{\text{corrected}} = (\text{Calcium}_{\text{serum}} + [\text{Albumin}_{\text{normal}} - \text{Albumin}_{\text{serum}}]) \times 0.8$$

Treatment strategies

First-line therapies

Mild hypercalcemia (corrected calcium ≤11.9 mg/dL)

- Treat underlying malignancy
- Oral or IV hydration with 0.9% sodium chloride
- Patient mobilization
- Bisphosphonates: pamidronate or zoledronic acid IV x1 dose (dose based on renal function)
- Onset of action: 3 days
- Reassess symptoms and calcium level, may repeat in 10–14 days
- Discontinue medications that may increase calcium levels (e.g., thiazide diuretics)

Moderate to severe hypercalcemia (corrected calcium ≥12 mg/dL)

- Aggressive IV hydration: 200–500 mL/hr of 0.9% sodium chloride
- Loop diuretics (e.g., furosemide 20–40 mg every 12 hours)
- Bisphosphonates: pamidronate or zoledronic acid IV x1 dose (dose based on renal function)
  - Onset of action: 3 days
  - Reassess symptoms and calcium level, may repeat in 10–14 days
- Discontinue medications that may increase calcium levels (e.g., thiazide diuretics)
- Treatment of hypophosphatemia (≤3 mg/dL; e.g., NeutraPhos 250 mg 4 times daily until serum phosphorus level >3 mg/dL)
  - Monitor calcium phosphate product

Second-line therapies

- Glucocorticoids: prednisone 60 mg PO daily for 10 days or hydrocortisone 200–400 mg IV daily for 3–5 days
  - Onset of action: 7–14 days
- Plicamycin 25 mcg/kg IV every 48 hours for 3 doses
  - Onset of action: 12 hours
- Calcitonin 4–8 units/kg SC or IM every 6–12 hours (especially if symptomatic)
  - Onset of action: 2 hours
- Gallium nitrate 200 mg/m^2/day continuous infusion for up to 5 days
- Onset of action: 2 days
- Dose is based on renal function
- Dialysis

Further reading

Higdon ML, Higdon JA (2006). Treatment of oncologic emergencies. *Am Fam Physician* **74**:1873–1880.

Stewart AF (2005). Hypercalcemia associated with cancer. *N Engl J Med* **352**:373–379.

Zojer N, Ludwig H (2007). Hematological emergencies. *Ann Oncol* **18**(Suppl.1):i45–i48.

Tumor lysis syndrome

Tumor lysis syndrome (TLS) is acute cell lysis caused by radiation and chemotherapy. This occurs from the rapid breakdown of tumor cells, causing the release of intracellular products and results in hyperuricemia, hyperphosphatemia, hypocalcemia, acute renal failure, and acidosis.

TLS is most common in hematologic malignancies or in patients with a high tumor burden (e.g., acute lymphoblastic leukemia and Burkitt's lymphoma). It usually manifests itself within 1 to 5 days after initiation of cytotoxic therapy.

Risk factors

- Leukemia
- Lymphoma
- High tumor burden
- High lactate dehydrogenase (LDH) (>1000 U/mL)
- Dehydration
- Elevated urea
- Renal impairment

Treatment strategies

Prophylaxis

- Aggressive fluid resuscitation with 0.9% sodium chloride (3 L/m^2/day); 24–48 hours prior to chemotherapy administration
- Urine alkalization with sodium bicarbonate to maintain pH between 7 and 8
- Loop diuretics to maintain urine output ≥100 mL/m^2/day
- Allopurinol PO or IV 300 mg daily (dose reduced in renal insufficiency); 24–48 hours prior to chemotherapy administration
- Rasburicase 0.2 mg/kg/day for 1–7 days in patients at highest risk for TLS or with existing TLS (e.g., elevated uric acid, high LDH, high tumor burden)
  - In adults, other dosing strategies for rasburicase have been used in clinical trials: 3–6 mg IV once (along with hydration and allopurinol, with or without urinary alkalinization)
  - Contraindicated in patients with glucose-6-phosphate dehydrogenase (G6PD) deficiency because of increased risk of severe hemolysis (see Chapter 10, p. 220)
  - May cause falsely reduced uric acid levels in blood samples left at room temperature. Thus prechilled heparin-anticoagulant tubes must be immersed and maintained in an ice-water bath. Blood samples assays must be completed within a 4-hour time frame.
  - Serious adverse effects include anaphylaxis and methemoglobinemia.

Common complications of TLS include hyperphosphatemia, hyperkalemia, hypocalcemia, and hyperuricemia. Treatments can be directed toward specific symptoms. Treatment recommendations include the following:

- For hyperphosphatemia: hydration, forced diuresis, oral phosphate binders, hemodialysis

- Monitor calcium phosphate product (see Management of Phosphate Disorders unit in this chapter, p. 432)
- Hyperkalemia; hydration, forced diuresis, potassium binders, glucose and rapid-acting insulin, aerosol beta$_2$ agonist, IV calcium, hemodialysis (see Management of Potassium Imbalance unit in this chapter, p. 434)

Several medications should be avoided, if possible, in patients with TLS. This avoidance strategy may help prevent renal dysfunction.

- Nephrotoxic drugs (e.g., aminoglycosides, tacrolimus, cyclosporine)
- Drugs that inhibit uric acid excretion (e.g., hydrochlorothiazide)

Further reading

Higdon ML, Higdon JA (2006). Treatment of oncologic emergencies. *Am Fam Physician* **74**:1873–1880.

McDonnell AM, Lenz KL, Frei-Lahr, et al. (2006). Single dose rasburicase 6 mg in the management of tumor lysis syndrome in adults. *Pharmacotherapy* **26**:806–812.

Zojer N, Ludwig H (2007). Hematological emergencies. *Ann Oncol* **18**(Suppl. 1):i45–i48.

Pain: a definition

The International Association for the Study of Pain defines *pain* as "an unpleasant sensory and emotional experience associated with actual or potential tissue damage, or described in terms of such damage. Pain is always subjective." Individuals learn the relevance of the term through early life experiences resulting in injury.

Pain is the experience we associate with actual or potential tissue damage. Pain is always an unpleasant sensation, which makes it an emotional experience as well.

Certain experiences resemble pain, e.g., pricking, but because they are not unpleasant these should not be termed pain. Unpleasant abnormal experiences such as dysesthesias may not be subjectively described as pain because they lack the typical sensory qualities of pain.

For psychological reasons, people may report pain in the absence of tissue damage or other pathophysiological cause. There usually is no way to distinguish their report of pain from that due to tissue damage. Relying on subjective report, we must regard their experience as pain if they describe it as such. This definition of pain avoids tying the sensation to a stimulus. Considering this, pharmacists should be cautious about expressing opinions about whether a patient is in pain or not.[1]

Types of pain

Nociceptive pain

Nociceptive pain occurs when pain receptors (nociceptors) are stimulated by the transmission of noxious stimuli from the site of injury to the central nervous system. It acts as an alarm system that indicates the presence of a potentially damaging stimulus.

This is a functional type of pain in that it discourages the use of injured body parts, reducing the risk of further injury. This pain responds well to acetaminophen, NSAIDs, and opioid analgesics (see Fig. 15.7).

Neuropathic pain

Neuropathic pain describes painful syndromes that are "initiated or caused by a primary lesion or dysfunction in the nervous system."[1] Neuropathic pain may be described as peripheral or central, although both components of the nervous system are involved.

This is a maladaptive type of pain. It is as if the alarm system were constantly turned on despite no imminent threat or repeated false alarms occurring. The quality of the pain is often described as burning, stabbing, or electric shock.

The pain may be evoked by stimuli otherwise considered benign, e.g., light touch, pressure of clothing, wind, hot, or cold. It may also occur spontaneously. Neuropathic pain may be constant, intermittent, or paroxysmal. It may not respond well to classic analgesics but frequently responds to unconventional analgesic treatments, including antidepressants, anticonvulsants, and other therapies such as clonidine and capsaicin (see Fig. 15.7).

1 International Association for the Study of Pain. www.iasp-pain.org

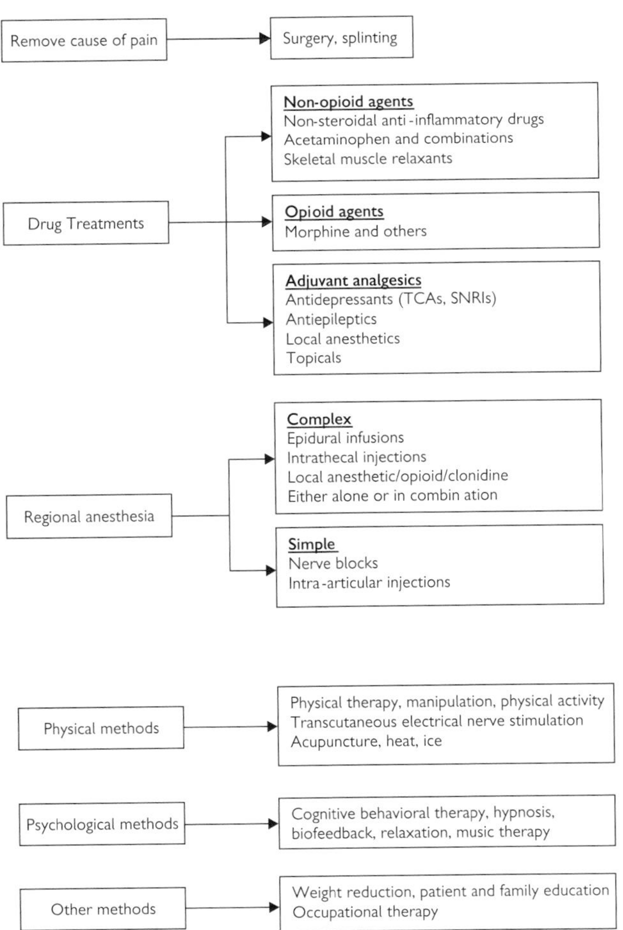

Figure 15.7 Methods available for treating pain.

Assessment of pain

Assessment of pain should include a description of the location, quality, and intensity of the pain. Many good, validated tools are available to assess pain.

Unidimensional tools such as the numerical scale, visual analog scales (VASs; a line moving from "no pain" to "worst possible pain"), or categorical scale (in which words such as *none, slight, moderate,* or *severe* are used) describe only pain intensity (see Fig. 15.8) They can be used to quickly assess current pain level and response to analgesic therapy.

Categorical scales

In categorical scales, words are used to describe the magnitude of the pain; the patient picks the most appropriate word. Most research groups use four words for pain intensity (*none, mild, moderate,* and *severe*). Scales to measure pain relief were developed later and commonly use a five-category scale (*none, slight, moderate, good,* and *complete*).

For analysis, numbers are given to the verbal categories (for pain intensity: none = 0, mild = 1, moderate = 2, severe = 3; and for relief: none = 0, slight = 1, moderate = 2, good = 3, complete = 4).

The main advantages of categorical scales are that they are quick and simple. However, the small number of descriptors could force the scorer to choose a particular category when none describes the pain satisfactorily.

Visual analog scales

VASs consisting of lines with the left end labeled "no relief of pain" and the right end labeled "complete relief of pain" seem to overcome the limit of descriptors. The standard VAS is 10 cm long. Patients mark the line at the point that corresponds to their pain. The scores are obtained by measuring the distance between the "no relief" end and the patient's mark, usually in centimeters.

The main advantages of VASs are that they are simple and quick to score, they avoid imprecise descriptive terms, and they provide many points from which to choose. More concentration and coordination are needed on the part of the scorer, which can be difficult postoperatively or with neurological disorders.

Pain-relief scales are perceived as more convenient than pain-intensity scales, probably because patients have the same baseline relief (zero), whereas they could start with different baseline intensity (usually moderate or severe). Relief-scale results are then easier to compare. They can also be more sensitive than intensity scales. A theoretical drawback of relief scales is that the patient has to remember what the pain was like to begin with.

Global subjective efficacy ratings, or simply "global scales," are designed to measure overall treatment performance. Patients are asked questions such as "How effective do you think the treatment was?" and then answer using a labeled numerical or categorical scale. Although these judgments probably include adverse effects, they can be the most sensitive way to discriminate between treatments.

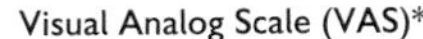

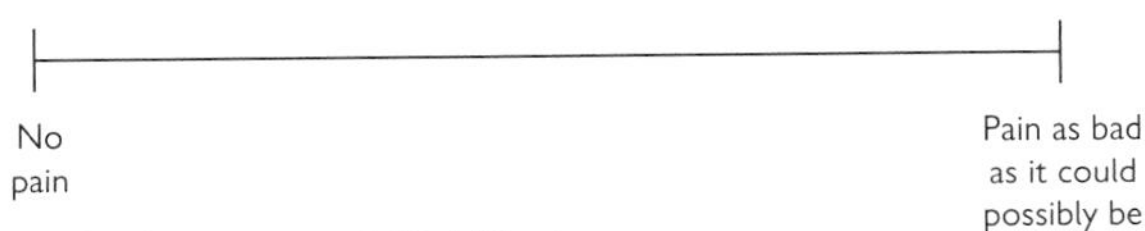

*A 10-cm baseline is recommended for VAS scales.
From: Acute Pain Management: Operative of Medical Procedures and Trauma, Clinical Pracice Guideline No. 1AHCR Publication No. 92-0032; February 1992. Agency for Healthcare Reasearch & Quality, Rockville, MD; Pages 116-117.

Simple Descriptive Pain Intensity Scale*

No pain — Mild pain — Moderate pain — Sever pain — Very severe pain — Worst possible pain

*If used as a graphic rating scale, a 10-cm baseline is recommended.

Figure 15.8 Unidimensional pain assessment scales.
From: Acute Pain Management: Operative or Medical Procedures and Trauma, Clinical Practice Guideline No. 1. AHCPR Publication No. 92–0032, February 1992. Rockville, MD: Agency for Healthcare Research & Quality, pp. 116–117.

Judgment of pain by the patient, rather than by a caregiver, is the ideal. Caregivers tend to overestimate the pain relief actually experienced by the patient.

Ancillary tools used in conjunction with unidimensional tools include pain diaries, pain diagrams (patient shades the area in pain on a picture of a person), and medication side-effect rating. Pain diaries are good for characterizing breakthrough pain. Figure 15.9 shows an example of a pain diary.

Multidimensional tools developed to assess the impact of pain on mood, activities, and quality of life are more time consuming and can be difficult for some patients to complete. These include the McGill Pain Questionnaire, Brief Pain Inventory, and Wisconsin Brief Pain Questionnaire.

Pain Management Log

Please use this pain assessment scale to fill out your pain control log.

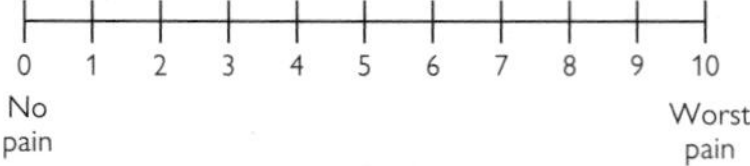

Date	Time	How severe is the pain?	Medicine or non-drug pain control method	How severe is the pain after one hour?	Activity at time of pain

Figure 15.9 Pain management log.

From: Management of Cancer Pain, Clinical Guideline No. 9. AHCPR Publication No. 94–0592, March 1994. Rockville, MD: Agency for Healthcare Research & Quality.

Acute pain

Acute pain is defined as pain that has been present for less than 3 to 6 months. It is very common, with more than half the population reporting pain or discomfort at any one time.

Initial therapy

- Nonsteroidal anti-inflammatory drugs (NSAIDs) and acetaminophen
- Aspirin is an effective analgesic for acute pain, but because of its lack of superiority over acetaminophen and other NSAIDs and its poor safety profile, it is not recommended.

Traditional NSAIDs are excellent analgesics with no clinically important differences in efficacy among specific agents. NSAIDs have demonstrated equal analgesia to starting doses of opioids in many acute-pain settings. NSAIDs do have a ceiling dose above which no further analgesia is achieved, and risk of side effects may limit their use.

Higher doses of NSAIDs are needed for anti-inflammatory effects. With higher doses comes a higher risk of side effects, especially gastrointestinal (GI) toxicity, renal dysfunction, and platelet dysfunction. Data support the use of ibuprofen 400 mg first, as its GI safety profile is similar to that of placebo.

Histamine 2 blockers, misoprostol, and proton pump inhibitors have demonstrated a reduction in duodenal ulcers with daily NSAID use and should be considered in at-risk patients and with long-term use. Be cautious when initiating NSAIDs in patients with pre-existing kidney disease, as NSAIDs can precipitate acute renal failure requiring dialysis.

Although many NSAIDs may be given rectally or by injection, there is no evidence to support these routes being faster or more effective than the oral route. If the patient can swallow, the medicine should be given orally.

The belief that NSAIDs should not be given after orthopedic surgery because they inhibit healing is a myth.

COX-2 inhibitors have not been proven to be more or less effective than traditional NSAIDs. Data do not support a decrease in significant adverse effects. Celecoxib is the only COX-2 inhibitor currently available in the United States; others were withdrawn for cardiovascular concerns. Less-frequent dosing appears to be the only advantage over traditional NSAIDs.

Acetaminophen is a unique analgesic without clear anti-inflammatory properties. Evidence has shown acetaminophen in doses up to 1000 mg to be as effective as NSAIDs in some conditions (e.g., orthopedic surgery and tension headache) while being less effective for other types of acute pain (e.g., dental and menstrual pain). It is a reasonable initial choice for patients with mild to moderate acute pain. Acetaminophen and NSAIDs can be used in combination to enhance pain relief.

Other treatment options

Opioids

- Appropriate for moderate to severe acute pain
- Patient-controlled analgesia preferred to provide consistent, effective relief
- No ceiling dose; titrate until pain relief is achieved or intolerable side effects occur
- Dependence is not a problem in acute pain; respiratory depression is only a problem if the patient is not in pain or is given a dose larger than that needed to control pain.
- Select one opioid for the treatment of acute pain, so that everyone is familiar with its profile. In most situations, morphine is a good choice.
- The metabolite of morphine (morphine-6-glucuronide) can accumulate in renal disease, prolonging the action of morphine, but with appropriate dosing and monitoring this should not be a problem.
- Meperidine should be avoided because of its toxic metabolites that accumulate in renal dysfunction and may lead to CNS stimulation and seizures.
- Codeine, propoxyphene, and tramadol have demonstrated poor analgesic activity and significant side effects. They are not recommended for routine use.
- At therapeutically equivalent doses, different opioids are likely to produce similar side effects (constipation, nausea, sedation, respiratory and cardiovascular depression, and pruritus). Persons vary greatly in their tolerance of these side effects.

Topical agents

Topical agents may be useful in treating acute injuries such as strains, sprains, and soft tissue trauma. There is limited evidence to support the use of counter-irritants such as menthol to relieve musculoskeletal pains. A systematic review has demonstrated that topical NSAIDs are effective, including ketoprofen and ibuprofen.

Chronic pain

Chronic pain is persistent pain that can be either consistent or recurrent and of sufficient duration and intensity to adversely affect a person's well-being, level of function, and quality of life. Intensity of chronic pain is often out of proportion to the observed pathology and is associated with both physical and psychological functional impairment.

A report from the CDC in 2006 showed that 1 in 4 U.S. adults reported suffering a day-long bout of pain in the previous month, while 1 in 10 reported pain lasting a year or more. Low back pain is the most common complaint, along with migraine or severe headache, and joint pain, aching, or stiffness.

Reports of severe joint pain increased with age and occurred more in women. The percentage of adults who took a narcotic drug to alleviate pain in the past month increased from 3.2% in 1988–1994 to 4.2% in 1999–2002.

Analgesics

In treating chronic pain, it is most logical to start with traditional treatments first. NSAIDs and acetaminophen should be tried early. The combination of NSAIDs and acetaminophen can be effective and decrease the dose of the NSAID needed. It is not necessary to make rapid adjustments in therapy initially.

The addition of a weak opioid can help in relieving chronic pain. Opioids should not necessarily be the first or only agent used for pain management in a patient with chronic pain.

Take time to develop a multimodal approach to managing the pain. Patients should be encouraged to initiate, maintain, or increase aerobic and strengthening activity to reduce their pain and improve functional ability. Patients on long-term NSAIDs should be given gastric protection and be educated on the need for this. Proton pump inhibitors are preferred in most patients.

For patients not gaining sufficient response from initial therapy a stronger opioid may be considered or adjunctive agents may be added, such as antidepressants or anticonvulsants.

Nonpharmacological therapies are important components of chronic pain management. Overweight patients with arthritis can see benefit from weight loss. Physical therapy, transcutaneous electronic nerve stimulation (TENS), exercise, cognitive-behavioral therapy (CBT), massage and thermal therapy, and adaptive devices have all demonstrated benefit in management of chronic pain. These may be used alone or in combination with each other and with pharmacological therapies.

Specialist clinics may provide nerve blocks or epidural injections, which may also be helpful.

Potential adjunctive agents

- Amitritptyline or other tricyclic antidepressants (TCAs)
- Carbamazepine
- Gabapentin
- Pregabalin

- Other anticonvulsants, such as, lamotrigine, topiramate, divalproex sodium, phenytoin
- Duloxetine or other serotonin norepinephrine reuptake inhibitors (SNRIs)
- Baclofen or other skeletal muscle relaxants
- Lidocaine topical
- SSRIs can also be beneficial but evidence for this is limited.

Cancer pain

Typically, cancer pain has a limited time frame permitting aggressive pain management. The World Health Organization's analgesic ladder (see Fig. 15.10), originally designed for management of cancer pain, has been broadly applied to any pain condition. The WHO recommends the use of gradually more potent agents with increasing intensity of a patient's pain. Adjuvant agents in addition to opioids are suggested. The selection of opioid is at the prescriber's discretion.

The National Comprehensive Cancer Network (NCCN)'s Clinical Practice Guidelines in Oncology for Adult Cancer Pain recommend the combination of short-acting agents with long-acting agents, because symptoms may worsen temporarily or with advancing disease.

Morphine is still considered a benchmark because of extensive clinical experience and proven analgesia. An advantage is the availability of multiple dosage forms. It is not always ideal, with wide inter-individual response and tolerability and accumulation of active metabolites in renal failure.

Oxycodone and methadone are alternatives. Methadone must be used cautiously because of its long and unpredictable half-life and often underestimated potency. Fentanyl transdermal has become popular as a long-acting agent with improved tolerability due to less constipation and drowsiness compared to that with other agents.

Dealing with breakthrough pain

Cancer pain is usually moderate to severe in intensity and persistent with flares of pain that "break through" the analgesia controlling the baseline pain. An average of 65% of patients with cancer pain report this type of pain up to 7 times a day. Each episode lasts about 30 minutes.

Breakthrough pain is typically managed with as-needed dosing every 2–4 hours of an immediate-release product that may or may not be the same as the controlled-release agent to manage baseline pain.

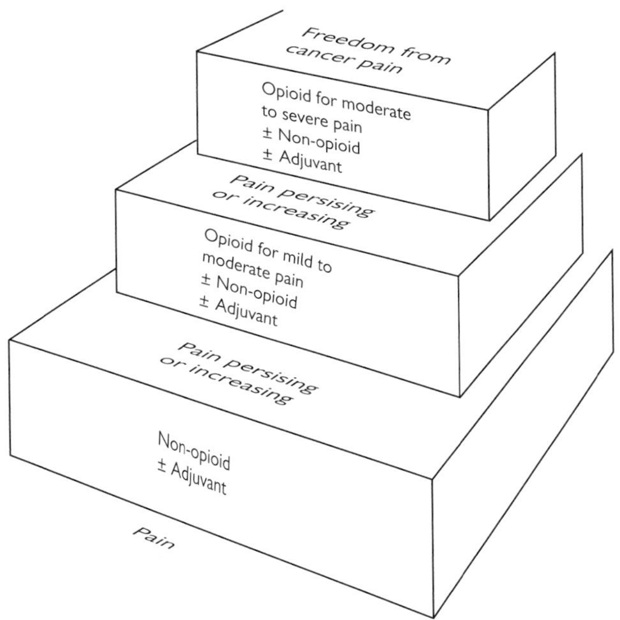

Figure 15.10 World Health Organization analgesic ladder.

Neuropathic pain

Neuropathic pain refers to a group of painful disorders characterized by pain caused by dysfunction or disease of the nervous system at a peripheral level, a central level, or both. It is a complex entity, with many symptoms and signs that fluctuate in number and intensity over time. The three common components of neuropathic pain are allodynia, dysesthesias, and hyperalgesia.

First-line agents in the treatment of neuropathic pain are antidepressants (tricyclic antidepressants, serotonin–norepinephrine reuptake inhibitors), anticonvulsants (gabapentin, pregabalin), lidocaine, opioids, and tramadol. Specific agents listed have demonstrated efficacy in controlled trials.

Second-line agents have either not been studied, not been studied in a controlled fashion, have few controlled studies, or have shown inconsistent results. These agents include carbamazepine, lamotrigine, and SSRIs.

Topical capsaicin, clonidine, dextromethorphan, and mexiletine cannot be recommended at this time because of lack of data.

Patients with chronic neuropathic pain may need frequent pharmacological adjustments until an optimal regimen with adequate pain control is achieved. Recommendations for modifying therapy when a patient has had an inadequate response to or intolerable side effect from a first-line agent include the following:

- Change to another first-line agent with a different mechanism of action.
- Change to a second-line agent with a different mechanism of action.
- Add a different first-line or second-line agent, using principles of rational polypharmacy (optimize synergistic effects, avoid adverse effects).

Osteoarthritis

Osteoarthritis is the most common joint disorder. Primary joints affected are spine, hand, hip, knee, and foot. It is characterized by increased degeneration and loss of cartilage, which results in alteration of subchondral bone and soft tissue changes. In addition to pain, these structural changes lead to decreased or altered motion of the joint, crepitus, and local inflammation. An algorithm for the treatment of osteoarthritis is shown in Figure 15.11.

Acetaminophen

Acetaminophen is the first-line drug of choice for management of osteoarthritis pain. It has analgesic properties but is not anti-inflammatory. Studies have shown that when dosing is scheduled every 6–8 hours, comparable pain relief to that with aspirin and NSAIDs is achieved for mild to moderate osteoarthritis pain.

While it is one of the safest and well-tolerated drugs, it can cause hepatotoxicity in large doses and renal toxicity with prolonged use. Limit the total daily dose of acetaminophen to 4 g/day in healthy individuals and 2 g/day in those with liver disease or a history of alcohol abuse, and in elderly patients.

Topicals

Capsaicin cream may be used alone or in combination with oral analgesics. For best results it should be regularly applied to the affected joints 2 to 4 times daily. It may take up to 2 weeks to see full benefit.

The burning sensation that patients initially experience when applying capsaicin should subside over 1–2 weeks with regular use.

Nonsteroidal anti-inflammatory drugs

NSAIDs may be considered if acetaminophen is ineffective. Efficacy is similar across NSAIDs, although patients may report preference for one NSAID over another. Higher doses are needed for anti-inflammatory effects (e.g., ibuprofen >1800 mg/day).

Proton pump inhibitors are preferred for prevention of GI toxicity. It is unclear if the COX-2 inhibitor celecoxib offers a superior GI side-effect profile. NSAIDs may precipitate renal failure, especially in patients with pre-existing kidney disease.

Opioids

Opioids alone or in combination with acetaminophen are recommended for treatment of moderate to severe pain, especially in those with cardiovascular, gastrointestinal, or renal risk factors. Combination products should be used initially, but if adequate pain control is not reached consider adding a long-acting opioid agent.

Constipation should be anticipated with the use of chronic opioid therapy and managed with an appropriate bowel regimen.

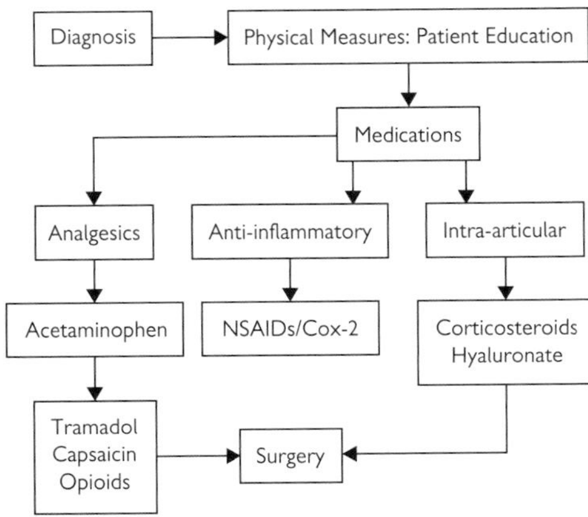

Figure 15.11 Osteoarthritis treatment algorithm. Adapted from American College of Rheumatology Subcommittee on Osteoarthritis Guidelines (2000). Recommendations for the medical management of osteoarthritis of the hip and knee. *Arthritis Rheum* **43**:1905–1915, with permission of John Wiley & Sons, Inc.

Intra-articular injections

Intra-articular glucocorticoid injections are beneficial for managing osteoarthritis when local inflammation or effusion is present. Data are lacking for the optimal number and frequency of injections, but therapy is generally limited to 3 to 4 injections per year. Systemic steroids are not recommended for management of osteoarthritis.

Intra-articular hyaluronic acid is approved for treatment of osteoarthritis of the knee for patients not responding to nonpharmacological treatments or acetaminophen. Studies have shown that hyaluronan therapies provide pain relief comparable to or greater than that observed with NSAIDs or glucocorticoid injections. The onset of pain relief is slower than that of glucocorticoid injections, but pain relief may last considerably longer.

Glucosamine and chondroitin

The efficacy of glucosamine and chondroitin in the treatment of osteoarthritis is still debatable. There may be small to moderate symptomatic efficacy. Continuous therapy for 4–8 weeks is needed before patients notice a difference.

Equianalgesic dosing of opioids

Calculating equianalgesic doses is not an exact science; special care and monitoring are necessary. There is great variation in published tables, which is probably due to extrapolations from single-dose kinetic studies. Key points to consider when converting patients from one opioid analgesic to another are as follows:

- Acute pain ratios may not be the same as chronic pain ratios.
- Ratio tables should only be used as a guide. Individual responses will vary. Doses should be started cautiously and titrated to effect.
- Monitor pain, pain relief, and adverse effects.
- In opioid-tolerant patients it is recommended that the calculated dose of the new opioid be reduced 25%–33% to account for incomplete cross-tolerance among opioids.
- Caution is advised in treating patients with renal impairment, as active metabolites may accumulate.
- Fentanyl and methadone are special cases. Manufacturer-suggested conversion of fentanyl may result in underdosing up to half of patients. Methadone's complex pharmacokinetic properties must be considered especially when switching a patient from methadone to another opioid.

Further reading

Anderson R, Saiers JH, Abram S, et al. (2001). Accuracy in equianalgesic dosing: conversion dilemmas. *J Pain Sympt Manage* **21**(5):397–406.

Global Rph online opioid conversion calculator: http://www.globalrph.com/narcoticonv.htm

Regnard C (1998). Conversion ratios for transdermal fentanyl. *Eur J Palliat Care* **5**(6):204.

Ripamonti C, Groff L, Brunelli C, et al. (1998). Switching from morphine to oral methadone in treating cancer pain: what is the equianalgesic dose ratio? *J Clin Oncol.* **16**:3216–3221.

Compatibility of drugs in pain and palliative care

It is common to mix opioids with other drugs such as baclofen, midazolam, or local anesthetics.

Chemical and physical compatibilities are commonly differentiated. In practice, it is often hard to find information on chemical compatibilities. Some information is available in the peer-reviewed pharmacy literature, and a search of International Pharmaceutical Abstracts (IPA) can be helpful.

Time and temperature are two key components affecting chemical reactions. It is recommended that mixtures not sit in syringes for many hours in a warm room. The risk of incompatibility increases with an increasing number of drugs mixed together.

The majority of recommendations are derived from physical compatibility—i.e., drugs are mixed and no obvious color change or precipitation occurs, even when examined microscopically. Additionally, no change in pharmacological effect is seen when the drugs are administered.

Further reading

Useful sources for information on common opioid mixtures are the following:

Dickman A, Schneider J, Varga J (2005). *The Syringe Driver: Continuous Subcutaneous Infusions in Palliative Care*. Oxford, UK: Oxford University Press.

Trissel L. (2005) *Trissel's Stability of Compounded Formulations*, 3rd edition. Washington, DC: American Pharmacists Association Publications.

Trissel L. (2007). *Handbook on Injectable Drugs*, 14th edition. Bethesda, MD: American Society of Health-System Pharmacists.

Twycross R, Wilcock A (2002). *Palliative Care Formulary*. Oxford, UK: Radcliffe Medical Press.

General psychiatry

Psychiatry is the medical specialty that focuses on diagnosing, treating, and preventing mental illness and substance use disorders. Psychiatry focuses on the relationship between emotional and physical illness. In a given year, just over 25% of the adult U.S. population suffers from a diagnosable mental illness.

Unlike many medical disorders, for which there is a battery of tests (labwork, ECG, MRI, etc.) used in diagnosis, the mainstay of diagnosing a mental illness is by using the Mental Status Exam (MSE). Not to be confused with the Mini Mental State Exam (MMSE) used to screen for dementia, the MSE comprises the components of a psychiatric interview.

This chapter reviews the components of the MSE, the Multiaxial Evaluation Report Form, and general psychiatry references.

Mental status exam (MSE)

- Appearance—brief description of the patient's appearance, grooming, and behavior
- Speech—description of rate, rhythm, and volume
- Mood—the patient's report of how they feel (subjective)
- Affect—the interviewer's perception of displayed emotions (objective)
- Thinking/perception—description of thought content; discuss presence of delusions or hallucinations
- Sensorium—assessment of orientation, concentration, memory, fund of knowledge, ability to abstract, insight, and judgment

The multiaxial evaluation report

- Axis I: psychiatric diagnosis (e.g., schizophrenia, major depressive disorder [MDD], general anxiety disorder [GAD])
- Axis II: mental retardation or personality disorders (e.g., borderline, dependent, antisocial)
- Axis III: general medical conditions (e.g., hypertension, diabetes, cancer)
- Axis IV: psychosocial and environmental stressors (e.g., homeless, divorced, financial situation, legal problems)
- Axis V: global area of functioning (GAF) score from 0 (impaired functioning) to 100 (highest functioning)

State-specific laws

Depending on the state you practice in, it is imperative to be aware of the laws that govern the commitment process and the ability to administer medications with a forced legal order against a patient's will.

Further reading

American Psychiatric Association (1994). *Diagnostic and Statistical Manual on Mental Disorders, fourth edition Text Revision (DSM-IV-TR)*. Washington, DC: American Psychiatric Press.

Sadock BJ, Sadock VA (2007). *Kaplan & Sadock's Synopsis of Psychiatry Behavioral Sciences/Clinical Psychiatry*, 10th ed. Philadelphia: Lippincott Williams & Williams.

Useful Websites

American Psychiatric Association: www.psych.org *or* www.psychiatryonline.com
College of Psychiatric and Neurologic Pharmacists: www.cpnp.org
National Institute of Mental Health: www.nimh.nih.gov
National Alliance on Mental Illness: www.nami.org
Texas Department of State Health Services: http://www.dshs.state.tx.us/mhprograms/ tmapover.shtm

Anxiety disorders

Anxiety disorders are a spectrum of disorders characterized by an intense fear of and a maladaptive response to psychological stressors. Generalized anxiety disorder (GAD), social anxiety disorder (SAD), specific phobia (SP), panic disorder, post-traumatic stress disorder (PTSD), and obsessive-compulsive disorder (OCD) encompass the anxiety spectrum disorders.

As high as 18% of Americans are affected by an anxiety disorder, with SP (8.7%) and SAD (6.8%) being the most prevalent and OCD (~1%) being the least common. GAD, panic disorder, and PTSD prevalence rates range from 2.7% to 3.5%. GAD and SP affect twice as many women as men, whereas SAD and OCD are likely to affect both genders equally. As veterans return from the Iraq war, diagnosis of PTSD is increasing.

Etiology

Genetics

- Play a role in GAD, phobias, panic disorder, and OCD, with rates of 20%–35%
- GAD, panic disorder, and OCD have a higher concordance rate in monozygotic twins (with GAD having an 80%–90% concordance rate)
- PTSD is not related to genetics

Biological

- Increased autonomic reactions and sympathetic tone
- Decreased GABA activity
- Serotonin dysregulation

Signs and symptoms (see Table 15.83)

Clinical features

- GAD is characterized by unrealistic and excessive worry or anxiety.
- SAD, also known as social phobia, is the fear of negative evaluation or embarrassment related to a social or performance situation.
- SP encompasses fear of an object or situation.

Table 15.83 Signs and symptoms of anxiety

Physical signs	Psychological symptoms
Shaking and trembling	Feelings of dread
Muscle tension	Inability to concentrate
Respiratory difficulties (shortness of breath or hyperventilation)	Hypervigilance
Startle response	Insomnia
Dizziness	Decreased libido
Difficulty swallowing	"Butterflies in stomach" or "lump in throat"
Paresthesias	
Autonomic hyperactitivty	
Flushing, tachycardia, palpitations, sweating, cold hands, diarrhea, dry mouth, urinary frequency or urgency	

- Panic disorder is characterized by panic attacks, which involve a response congruent to the person being in life-threatening danger (when in fact they are not), accompanied by a fear of having another panic attack. Patients can develop agoraphobia.
- PTSD requires exposure to a traumatic event. After the event, patients have re-experiencing, avoidance, and hyperarousal symptoms.
- OCD is characterized by obsessions and/or compulsions that cause significant distress and impairment in functioning. Most people suffer from both.

Diagnosis

Lab work-up

- Thyroid-stimulating hormone (TSH) level
- Urine drug screen

Screening tools for anxiety

- MSE
- Beck Anxiety Inventory
- Generalized Anxiety Disorder (GAD-7)
- Hamilton Anxiety Scale (HAM-A)
- PTSD checklist; civilian version (PCL-C), military version (PCL-M)
- Yale–Brown Obsessive Compulsive Scale (Y-BOCS)

Medications that can increase anxiety

- Antidepressants, fluoroquinolones, isoniazid, steroids, stimulants, sympathomimetics, levothyroxine

Rule out:

- Other anxiety disorders
- MDD
- Avoidant personality disorder
- Obsessive-compulsive personality disorder
- Substance abuse or dependence

Pharmacological treatment strategies

Antidepressants

Antidepressants will not be discussed in detail here; please refer to the Depression unit in this chapter (p. 674).

Antidepressants are first-line treatment for most anxiety disorders, except SP (see Table 15.84). Antidepressants may actually be harmful to patients with SP.

When initiating antidepressant therapy for most patients with anxiety spectrum disorders, start with half the dose recommended for depression. Patients with anxiety disorders tend to be more sensitive to the anxiety side effects of these medications; starting at a lower dose may help prevent them.

- Target doses of antidepressants (especially in PTSD and OCD) are higher than doses used in depression.
- Serotonin reuptake inhibitors (SRIs) are first-line for long-term management of GAD, SAD, panic disorder, and OCD.

- Serotonin–norepinephrine reuptake inhibitors (SNRIs) can be considered first-line for GAD. Venlafaxine can be considered for SAD in persons who do not respond to SRIs.
- Clomipramine can be considered in treating OCD.
- Imipramine is the most studied tricyclic antidepressant (TCA) used in treating panic disorder.
- Monoamine oxidase inhibitors (MAOIs) can be used in treatment-resistant SAD patients, and may be effective in ~77%.

Refer to Table 15.84 for the FDA indications of antidepressants in treating anxiety disorders.

Benzodiazepines
- Benzodiazepines are used in the treatment of most anxiety disorders (except OCD).
- Benzodiazepines are used for acute anxiety symptoms and acute panic attacks.
- All benzodiazepines have anxiolytic properties, but only seven of them are FDA approved for treating GAD (see Table 15.85).
- Identification of treatment goals will aid with benzodiazepine selection.
  - High-potency benzodiazepines (e.g., alprazolam and clonazepam) are frequently used in panic disorder.
  - Clonazepam is the most studied benzodiazepine for SAD.
  - Use lorazepam or oxazepam in patients with impaired hepatic function.
- When discontinuing benzodiazepines, be aware of the potential for rebound anxiety or withdrawal symptoms.

Other treatment options
- Buspirone may be an option to treat anxiety in benzodiazepine-naïve patients. Although it is FDA approved for GAD, it is considered second-line. It is ineffective for SAD and panic disorder.
- Prazosin may be considered to treat nightmares associated with PTSD.
- Propranolol decreases the autonomic symptoms of anxiety and is used in SAD taken 1 hour prior to a performance-related situation.

Augmentation strategies
- Augmentation with mood stabilizers can be considered in OCD.
- Augmentation with antipsychotics can be considered in PTSD and OCD.

Nonpharmacological treatment strategies
- Cognitive-behavioral therapy (CBT) is effective in treating SP, SAD, panic disorder, PTSD, and OCD. CBT may include exposure therapy, cognitive restructuring, response prevention, relaxation therapy, and stress management.
- Eye movement desensitization and reprocessing (EMDR) is effective for treatment of PTSD.
- Avoid substances that cause panic attacks or anxiety (e.g., caffeine, stimulants)

Table 15.84 FDA indications of antidepressants for treatment of anxiety

	GAD	SAD	SP	Panic disorder	PTSD	OCD
SRIs						
Escitalopram	√					
Fluoxetine				√		√
Fluvoxamine						√
Paroxetine	√	√		√	√	√
Sertraline		√		√	√	√
SNRIs						
Duloxetine	√					
Venlafaxine	√	√		√		
TCAs						
Clomipramine						√

Antidepressants are often used in the treatment of anxiety disorders. None of the agents listed here are FDA approved for specific phobia (SP), as they may be harmful to these patients.

Table 15.85 Benzodiazepines used in the treatment of anxiety

Generic	Brand name	Equivalent dose (mg)	Onset of action	Route of administration	Anxiety indications
Alprazolam	Xanax, Xanax XR Niravam	0.5	Rapid	PO Orally disintegrating	GAD, panic disorder
Chlordiazepoxide	Librium	10	Moderate	PO, IV, IM	GAD
Clonazepam	Klonapin Klonapin wafers	0.25–0.5	Slow	PO Orally disintegrating	GAD, panic disorder
Clorazepate	Tranxene	7.5	Rapid	PO	GAD
Diazepam	Valium	5	Rapid	PO, IV, IM*	GAD
Lorazepam	Ativan	1	Moderate	PO, IV, IM	GAD
Oxazepam	Serax	15	Slow	PO	GAD

Rapid = 30–60 minutes; moderate = 45–90 minutes; slow >90 minutes.

*IM diazepam has unpredictable absorption; IV is preferred.

Complications

- Depression (PTSD, SAD, GAD)
- Substance abuse (PTSD, SAD, GAD)
- Other anxiety disorders
- Suicide
- Cardiovascular disease

Further reading

Anxiety Disorders Association of America: www.adaa.org

Baldwin DS, Anderson IM, Nutt DJ, et al. (2005). Evidence-based guidelines for the pharmacological treatment of anxiety disorders: recommendations from the British Association for Psychopharmacology. *J Psychopharmacol* **19**(6):567–596.

Dell'Osso B, Altamura AC, Mundo E, et al. (2007). Diagnosis and treatment of obsessive-compulsive disorder and related disorders. *Int J Clin Pract* **68**(1):98–104.

Hoffman EJ, Mathew SJ (2008). Anxiety disorders: a comprehensive review of pharmacotherapies. *Mt Sinai J Med* **75**:248–262.

Depression

Depression is a mood disorder characterized by feelings of sadness or a loss of interest that affects social and occupational functioning. Depressive disorders include major depressive disorder (MDD) and dysthymia.

Depression affects approximately 9.5% of Americans and is one of the leading causes of disability in the United States and worldwide. Depression affects women more than men (2:1).

Etiologies (select)

Genetic

- Family history of depression: 1.5–3 times higher risk

Biological

- Deficiency or dysregulation of serotonin (5-HT), dopamine (DA), and/or norepinephrine (NE)

Signs and symptoms

- Depressed mood
- Loss of interest or pleasure in daily activities
- Weight changes or change in appetite
- Insomnia or hypersomnia
- Psychomotor agitation or retardation
- Fatigue or loss of energy
- Feelings of worthlessness or inappropriate guilt
- Inability to concentrate
- Suicidal ideation

Clinical features

- To be diagnosed as having major depression the person must have five symptoms present during a 2-week period, and one of the symptoms must be either depressed mood or loss of interest.
- For the full diagnostic criteria, refer to the *DSM-IV-TR*.

Diagnosis

Lab workup

- TSH level
- Urine drug screen

Screening tools for depression

- MSE
- Hamilton Rating Scale for Depression (HAM-D)
- Geriatric Depression Scale (GDS)
- Beck Depression Inventory
- Zung Self-Rating Depression Scale
- Montgomery–Asberg Depression Rating Scale (MADRS)

Rule out

- Bipolar disorder
- Mood disorder secondary to a general medical condition
- Substance-induced mood disorder
- Dysthymic disorder

- Schizoaffective disorder
- Dementia
- Adjustment disorder with depressed mood
- Bereavement
- Hypothyroidism

Pharmacological treatment strategies

- Antidepressants (see Table 15.86) remain the mainstay of treating depression.
- Serotonin reuptake inhibitors (SRIs), serotonin–norepinephrine reuptake inhibitors (SNRIs), bupropion, or mirtazapine are all reasonable first-line choices in treating depression.
- SRIs are considered first-line because of their tolerability and low risk of fatality in overdose. If a person fails one SRI it is reasonable to try a second SRI before trying a different class of antidepressants.
- Consider SRIs in most first-episode depressions, and in persons with many comorbidities (hypertension, diabetes, post-MI or post-stroke, seizure disorder).
- Consider SNRIs in persons with comorbid diabetic peripheral neurophathy or comorbid migraine disorders.
- Consider bupropion in persons who complain of weight gain or sexual dysfunction with SRIs or SNRIs.
- Consider bupropion in persons who may benefit from smoking cessation properties.
- Avoid bupropion in persons with seizure disorder, a history of head trauma, or alcohol or benzodiazepine abuse
- Consider mirtazapine in depression associated with decreased appetite and insomnia.
- Tricyclic antidepressants (TCAs) are not considered first-line, secondary to their intolerable side effects and potential for QTc prolongation and fatality in overdose. TCAs may be indicated in persons with comorbid insomnia, neuropathic pain, or migraine disorders.
- Monoamine oxidase inhibitors (MAOIs) are not first-line secondary to food and drug interactions, and risk of serotonin syndrome or hypertensive crisis. Selegiline, available as a transdermal system, may provide benefit in reducing food interactions.
- If a person has partial response but their depression is not in full remission, consider the following:
  - Augmentation with either lithium, liothyronine, buspirone, methylphenidate, or an atypical antipsychotic
  - Dual therapy—two antidepressants can be used concurrently if they have different mechanism of actions
    - SRI/SNRI + bupropion
    - SRI/SNRI + mirtazapine
    - Using two SRIs or an SRI + SNRI is not rational polypharmacy

Table 15.86 Available antidepressant agents

Class of antidepressant	Available agents (generic name)	Brand name	Neuro-transmitters
Serotonin reuptake inhibitors (SRIs)	Citalopram	Celexa	5-HT
	Escitalopram	Lexapro	
	Fluoxetine	Prozac	
	Fluvoxamine	Luvox	
	Paroxetine	Paxil, Paxil CR	
	Sertraline	Zoloft	
Serotonin–norepinephrine reuptake inhibitors (SNRIs)	Desvenlafaxine	Pristiq	5-HT, NE
	Duloxetine	Cymbalta	
	Venlafaxine	Effexor, Effexor XR	
Tricyclic antidepressants (TCAs)	*Tertiary amines*		5-HT, NE
	Amitriptyline	Elavil	
	Clomipramine	Anafranil	
	Doxepin	Sinequan	
	Imipramine	Tofranil	
	Trimipramine	Surmontil	
	Secondary amines		NE >> 5-HT
	Desipramine	Norpramin	
	Nortriptyline	Pamelor	
	Protriptyline	Vivactil	
Tetracyclic antidepressants	Amoxapine	Ascendin	NE >> 5-HT
	Maprotiline	Ludiomil	NE
Alpha-2 antagonists	Mirtazapine	Remeron	5-HT, NE
		Remeron Sol-tab	
5-HT2A receptor antagonist	Nefazodone	No longer available	5-HT
	Trazodone	Desyrel	
Dopamine–norepinehrine reuptake inhibitor (DNRI)	Bupropion	Wellbutrin	DA, NE
		Wellbutrin SR	
		Wellbutrin XL	
Monoamine oxidase inhibitors (MAOIs)	Phenelzine	Nardil	5-HT, DA, NE
	Selegiline transdermal system (TDS)	EMSAM	
	Tranylcypromine	Parnate	

5-HT, serotonin; DA, dopamine; NE, norepinephrine; TDS, transdermal system.

Pharmacological treatment strategies in special populations

Pregnancy

- Weigh risk vs. benefit
- Fluoxetine, sertraline, or bupropion preferred (most evidence)
- First-trimester exposure to paroxetine has been associated with cardiovascular malformations and is considered pregnancy category D.
- Third-trimester exposure to SRIs has been associated with persistent pulmonary hypertension and withdrawal syndrome in neonates.
- Reference: www.otispregnancy.org

Elderly

- Geriatric population accounts for ~16% of suicides annually; depression should not go untreated.
- SRIs or mirtazapine is preferred; avoid TCAs.
- Monitor for hyponatremia in elderly patients.
- Daily fluoxetine is on the Beer's List, secondary to its long half-life.
- Paroxetine is not first-line treatment, secondary to dose-dependent anticholinergic effects.

Nonpharmacological treatment strategies

- In combination with medications, cognitive-behavioral therapy (CBT) can improve outcomes in depression.
- Interpersonal psychotherapy (IPT)
- Electroconvulsive therapy (ECT)

Complications

- Suicide
- Absenteeism
- Substance abuse
- Psychotic depression

Further reading

Karasu TB, Gelenberg A, Merriam A, et al. APA Practice Guidelines: Practice Guideline for the Treatment of Patients with Major Depressive Disorder, 2nd edition. Available at www.psych.org or www.psychiatryonline.com

Mann JJ (2005). The medical management of depression. *N Engl J Med* **353**:1819–1834.

Suehs B, Argo TR, Bendele SD, et al. Texas Medication Algorithm Project Major Depressive Disorder Algorithms. Updated July 2008. Available at: http://www.dshs.state.tx.us/mhprograms/pdf/TIMA_MDD_Manual_080608.pdf

Counseling on antidepressants

Medication guides

All antidepressants should be dispensed with a medication guide regarding suicidal thinking in children, adolescents, and young adults.

Onset of action

In general, it takes 4–6 weeks to see a full effect from antidepressants. Some patients may feel an effect after 2 weeks. When antidepressants are used for anxiety spectrum disorders, it may take up to 12 weeks.

Side effects

SRIs and SNRIs

- Anxiety—transient, seen with initiation of therapy or dosage increases. Consider short-term use of benzodiazepines.
- Gastrointestinal upset—transient, usually subsides within 1–2 weeks. Consider taking medication with food.
- Insomnia—side effect of antidepressants and symptom of depression. Administer medication in the morning. Promote nonpharmacological strategies. Consider non-benzodiazepine hypnotics (e.g., zolpidem) or trazodone.
- Sexual dysfunction is a common cause of noncompliance. Males can experience decreased libido and delayed ejaculation; females may have decreased libido and anorgasmia. Consider bupropion or sildenafil.
- Weight gain is a side effect or may be associated with improved appetite with an improvement in the depression.
- Hypertension—venlafaxine is associated with dose-dependent HTN.
- Hyponatremia is a rare side effect, more common in elderly patients, and those taking thiazide diuretics (e.g., hydrochlorothiazide).

Mirtazapine

- Increased appetite results in weight gain; may need to monitor lipid profile, especially if taking in combination with an antipsychotic
- Sedation—lower doses, administer at bedtime

TCAs

- Anticholinergic side effects
- Sedation—administer at bedtime
- Orthostatic hypotension
- QTc prolongation—use caution with other QTc-prolonging medications
- Weight gain
- Seizure—TCAs lower the seizure threshold

Nefazodone

- Black box warning regarding hepatotoxicity—monitor LFTs

Drug interactions

SRIs and SNRIs

- Serotonergic agents such as MAOIs, tramadol, 5-HT agonist "triptans," and St. John's wort can increase the risk of serotonin syndrome; use with caution.
- Warfarin with SRIs or SNRIs can increase INR
- 1A2 substrates (e.g., clozapine, olanzapine)—fluvoxamine is a strong inhibitor of CYP 1A2
- 2D6 substrates (e.g., risperidone, haloperidol)—fluoxetine and paroxetine are strong inhibitors of CYP 2D6

MAOIs

- Most drug and food interactions with MAOIs can increase the risk of serotonin syndrome or a hypertensive crisis.
- Tyramine-containing foods (e.g., aged cheese, tap beers)—food restrictions are not required with transdermal selegiline at 6 mg dose
- Sympathomimetics (e.g., pseudoephedrine)
- Stimulants (e.g., amphetamine, methylphenidate)
- Serotonergic agents need a 2-week wash-out period prior to initiation; 5 weeks with fluoxetine
- Pain medications (e.g., tramadol, meperidine)

TCAs

- Serotonergic agents can increase the risk of serotonin syndrome; see SRIs and SNRIs
- QTc prolongation—use caution with other QTc-prolonging medications
- Weight gain
- TCAs lower the seizure threshold.

Stopping antidepressants

- Antidepressants **should not** be stopped abruptly.
- SRIs, SNRIs, and TCAs have been associated with a withdrawal syndrome.
- Symptoms include dizziness; nausea, vomiting, and diarrhea; headaches; lethargy; anxiety; tingling and numbness or electric shock–like sensations; tremors; sweating; insomnia, and irritability.
- Symptoms usually develop within 1–10 days of discontinuation. Medications with shorter half-lives (e.g., paroxetine, venlafaxine) are more likely to be associated with withdrawal symptoms than those with longer half-lives (e.g., fluoxetine).

Further reading

Spina E, Santoro V, D'Arrigo C (2008). Clinically relevant pharmacokinetic drug interactions with second-generation antidepressants: an update. *Clin Ther* **30**:1206–1227.

Labeling change request letter for antidepressant medications, issued by the FDA, October 2004. Available at: http://www.fda.gov/CDER/drug/antidepressants/SSRIlabelChange.htm

Schizophrenia

Schizophrenia is a psychotic disorder characterized by abnormal or bizarre thoughts, moods, and behaviors. Schizophrenia can manifest with hallucinations, delusions, disorganized thinking, an inappropriate affect, and/or an impairment in functioning.

Schizophrenia affects approximately 1% of Americans and 1% of adults worldwide. Schizophrenia affects women and men equally, with an average age of onset in the early to late 20s. Men are affected earlier than women.

Etiologies (select)

Genetic

- Risk is 10% with 1 parent, but 40% if both parents have schizophrenia. Monozygotic twins concordance rate is 45%–50%.

Biological

- Dopamine (DA) hypothesis: increased limbic DA activity is related to positive symptoms.
- Serotonin (5HT) hypothesis: antagonism of the 5-HT_2 receptor decreases psychotic symptoms and movement disorders associated with D_2 antagonism.
- Glutamate hypothesis involves hypofunctioning of glutamate N-methyl-D-aspartate (NMDA) receptors.
- Gamma-aminobutyric acid (GABA) hypothesis: Decreased GABA activity increases DA activity.

Signs and symptoms (see Table 15.87)

Clinical features

- Schizophrenia is characterized by hallucinations, delusions, disorganized speech, disorganized or catatonic behavior, and negative symptoms.
- To diagnose schizophrenia a person must have two or more of these symptoms significantly present during a 1-month period of time.
- Schizophrenia can be diagnosed with one criterion if the delusion is bizarre, or if the voices are either a running commentary or two or more voices are conversing together.

Table 15.87 Symptoms of schizophrenia

Positive	Negative
Hallucinations	Alogia
Delusions	Anhedonia
Disorganized thinking	Apathy
	Avolition
	Flat Affect
	Social Isolation

Diagnosis

Laboratory findings and monitoring

- Urine drug screen
- Consider an EEG, head CT, or head MRI
- When starting an SGA, recommend a baseline lipid panel, BP, fasting blood glucose, weight, family history of cardiovascular disease

Screening tools

- MSE
- Brief Psychiatric Rating Scale (BPRS)

Rule out

- Psychotic disorder not otherwise specified (NOS)
- Psychotic disorder secondary to general medical condition, delirium, or dementia
- Substance-induced psychotic disorder
- Schizoaffective disorder
- Mood disorder (bipolar or MDD) with psychotic features
- Schizophreniform disorder
- Brief psychotic disorder
- Delusional disorder
- Schizotypal, schizoid, or paranoid personality disorder

Pharmacological treatment strategies (see Tables 15.88, 15.89)

- Antipsychotics remain the mainstay of treatment in schizophrenia.
- Available options include the typical or first-generation antipsychotics (FGAs) and the atypical or second-generation antipsychotics (SGAs). Refer to Table 15.88 for a listing of available agents.
- FGAs work primarily through D_2 antagonism, whereas SGAs antagonize both 5-HT_2 and D_2.
- SGAs are considered first-line over the FGAs, secondary to decreased incidence of extrapyramidal symptoms (EPS) and other side effects.
- Choose an antipsychotic based on previous response, side-effect profile, patient comorbidities, and access to the medication.
- High-potency FGAs (e.g., haloperidol, fluphenazine) are associated with more EPS; low-potency FGAs (e.g., chlorpromazine) are associated with more sedation, hypotension, and anticholinergic side effects. SGAs (olanzapine and clozapine) have been associated with metabolic complications.
- For treatment-resistant patients, consider clozapine.
- For repeatedly noncompliant patients consider long-acting injections.
- For acute agitation associated with schizophrenia, consider management with a short-acting injectable antipsychotic (see Table 15.89).

Table 15.88 Available antipsychotic agents

First-generation antipsychotics		Second-generation antipsychotics	
Generic	**Brand**	**Generic**	**Brand**
Low potency			
Chlorpromazine	Thorazine	Clozapine	Clozaril, Fazaclo
Thioridazine	Mellaril	Risperidone	Risperdal, Risperdal Consta, Risperdal M-tab
		Olanzapine	Zyprexa, Zyprexa Zydis
Mid potency			
Molindone	Moban	Quetiapine	Seroquel, Seroquel XR
Loxapine	Loxitane	Ziprasidone	Geodon
Perphenazine	Trilafon	Aripiprazole	Abilify, Abilify Discmelt
		Paliperidone	Invega
High potency			
Haloperidol	Haldol	Iloperidone	Fanapt
Fluphenazine	Prolixin		
Thiothixene	Navane		
Trifluoperazine	Stelazine		

Table 15.89 Available antipsychotic dosage forms

Medication	RR	XR	ODT	PO Soln	SAI	LAI
First generation						
Chlorpromazine	√				√	
Haloperidol	√			√	√	√
Fluphenazine	√				√	√
Second generation						
Clozapine	√		√			
Risperidone	√		√	√		√
Olanzapine	√		√		√	
Quetiapine	√	√				
Ziprasidone	√				√	
Aripiprazole	√		√	√	√	
Paliperidone		√				

RR, regular release; XR, extended release; ODT, orally disintegrating; PO Soln, oral solution; SAI, short-acting injection; LAI, long-acting injection or decanoate.

Nonpharmacological treatment strategies

- ECT
- Psychotherapy
- Case management

Complications

- Suicide
- Substance abuse or dependence
- Nicotine dependence
- Metabolic syndrome
- Cardiovascular disease

Further reading

Argo TR, Crismon LM, Miller AL, et al. Texas Medication Algorithm Project Schizophrenia Treatment Algorithms. Updated June 2008. Available at: www.dshs.state.tx.us/mhprograms/pdf/schizophreniaManual 060608.pdf

Clozaril dosing, registry, and monitoring recommendations available at: www.clozaril.com.

Freedman R (2003). Schizophrenia. *N Engl J Med* **349**:1738–1749.

Lehman AF, Lieberman JA, Dixon LB, et al. Practice Guideline for the Treatment of Patients with Schizophrenia, 2nd ed., April 2004. Available at: www.psychiatryonline.com

Managing antipsychotic side effects

Extrapyramidal symptoms (EPS)

EPS are more common with high-potency FGAs (e.g., haloperidol, fluphenazine). Risperidone causes dose-dependent EPS.

Dystonia

- Symptoms: muscle contraction, torticollus, and oculogyric crisis
- Management: injectable anticholinergic medications (e.g., benztropine or diphenhydramine)

Psuedoparkinsonism

- Symptoms: bradykinesia, cogwheel rigidity, shuffling gait, and tremor
- Monitoring: Simpson–Angus Extrapyramidal Symptoms Rating Scale (SAS)
- Management: decrease dose of antipsychotic, anticholinergics (e.g., benztropine, trihexyphenidyl), or dopamine agonists (i.e., amantadine)

Akathisia

- Symptoms: internal restless, agitation, and an inability to sit still
- Monitoring: Barnes Akathisia Scale
- Management: decrease dose of antipsychotic, propranolol, or benzodiazepines; anticholinergics generally are ineffective

Tardive dyskinesia

- Associated with prolonged antipsychotic use
- Symptoms: abnormal, repetitive, involuntary movements, e.g., lip smacking, puckering, facial grimacing; can involve arms, legs, or trunk
- Monitoring: Abnormal Involuntary Movement Scale (AIMS) or Dyskinesia Identification System: Condensed User Scale (DISCUS)
- Management: switch to an SGA medication; there is no specific treatment to date. The best treatment is prevention.

Metabolic complications

Warning is related to SGAs; each medication carries its own metabolic profile (clozapine, olanzapine >> quetiapine ≥ risperidone, paliperidone > ziprasidone, aripiprazole).

Weight gain

- Symptoms: characterized by ≥5% weight gain from baseline
- Monitoring: weight at baseline, every 4 weeks ×4, then quarterly thereafter; monitor BMI and waist circumference
- Management: diet and nutrition education. If weight gain is excessive consider switching to an antipsychotic less likely to cause weight changes. There are minimal data on metformin and topiramate use.

Hyperglycemia

- Symptoms: FBG ≥126 mg/dL; polydipsia, polyuria, polyphagia
- Monitoring: FBG at baseline, 12 weeks later, then annually
- Management: diet and nutrition education. If there is new-onset hyperglycemia, consider switching to an antipsychotic less likely to cause metabolic changes; consider metformin.

Dyslipidemia

- Symptoms: elevated total cholesterol and triglycerides
- Monitoring: lipid panel at baseline, 12 weeks later, 5 years later
- Management: diet and nutrition education. If there is new-onset dyslipidemia, consider switching to an antipsychotic less likely to cause metabolic changes; consider a fibric acid derivative or a statin.

Hyperprolactinemia

- Associated with FGAs, risperidone, and paliperidone
- Symptoms: males may experience gynecomastia, decreased muscle mass, erectile dysfunction, infertility, and osteoporosis. Females may experience oligomenorrhea, amenorrhea, galactorrhea, decreased libido, infertility, habitual spontaneous abortion, osteoporosis
- Monitoring: serum prolactin level only if symptomatic
- Management: change to a medication less likely to increase prolactin levels, consider a dopamine agonist (e.g., bromocriptine or cabergolide).

Cardiovascular

Orthostatic hypotension

- Associated with α_1 antagonism—low-potency FGAs (e.g., chlorpromazine), clozapine, quetiapine, and risperidone
- Symptoms: dizziness, >20/10 mmHg drop in BP upon standing
- Monitoring: orthostatic BP changes
- Management: decrease dose of medication, slow titration

QTc prolongation

- Associated with FGAs (e.g., thioridazine, pimozide), ziprasidone
- Symptoms: dizziness, syncope
- Monitoring: baseline ECG, and after dosage increases or addition of medications that prolong QTc (e.g., erythromycin, levofloxacin)
- Management: decrease dose of medication, remove any interacting or other QTc-prolonging agent, or switch to a different antipsychotic.

Myocarditis

- Extremely rare side effect associated with clozapine
- Symptoms: fatigue, fever, tachycardia, chest pain, and dyspnea
- Management: stop clozapine, get cardiology consult

Blood dyscrasias

Agranulocytosis

- Associated with clozapine
- Symptoms: ANC <500/mm^3
- Monitoring: weekly CBC with differential the first 6 months of therapy, then every other week for the following 6 months, and yearly thereafter; Registration is required to dispense
- Management: refer to monitoring guidelines at: http://www.mylan-clozapine.com/PDFs/Treatment%20parameters%20table.pdf

Further reading

American Diabetes Association; American Psychiatric Association; American Association of Clinical Endocrinologists; North American Association for the Study of Obesity (2004). Consensus development conference on antipsychotic drugs and obesity and diabetes. *Diabetes Care* **27**:596–601.

Clozapine Web sites: www.clozaril.com or www.mylan-clozapine.com

Bipolar disorder

Formerly referred to as manic–depression, bipolar disorder is a mood disorder characterized by mood swings that alternate between periods of severe depression and extreme elation (mania).

Bipolar disorder affects approximately 2.6% of Americans, with bipolar I and bipolar II each affecting approximately 1% of the population. Men and women are affected equally.

Etiologies (select)

Genetic

- Risk is 15%–30% with 1 parent with bipolar disorder; 50%–75% with 2 parents having bipolar disorder

Biological

- Excess of NE and DA
- GABA deficiency or excess glutamate action
- Excess thyroid
- Circadian rhythm changes; mania recurs more frequently during the summer and depressive episodes occur during the spring

Signs and symptoms

Mania

- Inflated self-esteem, grandiosity
- Decreased need for sleep
- Pressured speech
- Flight of ideas
- Distractibility
- Increase in goal-directed activity
- Excessive involvement in pleasurable activities

Depression

- See signs and symptoms discussed under Depression, p. 674

Clinical features

- Bipolar I: symptoms of mania—elation, irritability, or expansiveness, and three or more of the above symptoms for 1 week causing impairment in functioning
- Bipolar II: symptoms of hypomania—symptoms lasting for 4 days with no impairment in functioning; individual may actually be more productive or creative
- Bipolar depression: characterizes the depressive phase, occurs in both bipolar I and II
- Mixed episode: meets the criteria for mania and major depression nearly every day for 1 week
- Refer to the *DSM-IV-TR* for the full diagnostic criteria

Diagnosis

Lab workup

- TSH level
- Urine drug screen (cocaine, PCP, amphetamines)

Screening tools for mania

- MSE
- Young Mania Rating Scale (YMRS)
- Goldberg Mania Questionnaire (self-rated)
- Mood Disorder Questionnaire

Recent addition of a medication that can induce mania

- Antidepressants
- Baclofen
- Decongestants
- Steroids
- Stimulants

This list is *not* all-inclusive.

Rule out

- Hypo- or hyperthyroidism
- Mood disorder due to a general medical condition
- Substance-induced mood disorder
- MDD
- Cyclothymic disorder
- Psychotic disorder
- Schizoaffective disorder

Pharmacological treatment strategies

When starting a mood stabilizer, refer to the Monitoring of Mood Stabilizers unit in this chapter (p. 690) for baseline workup. When starting a second-generation antipsychotic (SGA), assess the patient's baseline lipid panel, BP, fasting blood glucose, and weight and whether there is a family history of cardiovascular disease.

Acute mania

- First-line options include lithium (Li), valproic acid (VPA), or an SGA (except clozapine)
- Alternate options include carbamazepine (CBZ)
- For a severe episode consider starting two agents initially:
  - Li + VPA
  - Li + SGA
  - VPA + SGA
  - Two antipsychotics in combination is NOT recommended
- Adjunctive treatment with benzodiazepines and hypnotics help with insomnia, anxiety, and irritability

Mixed-episode mania

- First-line options include VPA or an SGA (ziprasidone, aripiprazole, or risperidone)
- Alternate options include CBZ or olanzapine

Acute mania with psychotic features

- Treat with a mood stabilizer (Li or VPA) plus an SGA

Depressed phase

- Optimize current mood stabilizer
- Consider addition of lamotrigine (LMT)
- Antidepressants should be used cautiously in treating bipolar disorder
  - Never treat with antidepressant monotherapy
  - Antidepressants increase risk of switch to mania, or rapid cycling
  - Risk of switch is higher with TCAs and venlafaxine
- Olanzapine/fluoxetine (Symbyax) and quetiapine have been FDA approved for bipolar depression

Maintenance phase

- The goal is to prevent relapse
- Focus on treatment adherence
- First-line options (most evidence) are Li and VPA
- Alternate options include CBZ, LMT, oxcarbazepine, or an SGA
- Olanzapine and aripiprazole have been FDA approved for bipolar maintenance, and quetiapine for adjunct maintenance treatment

Nonpharmacological treatment strategies

- ECT

Complications

- Suicide (rate 10–20× higher than for general population)
- Absenteeism
- Substance abuse
- Psychotic mania

Further reading

American Psychiatric Association Bipolar Guidelines, April 2002. Guideline watch update November 2005. Available at: www.psych.org or www.psychiatryonline.com

Belmaker RH (2004). Bipolar disorder. *N Engl J Med* **351**(5):476–486.

Crisman ML, et al. Texas Medication Algorithm Project—TIMA Bipolar DO. Last updated July 2007. Available at: http://www.dshs.state.tx.us/mhprograms/TIMABDman2007.pdf

Keck PE Jr, Perlis RH, Otto MW, Carpenter D, et al. The Expert Consensus Guidelines®: Treatment of Bipolar Disorder 2004. *Postgrad Med Special Report*. 2004(December):1–120.

Marken PA, Pies RW (2006). Emerging treatments for bipolar disorder: Safety and adverse effect profiles. *Ann Pharmacother* **40**:276–285.

Monitoring of mood stabilizers

Lithium carbonate/lithium citrate (Li)

- Carbolith, Eskalith, Eskalith CR, Lithobid

Pre-workup

- Renal function
- Electrolytes
- TSH
- Pregnancy test (if applicable)
- ECG (if applicable)

Level monitoring

- Draw morning serum trough levels (12 hours post-dose)
- Acute mania: 0.5–1.2 mEq/L; some titrate up to 1.5 mEq/L
- Maintenance: 0.6–1.0 mEq/L

Drug interactions

- Drugs that increase Li levels: NSAIDs (except sulindac and aspirin), ACE inhibitors, ARBs, thiazide diuretics
- Drugs that decrease Li levels: theophylline, caffeine, cisplatin
- Loop diuretics can either increase or decrease Li levels

Adverse effects

- Diarrhea, fine tremor, polydipsia, polyuria, nausea, weight gain

Signs of toxicity

- *Mild*—levels >1.5 mEq/L: fine tremors, fatigue, GI symptoms (nausea and vomiting), muscle weakness
- *Moderate*—levels 1.5–2.5 mEq/L: ataxia, dysarthria, coarse tremor, nystagmus, headaches, increased temperature, lethargy, sedation, changes in mental status, increased deep tendon reflexes (DTRs)
- *Severe*—levels >2.5 mEq/L: coarse tremors, delirium, respiratory impairment, seizures, coma, death

Valproic acid and derivatives (VPA)

- Depakene, Depakote, Depacon

Pre-workup

- Hepatic function (LFTs)
- CBC (specifically platelets)
- Pregnancy test (if applicable)

Level monitoring

- Draw morning serum trough levels (12 hours post-dose)
- Levels 50–125 mg/L

Drug interactions

- Drugs that increase VPA levels: felbamate
- Drugs that decrease VPA levels: carbamazepine (CBZ), phenytoin (PHT), phenobarbital (PB), primidone (PRM)
- Drugs that VPA increases levels of: CBZ-epoxide metabolite, LMT, felbamate, PHT, PB, PRM

Adverse effects

- Alopecia, GI symptoms (nausea, vomiting, diarrhea), polycystic ovarian syndrome, rash, tremor, weight gain

Signs of toxicity

- CNS toxicity (levels >175 mg/L)
- GI disturbances (nausea, vomiting, diarrhea), hepatotoxicity, thrombocytopenia, tremor

Carbamazepine (CBZ)

- Carbatrol, Equetro, Tegretol, Tegretol XR

Pre-workup

- Hepatic function (LFTs)
- Electrolytes (baseline sodium)
- CBC (specifically WBC)
- Pregnancy test (if applicable)

Level monitoring

- Levels 4–12 mg/L

Drug interactions (not all-inclusive)

- Drugs that increase CBZ levels: 3A4 inhibitors (e.g. cimetidine, erythromycin, fluconazole, ritonavir), felbamate, VPA
- Drugs that decrease CBZ levels: CBZ, PHT, PB, PRM
- Drugs that CBZ decreases levels of: aripiprazole, benzodiazepines that undergo oxidation (e.g., diazepam, alprazolam), CBZ, felbamate, haloperidol, LMT, olanzapine, oral contraceptives, PHT, PRM, quetiapine, risperidone, theophylline, VPA, warfarin

Adverse effects

- Aplastic anemia, GI disturbances, hyponatremia, increased LFTs, leukopenia, neutropenia, rash

Signs of toxicity

- Ataxia, blurred vision, confusion, diplopia, drowsiness, headache

Lamotrigine (LMT)

- Lamictal

Pre-workup

- History of rash

Level monitoring

- Not indicated

Drug interactions

- Drugs that increase LMT levels: VPA, oral contraceptives
- Drugs that decrease LMT levels: CBZ, PHT, PB, PRM

Adverse effects

- Steven–Johnson's syndrome—risk is increased with rapid dose titration and drug interactions (namely VPA)

Further reading

Harden CL (2000). Therapeutic safety monitoring: what to look for and when to look for it. *Epilepsia* **41**(Suppl 8):S37–44.

Murphy JE (2005). *Clinical Pharmacokinetics Pocket Reference*, 3rd ed. Bethesda, MD: American Society of Health System Pharmacists.

Long-term asthma management in adults

Asthma is a chronic inflammatory disorder of the airways in which many cells and cellular elements play a role—in particular, mast cells, eosinophils, T lymphocytes, macrophages, neutrophils, and epithelial cells. In susceptible individuals, this inflammation causes recurrent episodes of wheezing, breathlessness, chest tightness, and coughing, particularly at night or in the early morning.

These episodes are usually associated with widespread but variable airflow obstruction that is often reversible either spontaneously or with treatment. However, reversibility of airflow limitation may be incomplete in some patients. The inflammation also causes an associated increase in the existing bronchial hyperresponsiveness to various stimuli.

Statistics

- It is estimated that 20 million Americans suffer from asthma
- During childhood, more boys than girls are affected by asthma, but in adulthood, more females suffer from asthma than males.
- Asthma is regarded as the most common chronic childhood disease, affecting more than 1:20 children.
- Annually, asthma is responsible for more than 10 million outpatient visits and over 500,000 hospitalizations.
- It is estimated that 11 Americans die from asthma-related complications daily.
- Each year it is estimated that asthma accounts for 18 billion dollars in direct and indirect costs.

Causes

- Innate immunity
- Genetics
- Environmental factors such as airborne allergens and viral respiratory infections

Symptoms

- Wheezing
- Coughing (especially with worsening at night)
- Recurrent difficulty breathing
- Recurrent chest tightness
- Any of the above occurring during or in the presence of the following:
  - Exercise
  - Viral infections
  - Allergens (e.g., animal fur, dust mites, pollen, mold)
  - Noxious stimuli (e.g., tobacco smoke, airborne chemicals, wood-burning furnace)
  - Changes in weather
  - Emotional stress
  - Menses

Diagnosis

- Gold standard: spirometry
- Before and after administration of a short-acting beta$_2$-agonist (SABA), an improvement in forced expiratory volume in 1 second (FEV_1) of >200 mL and >12% from baseline measure suggests reversibility of airway obstruction.

Goals of therapy: CONTROL asthma symptoms

Reduce impairment

- Prevent daytime and nighttime symptoms (e.g., coughing or dyspnea).
- Minimize use of rescue medication (e.g., SABA) for quick relief.
- Maintain the best pulmonary function possible.
- Have no limitations in ability to perform usual physical activities (e.g., exercise, attendance of school or work).
- Achieve expectations and satisfaction of asthma control set forth by patients and families.

Reduce risk

- Prevent recurrent asthma exacerbations and necessity for emergency care or hospitalizations.
- Prevent decline in lung function.
- Use optimal pharmacotherapy with little or no adverse effects.

Treatment

- Determine the severity of asthma (e.g., intermittent, mild persistent, moderate persistent, or severe persistent; see Fig. 15.12).
- Initiate therapy at the most appropriate step as it relates to severity (see Fig. 15.13).
- Evaluate asthma control 2–6 weeks after treatment initiation to determine if an adjustment in therapy is needed.
    - Before going to a higher "step," assess patient's inhaler technique, compliance to medication regimen, and possible environmental triggers.
    - If add-on therapy is not providing better control after 2–6 weeks, depending on severity, stop therapy.
- If patients are well controlled for >3 months, consider gradually stepping down therapy.

Further reading

National Heart, Lung, and Blood Institute. Expert Panel 3: Guidelines for the Diagnosis and Management of Asthma. Bethesda, MD: U.S. Department of Health and Human Services, National Institutes of Health, NHLBI;2007. NIH publication 08–5846. Available at: http://www.nhlbi.nih.gov/guidelines/asthma/asthgdln.pdf

— Assessing severity and initiating treatment for patients who are not currently taking long-term control medications

Components of Severity		Classification of Asthma Severity $\geq$ 12 years of age			
			Persistent		
		Intermittent	Mild	Moderate	Severe
Intermittent	Symptoms	≤2 days/week	>2 days/week but not daily	Daily	Throughout the day
	Nighttime awakenings	≤2x/month	3–4x/month	>1x/week but not nightly	Often 7x/week
	Short-acting beta2-agonist use for symptom control (not prevention of EIB)	≤2x/week	>2 days/week but not daily, and not more than 1x on any day	Daily	Several times per day
Normal FEV1/FVC: 8–19 yr 85% 20–39 yr 80% 40–59 yr 75% 60–80 yr 70%		None	Minor limitation	Some limitation	Extremely limited
	Lung function	• Normal FEV_1 between exacerbations • FEV_1 >80% predicted • FEV_1/FVC normal	• FEV_1 >80% predicted • $FFEV_1$/FVC normal	• FEV_1 >60% <80% predicted • FEV_1/FVC reduce 5%	• FEV_1 >60% predicted • FEV_1/FVC reduced >5%
Risk	Exacerbations requiring oral systemic corticosteroids	0–1/year (see note)	>2/year (see note) →		
		← Consider severity and interval since last exacerbation. → Frequency and severity may fluctuate over time for paients in any severity category. Relative annual risk of exacerbations may be related to FEV_1			
Recommended step for Initiating Treatement		Step 1	Step 2	Step 3	Step 4 or 5
				and consider short course of oral systemic corticosteroids	
(see figure 4–5 for treatmet steps.)		In 2–6 weeks, evaluate level of asthma control that is achieved and adjust therapy accordingly			

Key: FEV_1 forced expiratory volume in 1 second; FVC forced vital capacity; ICU intensive care unit

Notes:

- The stepwise approach is meant to assist, not repace, the clinical decisionmaking required to meet individual patient needs.
- Level of severity is determined by assessment of both impairment and risk. Assess impairment domain by patent's/caregiver's recall of previous 2–4 weeks and spirometry. Assign severity to the most severe category in which any feature occurs.
- At present, there are inadequate data to correspond frequencies of exacerbations with different levels of asthma severity. In general, more frequent and intense exacerbations (e.g., requiring urgent, unscheduled care, hospitalization, or ICU admission) indicated greater underlying diseases severity. For treatment purposes, patients who had ≥2 exacerbations requiring oral systemic corticosteroids in the past year may be considered the same as patients who have persistent asthma, even in the absence of impairment levels consistent with persistent asthma.

Figure 15.12 Classifying asthma severity and initiating treatment in youths >12 years of age and in adults.

From: National Heart, Lung, and Blood Institute. Expert Panel 3: Guidelines for the Diagnosis and Management of Asthma. Bethesda, MD: U.S. Department of Health and Human Services, National Institutes of Health, NHLBI; 2007. NIH publication 08–5846. Accessed June 13, 2008, from: http://www.nhlbi.nih.gov/guidelines/asthma/asthgdln.pdf.

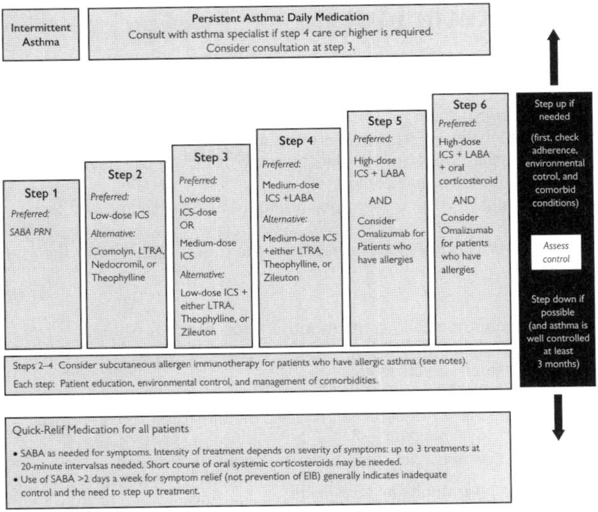

Intermittent Asthma
Persistent Asthma: Daily Medication
Consult with asthma specialist if step 4 care or higher is required.
Consider consultation at step 3.
Step 1
Preferred:
SABA PRN
Step 2
Preferred:
Low-dose ICS
Alternative:
Cromolyn, LTRA, Nedocromil, or Theophylline
Step 3
Preferred:
Low-dose ICS-dose OR Medium-dose ICS
Alternative:
Low-dose ICS + either LTRA, Theophylline, or Zileuton
Step 4
Preferred:
Medium-dose ICS +LABA
Alternative:
Medium-dose ICS +either LTRA, Theophylline, or Zileuton
Step 5
Preferred:
High-dose ICS + LABA
AND
Consider Omalizumab for Patients who have allergies
Step 6
Preferred:
High-dose ICS + LABA + oral corticosteroid
AND
Consider Omalizumab for patients who have allergies
Step up if needed
(first, check adherence, environmental cotrol, and comorbid conditions)
Assess control
Step down if possible
(and asthma is well controlled at least 3 months)
Steps 2–4 Consider subcutaneous allergen immunotherapy for patients who have allergic asthma (see notes).
Each step: Patient education, environmental control, and management of comorbidities.
Quick-Relif Medication for all patients
• SABA as needed for symptoms. Intensity of treatment depends on severity of symptoms: up to 3 treatments at 20-minute intervalsas needed. Short course of oral systemic corticosteroids may be needed.
• Use of SABA >2 days a week for symptom relief (not prevention of EIB) generally indicates inadequate control and the need to step up treatment.

Key: **Alphabetical order is used when more than one treatment option is listed wihtin either preferred or alternative therapy.** EIB, exercise-induced bronchospasm; ICS inhaled corticosteroid; LABA, long-acting inhaled beta2-agonist; LTRA, leukotriene receptor antagonist, SABA, inhaled short-acting beta2-agonist

Notes:

- The stepwise approach is meant to assist, not replace, the clinical decisionmaking required to meet individual patient needs.
- If alternative treatment is used and response is inadequate, discontinue it and use the preferred treatment before stepping up.
- Zileuton is a less desirable alternative due to limited studies as adjunctive therapy and the need to monitor liver function. Theophylline requires monitoring of serum concentration levels.
- In step 6, before oral systemic corticosteroids are introduced, a trial of high-dose ICS + LABA + either LTRA, theophylline, or zileuton may be considerd, although this approach has not been studied in clinical trials.
- Step 1, 2, and 3 preferred therapies are based on Evidence A; step 3 alternative therapy is based on Evidence A for LTRA, Evidence B for theophylline, and EVidence D for zileuton, Step 4 preferred therapy is based ib Evudebce B, and alternative therapy is based on Evidence B for LTRA and theophylline and Evidence D for zileuton, Step 5 preferred therapy is based on Evidence B. Step 6 preferred therapy is based on (on (EPR-2 1997) and Evidence B for omalizumab.
- Immunotherapy for steps 2–4 is based on Evidence B for house-dust mites, animal danders, and pollens; evidence is weak or lacking for molds and cockroaches. Evidence is strongest for immunotherapy with single allergens. The
- Clinicians who administer immunotherapy or omalizumab should be prepared and equipped to identify and treat anaphylaxis that may occur.

Figure 15.13 Stepwise approach for managing asthma in youths ≥12 years of age and in adults.

From: National Heart, Lung, and Blood Institute. Expert Panel 3: Guidelines for the Diagnosis and Management of Asthma. Bethesda, MD: U.S. Department of Health and Human Services, National Institutes of Health, NHLBI; 2007. NIH publication 08–5846. Accessed June 13, 2008, from: http://www.nhlbi.nih.gov/guidelines/asthma/asthgdln.pdf

Inhaler techniques

Metered dose inhalers (MDI)

The steps for using a pressurized MDI are as follows:

- Sit or stand in an upright position.
- Shake the inhaler vigorously 3–4 times and remove cap.
- Make sure that there are no objects in the mouth of the device.
- Breathe out slowly and completely.
- Hold the inhaler in an upright position between the thumb and the index finger.
- Place inhaler about 2 inches away from the mouth, aiming into the mouth.

  OR
- Place the mouthpiece into the mouth on top of the tongue.
- Simultaneously depress the canister and breath in slowly and deeply.
- Remove inhaler and close lips.
- Hold breath for 10 seconds or longer, then exhale slowly.
- If a second dose is needed, wait for 1–2 minutes then repeat above steps.
- If the MDI contains corticosteroids, rinse mouth after use.

Points for the pharmacist or technician

- Demonstrate the correct method using a placebo inhaler and ask the patient to demonstrate how they would use the inhaler.
- Most patients are on long-term therapy and may have developed bad habits.
- Patients with anything other than mild, occasional attacks gain substantial benefit from learning about their disease and management of their disease.
- Measure peak-expiratory flow rates regularly and keep a dairy of the results.
- Emphasize that synchronization of the initiation of breathing with the release of medication is very important and can require practice to maximize benefit.

Advice to the patient

- Keep the device clean and replace the mouthpiece cap after each use.
- The plastic housing can be cleaned with warm, mild detergent solution; ensure that it is dry before use.

Dry-powder inhalers

Several devices are now available to deliver medication in the form of a dry powder. These medications must be inhaled fast enough so that the medicine is released from the device.

The basic technique for using a dry-powdered inhaler is as follows:

- Sit or stand in an upright position.
- Exhale away from the inhaler.
- Make sure that there are no objects in the device.
- Remove cap, DO NOT SHAKE.

- Put mouthpiece in mouth, making a seal with the lips.
- Breathe in quickly and deeply.
- Hold breath for 10 seconds or longer.
- If the dry powder contains corticosteroids, rinse mouth after use.

Diskhaler®

A Diskhaler® is a dry-powder inhaler that holds small blisters, each containing a dose of medication, on a disk. The Diskhaler® punctures each blister so that the medication can be inhaled.

The basic technique for using the Diskhaler® is as follows:

- Remove the cover on the mouthpiece.
- Check to make sure the device and mouthpiece are clean.
- If a new medication disk is needed, pull the corners of the white cartridge out as far as it will go, then press the ridges on the sides inward to remove the cartridge.
- Place the medication disk with its numbers facing upward on the white rotating wheel. Then, slide the cartridge all the way back into the device.
- Pull the cartridge all the way out, then push it all the way in until the highest number on the medication disk can be seen in the indicator window.
- With the cartridge fully inserted and the device kept flat, raise the lid as far as it goes to pierce both sides of the medication blister.
- Move the Diskhaler® away from mouth and breathe out.
- Place the mouthpiece between the teeth and lips, making sure not to cover the air holes on the mouthpiece.
- Inhale quickly and deeply.
- Move the Diskhaler® away from mouth and continue holding breath for 10 seconds or longer.
- Breathe out slowly.
- If another dose is needed, pull the cartridge out all the way and then push it back in all the way. This will move the next blister into place. Repeat the above steps.

Advice to the patient

- When finished using the Diskhaler® put the cap back on.
- If the device is dropped after a dose is loaded, the dose may be lost and another dose needs to be loaded before inhalation of medication.
- The device should be cleaned before insertion of each new medication disk.

Turbuhaler®

The Turbuhaler® is a dry-powder inhaler that features a dose counter.
The basic technique for using the Turbuhaler® is as follows:

- Remove the cap from the Turbuhaler® by unscrewing it.
- Hold the Turbuhaler® with the mouthpiece in an upward position.
- Turn the bottom of the Turbuhaler® all the way to the right and back to the left until it "clicks."
- Hold the Turbuhaler® away from mouth and breathe out.

- Put the mouthpiece between the teeth and seal lips around the mouthpiece.
- Inhale rapidly and deeply.
- Remove the Turbuhaler® from mouth before breathing out.
- Repeat the above steps if more than one dose is prescribed.

Advice to the patient

- Keep the Turbuhaler® cap on when the device is not in use.
- A red dot indicates that there are 20 doses or less remaining.
- To clean the Turbuhaler® wipe the mouthpiece with a dry tissue or cloth. Never get this device wet, or it will not work properly.

Diskus®

- The Diskus® is a dry-powder inhaler that holds 60 doses and features a built-in dose counter.
- The basic technique for using the Diskus® is as follows:
- Open the Diskus® by holding the case in the palm of one hand and putting the thumb of the other hand on the thumb grip; push thumb away as far as it will go, until it "clicks."
- Release the dose by sliding the lever to the right of the mouthpiece away from the mouthpiece.
- After the release of medication the inhaler must be held level, not tilting the device.
- Hold the Diskus® away from the mouth and breathe out; remember, never breathe into the Diskus®.
- Put mouthpiece to lips; breathe in quickly and deeply, taking a full breath.
- Remove the Diskus® from the mouth; hold breath for 10 seconds or longer.
- Close the Diskus® by sliding the thumb grip back toward the mouthpiece; it should click shut.

Advice to the patient

- If Diskus® is dropped or tilted after the dose is loaded, then the dose is lost and must be reloaded before inhalation of medication.

Chronic obstructive pulmonary disease

Chronic obstructive pulmonary disease (COPD) is characterized by airway obstruction or airway limitations that are not fully reversible. The airway obstruction is most often progressive and related to an abnormal inflammatory response of the lung to noxious particles or gases (e.g., cigarette smoke).

Currently, COPD is the fourth leading cause of morbidity and mortality in the United States, and mortality continues to increase. It is estimated that over 12 million Americans have the diagnosis of COPD and it is projected that another 12 million people may have COPD but are not currently diagnosed. In the United States it has proven to be a costly disease. In 2002, the direct costs of COPD were $18 billion dollars and the indirect costs were $14.1 billion dollars.

Risk factors

Host factor

- Alpha$_1$-antitrypsin deficiency

Environmental factors

Inhalation exposures

- Cigarette smoking (active and passive smoke)
- Occupational dusts and chemicals
- Indoor and outdoor air pollution
- History of severe respiratory infections during childhood

Diagnosis and severity classification

- Spirometry is the gold standard for diagnosing COPD.
- Consider diagnosis if patient has had dyspnea, chronic cough or sputum production, and/or a history of exposure to risk factors for COPD. Spirometry should be performed if person is over age 40 years.
- Reduction in FEV$_1$/forced vital capacity (FVC) ratio <70% is the cutoff point used to define COPD (not clinically validated).
- Severity is characterized by the extent FEV$_1$ is affected.

Goals of chronic stable COPD management

Nonpharmacological

Prevention of disease progression

- Smoking cessation (most effective therapy in reducing progression of COPD)
- Nicotine replacement, bupropion, clonidine, nortriptyline, varenicline (see Tobacco Cessation unit in this chapter, p. 716)
- Reduce exposure to other noxious substances

Patient education

- Pathophysiology of COPD
- Avoidance of risk factors and smoking cessation
- Importance of immunizations
- Proper skills on how to use various inhalation devices (see Inhaler Techniques unit in this chapter, p. 698).

- Strategies to minimize dyspnea
- Develop a plan to recognize and manage symptoms and exacerbations.
- Advance directives and end-of-life issues
- Pulmonary rehabilitation
  - Improve exercise tolerance through exercise training.
  - Improve quality of life by helping patient to cope with social isolation and psychosocial issues (e.g., depression).
- Oxygen therapy
  - Shown to increase survival
  - Goal to increase baseline arterial oxygen pressure (PaO_2) to >60 mmHg at sea level at rest and/or to produce an arterial oxygen percent saturation (SaO_2) of >90%
- Surgery
  - Bullectomy
  - Lung volume reduction surgery
  - Lung transplantation

Pharmacotherapy for chronic stable COPD (see Fig. 15.14)

The goal is to prevent and control symptoms, reduce exacerbation frequency and severity, and improve exercise tolerance and overall health status.

Bronchodilators

- Mainstay of COPD treatment
- β_2-agonists and anticholinergics
- Methylxanthines (e.g., theophylline used only in rare instances; no longer preferred in COPD management)
- Combinations of bronchodilators may provide increased efficacy over a single agent.

Inhaled glucocorticosteroids (ICS)

- Used in stages III and IV COPD and those patients with repeated exacerbations (e.g., 3 exacerbations in last 3 years)
- May reduce exacerbation frequency
- Combination of ICS and β_2-agonists (e.g., fluticasone/salmeterol) improves spirometry more than either agent alone
- ICS increases risk for pneumonia

Oral glucocorticosteroids

- Not recommended for long-term management of COPD

Vaccinations

- Influenza vaccination can reduce morbidity and mortality in COPD patients by ~50%
- Consider influenza vaccination in patients <65 years old with FEV_1 <40% predicted
- Intranasal formulation of influenza vaccination is not recommended.
- Pneumococcal polysaccharide vaccine is recommended for those patients age 65 years or older.

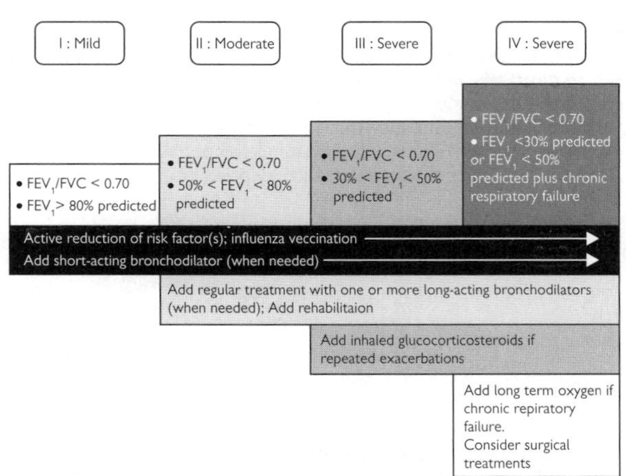

**Postbronchodilator FEV_1 is recommended for the diagnosis and assessment of severity of COPD.*

Figure 15.14 Therapy at each stage of COPD.

From the Global Strategy for the Diagnosis, Management, and Prevention of Chronic Obstructive Pulmonary Disease, Global Initiative for Chronic Obstructive Lung Disease (GOLD) 2008. Available from: http://www.goldcopd.org

Management of COPD exacerbations

Exacerbations of COPD occur as the disease naturally progresses and are characterized by a worsening of daily variations of symptoms including changes in baseline dyspnea, cough, and/or sputum production. These changes are often acute in onset and may necessitate changes in regular medication regimens and/or higher levels of care (e.g., intensive care setting).

Causes

- Viral infections
- Bacterial infections (e.g., *H. influenzae, S. pneumoniae, M. catarrhalis, M. pneumoniae,* and *C. pneumoniae*)
- Air pollution
- Unknown (about 30% of cases have no defined etiology)

Treatment

- Short-acting bronchodilators (e.g., albuterol)
  - Increase dose and/or frequency
  - May add short-acting anticholinergic agent (e.g., ipratropium) if symptoms are not improving
- Use nebulizer if patient is in distress and unable to properly execute metered dose inhaler

- Methylxanthines are not recommended first-line treatment.
- Do not use tiotropium for management of exacerbation (since it is a long-acting agent).
- Systemic glucocorticosteroids
  - Improves lung function, expedites recovery, and reduced relapse
  - Use of 30–60 mg oral prednisone daily is often employed
  - Duration: 7–14 days

Antibiotics

- Controversial
- May be beneficial in patients with the following clinical symptoms:
  - Increased dyspnea,
  - Increased sputum volume, and
  - Increased sputum purulence
- Two of the above symptoms, if one of the two includes increased sputum purulence
- And/or patient requires mechanical ventilation

Further reading

American Thoracic Society / European Respiratory Society Task Force. Standards for the Diagnosis and Management of Patients with COPD. Version 1.2. New York: American Thoracic Society; 2004 [updated 2005 September 8]. Available from: http://www.thoracic.org/go/copd

Global Initiative for Chronic Obstructive Pulmonary Diseases. Global Strategy for the Diagnosis, Management, and Prevention of Chronic Obstructive Pulmonary Disease. NHLBI/WHO Workshop. Updated 2007. Available at: www.goldcopd.com.

Cystic fibrosis

Cystic fibrosis (CF) is an autosomal recessive disorder caused by a mutation in the CF transmembrane conductance regulator (CFTR) gene prominently found in Caucasians. The most prevalent mutation occurs at position 508 of the CFTR protein (Delta F508).

CF affects many organ systems, with respiratory failure accounting for over 85% of its mortality. It is estimated that 1000 new cases of CF are diagnosed annually. In 2006, the median expected survival age was 37 years.

Clinical manifestations of CF

Respiratory disease

- Airway obstruction
- Infection
- Inflammation
- Chronic bronchitis/bronchiectasis
- Chronic sinusitis
- Nasal polyps
- Acute pulmonary exacerbations

Gastrointestinal disease

- Malabsorption and malnutrition
- Vitamin deficiency (e.g., fat soluble)
- Pancreatitis
- Gastroesophageal reflux disease
- Meconium ileus and distal intestinal obstruction
- Hepatobiliary disease

Genitourinary (male)

- Absence of vas deferens (e.g., azoospermia)

Endocrine disease

- Diabetes mellitus
- Bone disease (e.g., osteoporosis)
- Hypogonadism

Diagnosis criteria

Diagnosis is made with one or more clinical features of CF **OR** a history of CF diagnosis in a sibling **OR** a positive newborn screening test **AND** at least one of the following:

- Positive sweat chloride test by pilocarpine iontophoresis on two or more occasions (result >60 mmol/L suggests CF diagnosis)
- Two gene mutations known to cause CF
- Abnormal nasal epithelial ion transport

Treatments and medications used in management of chronic CF

Pulmonary

- Chest physiotherapy to mobilize thick secretions (e.g., chest percussion, chest wall oscillation vest)

For patients with CF >6 years of age

- Dornase alpha 2.5 mg daily via nebulizer, especially in moderate–severe lung disease
- Hypertonic saline (7%) via nebulizer 4 mL twice daily (consider use of short-acting beta$_2$-agonist pretreatment to minimize bronchospasm)
- Inhaled beta$_2$-agonists
- Oral azithromycin if *Pseudomonas aeruginosa* persistently present in sputum cultures
    - If patient's weight 25–40 kg: 250 mg three times weekly
    - If patient's weight >40 kg: 500 mg three times weekly
- Aerosolized tobramycin 300 mg twice daily in 28-day cycles if *Pseudomonas aeruginosa* persistently present in sputum cultures (especially in moderate–severe lung disease)
- Oral nonsteroidal anti-inflammatory agents if FEV$_1$ >60% predicted (e.g., ibuprofen). It is recommended that serum concentrations be monitored with the goal of 50–100 mcg/mL, which is usually a "send out" laboratory measurement. Concern for adverse effects such as bleeding and renal failure have limited use of nonsteroidal agents.

Gastrointestinal disease

- Pancreatic enzymes
    - Usual doses: 1000–2500 lipase/kg/meal
    - Maximum dose 2500 units lipase/kg/meal or 10,000 units lipase/kg/day
    - Generic products are not bioequivalent and patients should use one brand consistently.
    - Optimize nutritional status and body weight (goal: >90% IBW and/or BMI percentile >25th)
- Vitamin supplementation (A, D, E, K)
- Ursodeoxycholic acid (Ursodiol) for hepatobiliary disease or cirrhosis (15–30 mg/kg/day)
- Prokinetic agents (e.g., metoclopramide) and/or anti-acid (e.g., H2 blockers, PPI) medications for reflux

Endocrine disease

- Insulin
- Calcium and vitamin D
- Minimize glucocorticoid exposure
- Encourage weight-bearing exercise

Microorganisms and fungi implicated in colonizing and infecting CF airways

- *Pseudomonas aeruginosa* (non-mucoid and mucoid)
- *Staphylococcus aureus* (including methicillin-resistant *Staphylococcus aureus*)
- *Haemophilus influenzae*
- *Stenotrophomonas maltophilia*
- *Burkholderia cepacia*
- *Alcaligenes xylosoxidans*
- Nontuberculous mycobacteria
- *Panoraea apista*
- *Aspergillus fumigatus*
- *Scedosporium apiospermum*

Acute pulmonary exacerbations (necessitating hospitalization)

Infection management (see Table 15.90)

- IV antibiotics based on culture and sensitivity of sputum sample (if current sample unavailable, empiric therapy based on last available culture and sensitivity data)
- Two antipseudomonal agents with different mechanisms of action are recommended for synergy (preferably one agent being an aminoglycoside)
- Synergy testing may be useful for multidrug-resistant organisms; however:
  - Usually has long turnaround time for results
  - Treatment outcomes not well correlated with antibiotics chosen by synergy test results
- Usual treatment course: 10–21 days (usual 14 days), may be completed at home
- Patient should return to baseline pulmonary function 3–4 days prior to treatment discontinuation

Pharmacokinetics and antibiotic dosing in CF

- Increase total body clearance (CL) and volume of distribution (Vd)
- Often higher doses and/or more frequent dosing required
- Controversy exists over high-dose extended-interval dosing of aminoglycosides and the efficacy in CF patients.

Table 15.90 Common IV antibiotics and dosing recommendations for pulmonary exacerbations in CF

Antibiotic	Pediatric dosing*	Adult dosing*	Comments
Amikacin	10mg/kg/dose every 8 hours	10 mg/kg/dose every 8 hours	Dose based on ideal body weight (IBW); requires serum concentration measurements; goal peak: 20–30 mcg/mL with troughs <10 mcg/mL
Aztreonam	50 mg/kg dose every 6–8 hours (max: 8 g/day)	2 g every 6–8 hours	
Cefepime	50 mg/kg/dose every 8 hours	2 g every 8 hours	
Ceftazidime	50 mg/kg/dose every 8 hours	2 g every 8 hours	
Ciprofloxacin (IV)	30 mg/kg/day divided every 8 hours (max: 1.2 g/day)	400 mg every 8 hours	
Ciprofloxacin (oral)	40 mg/kg/day divided every 12 hours (max: 2 g/day)	750–1000 mg every 12 hours	
Colistimethate	3–8 mg/kg/day divided every 8–12 hours (max dose: 70 mg)	3–8 mg/kg/day divided every 8–12 hours (not to exceed 160 mg every 8 hours)	Monitor for nephrotoxicity and neurotoxicity
Gentamicin	2.5– 3.3 mg/kg/dose every 8 hours (traditional dosing) or 10 mg/kg/dose every 24 hours (high-dose extended-interval dosing)	2.5–3.3 mg/kg/dose every 8 hours (traditional dosing) or 10 mg/kg/dose every 24 hours (high-dose extended-interval dosing)	Dose based on IBW; requires serum concentration measurements; goal peak: 10–12 mcg/mL with troughs <2 mcg/mL with traditional dosing High-dose extended-interval monitoring: goal peak: 20–30 mcg/mL (2 hours post-dose initiation) and trough ≤1 mcg/mL

Table 15.90 (*Contd.*)

Antibiotic	Pediatric dosing*	Adult dosing*	Comments
Imipenem/ cilastatin	20–25 mg/kg/dose every 6 hours	1 g every 6 hours	Use caution in patients with seizure disorder
Meropenem	40 mg/kg/dose every 8 hours	2 g every 8 hours	
Piperacillin ± tazobactam	350–450 mg/kg/ day divided every 6 hours†	4.5 g every 6 hours	†Based on piperacillin component
Ticarcillin ± clavulanate	300 mg/kg/day divided every 4–6 hours† (Max: 18–24 g ticarcillin/day)	3.1 g every 4 hours	†Based on ticarcillin component
Tobramycin	2.5–3.3 mg/kg/ dose every 8 hours (traditional dosing) or 10 mg/kg/dose every 24 hours (high-dose extended-interval dosing)	2.5–3.3 mg/kg/ dose every 8 hours (traditional dosing) or 10 mg/kg/dose every 24 hours (high-dose extended-interval dosing)	Dose based on IBW; requires serum concentration measurements; goal peak: 10–12 mcg/mL with troughs <2 mcg/mL High-dose extended-interval monitoring: goal peak: 20–30 mcg/mL (2 hours post-dose initiation) and trough ≤1 mcg/ mL
Trimethoprim/ sulfamethoxazole	15–20 mg/kg/ day TMP divided every 6–8 hours	15–20 mg/kg/day TMP divided every 6–8 hours	Monitor for hyperkalemia and renal dysfunction
Vancomycin	15mg/kg/dose every 6–8 hours	15 mg/kg/dose every 6–8 hours	Dose based on total body weight (TBW); serum trough concentrations should be measured to maintain levels of 15–20 mcg/mL

* Dosages assume normal renal function.

Further reading

Cystic Fibrosis Foundation (1997). Clinical Practice Guidelines for Cystic Fibrosis. Bethesda, MD: Cystic Fibrosis Foundation.

Flume PA, O'Sullivan BP, Robinson KA, Goss CH, Mogayzel PJ, Willey-Courand DB, et. al. (2007). Cystic fibrosis pulmonary guidelines chronic medications for maintenance of lung health. *Am J Resp Crit Care Med* **176**:957–969.

Parameswaran GI, Murphy TF (2007). Infections in chronic lung disease. *Infect Dis Clin North Am* **21**:673–695.

Acute respiratory distress syndrome

Acute respiratory distress syndrome (ARDS) is a rare but serious complication in pediatric and adult critically ill patients on mechanical ventilation. A more severe form of acute lung injury (ALI), ARDS is characterized by diffuse alveolar damage resulting in respiratory distress and hypoxemic respiratory failure.

ARDS further consists of inflammatory and coagulation processes, pulmonary edema, pulmonary hypertension, ventilation–perfusion mismatching, and possibly pulmonary fibrosis. ARDS occurs in 7.1% of ICU patients and 16.1% of mechanically ventilated patients with an estimated mortality of up to 40%.

Common etiologies

Direct lung injury

- Pneumonia/aspiration pneumonia
- Fat emboli
- Near drowning
- Inhalation injury
- Lung/bone marrow transplantation
- Reperfusion injury after lung transplantation or pulmonary embolectomy

Indirect lung injury

- Sepsis
- Severe trauma and shock with multiple transfusions
- Cardiopulmonary bypass
- Drug overdose
- Acute pancreatitis
- Chronic alcoholism
- Acidemia
- Blood product transfusions

Diagnosis

- Acute onset
- New-onset bilateral infiltrates
- Ratio of partial pressure of arterial oxygen to the fraction of inspired oxygen (PaO_2/FiO_2) ratio ≤300 mmHg (ALI) or ≤200 mmHg (ARDS)
- Pulmonary capillary wedge pressure (PCWP) ≤18 mmHg or the absence of clinical evidence of left arterial hypertension

Treatment options in ARDS

Currently there are no established pharmacological therapies for ARDS. Treatment should focus on identifying and treating the underlying cause of the disease.

Anti-inflammatory agents

- Initially thought to be a useful treatment of ALI and ARDS due to the release of proinflammatory mediators (e.g., interleukin [IL]-1, IL-6, IL-8 and tumor necrosis factor (TNF-α)
- Currently no evidence supports use of corticosteroids in ALI or ARDS.
- Potential patient harm secondary to adverse effects (hyperglycemia, poor wound healing, pancreatitis, prolonged muscle weakness, and increased risk of infection)

Inhaled nitric oxide

- Potent vasodilator and smooth muscle relaxant
- Randomized, double-blinded trials have shown no difference in mortality or duration of mechanical ventilation.
- Limited role in short-term treatment of acute hypoxemia or severe elevated pulmonary artery pressures
- No other vasodilators have been shown to be beneficial.

Surfactant replacement

- Prevents alveolar collapse, reduces alveolar surface tension, and enhances host immune defenses
- Has shown no effect on mortality, duration of mechanical ventilation, or oxygenation
- No current evidence to support use in ALI or ARDS

Diuretics (e.g., furosemide)

- Used in volume overloaded patients with adequate systemic intravascular volume
- Improves pulmonary edema

β-Adrenergic agonists

- Decrease airflow resistance
- Bronchodilate and stimulate sodium and water transport by alveolar epithelial cells
- Reduce peak airway pressures and improve respiratory compliance
- May improve pulmonary edema, reduce pulmonary epithelial permeability, and decrease epithelial injury

Nonpharmacological treatments

Mechanical ventilation

- Maintain low tidal volumes (≤6 mL/kg)

Fluid and hemodynamic support

- Minimize fluid overload, but ensure adequate tissue perfusion
- Conservative fluid administration has shown improved oxygenation and decrease duration of mechanical ventilation.

Respiratory syncytial virus

Respiratory syncytial virus (RSV) is the leading cause of acute respiratory illness in infants and children worldwide. In the United States, 100,000–250,000 hospitalizations and approximately 450 deaths are attributed to RSV infection annually. Almost all children are infected with RSV by the age of 2 years. Annual outbreaks of RSV infection occur between November and April, with December, January, and February being the months of peak incidence.

RSV is an enveloped RNA paramyxovirus transmitted between humans via close contact with contaminated droplets. The incubation period of the virus is usually 4–6 days, and period of viral shedding is usually 3–8 days. Viral shedding may be prolonged up to 4 weeks in younger infants and immunocompromised individuals.

Although the primary population affected by this illness is children under the age of 12 months, acute RSV infection may also occur in immunocompromised individuals and the elderly.

Clinical manifestations

Infants commonly develop lower respiratory tract infection within 2–3 days of the appearance of upper respiratory tract infection signs and symptoms. These symptoms and other clinical features of RSV infection are highlighted below.

- Lethargy*
- Poor feeding*
- Apnea*
- Bradycardia*
- Hypoxemia*
- Dehydration*
- Mild to moderate nasal congestion
- Low-grade fever
- Productive cough (may be severe)
- Copious secretions
- Pharyngitis
- Respiratory distress (e.g., tachypnea, nasal flaring)
- Vomiting

* These signs and symptoms are more likely to occur in very young or preterm infants.

Indications for hospitalization

- Age <3 months
- Cardiopulmonary disease
- Immunodeficiency
- Respiratory rate >70 breaths per minute
- Lethargic appearance
- Pulse oximetry reading <93% on room air
- Indications of uncontrolled vomiting and/or dehydration
- Signs of apnea or respiratory failure
- Hypercarbia
- Atelectasis or consolidation on chest radiography

Diagnosis

RSV is diagnosed by the presence of clinical signs and symptoms and the use of a rapid diagnostic assay for detection of nasopharyngeal specimens. Although these assays are generally reliable, with sensitivities in the 80%–90% range, the decision to initiate prophylactic measures or treatment for RSV infection should not be solely based on their results.

Treatment

Treatment of RSV infection is primarily supportive, as there is no cure to this viral illness. Many previously healthy hospitalized infants improve with supportive care and are typically discharged in ≤5 days. Medications such as ribavirin, beta-adrenergic agents, corticosteroids, and antimicrobial agents are not indicated or recommended for routine treatment of RSV infection.

Supportive care

- Hydration
- Supplemental oxygen
- Upper airway suctioning
- Intubation (if necessary)

Prevention of RSV infection

Palivizumab is a monoclonal antibody indicated for the prevention of RSV lower respiratory tract disease in infants and children with chronic lung disease of prematurity (CLD), history of preterm birth (<35 weeks' gestation), or congenital heart disease. The dosing is 15 mg/kg administered intramuscularly every 30 days, beginning in early November, with 4 subsequent monthly doses.

The American Academy of Pediatrics also recommends palivizumab prophylaxis for children between 32 and 35 weeks of gestation with two or more of the following risk factors:

- Child care attendance
- School-aged siblings
- Exposure to environmental air pollutants
- Congenital airway abnormalities
- Severe neuromuscular disease

Additional preventative measures are influenza vaccination for all high-risk infants and their contacts and proper hand-washing techniques in pediatric wards during peak RSV season to prevent nosocomial infection.

Further reading

American Academy of Pediatrics (2006). Respiratory syncytial virus. In: Pickering LK,, ed. *Red Book: 2006 Report of the Committee on Infectious Diseases*, 27th ed. Elk Grove Village, IL: American Academy of Pediatrics, pp. 560–566.

Black CP (2003). Systematic review of the biology and medical management of respiratory syncytial virus infection. *Respir Care* **48**:209–231.

Steiner RWP (2004). Treating acute bronchiolitis associated with RSV. *Am Fam Physician* **69**:325–330.

Tobacco cessation

Tobacco dependence is a chronic disease that usually requires multiple quit attempts and repeated intervention. Tobacco dependence includes smokeless tobacco (snuff and chewing tobacco).

Tobacco use is the single leading preventable cause of premature death in the United States, accounting for 1 in 5 deaths yearly. Tobacco use contributes to deaths from COPD, heart disease, and stroke and contributes to 30% of all cancer-related deaths.

Annually, 70% of all smokers visit a practitioner and 70% of all smokers would like to quit.

Behavior management

- All health care providers are in the position to ask patients, "Do you smoke?" and "Would you like to quit?"
- Counseling and medications are both effective, but in combination they are more effective than either alone.
- Individual, telephone, group, and telephone quit-line counseling have all been shown to be effective and should be encouraged by all providers.
- 7% of smokers achieve long-term abstinence on their own; with clinician intervention this increase to 30%.
- For all patients, consider the five A's for every visit:
  - Ask about tobacco use at each visit or encounter
  - Advise all smokers to quit
  - Assess interest in quitting
  - Assist patients in quitting
  - Arrange for follow-up

Recognize the five stages of change or readiness to change:

- *Precontemplation:* behavior change is not an option; patient answers 'No" to "Do you plan to quit"?
- *Contemplation:* behavior change is considered in the near future; patient answers "Yes" to "Do you plan to quit in the next 6 months"?
- *Preparation:* serious attempt at behavior change is imminent; patient answers "Yes" to "Do you plan to quit in the next month"? The patient picks a quit date.
- *Action:* the first 6 months after quitting, when risk of relapse is highest
- *Maintenance:* when behavior change persists past the first 6 months

Patients can move at any time from one stage to another. Goals are to promote motivation, provide treatment, prevent relapse, and encourage continued abstinence.

Patients not ready to quit may need additional motivational counseling, such as the "five R's."

- *Relevance:* Encourage the patient to indicate why quitting is relevant.
- *Risks:* The clinician should ask the patient to identify potential negative consequences of tobacco use.
- *Rewards:* The clinician should ask the patient to identify potential benefits of stopping tobacco use.

- *Roadblocks:* The clinician should ask the patient to identify barriers to quitting and note ways to address barriers.
- *Repetition:* Repeat the intervention at every opportunity (telephone and visits) and regularly.

Motivational interviewing (MI)

MI has been shown to be effective in increasing quit attempts and is beneficial in uncovering any ambivalence about tobacco use. Its premise is based on examining the tobacco user's beliefs, ideas, values, and feelings about tobacco. A patient-centered approach and allowing the patient to use their own words or "change talk," instead of the provider lecturing, has been shown to increase patients' willingness to change.

The four principles of MI are as follows:

- Express empathy: use open-ended questions and reflective listening, support the patient's decision to embark on change or not.
- Develop discrepancy: emphasize the difference in the patient's current behavior and values, goals, or priorities identified.
- Roll with the resistance: reflect, express empathy, and ask permission to provide information. Do not argue with or lecture the patient.
- Support self-efficacy: offer support by helping the patient to build on past successes. Offer options to help achieve small goals or steps toward change, such as identifying triggers and offering support for addressing physical dependence and behavioral and psychological aspects of tobacco use, and helping the patient to work out their plan.

Pharmacotherapy for tobacco cessation

Nicotine replacement therapy (NRT)

Precautions

- Pregnancy (category D)
- Recent (≤2 weeks) myocardial infarction
- Serious underlying arrhythmias
- Serious or worsening angina

Transdermal patches

- Available over the counter; 7 mg. 14 mg, and 21 mg patches
- Duration: 8–10 weeks
- Step-down dosage :>10 cigarettes/day
  - 4–6 weeks: 21 mg/24 hours, then
  - 2 weeks: 14 mg/24 hours, then
  - 2 weeks: 7 mg/24 hours
- Patient instructions: At the start of each day, the patient should place a new patch on a relatively hairless location, typically between the neck and waist, rotating the site to reduce local skin irritation.
- Adverse effects include local skin reactions (up to 50% will experience; self-limiting; <5% of patients have to discontinue), insomnia and/or vivid dreams, and headache.

NRT lozenges

- Available over the counter; 2 mg and 4 mg
- Duration is 12 weeks
- Dosage depends on level of addiction:

  - If first cigarette ≤30 minutes after waking, use 4 mg
  - If first cigarette ≥30 minutes after waking, use 2 mg
  - Week 1–6: 1 lozenge every 1–2 hours
  - Week 7–9: 1 lozenge every 2–4 hours
  - Week 10–12: 1 lozenge every 4–8 hours
  - Maximum, 20 lozenges per day
- Patient instructions: allow lozenge to dissolve slowly; do not chew or swallow. Take in no food or beverage for15 minutes before or during use.
- Allows for flexible dosing and addresses behavioral component (satisfies oral craving)
- Adverse effects include nausea, heartburn, and hiccups.

NRT gum

- Available over the counter; 2 mg and 4 mg
- Duration is 12 weeks
- Dose: maximum is 24 pieces/day
  - <25 cigarettes/day: use 2 mg
  - >25 cigarettes/ day: use 4mg
  - Weeks 1–6: 1 piece every 1–2 hours
  - Weeks 7–9: 1 piece every 2–4 hours
  - Weeks 10–12: 1 piece every 4–8 hours
- Patient instructions: chew gum slowly until it tingles, then park it between the cheek and gum. When the tingle is gone, begin chewing again until the tingle returns. Repeat the process until most of the tingle is gone (about 30 minutes). Food and drink should be avoided for 15 minutes before chewing or while chewing the gum.
- Allows for flexible dosing and addresses behavioral component (satisfies oral craving).
- Adverse effects include belching, increased salivation, mild jaw muscle pain, and sore throat. It is difficult to use with dentures or dental work.

NRT nasal spray

- Prescription only; 0.5 mg/spray
- Duration: 3–6 months
- Dose: 1 mg of nicotine (2 sprays, 1 in each nostril) 1–2 times per hour
  - Minimum = 8 doses/day
  - Maximum = 40 doses/day
- Allows for flexible dosing and addresses behavioral component (satisfies oral craving)
- Adverse effects: nasal, throat irritation; sneezing; coughing; rhinitis; headache
- Patients with severe reactive airway disease should not use spray.
- Dependence may occur.

NRT inhaler

- Prescription only; 10 mg cartridge that delivers 4 mg of nicotine
- Duration 3–6 months
- Dose: initial dosage is individualized.
  - 6–18 cartridges/day
  - At least 6 cartridges/day for the first 3–6 weeks of treatment

- Patient instructions: puff continuously for 20 minutes for best results; inhale into back of throat or puff in short breaths
- Open cartridges are stable for 24 hours.
- Allows for flexible dosing
- Addresses behavioral component (satisfies oral craving)
- Adverse effects include mouth or throat irritation, coughing, rhinitis

Non-nicotine drugs for tobacco cessation

Bupropion sustained release

- Prescription only; 150 mg tablets
- Duration is 7–12 weeks
- Dose: begin treatment 1–2 weeks prior to quitting
    - 150 mg on days 1–3, then
    - 150 mg twice daily with at least an 8-hour interval between doses
- Avoid bedtime dosing to minimize possible insomnia
- Can be used in combination with NRT
- Oral therapy may be more appealing
- Contraindications: history of seizures or eating disorders; within 14 days of using MAO inhibitor; with excessive alcohol; if taking another form of bupropion; pregnancy category C
- Adverse effects include insomnia and dry mouth, may cause agitation

Varenicline

- Prescription only; 0.5 mg, 1 mg tablets
- Duration is 12 weeks; may be dosed for an additional 12 weeks
- Dose: start 1 week prior to tobacco cessation
    - Days 1–3: 0.5 mg once daily
    - Days 1–4: 0.5 mg twice daily
    - Day 8 to end of treatment: 1 mg twice daily
    - For Crcl <30 mL/min: start 0.5 mg daily, may titrate to twice daily
    - If on hemodialysis: maximum dose is 0.5 mg daily if tolerated
- Patient instructions: take with a full glass of water after meals
- Offers an oral option
- Adverse effects include insomnia, abnormal dreams, nausea, vomiting, flatulence, and constipation.
- Pregnancy category C
- Warnings: Depressed mood, agitation, changes in behavior, suicidal ideation, and suicide have been reported in patients attempting to quit smoking while using varenicline. Patients should tell their health-care provider about any history of psychiatric illness before starting varenicline. Clinicians should monitor patients for changes in mood and behavior when prescribing it and elicit patient psychiatric histories.

Further reading

Fiore MC, Jaén CR, Baker TB, et al. (2008). Treating Tobacco Use and Dependence: 2008 update. Clinical Practice Guideline. Rockville, MD: U.S. Department of Health and Human Resources. Public Health Service.

NIH State-of-the-Science Panel (2006). Conference statement: tobacco use: prevention, cessation, and control. *Ann Intern Med* **145**:839–844.

U.S. DHHS Public Health Guideline for Treating Tobacco Use and Dependence, May 2008.

Solid organ transplantation

Solid organ transplantation is a life-saving treatment for patients with end-stage organ failure. The kidney is the most commonly transplanted organ. Heart, lung, liver, heart–lung, pancreas, kidney–pancreas, and intestine transplants are also performed.

Care of the transplant patient requires balancing immunosuppression therapy to positively impact graft and patient survival while minimizing adverse effects.

Immunosuppression

There have been many advances in the prevention of acute and chronic rejection in patients who have received a solid organ transplant that have improved patient and graft survival. Contemporary immunosuppressant regimens continuously evolve based on new evidence. They differ according to the type of organ transplanted, individual patient variability, time since transplant, and institution protocol.

The goal of immunosuppressive agents is to promote acceptance of a foreign organ while limiting adverse effects. By using multiple immunosuppressive agents in combination, graft survival can be improved while doses of individual agents can be minimized to reduce the incidence of adverse effects. The general phases of immunosuppressant use are

- Induction therapy is used intraoperatively and immediately post-operatively to reduce the incidence of rejection in the first 6 months.
- Maintenance therapy is lifelong and used to prevent rejection.
- Treatment of rejection is used to reverse acute rejection.

Polyclonal and monoclonal antibodies

Anti-thymocyte globulin

Polyclonal anti-thymocyte globulin is thought to bind circulating T lymphocytes causing T-cell depletion. Anti-thymocyte globulin has been used for induction therapy in kidney, pancreas, kidney–pancreas, liver, and heart transplantation and for treatment of acute rejection, but it is FDA approved only for treatment of acute rejection in kidney transplant recipients. Thymoglobulin® (anti-thymocyte globulin, rabbit) is widely used, but Atgam® (anti-thymocyte globulin, equine) is also available.

Adverse reactions include infusion-related reactions (fever, chills, headache, nausea and vomiting, diarrhea, hypotension), leukopenia, thrombocytopenia, infections, and serum sickness.

Premedication with corticosteroids, acetaminophen, and/or an antihistamine is used to reduce infusion-related side effects. Side effects, including leukopenia and thrombocytopenia, may warrant dosage reduction or discontinuation.

Depleting monoclonal antibodies

Muromonab-CD3 (OKT3®) is a mouse derived monoclonal antibody that binds the CD3 receptor on mature T-cells, causing T-lymphocyte depletion. Its use is now limited because of adverse effects and the availability of other options. It was primarily used as induction treatment and for the treatment of acute rejection.

- Adverse effects: cytokine release syndrome (fever, chills, dyspnea, headache, nausea, and vomiting), pulmonary edema, infection, rash, aseptic meningitis, encephalopathy, and post-transplant lymphoproliferative disorder
- Monitoring: CD3 count and anti-OKT3 antibodies during and after OKT3 therapy

Alemtuzumab (Campath®) is a humanized anti-CD52 monoclonal antibody approved for use in the U.S. for B-cell chronic lymphocytic leukemia but has been recently used off-label for induction therapy and acute rejection. It exerts its lymphocytic action by binding to the CD52 surface antigen on T and B lymphocytes, natural killer cells, monocytes, and macrophages causing cell lysis.

- Adverse effects: infusion-related side effects (fever, chills, hypertension, hypotension), profound lymphopenia, neutropenia, thrombocytopenia, and infection

Non-depleting monoclonal antibodies

Daclizumab (Zenapax®) and basiliximab (Simulect®) are interleukin-2 (IL-2) receptor antagonists that inhibit IL-2-mediated activation of lymphocytes. Both are FDA approved for use as induction therapy for kidney transplant recipients, but have also been used in recipients of other solid organ allografts.

- Adverse effects: These agents are generally well tolerated, but acute hypersensitivity reactions including anaphylaxis have been reported.

Calcineurin inhibitors

Cyclosporine and tacrolimus inhibit the transcription of IL-2 and other cytokines, thereby inhibiting T-lymphocyte proliferation and activation. They are used as maintenance immunosuppressive therapy. The recommended starting dose for both agents is based on weight, type of organ transplanted, renal function, and use of other immunosuppressants.

They are substrates of cytochrome P450 3A4 and the P-glycoprotein efflux pump, resulting in a number of significant drug interactions (see Table 15.91). Concurrent nephrotoxic agents should be minimized.

Cyclosporine

- Available in an oil-based formulation (Sandimmune) and as a microemulsion (Gengraf®/Neoral®). The oil-based formulation has much greater variability in its absorption.
- Monitoring: target trough level 100–400 ng/mL
- Adverse effects: nephrotoxicity, hypertension, hyperlipidemia, hirsutism, gingival hyperplasia, GI disorders, tremor, hepatotoxicity, and diabetes mellitus

Tacrolimus (Prograf®)

- Adverse effects are similar to those for cyclosporine except tacrolimus is less likely to cause hyperlipidemia, hypertension, hirsutism, and gingival hyperplasia but more likely to cause diabetes mellitus and lymphoproliferative disorders.
- Monitoring: Whole blood concentration with a target trough level of 5–20 ng/mL

Table 15.91 Selected drug interactions with cyclosporine and tacrolimus

Interacting medication	Effect
Anticonvulsants (carbamazepine, phenobarbital, phenytoin)	Decreased cyclosporine and tacrolimus levels due to CYP450 metabolism induction
Azole antifungals (voriconazole, fluconazole, itraconazole, posaconazole)	Increased cyclosporine and tacrolimus levels due to CYP450 metabolism inhibition. Decrease tacrolimus dosage by 66% when initiating voriconazole. Decrease cyclosporine dosage by 50% when initiating voriconazole.
Non-dihydropyridine calcium channel blockers (diltiazem, verapamil)	Increased cyclosporine and tacrolimus levels due to CYP450 metabolism inhibition
Digoxin	Cyclosporine may increase the levels and effects of digoxin
Grapefruit juice	Increased cyclosporine and tacrolimus levels due to CYP450 metabolism inhibition. Advise patients to avoid grapefruit.
Protease inhibitors (indinavir, nelfinavir, ritonavir, saquinavir)	Increased cyclosporine and tacrolimus levels due to CYP450 metabolism inhibition
HMG-CoA reductase inhibitors (simvastatin, lovastatin, atorvastatin)	Increased HMG-CoA reductase levels due to competitive inhibition of CYP450
Macrolide antibiotics (clarithromycin, erythromycin)	Increased cyclosporine and tacrolimus levels due to CYP450 metabolism inhibition
Rifampin, rifabutin	Decreased cyclosporine and tacrolimus levels due to CYP450 metabolism induction
Sirolimus	Sirolimus and cyclosporine oral solution and capsules should be separated by 4 hours to avoid increases in sirolimus bioavailability.
St. John's wort	Decreased cyclosporine and tacrolimus levels due to CYP450 metabolism induction

Mammalian target of rapamycin (mTOR) inhibitors

Sirolimus and everolimus block the regulatory kinase mTOR, preventing T-cell progression from G1 to the S phase of the cell cycle and thus blocking cytokine-mediated T-cell proliferation. Sirolimus is used in maintenance immunosuppression regimens in patients receiving renal transplants in combination with corticosteroids and cyclosporine, or in regimens to minimize the need for calcineurin inhibitors and corticosteroids to reduce associated side effects.

Everolimus has been studied as maintenance immunosuppression for kidney and heart transplant recipients. Both are substrates and inhibitors of CYP450 3A4, and drug interactions are similar to those of cyclosporine and tacrolimus. There is an increased risk of nephrotoxicity when used in combination with tacrolimus and cyclosporine.

Sirolimus (Rapamune®)

- Adverse effects: hypertension, hyperlipidemia, thrombocytopenia, anemia, leukopenia, peripheral edema, diarrhea, acne, rash, hepatic artery thrombosis, interstitial pneumonitis, and delayed wound healing. Most effects are dose dependent.
- Monitoring: LFTs, CBC, serum cholesterol and triglycerides, BP, and serum creatinine. Serum drug concentration should be monitored in all patients. Target trough levels are 4–24 ng/mL depending on concomitant immunosuppressant use and time after transplant.

Everolimus (Certican®)

- Adverse effects: similar to those of sirolimus
- Monitoring: similar to sirolimus. Monitor whole blood concentration and target trough levels of 3–8 ng/mL.

Antiproliferative agents

Azathioprine and mycophenolate mofetil (MMF) inhibit the synthesis of guanosine monophosphate nucleotides by blocking purine synthesis and preventing B- and T-cell proliferation. MMF has supplanted azathioprine as the antiproliferative agent of choice since its introduction and is used as part of maintenance immunosuppression regimens in patients receiving kidney, heart, and liver transplants.

Women must use adequate contraception because of the risk of teratogenicity. Patients are at higher risk of infection and malignancy.

Azathioprine (Imuran®)

- Adverse effects: dose-related bone marrow suppression, GI disorders (diarrhea, constipation, nausea, vomiting), hepatotoxicity, and pancreatitis
- Drug interactions: allopurinol can increase the toxicity of azathioprine by inhibiting an active metabolite. Azathioprine dose should be reduced to 25%–33% of the usual dose. Concomitant use of azathioprine and ACE inhibitors may cause severe anemia.
- Monitoring: CBC and LFTs

Mycophenolate mofetil and sodium (CellCept® and Myfortic®)

- Adverse effects: bone marrow suppression and GI disorders. These may warrant dose reduction.
- Drug interactions: antacids, cholestyramine, or sevelamer should not be used concomitantly with MMF.
- Monitoring: frequent monitoring of CBC is recommended

Corticosteroids

Corticosteroids reduce inflammation and cause immunosuppression through a number of mechanisms. Corticosteroids are used as induction therapy and maintenance therapy and for treatment of acute rejection.

The dose is highest perioperatively and immediately postoperatively to minimize the risk of rejection, and is slowly tapered to minimize the risk of numerous adverse effects. Steroid withdrawal and steroid avoidance are strategies being studied to reduce effects of corticosteroid toxicity.

Adverse effects include psychosis, weight gain, fluid retention, hyperglycemia, hypertension, hyperlipidemia, osteoporosis, osteonecrosis, glaucoma, cataracts, Cushing's syndrome, peptic ulcers, growth impairment in children, muscle weakness, and thinning of the skin.

Common infections in transplant recipients

While immunosuppressants have improved graft and host survival, higher states of immunosuppression have caused opportunistic infections to become increasingly common. Transplant recipients with compromised immune defense systems may present differently with an infectious complication compared to patients with normal immune function. Furthermore, systemic signs and symptoms often associated with infections, such as fever, may be present in transplant recipients because of noninfectious etiologies.

The common pathogens that transplant recipients are likely to experience vary according to the time since transplantation. Early after transplantation (<1 month), most infections are nosocomial in origin. Efforts to reduce nosocomial infections that occur in all hospitalized patients, such as *Clostridium difficile*–associated disease and those associated with mechanical ventilation, vascular-access devices, urinary catheters, and surgical sites, are similarly successful in transplant recipients. Screening for and treatment of certain infections in the donor or recipient before transplantation are also important.

From 1 to 6 months after transplantation, in addition to potential nosocomial infection, the incidence of viral pathogens and other opportunistic infections increases. Important viral pathogens include hepatitis B and C virus, herpes viruses (e.g., cytomegalovirus, Epstein–Barr virus, varicella-zoster virus, herpes simplex viruses), respiratory syncytial virus, adenovirus, and polyomavirus BK. Other infections that appear during this time period may be due to *Pneumocystis jirovecii* (formerly *Pneumocystis carinii*), *Listeria monocytogenes, Nocardia asteroides, Toxoplasma gondii, Cryptococcus neoformans, Mycobacterium tuberculosis, Aspergillus* species, and endemic fungi (e.g., blastomycosis, histoplasmosis, coccidioimycosis). Antiviral and antibacterial prophylaxis has reduced the risk of many of these infections.

The risk of infection is reduced 6 months after transplantation owing to decreasing immunosuppression requirements. However, transplant recipients are more vulnerable to community-acquired infections (e.g., community-acquired pneumonia) than the general population. If allograft rejection necessitates intensified immunosuppression, the risk of opportunistic infection increases (see Opportunistic Infections unit in this chapter, p. 570).

Trimethoprim-sulfamethoxazole (TMP-SMX) is given to all transplant recipients without a contraindication, primarily because of its activity against *Pneumocystis jiroveci, Toxoplasma gondii*, and many community-acquired pathogens. It is usually given as one single-strength tablet once daily or one double-strength tablet once daily to three times weekly. Prophylaxis with TMP-SMX is continued for up to 1 year and longer in certain patients (e.g., those with intense immunosuppression or chronic viral infections) (see Opportunistic Infections unit in this chapter, p. 570)

The most common opportunistic pathogen in transplant recipients is cytomegalovirus (CMV). Transplant recipients at highest risk for active infection are those who are seronegative for CMV and receive an allograft from a donor who is seropositive (D+/R–). The most effective agents for prophylaxis are ganciclovir and valganciclovir, but acyclovir and valacyclovir may also be used. Prophylaxis for CMV is usually given for 3 to 12 months (see Opportunistic Infections unit in this chapter, p. 570)

Herpes simplex virus infections (HSV) occurring after transplantation are often the result of reactivation of a previous infection. Prophylaxis with low-dose oral acyclovir delays the development of HSV infections.

Management of poisoning inquiries

Poisoning is a leading cause of hospitalization and death due to unintentional injuries. In the United States, most poisoning exposures are acute, unintentional, occur at home, involve the ingestion of a single substance, and can safely be treated at home with poison center direction. Poisoning exposures can be caused by the following means:

- Unintentional poisoning
  - Small children eating tablets or berries
  - Adverse reactions to drugs or food
  - Drug–drug or drug–food interactions
  - Envenomations
  - Therapeutic drug errors
- Intentional poisoning
  - Intentional self-poisoning—e.g., tablets or chemicals are ingested intentionally, sometimes to manipulate family or friends, or with the intention of suicide.
  - Deliberate poisoning—e.g., Munchausen's syndrome by proxy (one person creates symptoms in another by, e.g., administering drugs)
  - Product tampering
  - Substance misuse or abuse

Any inquiry regarding a possible acute poisoning incident should be treated as potentially serious and urgent. Questioning can often establish if there is little possibility of harm, but consultation with a poison control center is recommended. The poison center specialist can help determine if the patient should be referred to the nearest emergency department (ED).

Some misconceptions

Members of the public might not be aware of the following misconceptions.

Alcohol poisoning can be potentially fatal, especially in children and adolescents. In children, if there are any signs of altered mentation or behavior, including intoxication, the patient should be referred to an ED.

Some forms of poisoning might not cause symptoms initially (e.g., acetaminophen overdose, ingestion of sustained-release tablets and capsules, some toxic alcohols). This can create the impression that there is no intoxication. Referral to an ED should be made if sufficient tablets have been taken, even in the absence of symptoms, or for any patient who has attempted self-harm.

Be aware that some over-the-counter (OTC) preparations have similar brand names but different ingredients, e.g., Tylenol® and Tylenol-PM®, Anacin (aspirin) and Anacin-3 (acetaminophen), and different versions of Coricidin®, Triaminic®, or Robitussin® products. Ensure that you and other health-care professionals are clear about what product is involved.

Sources of information

Consumers are encouraged to seek drug information from their pharmacist or physician. Numerous consumer-oriented books and Web sites (e.g., drugs.com) contain information on drug pharmacology, dosage, administration, adverse reactions, and identification.

Micromedex's Healthcare Series® is the poison and drug database used by most poison control centers in the United States. Information on drugs, chemicals, plants, mushrooms, venomous creatures, teratogenicity, occupational and environmental exposures, alternative medicines, and some foreign drugs can be found in this collection of electronic databases.

Poison control centers (or just poison centers) provide immediate, confidential, 24-hour telephone advice. If there is any cause for concern in an acute or chronic poisoning incident, consumers should contact a poison center immediately.

Since 2001, all U.S. poison centers can be reached through a nationwide toll-free number: **(800) 222–1222**. Calls are routed to the nearest poison center based on the area code and exchange of the caller. It is inappropriate to cause unnecessary delay in what might be a life-threatening situation by looking elsewhere for information.

Physicians or other health-care providers dealing with a (potential) poisoning exposure should also contact the poison center directly so that first-hand information is given and received. It is entirely appropriate for pharmacists to consult poison centers for information regarding any type of poisoning or adverse drug reaction information.

Information required when managing a poisoning inquiry

Eliciting as much information as possible about a poisoning incident can facilitate speedy management. It is especially important to have the relevant information available when contacting a poison center:

- Identity—brand name and active ingredients
- Timing—when did the incident occur relative to the time of the enquiry
- Quantity—number of tablets or volume of liquid. An estimate is better than no information. Checking the quantity left in a container instead of its full volume may give an estimate of maximum quantity ingested.
- If tablets or capsules—are these sustained release?
- Age and weight of the patient
- Any pertinent medical history and medication history?
- Any signs and symptoms observed?
- If the patient has vomited, is there any sign of the poison, e.g., colored liquid, undigested plant material, or tablet fragments?
- Any treatments or first aid already administered and the outcome?
- It should be noted that poison control centers are considered health-care providers under HIPAA privacy regulations (Federal Register Vol. 65, No. 250, December 28, 2000, p. 82626).

If the poison specialist recommends referral to an ED, the caller should be advised to take any containers or plant material with them that could help with identification (taking suitable precautions to avoid skin or clothing contamination with the poison).

First aid for poisoning incidents

- If the patient is unconscious or has difficulty breathing, chest pain, or seizure activity **call 911** immediately.
- If the patient is unconscious, check airway, breathing, circulation (ABC). As needed, perform the following:
- Perform CPR but not mouth-to-mouth resuscitation, except with a face shield (because of the risk of contaminating the first-aider).
- Place patient in a supine position.
- Do not induce vomiting.
- Safely remove contaminated clothing and poison from skin.
- Move patient to fresh air if needed.
- Call poison center for further instructions.

General management of poisoned patients

- Establish ABCs.
- Treat emergent complications such as convulsions, hypotension, and hyperthermia.
- Decontaminate the GI tract as soon as possible after overdose. Administration of activated charcoal is the preferred method; induction of emesis is no longer recommended, and gastric lavage has limited effectiveness and is potentially harmful.
- The need to employ a method to enhance elimination of toxins is rare. Toxins in which clinically significant improvement have been established following hemodialysis (under the right circumstances) include ethylene glycol, methanol, lithium, salicylate, and theophylline.
- Only a handful of drugs and toxins have specific antidotes. Each case should be assessed for the need for antidotal therapy.

Treatment of alcohol withdrawal

Alcohol-withdrawal syndromes are typically characterized as mild, moderate, or severe depending on the onset and severity of symptoms. Many alcohol-dependent patients might not be obvious "alcoholics."

Mild withdrawal

Mild withdrawal symptoms occur within 24 hours (6–12 hours) of cessation of alcohol use and may include diaphoresis, anxiety, tremor, nausea and/or vomiting, and mild tachycardia. Symptoms may occur with alcohol still detectable in the blood.

Moderate withdrawal

Moderate symptoms include alcoholic hallucinosis (auditory, visual, or tactile), withdrawal seizures, and/or mild to moderate autonomic hyperactivity (tachycardia, hypertension, fever). Half of patients who experience a seizure only suffer a single seizure. Hallucinations and autonomic effects occur 12–24 hours after alcohol use, followed by risk of seizures 24–48 hours after use.

Severe withdrawal

Severe withdrawal is characterized by altered mental status (disorientation, agitation), hallucinations, and autonomic toxicity (tachycardia, hypertension, hyperthermia). Some patients with severe withdrawal will progress to delirium tremens. Severe effects are usually delayed by at least 24 hours after last alcohol use, and can last for days to weeks.

Many alcohol-dependent people require no medication when withdrawing from alcohol. Supportive care, recognition, and treatment of dehydration and glucose and electrolyte imbalances, monitoring, reassurance, and a low-stimulus environment are effective in reducing withdrawal severity.

If medication is required, treatment can be given using cross-tolerant drugs on either a fixed schedule or based on symptoms (symptom-triggered loading). Relatively long-acting benzodiazepines are generally considered the drugs of choice.

Benzodiazepines reduce anxiety, reduce autonomic symptoms, and elevate the seizure threshold. Using symptom-triggered loading, the patient is given repeated doses until symptoms have diminished to an acceptable level.

Diazepam or chlordiazepoxide are long-acting drugs with active metabolites and are effective in the prevention and treatment of acute alcohol-withdrawal seizures. Because of the relatively large doses usually given, and the long half-lives, it might not be necessary to give any further medication for withdrawal relief. If symptoms reappear, however, further doses should be administered, with doses titrated according to symptom severity.

Suggested withdrawal regimen

Treatment of mild withdrawal symptoms should be started as soon as the patient can tolerate oral medication. Administer diazepam 10–20 mg by mouth every 1–2 hours until symptoms resolve or are significantly improved. For patients with mild symptoms who cannot tolerate oral intake, reduce the diazepam dose to 5–10 mg intravenously.

Symptom-triggered therapy has been shown to reduce total amounts of drug needed and decreased risk of delirium tremens. Sedative drugs such as benzodiazepines are more effective and safer than use of neuroleptics. Use of barbiturates should be reserved for refractory cases. In the absence of delirium, treatment duration is usually 5–7 days.

Patients with moderate or greater symptoms, particularly those with abnormal vital signs and those requiring inpatient care, should generally receive intravenous dosing. Diazepam 5–10 mg can be given every 10–15 minutes, not exceeding 100 mg/hr.

Rapid-acting benzodiazepines (e.g., diazepam, lorazepam) are the drugs of choice to terminate seizures. Avoid the use of phenytoin. Keep in mind that seizures can occur with any degree of alcohol withdrawal.

Review dose daily and titrate on individual patient basis

There is a clinical opinion that patients given the recommended maximum dose and still suffering symptoms of withdrawal should be given further doses every 2 hours until symptoms are controlled or patients are obviously too drowsy to swallow any more.

Cautions

- Patients might experience seizures as the dose of benzodiazepine is tapered off.
- Patients who are oversedated or sedated for too long are at risk for pulmonary aspiration.
- The dose should be adjusted to provide effective sedative and anticonvulsant end points while preventing oversedation, respiratory depression, and hypotension.
- Doses of diazepam or chlordiazepoxide should be reduced in severe liver dysfunction. Alternatively, a shorter-acting benzodiazepine, e.g., lorazepam, can be used (seek specialist advice). Patients with chronic liver disease should have their dose assessed twice daily to avoid oversedation.
- A maximum 24-hour dose (10 mg twice daily) should only be prescribed on discharge from the hospital, if necessary.

Thiamine and vitamin supplements

In patients who drink, poor nutrition is common for the following reasons:

- Inadequate intake of food
- Associated chronic liver disease
- Chronic pancreatitis
- Malabsorption (water-soluble and fat-soluble vitamins should be replaced and severely malnourished patients should be considered for enteral feeding)

Vitamin deficiency can lead to serious illnesses such as anemia, Wernicke–Korsakoff syndrome, and psychosis. Consider multivitamin (including thiamine and folate) administration in all alcohol abusers unless there is documentation of recent supplementation.

Thiamine

Thiamine deficiency leads to polyneuritis with motor and sensory defects. Ophthalmoplegia (paralysis of the eye muscles), nystagmus, and ataxia are associated with Wernicke's encephalopathy, in which learning and memory are impaired; there is an estimated 10%–20% mortality. Korsakoff's psychosis is characterized by confabulations (the patient invents material to fill memory blanks) and is less likely to be reversible once established.

Parenteral thiamine replacement

Give 100 mg intramuscularly or intravenously to all patients suspected of alcohol withdrawal. Continue at doses of 50–100 mg/day (up to 300 mg for severe symptoms) until the patient resumes a normal diet. Intravenous thiamine must be diluted prior to administration and is incompatible with alkaline solutions.

Oral thiamine replacement

If symptoms of withdrawal are not severe, the following regimen is recommended:

- Oral thiamine, 10–30 mg daily should be given until withdrawal is complete.

Other vitamins

- Consider oral multivitamin, including folic acid, supplementation as needed.
- Replenish hypokalemia or hypomagnesemia as needed.

At discharge

Oral supplements should be continued at discharge in patients who are malnourished or have inadequate diets. Thiamine should be continued long term if there is cognitive impairment or peripheral neuropathy (100 mg twice daily).

Consideration should also be given to the setting in which withdrawal occurs. In all cases, careful monitoring of withdrawal severity is essential, whereas more severe withdrawal requires inpatient care. Specialist alcohol treatment services and most hospitals can provide charts to be used in the monitoring of symptom severity.

Treatment of selected overdoses

Substances most frequently involved in poisoning exposures reported to U.S. poison centers include analgesics (OTC and prescription), cleaning substances, personal care products, CNS medications, cough and cold preparations, foreign bodies, pesticides, and envenomations (bites and stings).

All of these substances are commonly available in homes. Substances with the highest fatality rate include CNS medications (sedatives, hypnotics, neuroleptics), opioid analgesics, cardiovascular drugs, combination products that contain acetaminophen, and antidepressants.

Acetaminophen

Acetaminophen (APAP) is one of the most commonly consumed drugs in the world, and it has an excellent safety profile when used as directed. Overdose or excessive "therapeutic" doses can result in hepatotoxicity.

Clinical toxicology

Hepatotoxicity is caused by a toxic intermediate (NAPQUI), formed via acetaminophen metabolism by cytochrome 2E1 isoenzymes. This metabolite accumulates following excessive doses, with subsequent depletion of glutathione, which normally reduces NAPQUI to inactive metabolites. The presence of centrilobular necrosis is essentially pathonogmonic for acetaminophen toxicity.

Presentation

Most patients develop nausea, vomiting, and abdominal pain within 6 hours of ingestion, which may be followed by a latent period in which patients look and feel better. Hepatic transaminases become elevated approximately 24 hours out, and peak at 72–96 hours.

In uncomplicated cases, hepatic enzymes drop quickly and organ dysfunction does not occur. Patients who progress to fulminant hepatic failure typically have right upper quadrant tenderness, jaundice, coagulopathy, renal failure, hypoglycemia, altered mental status, cerebral edema, coma, and death.

Patient evaluation

All patients who present to an emergency department with overdose or suicidal gesture should have serum acetaminophen levels assessed. Patients who ingest >7.5 g (200 mg/kg in children) at one time or exceed maximum daily doses for 3 or more days should be referred to an emergency department for evaluation.

Serum APAP concentration should be obtained as soon as possible, but at least 4 hours after an acute ingestion. Risk for hepatotoxicity is assessed by plotting the serum level vs. time on the Rumack–Matthew nomogram (acute ingestions only). If the time of ingestion is unknown, check serum APAP level and hepatic transaminases. If either the serum APAP, AST or ALT are elevated, then empiric therapy with N-acetylcysteine should be initiated.

Patients with evidence of APAP toxicity should have coagulation, electrolytes, and renal function assessed.

Management

Activated charcoal may be of benefit in reducing the 4-hour serum level and should be administered as soon as possible.

No further medical treatment is needed if the serum APAP level falls below the lower line on the Rumack–Matthew nomogram. Begin treatment with N-acetylcysteine (NAC) for any of the following:

- The serum APAP level obtained between 4 and 24 hours after an acute overdose is above the lower line on the nomogram.
- The serum APAP level is elevated (e.g., >20 mg/L) and no history of APAP ingestion is available.
- The patient has unexplained evidence of hepatic injury (e.g., AST or ALT are >50 IU/L).

Prophylactic dosing of NAC in patients at risk for hepatotoxicity:

- Oral: 140 mg/kg loading dose, followed by 70 mg/kg every 4 hours for 72 hours. Administer as a 5% solution. Shorter courses of oral NAC may be acceptable after consultation with a poison center or clinical toxicologist.
- Intravenous: 150 mg/kg infused over 1 hour, then 50 mg/kg infused over 4 hours, then 100 mg/kg infused over 16 hours.

For patients with evidence of hepatic injury or dysfunction, treat with either oral or intravenous doses as above, but continue treatment until the patient is improved, showing normal mental status, resolved coagulopathy, and transaminase levels below 500–1000 IU/L.

Anticholinergics

Medications with anticholinergic effects include atropine and other belladonna alkaloids, H1 antihistamines, cyclic antidepressants, phenothiazines, antiparkinson drugs (benztropine, trihexyphenidyl), GI drugs (dicyclomine, glycopyrrolate, propantheline), urinary tract drugs (oxybutynin), and ipatropium. Other sources include natural products such as nutmeg, jimson weed (datura stramonium), and deadly nightshade (atropa belladonna).

Clinical toxicology

Drugs and chemicals with anticholinergic properties competitively antagonize the effects of acetylcholine at muscarinic and/or nicotinic receptors. Muscarinic receptors are primarily found in cardiac, smooth muscle, and exocrine gland cells. Nicotinic receptors are predominantly found in autonomic ganglia, striated muscle, and adrenal medulla.

Presentation

Anticholinergic drugs and chemicals usually affect both the central and peripheral nervous systems, but occasionally can affect either one alone. Common effects include tachycardia, mydriasis, sedation, delirium, and warm, dry skin. Constipation (decreased bowel sounds) and/or urinary retention may also occur.

Serious effects include psychosis, seizures, coma, hyperthermia, hypertension or hypotension, QTc prolongation, and ventricular dysrhythmias. The anticholinergic toxic syndrome (toxidrome) is one of the most recognizable of all toxidromes and includes the following:

- Blind as a bat
- Red as a beet
- Dry as a bone
- Hot as hades
- Mad as a hatter (or mad as a wet hen)

Patient evaluation

Patients should have frequent monitoring of vital signs and mental status. Further evaluation should include an ECG, cardiac monitoring, and serum electrolytes. Determination of acid–base status and CPK is useful in patients with seizures, coma, or altered hemodynamics. Serum drug levels are not helpful in assessment of toxicity or to guide management.

Management

Provision of supportive care is of primary importance. All patients should be monitored in an intensive care setting with intravenous access, frequent vital signs, seizure precautions, and continuous monitoring of cardiac rhythm and pulse oximetry.

Oral activated charcoal, if tolerated, should be given to patients presenting with acute overdose, and may be helpful for several hours after ingestion because of slowed gastric emptying and motility. Comatose patients require airway support.

Most patients with anticholinergic toxicity do well with only supportive care and gastric decontamination. More definitive therapy may be needed in patients with seizures, severe agitation or delirium, symptomatic tachycardia, or significant hyperthermia. A benzodiazepine (lorazepam or diazepam) is reasonable initial therapy in these patients.

Physostigmine is a specific antidote for (severe) anticholinergic toxicity. Physostigmine is a tertiary amine carbamate derivative that reversibly inhibits plasma acetylcholinesterase, thereby decreasing the breakdown of acetylcholine and increasing the amount of acetylcholine available at muscarinic and nicotinic receptors.

The usual initial dose is 1–2 mg given intravenously by slow injection over 5–10 minutes. The dose may be repeated in 30 minutes if needed. A therapeutic response usually occurs within minutes and can confirm the diagnosis. Adverse effects include seizures and bradycardia. Physostigmine should be used with caution, if at all, to treat anticholinergic effects associated with TCA poisoning.

Ventricular dysrhythmias can be treated with lidocaine, phenytoin, amiodarone, and/or magnesium. Drugs that prolong atrioventricular (AV) conduction (Class IA and IC) are contraindicated.

Hypotension should be treated with intravenous fluids and vasopressors as needed. Norepinephrine is generally considered the vasopressor of choice since it is direct acting.

Prolonged intraventricular conduction (widened QRS complex) may respond to intravenous sodium bicarbonate (100–150 mEq in 1 L D5W) or intermittent 50 mEq boluses (preferred by most toxicologists).

Patients should be monitored until resolution of significant effects. Mild tachycardia and/or mild CNS effects (agitation, confusion, hallucinations) can rarely persist for 3–4 days, even up to a week.

Benzodiazepines

Benzodiazepines are among the most widely prescribed class of medications and thus are frequently misused or abused. Benzodiazepines have largely replaced barbiturates as sedative/hypnotics, and are also used as anxiolytics, muscle relaxants, and anticonvulsants (particularly in children).

Fortunately, and compared to barbiturates, benzodiazepines have relatively low toxicity when taken orally. However, intravenous administration and ingestions combined with other CNS depressants, including ethanol, can have serious toxicity.

Clinical toxicology

Benzodiazepines are thought to work primarily by enhancing the actions of gamma aminobutyric acid (GABA), the primary inhibitory neurotransmitter in the CNS. The various pharmacologic effects of benzodiazepines result from GABA-ergic effects in different parts of the CNS: cerebral cortex, cerebellum, basal ganglia, thalamus, etc.

Benzodiazepines produce dose-dependent sedation of the CNS— drowsiness to hypnosis to stupor—but rarely produce coma when ingested alone. All benzodiazepines are capable of producing tolerance with repeated use, and symptoms of withdrawal upon sudden discontinuance.

Presentation

Patients with benzodiazepine ingestion are commonly reported to poison centers and seen in emergency departments. Frequent effects include mild–moderate CNS depression, slurred speech, ataxia, and disinhibition. Less common effects that occur, particularly with very high doses or presence of additional CNS depressants, include stupor, respiratory depression, hypotension, bradycardia, and hypothermia.

Retrograde amnesia is relatively common. Pupil size is not diagnostic, since either miosis or mydriasis can occur. Paradoxical excitation and agitation, usually associated with therapeutic doses, have also been reported, especially in children and the elderly.

Patient evaluation

All patients should be evaluated as having potentially life-threatening toxicity, with continuous monitoring of cardiac rhythm and pulse oximetry. Serum levels of benzodiazepines are not useful to judge toxicity or guide therapy. Most urine "drug abuse" screens are qualitative immunoassays that detect oxazepam and nordiazepam.

All urine screens are subject to drug concentrations, which must exceed a certain cutoff value for the test to be positive. Variations exist among the different assay brands, therefore, clinicians should consult their clinical laboratory for test-specific issues.

Management

Most patients who ingest only benzodiazepines do well with provision of supportive care and usually do not require mechanical airway support. All patients should initially be monitored in an intensive care setting with intravenous access, at least until the peak effects have passed (usually less than 24 hours).

Oral activated charcoal, if tolerated, should be given to patients presenting soon (within first few hours) following acute overdose. Procedures to enhance elimination are not indicated.

Flumazenil (Romazicon®) is a competitive benzodiazepine antagonist that may be indicated in patients with respiratory depression or an unstable airway, and intubation is not desirable. Flumazenil generally reverses benzodiazepine effects in the reverse order in which they occurred. Thus respiratory depression would be reversed before anxiolysis.

Flumazenil is indicated for reversal of excessive sedation, respiratory depression, or hypotension associated with known benzodiazepine use. It should not be used routinely as empiric therapy in emergency department patients who present in a coma.

The recommended initial dose of flumazenil is 0.2–0.3 mg administered intravenously over 15–30 seconds. If there is no effect the dose may be repeated every 1 minute until a total dose of 1 mg. Patients must be monitored for resedation and for symptoms of withdrawal. If needed, an intravenous infusion can be started at 1 mg/hr and titrated to effect.

A positive response to flumazenil is consistent with benzodiazepine or benzodiazepine analog toxicity, although reports of response in ethanol-intoxicated patients who tested negative for benzodiazepines have been published.

Beta-adrenergic blockers

Beta-adrenergic blocking drugs (beta-blockers) are used in the treatment of a variety of diseases, including ischemic heart disease, hypertension, and tachydysrhythmias. Most beta-blockers share structural similarity, with various (ring) substitutions resulting in receptor selectivity, intrinsic agonist activity, lipid solubility, or concomitant antagonism of alpha-adrenergic receptors.

Over 18,000 exposures to beta-blockers (regardless of severity) were reported by U.S. poison centers in 2006, with four reported deaths in patients with beta-blocker-only ingestions.

Clinical toxicology

All beta-blockers competitively bind to beta-adrenergic receptors and prevent the action of agonists such as norepinephrine. Little change in hemodynamics occurs in healthy subjects with therapeutic doses. However patients with increased sympathetic tone (e.g., exercise) or cardiovascular disease may have more pronounced effects. Bradycardia and hypotension resulting from excessive beta-blockade are the hallmarks of toxicity following overdose.

Blockade of beta-receptors in noncardiac tissue such as bronchial smooth muscle rarely produces significant toxicity, but patients with asthma or COPD are at increased risk. Likewise, beta-blockers can inhibit catecholamine-induced glycogenolysis. However, beta-blockade overdose rarely causes hypoglycemia in healthy patients, but can mask the symptoms of hypoglycemia and delay glucose response to hypoglycemia in insulin-dependent diabetics. It should also be noted that beta-blockers typically lose selectivity with increasing doses, such that overdose from most beta-blockers has similar toxicity.

Presentation

Principle effects in patients with beta-blocker toxicity are bradycardia and hypotension. Other cardiovascular effects include AV block, prolonged intraventricular conduction (widened QRS), ventricular ectopy, idioventricular rhythm, and cardiac arrest. Common noncardiac effects may include nausea, dizziness, and lethargy. Stupor, acute lung injury, seizures, metabolic acidosis, or coma may occur in severe poisoning.

The onset of toxicity usually occurs within 3–4 hours following overdose, but may be delayed when sustained-release products are ingested. Patients with pre-existing cardiovascular disease or patients who co-ingest other cardioactive medications such as digitalis or calcium channel blockers are at highest risk for severe cardiac effects.

Patient evaluation

All patients should be evaluated as having potentially life-threatening toxicity, with continuous monitoring of vital signs and cardiac rhythm. Initial evaluation should include an ECG and monitoring for at least 4–6 hours. Blood glucose should be rapidly assessed in patients with altered mental status.

Assessment of serum electrolytes, renal function, hepatic function, and/or acid–base status is indicated in patients with symptomatic toxicity. Serum levels of beta-blockers are not useful to judge toxicity or guide therapy.

Management

All patients with known, impending, or suspected beta-blocker toxicity should be monitored in an intensive care setting with intravenous access and continuous cardiac monitoring. Monitor serum electrolytes and glucose in symptomatic patients.

Oral activated charcoal, if tolerated, should be given to patients presenting soon (within first few hours) following acute overdose. Whole bowel irrigation may be of benefit if instituted prior to absorption of large numbers of sustained-release products.

Treatment of beta-blocker toxicity should be targeted to restore hemodynamic stability through improvement of heart rate and/or cardiac contractility. Atropine, beta-agonists, glucagon, and cardiac pacing can positively influence heart rate. Atropine is safe and readily available but has had inconsistent results.

- Atropine: 0.5–1.0 mg (0.02 mg/kg) intravenously, and repeat dose every 5–10 minutes as needed to a maximum dose of 1 mg (children) or 3 mg (adults)

- Beta-agonists: titrated doses of epinephrine, norepinephrine, or dopamine may be effective in increasing heart rate. Isoproterenol is generally avoided due to risk of worsening hypotension.
- Glucagon is a pancreatic hormone that has demonstrated efficacy in improving heart rate and contractility in beta-blocker poisoning. Its effects are likely mediated by increasing intracellular cAMP through mechanisms independent of the adrenergic nervous system. The initial dose is 5–10 mg (0.1–0.2 mg/kg) by intravenous bolus, with repeat doses of 5 mg every 15–30 minutes as needed for up to three doses. Intravenous infusions of 1–5 mg/min have also been successful in maintaining heart rate and tissue perfusion. Glucagon infusions should be prepared using saline rather than phenol diluent.

Patients with hypotension should receive intravenous crystalloid prior to vasopressor therapy. Administration of dopamine, norepinephrine, or epinephrine infusions titrated to effect all have been used successfully.

Intravenous calcium (1 g of 10% calcium chloride) has also been shown to increase blood pressure following some beta-blocker overdoses.

Phosphodiesterase inhibitors (inamrinone, milrinone) that inhibit the breakdown of cAMP have theoretical benefit in patients with refractory hypotension; however, successful use in humans is limited.

The use of high-dose insulin with dextrose, recently described to be of benefit in calcium-channel blocker poisoning, may also have a role in treating refractory toxicity in patients with beta-blocker toxicity. Infusions of 0.1–2 units/kg/hr of regular insulin, with supplemental dextrose and potassium to maintain euglycemia and eukalemia, respectively, have successfully reversed hypodynamic shock in animal studies and limited case reports of patients with calcium-channel blocker toxicity. Infusions may be preceded by a bolus dose of 1 unit/kg. The benefit in beta-blocker toxicity remains to be proven.

Extracorporeal methods to enhance elimination are generally not useful in beta-blocker poisoning, although several case reports of benefit in atenolol toxicity do exist.

Calcium channel blockers

Calcium channel blockers (CCB) are used in the treatment of a variety of diseases, including angina pectoris, hypertension, and tachydysrhythmias. Unlike beta-blockers, CCB drugs are derived from one of four distinct chemical classes, yet they share in common the ability to inhibit transmembrane calcium influx in many tissues.

Over 10,000 exposures to CCB (regardless of severity) were reported by U.S. poison centers in 2006, with 13 reported deaths in patients with CCB-only ingestions.

Clinical toxicology

Depolarization results in the movement of extracellular calcium into cardiac and smooth muscle cells through L-type (slow) calcium channels. The increase in intracellular calcium triggers contraction and/or release of calcium from intracellular stores. Blockade of calcium influx in vascular smooth muscle results in vasodilatation, and negative inotropy, chronotropy, and dromotropy (conduction velocity) in cardiac muscle cells and conduction tissue.

The pharmacology of CCB in therapeutic doses differs by chemical class. Dihydropyridines (e.g., nifedipine, amlodipine, nicardipine, felodipine) act primarily on vascular smooth muscle. Verapamil (phenylalkylamine class) is the most potent negative inotrope, and diltiazem (benzothiazepine class) has less vasodilating effects than dihydropyridines and is similar to verapamil with respect to heart rate and conduction velocity. Many of these therapeutic nuances disappear with high doses, such that all CCB produce similar severe toxicity.

Hyperglycemia is frequently reported in CCB poisoning, as pancreatic insulin release is mediated by L-type calcium channels.

Metabolic acidosis that occurs in severe poisoning results from decreased tissue perfusion (shock), mitochondrial dysfunction, and decreased glucose utilization.

Presentation

Similar to beta-blocker poisoning, bradycardia and hypotension are the hallmarks of CCB toxicity. Other cardiovascular effects include impaired atrioventricular conduction, junctional rhythms, congestive heart failure with pulmonary edema, asystole, and cardiovascular collapse.

Noncardiac effects include nausea, hyperglycemia, CNS depression, and metabolic acidosis. Seizures are not common and likely are secondary to insufficient cerebral perfusion. Hypocalcemia is not an expectant finding but has been reported.

The onset of toxicity usually occurs within 3–4 hours following overdose, but may be delayed when sustained-release products are ingested. Patients with pre-existing cardiovascular disease or patients who co-ingest other cardioactive medications such as digitalis or beta-blockers are at highest risk for severe cardiac effects.

Patient evaluation

All patients should be evaluated as having potentially life-threatening toxicity, with continuous monitoring of vital signs and cardiac rhythm. Initial evaluation should include an ECG and monitoring for at least 4–6 hours (longer if sustained release product). Blood glucose should be rapidly assessed in patients with altered mental status.

Assessment of serum electrolytes, renal function, hepatic function, and/or acid–base status is indicated in patients with symptomatic toxicity. Symptomatic patients should be monitored for development of pulmonary edema. Serum levels of CCB are not useful to judge toxicity or guide therapy.

Management

All patients with known, impending, or suspected CCB toxicity should be monitored in an intensive care setting with intravenous access and continuous cardiac monitoring. Monitor serum electrolytes and glucose in symptomatic patients.

Oral activated charcoal, if tolerated, should be given to patients presenting soon (within first few hours) following acute overdose. Whole-bowel irrigation may be of benefit if instituted prior to absorption of large numbers of sustained-release products.

Treatment of CCB toxicity should be targeted to restore hemodynamic stability through improvement of heart rate and/or cardiac contractility. Reduced peripheral vascular resistance and decreased cardiac output both may contribute to hypotension.

Treatment of bradycardia/hypotension includes the following:

- Assure adequate, but not excessive, intravascular volume with intravenous crystalloid infusion.
- Atropine: 0.5–1.0 mg (0.02 mg/kg) intravenously, and repeat dose every 5–10 minutes as needed to a maximum dose of 1 mg (children) or 3 mg (adults)
- Calcium: 1 g of calcium chloride by slow intravenous push. This dose can be repeated every 10–15 minutes for 2–3 additional doses. Titrate to response and/or high range of normal for serum-ionized calcium. Calcium chloride contains three times the amount of elemental calcium contained in calcium gluconate.
- Glucagon is a pancreatic hormone that may also have efficacy in CCB poisoning, though it is more effective in improving blood pressure than heart rate. Its effects are likely mediated by increasing intracellular cAMP through mechanisms independent of the adrenergic nervous system. The initial dose is 5–10 mg (0.1–0.2 mg/kg) by intravenous bolus, with repeat doses of 5 mg every 15–30 minutes as needed for up to three doses. Intravenous infusions of 1–5 mg/min have also been successful in maintaining heart rate and tissue perfusion. Glucagon infusions should be prepared with saline rather than phenol diluent.
- Catecholamines: beta-adrenergic agonists such as isoproterenol have been used with mixed results to treat bradycardia. The increase in heart rate may be offset by vasodilatation. Administration of dopamine, norepinephrine, or epinephrine infusions titrated to desired blood pressure all have been used successfully.
- Administration of the phosphodiesterase inhibitor inamrinone has been effective in treating hypotension in several case reports.
- The use of high-dose insulin with dextrose (hyperinsulinemia/euglycemia) to reverse verapamil-induced hypodynamic shock has been documented in animal studies and several human case reports. Treatment can be initiated with a bolus of 1 unit/kg, followed by infusion of 0.1–2 units/kg/hr (usually 0.5–1 unit/kg/hr) of regular insulin, with supplemental dextrose and potassium to maintain euglycemia and eukalemia, respectively. The mechanism of this therapy has not been clearly identified, but the prevailing theory is that the primary energy source in the poisoned myocardium is carbohydrates and not free fatty acids.
- Patients with severe, refractory shock have been successfully supported with temporary mechanical methods (balloon counterpulsation, coronary by-pass) during peak toxic effects.
- It is unlikely that hemodialysis will produce a significant benefit in patients with CCB poisoning.

Cardiac glycosides

Digoxin, the most commonly used cardiac glycoside, is used in the treatment of congestive heart failure and to slow ventricular rate in patients with supraventricular dysrhythmias. Despite declining use, digoxin causes significant toxicity due to its narrow therapeutic index.

Of single drug exposures to cardiovascular drugs (n = 80,426) reported to U.S. poison centers in 2006, cardiac glycosides accounted for only 3.2% of exposures, but resulted in 16% of significant toxic effects and 51% of deaths. These numbers include the few exposures to digitoxin, but not plants that contain cardiac glycosides—foxglove, oleander, red squill, and lily of the valley.

Clinical toxicology

Digoxin is a positive inotrope that increases intracellular calcium through inhibition of the sodium-potassium-ATPase pump located on the cell membrane. Inhibition of this pump in turn decreases calcium expulsion from the cell. The elevated intracellular calcium triggers additional calcium release from the sarcoplasmic reticulum. With digoxin toxicity, potassium cannot enter the cell, and high intracellular calcium levels can cause electrical instability.

The negative chronotropic and dromotropic effects of digoxin are mediated through enhanced vagal tone. Toxic effects result in excessively slow heart rate and conduction, leading to heart blocks and bradydysrhythmias.

Hypokalemia, hypomagnesemia, hypercalcemia, or hypothyroidism each can increase the effects of digoxin.

Presentation

Clinical presentation of digoxin poisoning depends largely on the presence or absence of existing heart disease, poisoning history (acute overdose vs. chronic toxicity), and dose. Acute overdose is associated with GI effects (nausea and perhaps vomiting), CNS effects (dizziness, lethargy), and cardiac effects (tachydysrhythmias, AV block).

Patients with chronic digoxin toxicity often present with nonspecific complaints such as weakness, confusion, and malaise, as well as lethargy, nausea, abdominal pain, visual disturbances, and potentially life-threatening dysrhythmias. Complaints of seeing yellow–green spots or halos strongly suggest digoxin toxicity.

Patient evaluation

All patients should be evaluated as having potentially life-threatening toxicity. A 12-lead ECG should be obtained as soon as possible, with continuous cardiac monitoring. Immediate laboratory studies should include serum digoxin level, electrolytes (particularly potassium, magnesium, and calcium), and renal function tests.

Hyperkalemia (K >5.0 mEq/L) is associated with acute overdose (or renal failure) and should be immediately treated. Chronic digoxin toxicity is associated with normal or low potassium serum levels.

It should be recognized that a "normal" serum digoxin level does not rule out clinical digoxin poisoning.

Management

Provision of supportive care is of utmost importance. Oral activated charcoal, if tolerated, should be given to patients presenting with acute overdose and to patients with chronic toxicity who have significant renal dysfunction. Serum potassium should be determined; levels >5.0 mEq/L or <3.5 mEq/L should be corrected, especially in the presence of (new-onset) dysrhythmias.

The use of calcium in the treatment of digoxin-induced hyperkalemia is controversial and avoided by most clinicians, although human data to support this position are lacking.

Bradydysrhythmias should be treated with atropine, and temporary cardiac pacing if needed. Use caution with pacing, as the safety of pacing in patients with acute overdoses has been questioned.

Ventricular dysrhythmias can be treated with lidocaine, phenytoin, amiodarone, and/or magnesium. Beta-adrenergic blockers, calcium antagonists, or other drugs that slow AV conduction should generally be avoided.

Digoxin immune Fab (Digifab®, Digibind®) provides effective, definitive treatment for serious digoxin toxicity. Indications for immune Fab therapy include the following:

- Refractory symptomatic bradydysrhythmias
- Ventricular dysrhythmias requiring treatment
- AV dissociation
- Serum potassium >5.0 mEq/L following acute overdose
- Serum digoxin levels >10 ng/mL (approximately) following acute overdose after distribution
- Empiric treatment following ingestion of 10 mg (4 mg in a child) in the absence of digoxin levels. Data to support this manufacturer recommendation are lacking.

Digoxin immune Fab dosing is based on the amount of digoxin ingested (acute overdose) or steady-state digoxin concentration and body weight (chronic toxicity). Poison control centers are an excellent source of immediate, accurate dosing information.

Each vial of Digifab® or Digibind® binds 0.6 mg of digoxin. Digoxin immune Fab should be administered intravenously over 30 minutes (IV push in cardiac arrest), with therapeutic effect occurring within 15–30 minutes.

Only free (unbound) serum digoxin levels are useful for monitoring after treatment, as most assays detect total digoxin (including that bound to immune Fab, which is inactive).

Digoxin has a large distribution volume, thus hemodialysis or other extracorporeal methods to enhance elimination are not clinically effective.

Cyanide

Cyanide is an uncommon but potent toxin that resulted in 216 exposures reported to U.S. poison centers in 2006, yet had a 3.3% fatality rate. Perhaps the most common but least reported source of cyanide poisoning is smoke inhalation, particularly from burning plastics, wool, and silk, as well as tobacco smoke.

Other sources of cyanide include plants (prunus species seeds), laetrile, and acetonitrile. Exposures to cyanide can also occur during its use in metal polishes, rodenticides, fumigants, gold or silver ore extraction, electroplating, and chemical manufacturing. Of particular interest to pharmacists is the liberation of cyanide from nitroprusside.

Clinical toxicology

Cyanide poisoning occurs through ingestion of cyanide salts (potassium, sodium or calcium), cyanogens, or inhalation of hydrogen cyanide gas. The odor of bitter almonds is characteristic but reportedly not detectable in a significant percent of people. Cyanide is absorbed across all membranes, with respiratory significantly faster than gastrointestinal or dermal absorption.

The most significant toxic mechanism involves the binding of cyanide to ferric iron in mitochondrial cytochrome oxidase (a-a3 step). Inhibition of this enzyme system prevents oxidative phosphorylation and aerobic cellular metabolism. The inability to utilize oxygen results in anaerobic metabolism, lactic acidosis, and cell death. Other mechanisms of toxicity include GABA antagonism and lipid peroxidation.

Presentation

The route of exposure largely determines the clinical presentation and appearance of the patient. Inhalation of cyanide gas produces rapid decompensation and patients may present in cardiopulmonary arrest. Signs of significant toxicity include altered mental status (confusion, agitation, syncope, coma), respiratory depression, hypotension, seizures, metabolic acidosis, cardiovascular collapse, and cardiac arrest. Cyanosis is a relatively late finding.

Patients who ingest cyanide salts may present with gastrointestinal irritation, ranging from minor irritation to corrosive effects, followed by more subtle onset of cellular hypoxia. The lack of detection of bitter almond odor does not exclude the diagnosis of cyanide poisoning.

Patient evaluation

A history of exposure is an important determinant in suspecting cyanide poisoning. Cyanide exposure should be considered in all symptomatic patients with smoke inhalation, particularly those patients who remain comatose, hypotensive, or acidotic despite aggressive supportive care with 100% oxygen.

Cyanide levels are not readily available in most clinical laboratories; however, plasma lactate levels ≥10 mmol/L have been correlated with blood cyanide levels of ≥1 mg/L (40 µmol/L). In addition to lactate, tests in symptomatic patients should include ECG, arterial blood gas analysis, carboxyhemoglobin, methemoglobin, and measured oxygen saturation. Because tissue utilization of oxygen is impaired, venous blood may appear bright red as the difference between arterial and venous oxygenation decreases.

Management

All patients with (suspected) cyanide exposure should be monitored in an intensive care setting with intravenous access and continuous cardiac and pulse oximetry monitoring; 100% oxygen should be administered until the diagnosis is excluded

Oral activated charcoal, if tolerated, should be given to patients presenting soon (within first few hours) following acute overdose. Although charcoal is not known to readily bind cyanide, even small decreases in absorption may be helpful.

Definitive treatment of cyanide poisoning involves prevention or removal of cyanide from cytochrome oxidase. There are currently two different antidote kits available to treat cyanide toxicity.

Cyanide Antidote Kit (Lilly kit, Taylor kit)

This kit contains amyl nitrite perles, sodium nitrite, and sodium thiosulfate. Nitrites are administered to induce approximately 20% methemoglobin. Cyanide preferentially binds to methemoglobin rather than cytochrome oxidase. As cyanide is slowly released from cyanomethemoglobin, its metabolism to thiocyanate is facilitated by sodium thiosulfate.

Amyl nitrite perles are only administered initially if IV access has not been established. The dose of sodium nitrite is 300 mg (10 mL of 3% solution) intravenously over 5 minutes, followed by 12.5 g sodium thiosulfate (50 mL of 25% solution) intravenously.

Monitoring parameters include vital signs, acid–base status, and methemoglobin level. Use of nitrates in patients with concomitant carbon monoxide poisoning, hypotension, or hypoxemia should be carried out with extreme caution.

Cyanokit® (Dey Pharmaceuticals)

Cyanokit was approved in the United States in December 2006 and has become the drug of choice for cyanide poisoning. Each kit contains two 2.5-g vials of hydroxocobalamin (vitamin B_{12a}), which binds with cyanide to form cyanocobalamin (vitamin B_{12}), which can be renally excreted. The adult dose is 5 g infused intravenously over 15–30 minutes. The dose may be repeated one time in severe poisoning.

Hydroxocobalamin is not approved for use in children, but the recommended dose is 70 mg/kg by intravenous infusion.

Side effects are dose related and include reddish color of skin and urine, headache, mild injection-site irritation, and mild transient increase in blood pressure.

The use of hyperbaric oxygen to treat cyanide poisoning is controversial. It should probably be reserved for patients refractory to antidotal therapy (e.g., remain comatose or hypoxic) who can safely undergo the procedure.

Cyclic antidepressants

Cyclic antidepressants (tricyclic antidepressants, TCA) were the most widely prescribed class of antidepressants for many years, only recently being supplanted by selective serotonin reuptake inhibitors (SSRIs). During their widespread use, TCAs consistently had higher mortality than any other class of drugs. TCAs are used in the treatment of chronic pain syndromes, migraines, and enuresis as well as depression.

Clinical toxicology

The efficacy of TCAs is probably due to inhibition of neurotransmitter (norepinephrine, serotonin, dopamine) reuptake into presynaptic nerve terminals. Other pharmacological effects that contribute to toxicity include anticholinergic effects, sodium channel blockade, α-receptor blockade, potassium channel blockade, and perhaps GABA inhibition. Sodium channel blockade is the effect most associated with serious and fatal poisoning.

Tertiary amine compounds (amitriptyline, doxepin, imipramine) tend to have greater sedative and anticholinergic properties than do secondary amines (amoxpine, desipramine, nortriptyline).

Presentation

The most common effects following TCA overdose are lethargy, agitation, and sinus tachycardia. Other common effects include confusion and nausea. Most patients recover from these symptoms within 24 hours, though central and/or peripheral anticholinergic effects can last up to 3–4 days in some patients. Serious toxicity, which can occur suddenly and unexpectedly, includes hypotension, coma, seizures, ARDS, and ventricular dysrhythmias.

Patient evaluation

All patients should be evaluated as having potentially life-threatening toxicity. A 12-lead ECG should be obtained as soon as possible, with particular attention to intraventricular conduction (QRS duration). Patients with prolonged QRS intervals are at increased risk for seizures and ventricular ectopy.

Serum TCA levels do not correlate with toxicity but can confirm or rule out ingestion. Baseline and subsequent monitoring of serum electrolytes and acid–base status are needed for symptomatic patients.

Management

Provision of supportive care is of utmost importance. All patients should be monitored in an intensive care setting with intravenous access, frequent monitoring of vital signs, seizure precautions, and continuous monitoring of cardiac rhythm and pulse oximetry.

Early endotracheal intubation may be indicated to protect and secure the airway. Oral activated charcoal, if tolerated, should be given to patients presenting with acute overdose.

Sinus tachycardia usually results from anticholinergic effects and does not require treatment in most patients.

Ventricular dysrhythmias can be treated with lidocaine, phenytoin, amiodarone, and/or magnesium. Drugs that prolong AV conduction (class IA and IC) are contraindicated.

Hypotension should be treated with intravenous fluids, though excess volume can result in pulmonary edema and ARDS. Norepinephrine is generally considered the vasopressor of choice since it is direct acting.

Seizures and significant agitation should be treated with benzodiazepines (diazepam or lorazepam).

Sodium bicarbonate can be considered antidotal for severe TCA poisoning. Both exogenous sodium and alkalosis (to serum pH 7.45–7.5) help to overcome toxic sodium channel blockade. Indications for intravenous sodium bicarbonate include conduction delay (QRS >120 msec), hypotension, ventricular dysrhythmias, and seizures. Sodium bicarbonate can be administered by intravenous infusion (100–150 mEq in 1 L D5W) or intermittent boluses (preferred by most toxicologists).

Patients who remain asymptomatic for 6 hours following ingestion are not at risk for subsequent toxicity and do not require 24-hour hospitalization.

Narcotic analgesics

Analgesics represent the category of medications with the largest number of human exposures reported to U.S. poison centers. The category includes OTC and prescription drugs, and nonsteriodal anti-inflammatory agents and narcotics. The opiate and synthetic narcotics are responsible for most severe toxicity following acute exposure. Prescription narcotic medications have become the most widely misused and abused class of drugs.

Clinical toxicology

Opiates and opioid narcotics provide pain relief through stimulation of opiate receptors in the CNS. Analgesia, sedation, respiratory depression, reduced GI motility, and euphoria are believed to occur primarily through actions at mu (OP3, opiate peptide 3) receptors.

Pharmacological effects are typically dose related and follow a continuum of analgesia → drowsiness → lethargy → stupor → obtundation → coma → respiratory depression → apnea → death. All opiates are capable of producing tolerance with repeated use, and symptoms of withdrawal upon sudden discontinuance.

Presentation

Opioid toxicity is very common and is usually apparent with recognition of the opiate toxic syndrome: coma, respiratory depression, and miosis. Miosis, however, may not be present with some opioid drugs, such as meperidine and propoxyphene. The presence of these symptoms suggests but does not confirm opiate toxicity, since similar effects can be seen with barbiturates, clonidine, and other CNS depressants.

Other clinical findings may include constipation or decreased bowel sounds, bradycardia, hypotension, and acute lung injury including pulmonary edema. Patients found after prolonged periods of unconsciousness may have rhabdomyolysis, renal failure, skin ulcers or bullae, aspiration pneumonia, or sepsis.

Patient evaluation

All patients should be evaluated as having potentially life-threatening toxicity, with continuous monitoring of cardiac rhythm and pulse oximetry. Serum levels of opioids are not useful to judge toxicity or guide therapy, but an acetaminophen serum level should be checked to rule out coingestion.

Most urine "drug abuse" screens are qualitative tests for naturally occurring opiates (e.g., codeine, morphine, and some semi-synthetic compounds), and thus may not detect synthetic opioids such as meperidine, methadone, or fentanyl. Patients with severe toxicity should be evaluated for cardiac ischemia, acidosis, lung injury, and cerebral hypoxia.

Management

Provision of supportive care is of utmost importance. All patients should be monitored in an intensive care setting with intravenous access and maintenance of airway and respirations. Endotracheal intubation may be necessary to protect and secure the airway. Oral activated charcoal, if tolerated, should be given to patients presenting soon (within first few hours) following acute overdose. Most patients will recover with supportive care only.

Naloxone (Narcan®) is an opioid receptor antagonist that can reverse the CNS and respiratory depressant effects of opioids. If given early its use can prevent the need for intubation. Once a patient is intubated and is being successfully ventilated, the use of naloxone may result in a combative or uncooperative patient. Small doses of naloxone can also be used for diagnostic purposes in some patients with prolonged toxicity.

The usual initial dose of naloxone in adults or children with suspected opioid overdose is 1–2 mg intravenously. Lower doses (0.2–0.4 mg) can be used in patients with known or suspected opioid dependence. A positive response suggests but does not confirm opioid toxicity, since the effects of clonidine can also be reversed by naloxone.

Partial responses are commonly reported in patients with ethanol or benzodiazepine intoxication. However, the lack of response to ≥4 mg should reasonably exclude the diagnosis of opioid toxicity (as least as the sole cause of toxicity).

The effects of naloxone typically last 30–60 minutes, so patients often re-sedate as naloxone wears off. Patients who require multiple bolus doses to maintain the desired level of consciousness and/or ventilation may benefit from a naloxone infusion. The usual starting dose should be 2/3 of the awakening dose per hour, and titrated to desired effect. Patients should be monitored for signs of opioid withdrawal.

Opioid narcotics with atypical effects include the following:

- Meperidine: seizures are due to accumulation of metabolite normeperidine; serotonin syndrome occurs when combined with other serotonergic drugs.
- Propoxyphene: cardiac conduction disturbances due to sodium channel blocking effects of metabolite norpropoxyphene
- Tramadol: seizures
- Fentanyl: truncal rigidity

It should be noted that naloxone is not effective in treating complications associated with (non-opioid) metabolites.

Toxic alcohols/glycols—ethylene glycol

Ethylene glycol is the prominent ingredient in many (but not all) types of radiator antifreeze. Lower concentrations may be found in some solvents and brake fluids.

Clinical toxicology

Ethylene glycol itself causes little harm. It is metabolized via alcohol dehydrogenase to glycoaldehyde, and then sequentially to glycolic acid, glyoxylate and oxalic acid. Glycolic acid appears to be the primary toxin, and correlates with degree of acidosis. Oxalic acid in high concentrations can complex with calcium ions and result in significant hypocalcemia. Acute renal failure can occur with or without calcium oxalate deposition in renal tubules.

Presentation

Like methanol, the serious effects of ethylene glycol poisoning have a delayed onset (4–10 hours), pending formation of toxic metabolites. However, early signs of ingestion may include nausea, vomiting, abdominal pain, and mild inebriation. The hallmarks of serious toxicity are metabolic acidosis and acute renal failure. Other effects include hypotension, seizures, ARDS, and coma.

Patient evaluation

Diagnosis can be established or excluded with determination of a serum ethylene glycol level. However, as is the case with methanol, hospital clinical laboratories cannot perform this test, yet treatment cannot be delayed while the sample is sent out to a reference laboratory. The local poison center should be contacted to facilitate a more rapid assessment of ethylene glycol serum levels.

Pending the ethylene glycol level, blood ethanol level, basic metabolic panel (including blood glucose), measured serum osmolality, serum lactate, and arterial blood gas should be checked. Suicidal patients should also have a serum APAP concentration obtained.

Urine should be examined for presence of crystals—calcium oxalluria would be expected, but reports may indicate urate or hippurate crystals. Any of the three should be considered positive. The urine of patients who ingest a fluorescein-containing antifreeze may fluoresce under examination with a wood's lamp. Additional testing (ECG, chest X-ray, head CT) may be necessary in severe cases.

Ethylene glycol toxicity must be considered in patients who present with elevated osmol and anion gaps.

Management

Due to the extreme toxicity of ethylene glycol, suctioning of stomach contents via nasogastric tube may be of benefit in the first hour or two after ingestion. Activated charcoal does not effectively bind alcohols or glycols and should be withheld unless there are other drugs ingested. Sodium bicarbonate may be given for metabolic acidosis.

Therapy of ethylene glycol poisoning is similar to that for methanol and is based on 1) inhibition of ethylene glycol metabolism to toxic metabolites, and 2) removal of ethylene glycol and metabolites via hemodialysis. Like methanol, ethylene glycol metabolism can be inhibited using ethanol or fomepizole.

Ethanol is metabolized by alcohol dehydrogenase, which has a higher affinity for ethanol than ethylene glycol. Ethanol can be given orally, but intravenous infusion is preferred. However, titration to desired serum levels of 100–120 mg/dL is often difficult and requires a lot of nursing time and frequent blood sampling. Ethanol also causes CNS depression and may cause hypoglycemia.

- Loading dose: 8–10 mL/kg as a 10% solution in D5W over 30 minutes
- Maintenance dose: 1.4 ml/kg/hr (110 mg/kg/hr) and titrate to blood ethanol of 100–120 mg/dL. Begin as soon as the loading dose is complete. Dosage adjustment may be needed for chronic drinkers (higher dose) or for patients who never drink (lower dose).

Fomepizole (4-MP, Antizol®) competitively inhibits alcohol dehydrogenase and effectively inhibits formation of glycoaldehyde and glycolic acid. It has fewer adverse effects than ethanol, does not require serum level monitoring, can be dosed twice a day, and is significantly more expensive. Fomepizole is considered the drug of choice because of its ease of administration and low toxicity. Treatment should begin as soon as the diagnosis is suspected (do not wait for symptoms!).

The intravenous loading dose is 15 mg/kg, followed by 10 mg/kg every 12 hours for 4 doses, then 15 mg/kg every 12 hours until methanol is no longer detected (<10 mg/dL). Use of hemodialysis may decrease the duration of fomepizole therapy.

The administration of thiamine and pyridoxine may enhance the metabolism of glycoaldehyde to nontoxic metabolites, though outcome data are generally lacking. Both vitamins should be administered intravenously at 100 mg daily to patients with evidence of toxicity.

Hemodialysis provides definitive treatment of ethylene glycol poisoning. It is generally indicated in patients with significant acidosis renal failure, or serum ethylene glycol level above 50 mg/dL.

Toxic alcohols/glycols—methanol

Methanol (methyl alcohol, wood alcohol) is a prominent ingredient in Sterno, windshield washing fluid, and gasoline antifreeze and can also be found in lower concentrations in moonshine liquor, varnishes, and solvents.

Clinical toxicology

Methanol can directly cause mild inebriation and CNS depression, but serious toxicity results from its biotransformation (via alcohol and aldehyde dehydrogenases) to formaldehyde and formic acid. Formic acid is the primary toxic agent responsible for its toxic effects: metabolic acidosis and blindness.

Presentation

Patients who present soon after ingestion may complain of drowsiness and appear intoxicated. However, many patients may not seek medical attention until the onset of delayed (6–12 hours) effects that result from formic acid.

At this stage, patients may have nausea, vomiting, abdominal pain, tachycardia, tachypnea, blurred vision or other ocular complaints, and more significant altered mentation. Severe toxicity manifests as profound metabolic acidosis, seizures, coma, and/or hypotension.

Patient evaluation

Diagnosis can be established or excluded with determination of a serum methanol level. However, most hospital clinical laboratories do not perform this test, and send the sample to a reference laboratory. The local poison center should be contacted to facilitate a more rapid assessment of methanol serum levels.

Pending the methanol level, blood ethanol level, basic metabolic panel (including blood glucose), measured serum osmolality, serum lactate, and arterial blood gas should be checked. Suicidal patients should also have serum APAP concentration obtained. Additional testing (ECG, chest X-ray, head CT) may be necessary in severe cases.

Methanol toxicity must be considered in patients who present with elevated osmol and anion gaps.

Management

Due to the extreme toxicity of methanol, suctioning of stomach contents via nasogastric tube may be of benefit in the first hour or two after ingestion. Activated charcoal does not effectively bind alcohols and should be withheld unless there are other drugs ingested. Sodium bicarbonate may be given for metabolic acidosis.

Therapy of methanol intoxication is based on 1) inhibition of methanol metabolism to the more toxic formic acid, and 2) removal of methanol and metabolites via hemodialysis. Methanol metabolism can be inhibited using ethanol or fomepizole.

Ethanol is metabolized by alcohol dehydrogenase, which has a higher affinity for ethanol than methanol. Ethanol can be given orally, but intravenous infusion is preferred. However, titration to desired serum levels of 100–120 mg/dL is often difficult and requires a lot of nursing time and frequent blood sampling. Ethanol also causes CNS depression and may cause hypoglycemia.

- Loading dose: 8–10 mL/kg as a 10% solution in D5W over 30 minutes
- Maintenance dose: 1.4 mL/kg/hr (110 mg/kg/hr) and titrate to blood ethanol of 100–120 mg/dL. Begin as soon as the loading dose is complete. Dosage adjustment may be needed for chronic drinkers (higher dose) or for patients who never drink (lower dose).

Fomepizole (4-MP, Antizol®) competitively inhibits alcohol dehydrogenase and effectively inhibits formation of formic acid. It has fewer adverse effects than ethanol, does not require serum level monitoring, can be dosed twice a day, and is significantly more expensive. Fomepizole is considered the drug of choice because of its ease of administration and low toxicity. Treatment should begin as soon as the diagnosis is suspected (do not wait for symptoms!).

The intravenous loading dose is 15 mg/kg, followed by 10 mg/kg every 12 hours for 4 doses, then 15 mg/kg every 12 hours until methanol is no longer detected (<10 mg/dL). Use of hemodialysis may decrease the duration of fomepizole therapy.

The administration of folic acid may enhance the metabolism of formic acid. The recommended dose is 1 mg/kg every 4 hours for 6 doses. Symptomatic patients should receive leucovorin (the active form of folic acid, also known as folinic acid) rather than folic acid.

Hemodialysis provides definitive treatment of methanol poisoning. It is generally indicated in patients with significant acidemia, evidence of end-organ toxicity, or serum methanol level above 50 mg/dL.

Appendix

Susan B. Cogut

Pathology ranges and interpretation

Table A1 Common laboratory values and interpretation

	Increased by	Decreased by	Comments
Sodium (Na^+) 135–145 mmo/L	Water depletion, nephrogenic diabetes insipidus, (e.g., lithium toxicity), mineralocorticoid excess (e.g., Cushing's syndrome), corticosteroids, secondary aldosteronism, nephrotic syndrome, hepatic cirrhosis, uremia *Symptoms:* dry skin, postural hypotension, oliguria, cerebral dehydration, thirst, confusion, coma	Water excess, mineralocorticoid deficiency (e.g., Addison's, thyroid deficiency); thiazide and loop diuretics; burns; syndrome of inappropriate antidiuretic hormone (SIADH); excess sweating; diarrhea; vomiting; aspiration; atypical pneumonia; hemodilution caused by cardiac, hepatic, or renal failure; edema; infection; carcinoma *Symptoms*: headache, nausea, hypertension, cardiac failure, cramps, confusion convulsions, overhydration	Regulated by aldosterone
Potassium (K^+) 3.5–5 mmol/L	Mineralocorticoid deficiency, Addison's disease, acidosis, ACE inhibitors, K^+-sparing diuretics, renal failure, severe tissue damage (e.g., burns, surgery), hypoaldosteronism, diabetic ketoacidosis, red blood cell (RBC) transfusion *Symptoms*: muscle weakness and abnormal cardiac conduction (e.g., ventricular fibrillation, asystole)	Thiazide and loop diuretics, vomiting, diarrhea, ileostomy, fistula, steroids, glucose and insulin therapy, mineralocorticoid excess (e.g., Cushing's syndrome), beta-agonists, aspiration, metabolic alkalosis *Symptoms:* hypotonia, cardiac arrhythmias, muscle weakness, paralytic ileus	Regulated by aldosterone, insulin/glucose. For hypokalemia secondary to diuretics, increased bicarbonate is the best indication that hypokalemia is likely to be long-standing. Hypokalemia is often difficult to correct until magnesium normalizes.
Chloride (Cl^-) 95–105 mmol/L	Excessive ingestion, dehydration, hyperventilation, metabolic acidosis, renal disorders *Symptoms:* nonspecific	Vomiting, diarrhea, diuretics, dehydration, metabolic alkalosis, gastric suctioning, heat exhaustion, acute infection *Symptoms:* nonspecific	Cl^- follows Na^+ movement.

Bicarbonate (HCO_3^-) 22–30 mmol/L	Excessive antacid use, thiazide and loop diuretics, metabolic alkalosis, hypokalemia, vomiting, Cushing's syndrome, emphysema *Symptoms:* vomiting	Diarrhea, renal failure, diabetic acidosis, hyperventilation, salicylate toxicity *Symptoms:* headache, drowsiness, coma	Reflects renal, metabolic, and respiratory functions.
Blood urea nitrogen (BUN) 7–20 mg/dL	Renal failure, urinary tract obstruction, dehydration, corticosteroids, high-protein diet, increased catabolism, gastrointestinal (GI) bleed	Increased glomerular filtration rate (GFR), pregnancy, excessive IV infusion, low protein intake, anabolic states or synthesis, liver failure, diabetes insipidus, diuresis, overhydration	Derived from amino-acid metabolism in the liver; indicator of kidney function
Creatinine 0.6–1.1 mg/dL	Dehydration, renal failure, decreased GFR, urinary tract obstruction	Malnutrition, pregnancy, muscle wasting	Derived from muscle mass, determined by lean body mass and indication of renal insufficiency
Glucose 80–110 mg/dL	Diabetes mellitus, severe stress, corticosteroids, thiazides, Cushing's disease, pheochromocytoma, potassium deficiency, infection *Symptoms:* polyuria, polydipsia, polyphagia, ketoacidosis	Insulin overdose, Addison's disease, sulfonylureas, alcohol, hepatic failure *Symptoms:* dizziness, lethargy, sweating, tachycardia, agitation, coma	
Calcium (Ca^{2+}) 8.5–10.2 mg/dL	Hyperparathyroidism, malignancy, Hodgkin's disease, myeloma, leukemia, Paget's disease, vitamin A or D overdose, thiazides, estrogen, lithium, tamoxifen *Symptoms:* nausea, vomiting, constipation, abdominal pain, renal stones, cardiac arrhythmias, headache, depression, mental fatigue, psychosis	Hyperphosphatemia, hypermagnesemia, thyroid surgery, hypoparathyroid- ism, alkalosis, renal failure, osteomalacia, vitamin D deficiency, acute pancreatitis *Symptoms:* excitability, tetany, convulsions, muscle cramps, spasms, tingling, numbness of fingers, ECG changes	Regulated by parathyroid hormone calcitonin (1,25-dihydroxychole-calciferol). Apparent hypocalcemia may be caused by hypoalbuminemia. Calculate corrected calcium level: $0.8 \times (4\text{–albumin}) + Ca$

Table A1 (*Contd.*)

	Increased by	Decreased by	Comments
Magnesium (Mg^{2+}) 1.6–2.6 mg/dL	Renal failure, diabetic acidosis, excessive antacids, hypothyroidism, dehydration *Symptoms:* loss of muscle tone, lethargy, respiratory depression	Severe diarrhea, fistula, hemodialysis, alcohol abuse, pancreatitis, diuretics, hyperaldosteronism, hepatic cirrhosis, malabsorption *Symptoms:* tetany, arrhythmias, neuromuscular excitability secondary to hypocalcemia and hypokalemia	Deficiency can exacerbate digitalis toxicity. Mg^{2+} is excreted renally.
Phosphate (PO_4^{3-}) 2.5–4.5 mg/dL	Renal failure, uremia, hypoparathyroidism, diabetic ketoacidosis, increased vitamin D intake	Osteomalacia, hyperparathyroidism, alcohol abuse, antacids, respiratory alkalosis	Ca^{2+} and PO_4^{3-} metabolism are closely linked.
Zinc (Zn^{2+}) 70–130 mcg/dL	Zinc therapy, tissue injury, hemolysis	Cirrhosis, diarrhea, alcoholism, drugs, parenteral nutrition, inadequate diet, steroids, diuretics, malabsorption *Symptoms:* poor wound healing and growth, alopecia, infertility, poor resistance to infection	
Creatine kinase <250 U/L	MI, cardiovascular disease, skeletal muscle damage, muscular dystrophy, acute psychotic episodes, head injury, surgery, hypothyroidism, alcoholism		Found in heart, skeletal and smooth muscle, brain
Total cholesterol <200 mg/dL	Familial hypercholesterolemia, diet	Sepsis, severe weight loss, liver disease	Treatment depends on cardiovascular risk factors

Triglycerides 10–190 mg/dL	Alcoholic cirrhosis, anorexia, chronic renal failure, diabetes, hepatitis	Chronic obstructive pulmonary disease (COPD), hyperparathyroidism, hyperthyroidism, malnutrition	
High-density lipoprotein (HDL) Males: >40 mg/dL Females: >50 mg/dL	Exercise, alcoholism, cirrhosis, estrogens, nicotinic acid	Cystic fibrosis, smoking, diabetes, nephritic syndrome, acute infections	
Low-density lipoprotein (LDL) <160 mg/dL	Hyperlipoproteinemia, diabetes, hypothyroidism, nephritic syndrome, familial/idiopathic hyperlipidemia	Hypoproteinemia, severe illness, estrogens	Goal LDL determined by cardiovascular risk factors
White blood cell (WBC) 4–11 $\times 10^3/mm^3$	Drugs, infection, septicemia, malignancy, steroids, bacterial infection, alcohol hepatitis, cholecystitis	Drugs, bacterial infections, HIV, hypersensitivity reactions, surgery, trauma, burns, hemorrhage, leukemia, radiation, cytotoxics, decreased vitamin B_{12}, decreased folate	Produced in bone marrow and stimulated by granulocyte stimulating factor (GSF)
Hemoglobin Males: 13.5–18 g/dL Females: 11.5–16 g/dL	Polycythemia, burns, COPD, heart failure	Anemia, sickle cell disease, thalassemia, GI bleed, hemorrhage, iron deficiency, marrow depression, renal failure, hemolysis, pregnancy, chronic liver disease, hyperthyroidism	

Table A1 *(Contd.)*

	Increased by	Decreased by	Comments
Hematocrit Males: 40–52% Females: 34–46%	Erythrocytosis, COPD, shock, dehydration, polycythemia	Anemia, hemolysis, leukemia, cirrhosis, hemorrhage	Relative measure of cells in blood and packed cell volume
Platelets 150–450 x $10^3/mm^3$	Inflammatory disorders, bleeding, malignancy, splenectomy, polycythemia	*Decreased production:* bone marrow failure/suppression, leukemia, cytotoxic drugs, megaloblastic anemia, systemic lupus erythematosus (SLE), heparin *Increased consumption:* disseminated intravascular coagulopathy (DIC), splenomegaly, furosemide, idiopathic thrombocytopenia	Derived from megakaryocytes in bone marrow and destroyed in spleen
Prothrombin time (PT) 11–15 sec	Severe liver damage, cholestasis causing malabsorption of vitamin K		Used to monitor anticoagulant therapy and assess liver function
Thrombin time (TT) 17.5–23.5 sec	Heparin, DIC, urokinase, asparaginase		
Activated partial thromboplastin time (aPTT) 25–35 sec	Heparin, hemophilia, liver failure, DIC		Used to monitor heparin therapy
Fibrinogen 1.7–4.1 g/L	Nephrotic syndrome, pulmonary embolism (PE)	DIC, blood transfusion	

Total protein 6–8 g/dL	Myeloma, dehydration, liver disease, SLE	Catabolic states	
Albumin 3.9–5 g/dL	Dehydration, shock	Losses through skin (e.g., burns and psoriasis) liver disease, malnutrition, septicemia, nephrotic syndrome, late pregnancy *Symptoms:* edema, toxic effects of drugs normally bound to albumin (e.g., calcium, phenytoin)	$t_{1/2}$ = 20–26 days
Bilirubin Total: 0.3–1.2 mg/dL Conjugated: <0.5 mg/dL	Hepatocellular injury, cholestasis, gallstones, inflammation, malignancy, hemolysis *Symptoms:* jaundice		Derives from breakdown of red blood cells by monocyte macrophage system
Gamma-glutamyl transferase (GGT) Males: 0–85 U/L Females: 0–40 U/L	Cholecystitis, cholelithiasis, cirrhosis, enzyme inducers, alcoholism		Found in liver, kidneys, pancreas, and prostrate; released by tissue damage
Alkaline phosphatase 40–150 U/L	Renal failure, cholestasis, liver cell damage, osteomalacia, bone disease, hyperparathyroidism, Paget's disease, metastases, total parenteral nutrition (TPN), hyperphosphatemia	Hypophosphatemia, hypothyroidism, malnutrition	50% bone related, ~50% hepatic fraction, and ~2–3% intestinal fraction

Table A1 *(Contd.)*

	Increased by	Decreased by	Comments
Alanine aminotransferase (ALT) <65 U/L	Hepatocellular disease, cirrhosis, biliary obstruction, hepatitis, medications		Found in liver, heart, muscle, kidneys
Aspartate aminotransferase (AST) <35 U/L	Liver disease, cholestasis, severe hemolytic anemia, myocardial injury, trauma, surgery, pancreatitis	Acidosis in diabetes mellitus	Found in liver, heart, muscle, kidneys, erythrocytes
Amylase 20–100 U/L	Acute pancreatitis, abdominal trauma; diabetic ketoacidosis; chronic renal failure; cholecystitis; intestinal obstruction; mumps; carcinoma of ovaries, esophagus, lung	Hepatitis, pancreatic insufficiency	Produced in salivary glands, pancreas, liver, fallopian tubes
pH 7.35–7.45	Alkalosis	Acidosis	Reflects ratio of acid to base and not absolute concentration. May mask defect for which the body has compensated
PaO_2 80–90 mmHg	Artificial over-ventilation, hyperventilation, polycythemia	Chronic obstructive airway disease (COAD), hypoventilation, acute respiratory distress syndrome (ARDS), anemia	
$PaCO_2$ 34–46 mmHg	COAD, hypoventilation	Hypoxia, hyperventilation, anxiety, aspirin overdose, compensated metabolic acidosis, pulmonary embolism	Indicator of respiratory function

Normal ranges

Table A2 Normal ranges for common laboratory values

Laboratory test	Reference range	Laboratory test	Reference range
Sodium	135–145 mmo/L	WBC	4–11 x $10^3/mm^3$
Potassium	3.5–5 mmol/L	Hemoglobin	Males: 13.5–18 g/dL Females: 11.5–16 g/dL
Chloride	95–105 mmol/L	Hematocrit	Males: 40%–52% Females: 34%–46%
Bicarbonate	22–30 mmol/L	Platelets	150–450x$10^3/mm^3$
BUN	7–20 mg/dL	PT	11–15 sec
Creatinine	0.6–1.1 mg/dL	Thrombin time	17.5–23.5 sec
Glucose	80–110 mg/dL	aPTT	25–35 sec
Calcium	8.5–10.2 mg/dL	Fibrinogen	1.7–4.1 g/L
Magnesium	1.6–2.6 mg/dL	Total protein	6–8 g/dL
Phosphate	2.5–4.5 mg/dL	Albumin	3.9–5 g/dL
Zinc	70–130 mcg/dL	Bilirubin (total)	0.3–1.2 mg/dL
Creatine kinase	<250 U/L	Bilirubin (conjugated)	<0.5 mg/dL
Total cholesterol	<200 mg/dL	GGT	Males: 0–85 U/L Females: 0–40 U/L
Triglycerides	10–190 mg/dL	Alkaline phosphatase	40–150 U/L
HDL	Males: >40 mg/dL Females: >50 mg/dL	ALT	<65 U/L
LDL	<160 mg/dL	AST	<35 U/L
pH	7.35–7.45	Amylase	20–100 U/L
PaO_2	80–90 mmHg		
$PaCO_2$	34–46 mmHg		

Pediatric normal laboratory values

Table A3 Biochemistry

ALT	Neonate/infant	13–45 U/L
Albumin	Preterm Newborn (term) 1–3 months 3–12 months 1–15 years	25–45 g/L 25–50 g/L 30–42 g/L 27–50 g/L 32–50 g/L
Alkaline phosphatase	Infant 2–10 years	150–420 U/L 100–320 U/L
Amylase	Newborn	5–65 U/L
AST	Newborn Infant 1–3 years 4–6 years 7–9 years 10–11 years 12–19 years	25–75 U/L 15–60 U/L 20–60 U/L 15–50 U/L 15–40 U/L 10–60 U/L 15–45 U/L
Bilirubin (total)	0–1 day 1–2 days 3–5 days Older infant	<8 mg/dL <12 mg/dL <16 mg/dL <2 mg/dL
Calcium (total)	Preterm Term <10 days 10 days–2 months 2–12 years	6.2–11 mg/dL 7.6–10.4 mg/dL 9–11 mg/dL 8.8–10.8 mg/dL
Chloride		95–105 mmol/L
Creatine kinase	Newborn	10–200 U/L
Creatinine	Newborn Infant Child Adolescent	0.3–1 mg/dL 0.2–4 mg/dL 0.3–0.7 mg/dL 0.5–1 mg/dL
C-reactive protein		<0.5 mg/dL
GGT	Preterm 0–3 weeks 3 weeks–3 months 3–12 months 1–15 years	56–233 U/L 0–130 U/L 4–120 U/L 5–65 U/L 0–23 U/L
Glucose	Preterm Newborn Child	20–60 mg/dL 40–80 mg/dL 60–100 mg/dL
Lactate		<27 mg/dL
Magnesium		1.3–2 mEq/L
Phosphate	Newborn 10 days–2 years 2–12 years	4.5–9 mg/dL 4.5–6.7 mg/dL 4.5–5.5 mg/dL
Potassium	Newborn Infant Child	4.5–9 mg/dL 4.1–5.3 mg/dL 3.4–4.7 mg/dL

Table A3 (*Contd.*)

Protein (total)	Newborn–1 month 1–6 months 7 months–2 years 2–5 years	4.4–7.6 mg/dL 3.6–7.4 mg/dL 3.7–7.5 mg/dL 4.9–8.1 mg/dL
Sodium		135–145 mmol/L
BUN	Premature Newborn Infant/child	3–25 mg/dL 4–12 mg/dL 5–18 mg/dL

Table A4 Hematology

Age	Hb (g/dL) mean	MCV (f/L) mean	WBC (10^3/mm^3) range
Birth	16.5	108	9–30
1 month	14	104	6–18
6 months	11.5	91	6–15
1 year	12	78	6–15
6 years	12.5	81	6–15
12 years	13.5	86	4.5–13.5

Table A5 Respiratory rate

Newborn	40–50 breaths/min	Heart rate is usually four times the respiratory rate.
0–1 years	24–38 breaths/min	
1–3 years	22–30 breaths/min	
4–6years	20–24 breaths/min	
7–9 years	18–24 breaths/min	
10–14 years	16–22 breaths/min	
14–18 years	14–20 breaths/min	

Table A6 Blood pressure

	Mean (mmHg)	
	Systolic BP	**Diastolic BP**
Newborn–2 years	100	54
3–6 years	100	65
7–10 years	105	70
11–15 years	115	70

Drug interference with laboratory tests

Certain drugs may interfere with laboratory diagnostics, which can lead to wrong diagnoses or treatments and unnecessary additional tests.

Table A7 Select drug–laboratory test interferences

Drug	Laboratory test	Reaction	Mechanism
Amoxicillin-clavulanate; piperacillin-tazobactam	Galactomannan assay	False positive	Certain antibiotics contain galactomannan antigen
Ampicillin	Urine glucose (cupric sulfate); urine protein (Coomassie brilliant blue); serum protein (bromcresol green); serum uric acid (copper-chelate)	False positive or increased concentrations	
Ampicillin, ticarcillin-clavulanic acid	Direct antiglobulin (Coombs') test	False positive	
Ascorbic acid	Oxidation-reduction reactions	Varied	
Carbonic anhydrase inhibitors (IV)	Urinary protein test (bromophenol blue reagent, sulfosalicylic acid)	False positive	
Etanercept	Murine monoclonal antibody–based troponin assay	Increased concentrations of troponin	Potentially from cross-reactivity of antibodies
Heparin	Serum thyroxine	Increased thyroxine concentrations	Heparin interferes via competitive protein binding
Heparin	Aspartate aminotransferase (AST) via Ektachem dry-chemistry system analyzer	Increased AST concentrations	
Hydroxyzine	Urinary 17-hydroxycorticosteroids (Porter–Silber, Glenn–Nelson)	Increased concentrations	

Table A7 (*Contd.*)

Drug	Laboratory test	Reaction	Mechanism
Immune globulin	Blood glucose (glucose dehydrogenase pyrroloquinoline quinone–based tests)	Increased glucose concentrations	Maltose-containing immune globulin products falsely increase blood glucose concentrations with methods non-glucose specific.
Levofloxacin	Commercially available urine opiate screening tests	False positive	
Pegvisomant	Growth hormone assay	Falsely increases growth hormone levels	Pegvisomant is structurally similar to endogenous growth hormone. Monitoring and dose adjustments should be based on insulin-like growth factor-1.
Penicillin G	Urinary, CSF, serum protein; urinary glucose (cupric sulfate); serum uric acid (copper-chelate)	False positive or increased concentrations	
Phenazopyridine	Glucose oxidase reagent-based urinary glucose test	False negative	
Rasburicase	Uric acid concentration	Falsely low uric acid	Rasburicase degrades uric acid if sample is kept at room temperature.

Therapeutic drug monitoring (TDM) in adults

The aim of TDM is to provide an assessment of the drug concentration that will assist in achieving rapid, safe, and optimum treatment.

TDM is generally of value in the following situations:

- Good correlation between blood concentration and effect
- Narrow therapeutic index
- High risk of adverse effects

Table A8 lists commonly monitored drugs, and Table A9 lists antibiotics.

Table A8 Commonly monitored drugs

Drug	Therapeutic range	Ideal sampling time	Comments
Carbamazepine	4–12 mg/L	Trough 30 min prior to next dose	Adverse effects occur more commonly with levels 8–12 mg/L
Cyclosporine	100–200 ng/mL	Trough 30 min prior to next dose	Therapeutic range determined by the disorder or clinical situation being treated
Digoxin	0.5–0.8 ng/mL	Measure 6–12 hrs after dose	Risk of digoxin toxicity increases with levels >2 ng/mL
Lithium	0.6–1.2 mEq/L	Measure 12 hours after dose	Risk of toxicity increases with level >1.5 mEq/L
Phenytoin	10–20 mg/L Free phenytoin: 1–2 mg/L	Trough 30 min prior to next dose	Adverse effects occur more commonly with levels >20 mg/L
Phenobarbital	15–40 mg/L	Measurement can be taken without regard to timing of dose, due to long $t_{1/2}$ (3–5 days)	
Tacrolimus	5–15 ng/mL	Trough 30 min prior to next dose	

Table A8 *(Contd.)*

Drug	Therapeutic range	Ideal sampling time	Comments
Theophylline	10–20 mcg/L	Trough 30 min prior to next dose	Levels >15 mg/L more likely to produce adverse effects than produce benefit. If toxicity suspected, draw level at any time during IV infusion or 2 hours after oral dose
Valproic acid	50–100 mcg/mL	Trough 30 min prior to next dose	Toxic concentration >200 mcg/mL

Table A9 Commonly monitored antibiotics

Drug	Therapeutic range	Ideal sampling time	Comments
Gentamicin (traditional dosing)	Trough: <1–2 mg/L Peak: 3–10 mg/L (depending on indication)	Trough 30 min prior to third dose. Peak 30 min after completion of infusion	
Amikacin	Trough: <8 mg/L Peak: 25–35 mg/L	Trough 30 min prior to third dose. Peak 30 min after completion of infusion	
Vancomycin	Trough: 10–20 mg/L (depending on indication)	Trough 30 min prior to third dose	
Tobramcyin	Trough: <1–2 mg/L Peak: 3–10 mg/L (depending on indication)	Trough 30 min prior to third dose. Peak 30 min after completion of infusion	Peak for cystic fibrosis: 10–15 mg/L

Useful Web sites

Description	Web address (URL)
American College of Clinical Pharmacy (ACCP)	www.accp.com
American Journal of Health-System Pharmacy (AJHP)	www.ajhp.org
American Medical Association (AMA)	www.ama-assn.org
American Pharmacists Association (APhA)	www.pharmacist.com
American Society of Health-System Pharmacists (ASHP)	www.ashp.org
Annals of Internal Medicine	www.annals.org
The Annals of Pharmacotherapy	www.theannals.com
Archives of Internal Medicine	archinte.ama-assn.org
British Medical Journal	www.bmj.com
Centers for Disease Control and Prevention	www.cdc.gov
Centers for Medicare and Medicaid Services	www.cms.hhs.gov
Chest	www.chestjournal.org
Circulation	circ.ahajournals.org
Clinical Infectious Diseases	www.journals.uchicago.edu/CID/home.html
ClinicalTrials.gov	www.clinicaltrials.gov
Electronic Orange Book	www.fda.gov/cder/ob
Food and Drug Administration	www.fda.gov
FDA Postmarket Drug Safety Information for Patients and Providers	www.fda.gov/cder/drugSafety.htm
DailyMed	dailymed.nlm.nih.gov/dailymed/about.cfm
Drugs that prolong QT interval	www.azcert.org
Gluten-Free Drugs	www.glutenfreedrugs.com
Health Information Translations	www.healthinfotranslations.com
Institute for Safe Medication Practices	www.ismp.org
The Joint Commission	www.jointcommission.org
The Journal of the American Medical Association (JAMA)	www.jama.ama-assn.org
The Journal of Infectious Diseases	www.journals.uchicago.edu/toc/jid/current

Description	Web address (URL)
Journal Watch	www.jwatch.org
The Lancet	www.thelancet.com
MedWatch	www.fda.gov/medwatch
Merck Manual	www.merck.com/pubs/
National Association of Boards of Pharmacy (NABP)	www.nabp.net
National Cancer Institute Clinical Trials	www.cancer.gov/CLINICALTRIALS
National Comprehensive Cancer Network	www.nccn.org
National Institutes of Health	www.nih.gov
Natural Standard	www.naturalstandard.com
The New England Journal of Medicine	content.nejm.org
Pharmacotherapy	www.pharmacotherapy.org

Levels of evidence-based medicine

American College of Chest Physicians grading recommendations[1]

American College of Cardiology/American Heart Association classes of recommendations and levels of evidence[2]

Grade of recommendation	Methodological quality of supporting evidence
1A Strong recommendation, high-quality evidence	RCTs without important limitations or overwhelming evidence from observational studies
1B Strong recommendation, moderate-quality evidence	RCTs with important limitations or exceptionally strong evidence from observational studies
1C Strong recommendation, low-quality evidence	Observational studies or case series
2A Weak recommendation, high-quality evidence	RCTs without important limitations or overwhelming evidence from observational studies
2B Weak recommendation, moderate-quality evidence	RCTs with important limitations or exceptionally strong evidence from observational studies
2C Weak recommendation, low-quality evidence	Observational studies or case series

RCTs = randomized, controlled trials

1 Guyatt G, Gutterman D, Baumann MH, Addrizzo-Harris D, Hylek EM, Phillips B, et al. (2006). Grading strength of recommendations and quality of evidence in clinical guidelines: report from an American College of Chest Physicians task force. *Chest* **129**:174–181.

2 Gibbons RJ, Smith S, Antman E. (2003) American College of Cardiology/American Heart Association clinical practice guidelines: Part I: where do they come from? *Circulation* **107**:2979–2986.

I	Intervention is useful and effective
IIa	Weight of evidence or opinion is in favor of usefulness or efficacy
IIb	Usefulness or efficacy is less well established by evidence or opinion
III	Intervention is not useful or effective and may be harmful
A	Data from many large, RCTs
B	Data from fewer, smaller RCTs, careful analyses of nonrandomized studies, observational registries
C	Expert consensus

RCTs = randomized, controlled trials

Index

B

C

E

F

H

Q

T

Z